Clinical Immunodiagnostics
Laboratory Principles and Practices

Ian C. Clift, PhD MLS(ASCP)CM

Indiana University
Program Director, Clinical Laboratory Science
Indiana University South Bend
South Bend, Indiana
Scientific Consultant, Biomedical Associates

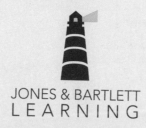

JONES & BARTLETT
LEARNING

World Headquarters
Jones & Bartlett Learning
5 Wall Street
Burlington, MA 01803
978-443-5000
info@jblearning.com
www.jblearning.com

Jones & Bartlett Learning books and products are available through most bookstores and online booksellers. To contact Jones & Bartlett Learning directly, call 800-832-0034, fax 978-443-8000, or visit our website, www.jblearning.com.

Substantial discounts on bulk quantities of Jones & Bartlett Learning publications are available to corporations, professional associations, and other qualified organizations. For details and specific discount information, contact the special sales department at Jones & Bartlett Learning via the above contact information or send an email to specialsales@jblearning.com.

Production Credits
VP, Product Management: Amanda Martin
Director of Product Management: Cathy L. Esperti
Product Assistant: Melina Leon
Product Specialist: Andrew LaBelle
Project Specialist: Nora Menzi
Digital Products Manager: Jessica deMartin
Marketing Manager: Suzy Balk
VP, Manufacturing and Inventory Control: Therese Connell
Composition and Project Management: Exela Technologies

Cover Design: Theresa Manley
Text Design: Kristin E. Parker
Senior Media Development Editor: Troy Liston
Rights Specialist: Rebecca Damon
Rights Specialist: Liz Kincaid
Cover Image (Title Page, Part Opener, Chapter Opener):
   © Science photo/Shutterstock
Printing and Binding: LSC Communications

Library of Congress Cataloging-in-Publication Data

Names: Clift, Ian C., author.
Title: Clinical immunodiagnostics : laboratory principles and practices / Ian C. Clift.
Description: First edition. | Burlington, MA : Jones & Bartlett Learning, [2021] | Includes bibliographical references and index. | Summary: "The purpose of this project is to provide a contemporary guide to the diagnostic principles and practices of immunology and serology in the clinical laboratory. This book will focus on an entry level understanding of clinical immunology, serology, and immunodiagnostics for use in the diagnostic clinical lab, it will also touch on conceptual overlaps with blood banking (immunohematology), transfusion medicine, infectious disease, cellular phenotyping, and oncology as they pertain to immunology-based clinical diagnostics. The book will be selective in its coverage; emphasizing entry-level knowledge and contemporary practical approaches. Content will also cover important historical and emerging concepts in the field"— Provided by publisher.
Identifiers: LCCN 2019033935 | ISBN 9781284173017 (paperback)
Subjects: MESH: Immunologic Tests
Classification: LCC RB46.5 | NLM QY 250 | DDC 616.07/56—dc23
   LC record available at https://lccn.loc.gov/2019033935

6048

Printed in the United States of America
24 23 22 21 20   10 9 8 7 6 5 4 3 2 1

To my family and all forward-looking laboratory professionals

© Science photo/Shutterstock

Brief Contents

Contents

Chapter 8 Immunophenotyping 155

Chapter 9 Viral Serology. 175

Step-by-Step Procedures

▶ **DAT and IAT Procedures**

▶ **HRP Antibody: Enzyme Conjugation with Succinimidyl Ester**

▶ **Ouchterlony Double Diffusion Assay**

▶ **Peripheral Blood Processing**

▶ **Preparing a Blood Control for Flow Cytometry Assays**

▶ **Rapid Plasma Reagin (RPR) Test for Syphilis**

▶ **Sensitization of Sheep RBCs for use in Complement Fixation**

▶ **Tube Typing for D**

Preface

The diagnostic clinical laboratory and the field of medical laboratory science, often called clinical laboratory science or medical technology, was a 20th-century invention that arose as an outgrowth of the massive clinical and scientific discoveries of that and previous eras. The field, in effect, was the application arm for biological and chemical investigations aimed at diagnosing disease in medical facilities. The practitioners of these skills were fundamentally biological scientists specifically experienced in the techniques and skills most suited to pathogenic identification. Their role in the healthcare team, although often unsung, is still pivotally important in increasing the overall efficacy of medical diagnosis and treatment. This text focuses not on the entire medical laboratorian profession but on several key technologies of continuing importance in the field, namely serology and immunology as they pertain to clinical diagnostics. The text is intended for both undergraduates and graduate students engaged in a condensed 8-week course or traditional 16-week course in clinical immunology, clinical serology, immunodiagnostics, or an advanced methods course taught within the medical laboratory science curriculum or within other programs focused on clinical diagnostics.

▶ Approach

This text departs from other texts in the field by attempting to establish a restructuring of the clinical laboratory science scholastic curriculum for use in the 21st century. It does so by focusing on the theoretical principles that underlie a diversity of diagnostic tests performed in the clinical lab instead of focusing only on studies in the historical demarcations provided by laboratory unit structuring.

While only 5 to 10% of the coverage in the American Society for Clinical Pathology's (ASCP) Board of Certification (BOC) generalist Medical Laboratory Scientist exam is specifically focused on immunology, immunodiagnostic tests are performed in every laboratory unit including the major areas of microbiology, blood bank, hematology, and chemistry; this suggests that a fundamental understanding of immune principles and theory is one of a few competency areas that are essential for future work in the profession.

In the 21st century, the models used to define competency will require significant remodeling if laboratory professionals are to compete well for healthcare jobs, which may go hand in hand with the remodeling of the lab itself around the key diagnostic techniques gaining traction—namely clinical immunodiagnostics, already taking up a significant market share of testing—and molecular diagnostics, with its rapidly growing utility. The laboratorian of the 21st century will also find an ever-increasing requirement to understand the mechanical and computer components of complex laboratory instrumentation. Therefore, a streamlined course curriculum would focus on the most important methodological principles underlying these evolved diagnostic tests.

Additionally, this text provides what I feel is a deeper analysis of the theoretical principles surrounding the development of the innate and adaptive immune system pertaining to the study of immunodiagnostics and may seem to expand on subjects traditionally found in other texts in the larger clinical laboratory field. For example, one will see within these pages a reference to microbiological testing by immunodiagnostic approaches, a subject often contained only in texts for microbiology; one will also see blood banking serology as it pertains to antigen and antibody interactions, as well as discussions of transfusion, cancer, virology, and autoimmune diseases as they pertain to immunodiagnostics. However, a fuller analysis of these other subject areas is outside the scope of the content and should not be neglected in generalized study.

▶ Organization

This text holds true to many of the immunodiagnostic areas that are traditionally covered in entry-level texts on serology and clinical immunology; early chapters begin by defining the specimens found in the serological lab, generalized immunodiagnostic testing methods and the fundamental knowledge in immunology, and the most common safety and operational practices. The text then proceeds with an examination of both the classical and contemporary methods used in

immunodiagnostics as they are described by the ASCP and through the American Society of Clinical Laboratory Sciences (ASCLS) entry-level curriculum (ELC) documents. Subsequent chapters discuss specific pathogenic testing through serology and immunodiagnostics, such as bacterial, viral, and fungal assays as well as immunohematology (blood banking) and transfusion medicine.

▶ Instructor Resources

The instructor who adopts this text can also request access to a robust set of ancillaries, including the following:

- **Test Bank** for each chapter
- **Slides in PowerPoint format** for each chapter
- **Instructor Manual**
- **Answers** to case study questions

Ian Clift, 2019

A Visual Walk-Through of Key Box Features

A Deeper Look boxes expand upon specific chapter concepts and define important key terms.

A DEEPER LOOK BOX 2–1

Bonds are chemical interactions between atoms to create molecules (intramolecular) or an interaction between molecules (intermolecular) to create macromolecular networks and structure.

Intramolecular forces are ionic or covalent bonds. Ionic bonds are electrostatic interactions between atoms of opposite charges that occur as a result of donation and acceptance of electrons. For example, sodium (Na) donates an electron to chlorine (Cl) to form sodium chloride (NaCl). In the process, Na becomes positively charged and Cl becomes negatively charged. Covalent bonds involve the sharing of electrons between atoms. Carbon (C) bonding is covalent and is abundant in biological molecules. Carbon can make single, double, and triple bonds, allowing it to create a multitude of interactions. In a single water molecule, the interaction between one oxygen (O) molecule and two hydrogen (H) molecules is a covalent bonds.

Intermolecular forces are weak bonds. These include Van der Waals forces and hydrogen bonds. Van der Waals forces are distance dependent and exist between temporary dipoles. Hydrogen bonds are electrostatic interactions between electronegative (electron pulling) atoms. Although water molecules are a result of electron sharing, the sharing is unequal between O and H. O is electronegative and pulls electrons toward itself in a H–O–H molecule, becoming slightly negatively charged, and H atoms adopt a slightly positive charge (dipole formation). The slightly negative charge on O in a water molecule can attract a slightly positive charge on H on a neighboring water molecule. Hydrogen bonding confers high surface tension to water. Such interactions can lend stability to a molecule. For example, DNA consists of two strands held together by stacking hydrogen bond interactions.

STEP-BY-STEP PROCEDURE 1–1 Peripheral Blood Processing

The general method of blood collection in the clinical laboratory is through the process of phlebotomy, specifically venipuncture, typically using one of the inner arm veins, but may also occur in other venous sites included in the hand, shoulder, and foot. Collection typically occurs using a needle associated with an evacuated blood collection tube. Additional processing is dependent on the blood component and tube type used.

Whole Blood Processing

1. Collect blood in an EDTA (or other) anticoagulant tube. Depending on use, as little as 1 mL and as much as 450 mL may be collected
2. Mix six to eight times by careful inversion
3. Depending on assay, blood may be used or processed further within 24 to 72 hours after collection
4. Stabilizers can be added to increase the shelf life of the specimen
5. Specimens expected to be kept longer than 24 hours should be kept at 4°C for no more than a week. *Typically for repeat testing. Lower temperature storage may produce hemolysis.*

Plasma Processing

1. Collect blood in an EDTA (or other) anticoagulant tube
2. Mix six to eight times by careful inversion
3. Within 24 hours postcollection, centrifuge the specimens at 1,300 to 1,800 × g for 10 to 15 minutes
4. Remove the plasma from the packed red cells using a transfer pipet and place in a polypropylene tube. *Smaller aliquots are advisable for multiple assays as freezing and thawing can affect results*
5. Carefully label the new tube with sample and patient identifiers per institutional protocol
6. Samples then may be stored at −20°C until assays are performed. Long-term storage occurs best at −80°C or lower

Serum Processing

1. Whole blood is collected in either a non-anticoagulant tube or serum-separator tube
2. Non-anticoagulant tubes can be stored at room temperature for 90 minutes, until a clot forms. *Lower temperature storage may produce hemolysis*
3. Use a wooden applicator stick to disrupt the clot and centrifuge at 1,300 to 1,800 × g for 10 to 15 minutes
4. Remove serum using a transfer pipet and place in a polypropylene tube. *Smaller aliquots are advisable for multiple assays as freezing and thawing can affect results*
5. Carefully label the new tube with sample and patient identifiers per institutional protocol
6. Samples then may be stored at −20°C until assays are performed. Long-term storage occurs best at −80°C or lower

Step-by-Step Procedures are provided in all chapters that contain a discussion of a specific procedure. These box features provide clear and easy to follow steps to help with student learning and retention.

Case Studies provide students with challenging real-world scenarios to test their knowledge and critical thinking skills.

CASE STUDY

Three Immune System Disorders
Case Study 1
This case has been adapted from Markert et al, *N Engl J Med*, 1999.[18]

The DiGeorge syndrome is a heritable disorder that prevents normal thymus development leading to a reduction of T-cell function. Five infants, from age 1 to 4 months with profound DiGeorge syndrome were treated with transplantation of postnatal thymus tissue. Follow-up tests involved immune phenotyping, proliferation assays of peripheral-blood mononuclear cells. Thymic production of new T cells was assessed in peripheral blood. Following transplantation, T-cell proliferative responses developed in four infants. Two patients survived and attained immune function. The remaining three patients died from infections or anomalies independent of transplantation. Biopsies of grafted thymus in the surviving patients showed normal morphologic features and active T-cell production. In one surviving patient, T-cell development occurred within the graft, leading to accumulation of recently developed T cells in the periphery and acquisition of normal T-cell function. In the second patient, thymus function and T-cell development was observed for more than 5 years after transplantation. This study led to the conclusion that in some infants with severe DiGeorge syndrome, transplantation of the thymus can lead to restoration of the T-cell compartment and function. However, it is likely that early thymus transplantation is essential, prior to any infections, to increase chances of survival.

Critical Thinking Question
With crucial knowledge about DiGeorge syndrome in hand, you diagnose it in a newborn. Suppose you are a physician. What treatment would you administer to restore T-cell function in the infant?

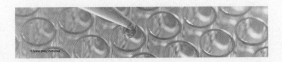
© Science photo/Shutterstock.

APPENDIX
Advanced Concepts

Appendix A: Advanced Concepts is a background guide on topics that aren't fully explored in the main chapters and also expands on several topics that are already included. This addition is a great way to expand on knowledge in these areas, which include properties of other chemical diluents and buffers used in serological testing, diagnostic polyclonal and monoclonal antibody development, expanded isolation considerations for blood products, and more.

Contributors

Barsha Dash, PhD (Chapter 2, 3)
Department of Immunology
Graduate School of Biomedical Sciences
Mayo Clinic
Rochester, Minnesota

Brittney Dinkel, PhD (Chapter 2, 3)
Assistant Professor
Biology Program
School of Science
Buena Vista University
Storm Lake, Iowa

Alexandra Greenberg-Worisek, PhD, MPH (Chapter 15)
Center for Regenerative Medicine
Mayo Clinic
Rochester, Minnesota

Shaheen Kurani, ScM (Chapter 15)
Graduate School of Biomedical Sciences
Mayo Clinic
Rochester, Minnesota

Annika Lee
School of Medicine
Emory University
Atlanta, Georgia

Diane Leland, PhD (Chapter 9)
Professor Emeritus
Department of Laboratory Medicine and Pathology
and
Program Director, Clinical Laboratory Science
Bachelor of Science Degree
School of Medicine
Indiana University–Purdue University
Indianapolis
Indianapolis, Indiana

Andrew McKeon, MD D(ABMLI) (Chapter 13)
Neurologist
Departments of Laboratory Medicine and
Pathology and Neurology
Mayo Clinic
Rochester, Minnesota

Barbara Spinda, MS, MLS(ASCP)CM (Chapter 10, 11)
Professor
Division of Clinical Laboratory Science
School of Applied Health Sciences
Vera Z. Dwyer College of Health Sciences
Indiana University South Bend
South Bend, Indiana

Rosalie Sterner, MD, PhD (Chapter 14)
Graduate School of Biomedical Sciences
Mayo Clinic
Rochester, Minnesota

Elitza S. Theel, PhD (Chapter 15)
Consultant, Division of Clinical Microbiology
and
Associate Professor
Department of Laboratory Medicine and Pathology
Mayo Clinic
Rochester, Minnesota

▶ Reviewers

Pamela B. Primrose, PhD, MLS(ASCP)
Faculty
Department of Medical Laboratory Technology
School of Health Sciences
Ivy Tech Community College–South Bend
South Bend, Indiana

Dick Y. Teshima, MPH, MT(ASCP)
Associate Professor and Chair
Department of Medical Technology
John A. Burns School of Medicine
University of Hawai'i at Mānoa
Honolulu, Hawaii

Patricia Tille, PhD, MLS(ASCP), FACSc
Instructor
Department of Medical Laboratory Science
College of Pharmacy and Allied Health Professions
South Dakota State University
Brookings, South Dakota

Reannon Wilkerson, BS, MS, MLS(ASCP)
Instructor
Medical Laboratory Assistant Program
Department of Health Sciences
Calhoun Community College–Huntsville Campus
Huntsville, Alabama

▶ Student Reviewers

Esther Boateng, BS
Indiana University South Bend CLS Graduate

James Dishman, BS
Indiana University South Bend CLS Graduate

RJ Dudash, BS
Indiana University South Bend CLS Graduate

Molly Feller, BS, MLS(ASCP)
Indiana University South Bend CLS Graduate

Brandie Morgan, BS, MLS(ASCP)
Indiana University South Bend CLS Graduate

Chantel Shores, BS, MLS(ASCP)
Indiana University South Bend CLS Graduate

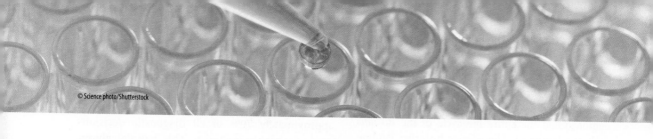

CHAPTER 1

The Serological Specimen

Ian Clift, PhD, MLS(ASCP)^{CM}

KEY TERMS

Antibody-antigen complex
Antibody titer
Antithrombin
Clot
D-dimer
Diluent
EDTA

Factor XIII
Fibrinogen
Immunogenicity
mRNA
Peripheral blood
Plasmin
Protein C

Protein S
Serial dilution
Serology
Serum
Solute
Thrombin

LEARNING OBJECTIVES

Upon completion of this chapter, the reader should be able to:

1. Based on understanding of biological fluids, define potential antigenic materials.
2. Associate the major cells within the peripheral blood with their immunological function.
3. Describe the four structural levels of protein biosynthesis.
4. Provide the correct terms for proteins associated with fats, sugars, and nucleic acid.
5. Map the association of antigen and antibody as a curve of observable reactions.
6. Explain the relationship between titer and dilution.
7. Calculate an antibody titer.

▶ The Roots of Immunodiagnostics

Immunodiagnostics has decidedly been a 20th century invention. However, the stage was first set for these discoveries in the late 1800s. It was in Germany where the new field of "experimental physiology" was first developed and expounded upon by scientists such as Johannes Muller and Matthias Schleiden, who wanted to find unity behind living things instead of simply subdividing them into categories, which had been the prevailing trend with the popular Linnaean classification system. Others, such as Ferdinand Cohn, developed classifications for simple plants and bacteria, which were followed by the work of Robert Koch who demonstrated the entire life cycle of the *Bacillus anthracis* (anthrax). The science historian Pauline Mazumdar, in her book *Species and Specificity*, contends that it is these two groups of scientists—those focused on unification and those focused on specification—that have contributed equally to establishing our current understanding of immune-mediated disease and diagnostics.[1] In 1880, Koch and his specificationists published an attack on the unificationists, including the famous Louis Pasteur. These two schools continued to thrive and produce great minds who would contribute to our current theoretical understanding. Despite notable unificationists, such as Karl Landsteiner who received the Nobel Prize for his work on defining blood groups, it would be the differences among bacteria that defined them within the immune system and be diagnostic within the field of serology.

Some of the earliest notables in the history of immunodiagnostics include Paul Ehrlich, whose pioneering staining work in the fields of hematology, immunology, and bacteriology allowed for the differentiation of cells, including immune cells and bacterial cells; Rudolf Krause, who was one of the first to describe the reaction of soluble antigens to antiserum; Gruber and Durham, who, in 1896, provided the first report of the antibody agglutination of bacterial cells; and Karl Landsteiner, who famously defined the ABO blood groups and later the Rh blood system. Later luminaries of the 20th century included Heidelberger and Kendall, who showed the first precipitin curve in 1929; Coons, who attached the first fluorochrome to an antibody in 1941; and Ouchterlony, who, in 1947, developed his now-standard Ouchterlony techniques for single and double diffusion of antibody and antigen complexes. Later, Statvitsky and Aquilamay performed the first contemporary labelled immunoassay in 1954 when they used antibodies bound to RBCs as labels to perform what is now known as hemagglutinin. Since these early works, the clinical aim has been to increase the number of clinical biomarkers, increase sensitivity and specificity, detect earlier, and reduce sample-volume necessities.

▶ Fundamentals

Laboratory medicine is thought to contribute to approximately 70% of all diagnostic decisions made in healthcare today. This has not always been the case. The history of medicinal diagnostics occurred in three stages. In the beginning, diagnosis relied only on the physical senses of the bedside doctor. In the second stage, a complete accounting of the patient history was collected in a hospital or healthcare setting. Finally, the laboratory came into its own, but not until the later part of the 19th century. In the beginning of the 19th century, doctors relied primarily on patient accounts and rudimentary observations to make a diagnosis. By the middle of that century, laboratory tests were available and being used to diagnose diseases such as typhoid, cholera, and diphtheria.[2] Fundamentally, these laboratory tests required a more exquisite examination of the cellular and subcellular level; they required the microscope for visualization and led to a whole host of serological and immunodiagnostic techniques that are the subject of this book. Indeed, serology and immunodiagnostics grew out of the need for a systematic set of methods of diagnosing cellular pathology involved in disease. First, scientists, physicians, and laboratorians had to define the components of the cellular and subcellular environment.

Arguably, the most important clinical diagnostic information has come from the analysis of blood and body fluids. Additionally, the basic methods of immunodiagnostics and serology revolve around the detection and quantitation of antigens and antibodies. Immunoassays, which are discussed in great detail in this textbook, were originally and still are commonly referred to as serological assays because they were conducted using antisera or serum, the liquid fraction of blood containing antibodies. The field of immunodiagnostics, at least a substantial part of it, is commonly called **serology**, from the study of antisera. Titration is a backbone of many immunoassays and is described later in this chapter. In addition to titration, the immunodiagnostician should be fully acquainted with the classical methods of precipitation and agglutination, still used in clinical assays today. These two methods allow for the visible expression of antigenic and antibody complexes. They are different in the way that the antigen-antibody complexes are visualized, with precipitation being used to assay the aggregation of soluble test antigens and agglutination focused on the aggregation of particulate test antigens. These two methods are commonly considered the classical methods of serology. More complex methods that employ instrumentation or involve labeled immunoreagents and/or complex interactions are described as manual and/or automated immunoassays. Furthermore, the fundamental methods of serology overlap significantly with other fields of clinical diagnostics such as chemistry, microbiology, and immunohematology. Advanced techniques involved in these types of testing are described in more detail in later chapters. The concepts presented below are meant to provide a primer to the student for further study. Terms are introduced and general concepts are provided below. More detailed study of these topics can be found in the subsequent chapters as they are related to clinical practice.

Blood and Other Body Fluids

Peripheral blood is the fluid with which most serological and immunological studies are performed. In the average adult, the liquid components of blood, i.e., plasma, make up one fourth of the total extracellular fluid in the body; the rest is contained in what is known as interstitial fluid the fluid between tissues.[3] All of the main components of blood—cells, proteins and metabolites—are powerful sources of diagnostic information. However, serology is named for an important protein component of blood, specifically, the antibodies.

From ancient times, blood products have been used in medical practice. Historically, however, blood usage for diagnostics was limited by rapid clotting and degradation time until storage procedures were optimized—for instance, the addition of discovered anticoagulants decreased product clotting, and the addition of glucose or

dextrose prolonged product stability. Temperature control and sterile procedures further aided blood stability. Further advances came from the work of specific investigators. For example, in 1940 Edwin Cohn successfully separated plasma proteins from blood via continuous flow, developing the first isolated blood product for use in transfusion,[2] and in 1965 Judith Pool discovered that the precipitate left behind when thawing frozen plasma contained coagulation factor, innovating a new way to deliver clotting factors to hemophiliacs and others with clotting disorders.[2] These discoveries and others cleared the way for an expanded use of blood products in medicine. Contemporarily, whole blood is frequently separated into isolated components: red blood cells (RBC), platelet concentrates, fresh frozen plasma (FFP), cryo-precipitated antihemophilic factor, peripheral blood progenitor cells, and granulocytes, depending on the blood's intended use. Today, the medical condition of an individual or group of individuals is commonly defined by the testing of blood products in diagnostic testing procedures called immunoassays. The components of blood are isolated and stored for medical therapy as well.

In general, blood can be separated into several components by various methods; many of these separation techniques have been systematized by the use of blood collection tubes, such as the serum separator tube (SST) or anticoagulant tubes collected by the phlebotomist. Separation steps are also used in the assay-specific stages of immunodiagnostics.

Phlebotomy is the practice of drawing blood and is often performed by trained phlebotomists, clinical laboratory professionals, nurses and physicians (**FIGURE 1–1**). Contemporary blood draws typically occur via two types of needles: multisample needles and winged infusion (butterfly) needles, commonly associated with evacuated tubes. Very specific tests can also be collected using specks of blood from finger and heel sticks. Less commonly, the hypodermic needle, as part of a syringe system, is used, especially for line draws and aspirates. Needles for blood collection must come attached with a safety closure feature according to OSHA regulations, to aid in avoiding unintended exposures. Importantly, additives

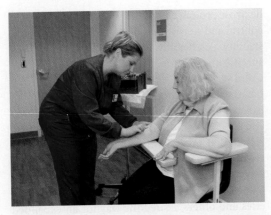

A

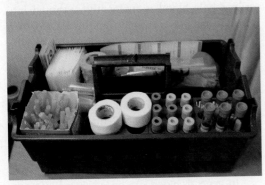

B

FIGURE 1–1 Phlebotomist performing venipuncture.
(A) Phlebotomist and patient **(B)** Phlebotomy supplies
for transport to patient.

(a) and (b) Courtesy of National Healthcareer Association (NHA).

Body Fluids

Like blood, other body fluids, such as cerebral spinal fluid (CSF) extracted from the spinal column, and amniotic fluid, extracted from the amniotic sac in pregnancy, are common sources for serological and immunodiagnostic testing. IgG is the major source of maternal antibodies found in fetuses and newborns, as it crosses the placenta. Another important source of specimen collection is the bone marrow, where significant information can be obtained regarding blood and immune-related cancers and other blood disorders. Fluids, such as seminal and vaginal fluids, are used in the diagnosis of sexually transmitted diseases (STDs). Finally, urine is commonly serologically tested. It is a source used for testing infectious diseases, such as bacterial infections. The properties of each fluid should be considered in the design of any laboratory assay; for example, urine may include high salt concentrations, which could act as an interferent to many clinical assays.

Cells

The study of cells within the bloodstream is called hematology and consists of examinations of the erythrocytes (red blood cells—RBCs), which transport oxygen throughout the body from the lungs via hemoglobin, and leukocytes (white blood cells, WBCs), the components of the innate and adaptive immune system.

General anatomical features of cells are often used for their diagnostic indications. The size, shape, and morphology using eosin and methylene blue, containing Wright or Wright-Giemsa stains, have been used for more than 100 years for microscopic examination of peripheral blood and bone marrow. Histological examinations of cells within tissue are often visualized using eosin, to detect the cytoplasm of cells, and hematoxylin, to detect the cell nuclei, in the common H & E stain. Both quantitative and qualitative changes in cell number and morphology can be visual indicators of pathophysiology. The complete blood count (CBC) and cell differentials, commonly performed in hematology labs, often provide clues for expanded serological and immunological testing

are typically added to evacuated tube systems to prevent the coagulation of blood by clotting factors. For example, citrates, such as sodium citrate, added to the tube to prevent the coagulation of blood through calcium chelation (binding). **EDTA** (ethylenediaminetetraacetic acid) is used to chelate calcium as well, and is preferred for hematology and many immunohematology tests. By definition, serological studies are the study of the extracellular components of the blood. For serological testing, often either plasma, the straw colored extracellular matrix of the blood or serum, the plasma with clotting factors removed, can be used. An EDTA tube or serum separator tube is used to collect plasma specimens for usage, while a clot tube is used to collect serum.

as well. Cells of the bloodstream may also be studied for surface markers in the process of cell differentiation, using a series of established surface markers categorized as the cluster of differentiation (CD) markers. In immunophenotyping, the use of antigens and antibodies for the differentiation of specific cell types is conducted, often as part of the testing profiles performed in either a hematology or immunology laboratory.

Like the patient's own cells, bacterial cells are also detectable using antigenic detection in common body fluids and specimens. Furthermore, these cells in a patient sample may shed proteins and other factors that are diagnostically relevant in infectious disease serology.

Types of Cells. Beyond initial hematological stratification of cells, more advanced methodologies have been developed to define both the physiological and pathophysiological nuances in blood cell populations. This is accomplished by the detection and quantitation of markers on the surface of cells, primarily through antibody binding. Cells are commonly divided into leukocytes

the white blood cells (WBCs), and erythrocytes, the red blood cells (RBCs) (**FIGURE 1-2**).

The classifications of leukocytes is further divided into two lineages, based on their progenitor stem-cell population, as either myeloid or lymphoid. Early on, the erythrocyte lineage branches off from the myeloid lineage, which goes on to form platelets, neutrophils, macrophages, eosinophils, and mast cells. These cells play a major role in the innate immune system as well as important roles in aspects of the adaptive immune system as well. However, pivotal to the story of serology and immunodiagnostics are the antibody producing and detecting cells called lymphocytes.

Lymphocytes are described as a heterogeneous collection of cells, which can be differentiated from other leukocytes based on morphological characteristics, surface markers, and functional characteristics. The terms, T-cell and B-cell come from earlier work on the origins of these cells. T cells were found to reside within the thymus, where they are now known to undergo selection to avoid autoimmune responses; known as thymic education. B cells, in turn, derived from the bone marrow, or

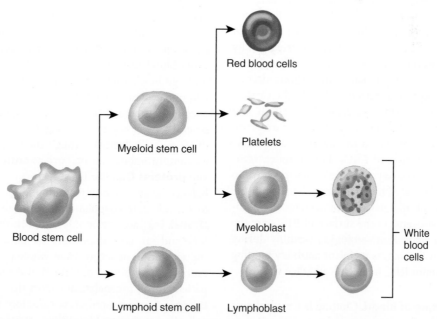

FIGURE 1-2 General Characteristics of WBC and RBC cells. WBC, RBC, and platelet development. Both RBCs and WBCs derive from a common hematopoietic (blood) stem cell, which splits into separate myeloid and lymphoid lineages before becoming either myelocytes, RBCs, and platelets or lymphocytes, respectively.

bursa in birds, where they were first described.[4] Lymphocytes differentiate into various types of effector immune cells when their antibody/antigen receptor is triggered. For example, CD8+ T cells become relatively short-lived cytotoxic lymphocytes that function to kill antigen-expressing cells and CD4+ T cells differentiate toward one of several different lineages of helper and/or regulatory T cells that secrete specific cytokines in order to coordinate and control all of the other immune cells. B cells become long-lived antibody-producing cells called plasma cells, which are a primary source of the antibodies found circulating in the peripheral blood as well as other body fluids. Other leukocytes include the monocyte, macrophage, eosinophil, and basophil. As members of the innate immune system, their role in traditional antigen-antibody serology is less well examined, but a discussion of their immune profile can be found in Chapter 8: Immunophenotyping. However, they are also known to interact with adaptive immune components to complete the lysis and destruction of pathogens.

Erythrocytes are also of practical importance in determining underlying anemias and iron and blood oxygenation disorders. Of fundamental importance to hematopoiesis; RBCs are developed in the bone marrow alongside WBCs. Erythropoiesis, the regeneration of RBCs, is triggered by oxygen tension and a response to erythropoietin upon the stem-cell population in the bone marrow to replace lost or damaged RBCs. As the carriers of hemoglobin, RBCs are critical to survival, and very often, the first laboratory tests performed on a patient are conducted to quantitate and determine the function of RBCs. Furthermore, serological immunoassays are one of several ways in which glycosylated hemoglobin is detected in the diagnosis and maintenance of diabetes.[5] In addition, the antigens on the surface of RBCs are the subject of significant serological scrutiny during blood transfusions, as recipient antibody binding leads to donor RBC hemolysis and vice versa.

The Clotting of Blood. Clotting is a natural process that begins as soon as blood is exposed to open air and is part of the innate immune system's defense against infection. This process can be seen after an incision or puncturing of the skin, culminating in the formation of a scab, which creates a temporary shield around an injury.

The clot contains the white and red blood cells as well as numerous clotting factors and other cellular debris. During serological testing, blood is typically centrifuged to accelerate the clotting process and to separate the serum for further testing. However, blood collected in a glass tube, which starts as a darkly translucent red fluid, will begin to clot, or coagulate, in a matter of minutes. Within 1 hour, the clot, which resembles a jelly-like mass, will retract, leaving behind the straw-colored serum fraction commonly used in immunodiagnostics. Left untouched, the process is complete within 24 hours but can be enhanced through the process of centrifugation and the use of serum-separator tubes. Clotting can be prevented by the addition of chemical anticoagulants, typically added to commercially available specimen collection tubes.

Coagulation. Hemostasis is the series of physical processes occurring between the blood vessels, platelet factors, and clotting (or coagulation) factors that lead to the blood clot. In vivo, the platelets aggregate at the site of injury by binding to collagen fibers that are exposed during vascular injury. The platelet plug temporarily prevents blood loss and stimulates the platelets to undergo biochemical changes and begin to expel additional platelet stimulation factors as well as coagulation factors. In a normal in vivo process, several factors counteract coagulation, including dilution of the factors through the flow of blood and antithrombotic agents such as **antithrombin** and **proteins C** and **S**. These factors maintain the balance between clotting and blood fluidity. Factors involved in coagulation and clot destruction (**FIGURE 1–3**) are commonly tested in the laboratory and are also important for understanding the separation of serum from whole blood. Diet, exercise, alcohol use, and medication use in the patient are all preanalytical factors that can affect the rate of coagulation, as are variations in sample collection including blood flow interruption and inadequate ratios of blood to tube additive.[6]

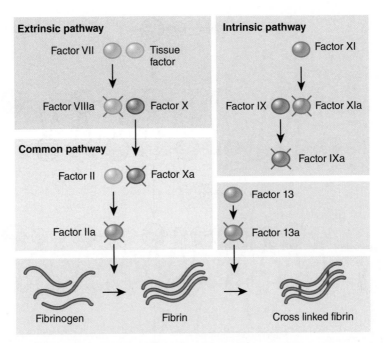

FIGURE 1-3 Pathways of Coagulation. The intrinsic and extrinsic pathways of the coagulation cascade ending with the production of cross-linked fibrin polymers.

Clotting Factors. Blood clotting occurs through the process of coagulation and leaves behind a liquid serum fraction. One of the most important and abundant clotting (or coagulation) factors is **fibrinogen**. Fibrinogen is depleted when blood is exposed to air. It is converted into fibrin through the enzyme **thrombin**. Fibrin lends structure to the clot in the form of a fine thread that weaves the white and red blood cells into a mesh. Thrombin also stimulates **Factor XIII**, of the coagulation cascade, which crosslinks the fibrin monomers into stable insoluble fibrin polymers.

Fibrin polymers are broken down by the presence of the fibrinolytic system. The degradation products of fibrinogen are widely used indicators of thrombosis, as are the levels of factors such as fibrinogen consumed during the process. **Plasmin** is the major effector of the fibrinolytic system and is generated from an inactive precursor called plasminogen. The breakdown products of polymeric fibrin are termed fragments X, Y, D, and E. However, only the fragments that are crosslinked via Factor XIII have an intact

covalent bond, creating the **D-dimer** fragment (**FIGURE 1-4**), commonly used in laboratory assessments of thrombosis.[7]

The study and artificial prevention of coagulation led to the other primary products used in the clinical immunodiagnostic laboratory, specifically anticoagulated whole blood and plasma, as well as the proliferation of commercially prepared anticoagulants. The differences and a general usage of these other blood products in serological and immunodiagnostics is described below.

Serum. The laboratory-based fractionation of blood into cellular and noncellular components begins with the natural process of blood clotting, which leads to the separation of the straw-colored fluid called serum. Serum and its subcellular molecules were one of the first and still a major body fluid studied. It is from serum that the study of serology gets its name.

During the process of coagulation, fibrinogen is converted to fibrin, which forms the matrix (or mesh) that binds all white and red blood cells

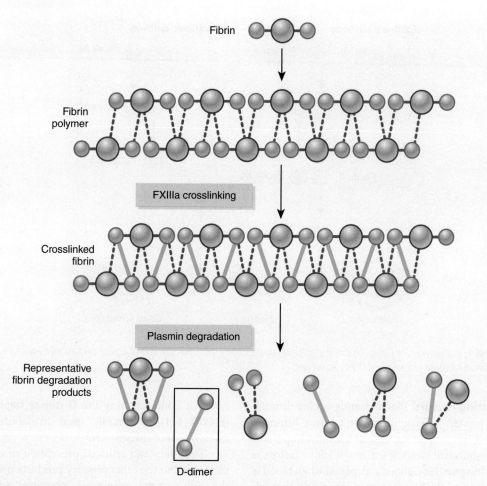

Fibrin

Fibrin polymer

FXIIIa crosslinking

Crosslinked fibrin

Plasmin degradation

Representative fibrin degradation products

D-dimer

FIGURE 1–4 D-dimer formation from fibrinogen (see Riley et al., Lab Medicine 2016).

together and leads to the subsequent clot. Serum can then be decanted or aspirated and used for testing. It contains antibodies and antigens but no clotting factors.

Plasma. In contrast to serum, plasma is found in circulation and also after the process of anticoagulation. In the presence of anticoagulating additives, the straw-colored substance that separates from the cellular components of blood is called plasma **SSP 1–1**. Plasma is also commonly used in immunodiagnostics. Like serum, it not only contains antibodies and antigens for detection, but also contains clotting factors that can be used for additional diagnosis, specifically the testing of the coagulation cascade.

Proteins and Subcellular Products

Proteins in all shapes and forms, whether free floating in the blood, attached to the surface of a cell (surface markers and receptors), or presented in association with an immune response, are the physiological source of **immunogenicity** (antibody-based detection) and one half of all of the components of serological diagnosis. Proteins and their components are defined by a multitude of names such as ligand, antigen, epitope, receptor, and marker, depending on their functional role. Proteins used in clinical immunodiagnostics are also defined by their associations: with fats, they are called lipoproteins; with sugars, they are called glycoproteins; with DNA or RNA, they are called

STEP-BY-STEP PROCEDURE 1–1 Peripheral Blood Processing

The general method of blood collection in the clinical laboratory is through the process of phlebotomy, specifically venipuncture, typically using one of the inner arm veins, but may also occur in other venous sites included in the hand, shoulder, and foot. Collection typically occurs using a needle associated with an evacuated blood collection tube. Additional processing is dependent on the blood component and tube type used.

Whole Blood Processing

1. Collect blood in an EDTA (or other) anticoagulant tube. Depending on use, as little as 1 mL and as much as 450 mL may be collected
2. Mix six to eight times by careful inversion
3. Depending on assay, blood may be used or processed further within 24 to 72 hours after collection
4. Stabilizers can be added to increase the shelf life of the specimen
5. Specimens expected to be kept longer than 24 hours should be kept at 4°C for no more than a week. *Typically for repeat testing. Lower temperature storage may produce hemolysis.*

Plasma Processing

1. Collect blood in an EDTA (or other) anticoagulant tube
2. Mix six to eight times by careful inversion
3. Within 24 hours postcollection, centrifuge the specimens at 1,300 to 1,800 × g for 10 to 15 minutes
4. Remove the plasma from the packed red cells using a transfer pipet and place in a polypropylene tube. *Smaller aliquots are advisable for multiple assays as freezing and thawing can affect results*
5. Carefully label the new tube with sample and patient identifiers per institutional protocol
6. Samples then may be stored at −20°C until assays are performed. Long-term storage occurs best at −80°C or lower

Serum Processing

1. Whole blood is collected in either a non–anticoagulant tube or serum-separator tube
2. Non–anticoagulant tubes can be stored at room temperature for 90 minutes, until a clot forms. *Lower temperature storage may produce hemolysis*
3. Use a wooden applicator stick to disrupt the clot and centrifuge at 1,300 to 1,800 × g for 10 to 15 minutes
4. Remove serum using a transfer pipet and place in a polypropylene tube. *Smaller aliquots are advisable for multiple assays as freezing and thawing can affect results*
5. Carefully label the new tube with sample and patient identifiers per institutional protocol
6. Samples then may be stored at −20°C until assays are performed. Long-term storage occurs best at −80°C or lower

nucleoproteins. The shape and form of a protein is defined by its genetic coding, assembly, and cellular processing. Therefore, inherited diseases can be defined by the presence, absence, structural alteration, or change in expression of proteins. Furthermore, infectious diseases lead to the upregulation and downregulation of a multitude of endogenous proteins as well as the novel expression of pathogen-associated proteins, all of which are of diagnostic utility. It is from a complex study of cellular physiology that the interactions between proteins, cells, and larger-order biological systems have been defined. These interactions and their alterations provide major hallmarks of disease.

Protein Structure

Proteins are highly structured polymeric molecules. This structure is broken into four levels: primary, secondary, tertiary, and quaternary (**FIGURE 1–5**). A protein's primary structure refers to the specific sequence of amino acid monomers that compose that protein. An amino acid is named for its chemical structure: It contains a central carbon attached

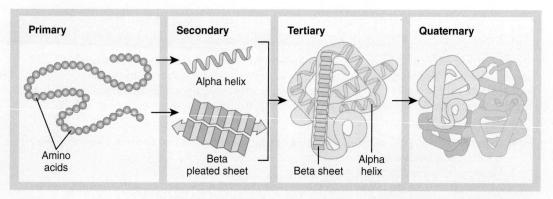

FIGURE 1–5 Protein structure from amino acid to protein. A protein is built in four panels. Amino acid polymers form the protein's primary structure. Charges in the amino acids determine several secondary structures, such as the beta pleated sheet and alpha helix, as well the more complex tertiary structure. Finally, polymers can come together to form dimers with similar polymers (homodimers) or with dissimilar polymers (heterodimers), which establishes the quaternary structure of a protein.

to one hydrogen group (—H), one amino group (—NH$_2$), one carboxyl group (—COOH), and one variable side chain (—R). Although any molecule with this structure could be considered an amino acid, there are only 20 amino acids that are naturally specified for when translating a system's nucleic acid messenger, **mRNA**, into a protein. Amino acids could also be one of two stereoisomers around the chiral carbon center, but naturally formed amino acids are always L-stereoisomers. To form a polymer, the cell links the carboxyl group of one amino acid to the amino group of the adjacent amino acid. This is a condensation reaction, which forms a covalent peptide bond and releases a water molecule. The variable group of each amino acid confers various chemical and stearic properties onto each amino acid; for example, the natural amino acids can be broken into positively charged, negatively charged, polar, aromatic, and nonpolar based on this side chain.

Secondary structure refers to regular, repeating structural motifs that are formed by regularly spaced hydrogen bonding between the atoms in the "main chain" of the peptide bond, as opposed to the side chain atoms. These structures include alpha helices and beta sheets.

Tertiary structure refers to binding between side groups in the polypeptide, i.e., disulfide bonds, hydrogen bonding, ionic bonds, hydrophobic/hydrophilic interactions, and van der Waals interactions. Tertiary structure is broadly separated into globular or fibrous proteins. Most proteins have a primary, secondary, and tertiary structure.

Quaternary structure refers to two or more distinct polymers (called subunits) that bind to form a functional unit—the classic example is hemoglobin: the oxygen-carrying protein found in RBCs (**FIGURE 1–6**).

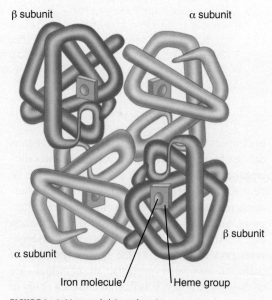

FIGURE 1–6 Hemoglobin subunits.

Data from Reisner, H. (2017). Crowley's an introduction to human disease, 10e. Jones & Bartlett Learning.

Amino acids have distinct chemical and stearic properties based on their side groups. These properties allow diagnosticians to distinguish between different proteins and define a protein's binding affinity for another substance. To detect proteins by their charged residue, one can use chromatography or isoelectric forcing. For ion-exchange chromatography, if the protein is rich in positive residues (lysine, arginine, and histidine), the protein would be run through a negatively charged column. For negative residues (aspartate, glutamate), the protein would be run through a positive column. This column will preferentially bind charged proteins, eluting noncharged proteins and purifying the charged protein for further use or analysis. Alternatively, one can run a charged protein on a gel by running an electric current through the gel, which will cause the protein to migrate toward its opposite charge. This clarifies the protein into a distinct band. These charged residues can define a protein's binding site for an oppositely charged substrate. This, in combination with the unique folding of the protein, often brings these charged residues into close proximity with the charged substrate, creating a specific binding for that substrate. To test if a residue is particularly important for binding, researchers will create a mutated protein at the proposed binding site, switching a charged reside for a noncharged residue, normally alanine. If binding is altered following mutation, it distinguishes that charged residue as particularly important. These charged residues are also used in the chemical synthesis of bound tracer molecules and are extremely important in the confirmation of a protein, leading to specific antigenicity. Change in protein structure leads to changes in binding affinity to specific antibodies, an important consideration in immunodiagnostic detection.

Fats, Sugars, and Metabolites

Hyperlipidemia and hypercholesterolemia are major risk factors for development of atherosclerosis, coronary artery disease, and myocardial infarction; some of the top killers of the current era. Hyperglycemia is a primary indicator of metabolic syndrome and diabetes. Therefore, the study of fats and sugars within the bloodstream provides important clinical correlation for disease prediction. Lipids, such as those used for treponemal infection titers,[8] have also historically been used in diagnostic serology. Cellular membranes not only consist of proteins but also lipid moieties such as phospholipids, polysaccharides, and cholesterol. Each of these products can be the source of an immune response when detected as foreign in a host system. Additionally, the levels of fats, sugars, and metabolites in a patient's specimen may alter the microenvironment and interfere with other laboratory tests including many serological assays.

Nucleic Acids

Genes and genetics are rapidly becoming the next paradigm in clinical diagnostics. Before the understanding of this process was complete, the study of genetic disease was much less refined. Genes, which are composed of nucleotides of DNA (Deoxyribonucleic acid), are the functional unit of inheritance controlling the transmission and expression of traits. These traits are transmitted from the genetic code to RNA, in a process known as transcription, before being converted, or translated, into proteins (**BOX 1-1**). Changes in the structure of DNA, RNA, and proteins, as well as communication between these states, can all lead to disease. The examination of the upregulation of mRNA (messenger RNA) is extensively studied as a hallmark in changing physiological or pathophysiological states as it typically acts as an indicator for a change in protein production. In other sections of this book, we will discuss the changes in protein levels that result from changes in the mRNA code.

Genetics is the study of the genes, coded as the DNA of most living cells, and provides evidence of heredity and genetic variation that occurs between individuals. Diagnostically, differences in genes between individuals can be the basis of many chronic and inborn diseases. The variations in genes may also account for the way in which we respond to infections and other acquired pathologies.

A DEEPER LOOK BOX 1–1 Central Dogma of Biology

- Central Dogma of Biology: DNA → RNA → Proteins
- Proteins consist of amino acids held together by covalent peptide bonds. Amino acids contain amine and carboxyl functional groups and a side chain (R group). There are 20 common amino acids (show peptide bond)
- Structures of proteins are critical for their functions and informed by the amino acid sequence. A string of amino acids is the primary structure of the protein. Amino acid functional groups (R groups) interact to give rise to secondary protein structures, which consists of α helices and β sheets (show cartoons). Proteins can have multiple subunits held together by weak forces such as hydrogen bonds, van der Waals force, and ionic interactions.

Genomics is the study of whole genomes. Variations in genomes are useful predictors of the causation of particular population-specific diseases. While examinations of single genes has been informative in the study of disease, it is also important to understand the relationship between genes, specifically when the disease is systemic. Many diseases occur as a result of more genes working together.

Although less common, antibodies can be used to detect DNA and RNA, most often in association with proteins called nucleoproteins. However, recent advancements in blood detection technologies have allowed for the isolation and analysis of genetic components in blood and body fluids through serological methods. Both directly and indirectly, these assays identify genetic variations and modifications that impact the body's response to disease conditions and therapeutics. For example, mRNA detection and concentration can be assessed through immunoassays. Additionally, changes in gene expression are indicated by changes in the opening and closing of reading frames within the chromosome, which are also detectable through immunoreagents.

Technical Underpinnings of Serodiagnosis

Serology is simply defined as the testing of serum. Serum is the most tested product of the blood. Serology is fundamentally useful in the evaluation of infectious diseases through the fluctuation in specific antibody titers that occur during the disease process. It is, therefore, central to the diagnosis and management of illness. Often, serologic testing is performed after a certain period of disease latency, as antibody titers rise and fall days to weeks after the first signs of illness. Both an acute, directly following infection and a convalescent titer of the disease biomarker are often collected. Thus, baseline readings of antibody titers are used as general guidelines for determining the presence of disease. Without the baseline values from an individual, the values of pooled titers are commonly utilized to establish a reference range for these fluctuations. Therefore, new assays must be carefully validated prior to adoption in the clinical lab. An additional utility of these serological values is in determining the efficacy of vaccination efforts, which also lead to subsequently increased antibody titers for the vaccine antigens.

Serological tests are performed by first collecting blood in a sterile tube, typically through the process of venipuncture, and allowing it to clot. Subsequently, the liquid component, the **serum**, is then separated from the solid cellular components of the blood, the **clot**. The serum would then ideally be tested immediately; however, various storage conditions have also been devised and experimentally verified to allow for the delay in testing that is sometimes necessary in clinical diagnostics.

Serological Classification

The sheer variety of immunoassays is a result of many decades of scientific and technical inquiry by both public and private sources. However, there was a time that serological testing was considered only for the examination of antibodies to microbial organisms; for example, the early examinations of sera for syphilis antibodies saw a steady increase from 1957 to 1967.[9] The patenting of immunodiagnostic technologies means that many processes are still not completely available for general laboratory usage except via specific agreements with commercial reagent and assay producers. However, a simple reaction between the antibody and the antigen (on analyte) is still the fundamental basis for all protocols and procedures described as serological or immunodiagnostic assays.

$$Ab + Ag = Ab - Ag$$
'free'   'bound'

Typically, a fixed amount of antibody combined with a varying concentration of antigen occurs to form an **antibody-antigen complex**. Although no consistent classification system has been adopted, in principle, one can divide the responses into three categories; 1) antibody in relative excess, 2) antibody and antigen in equal proportions, and 3) antigen in relative excess. This relationship can be visualized in the traditionally used precipitin curve (**FIGURE 1–7**),

which describes the relationship between a fixed amount of antibody with a varying amount of antigen.

Dilutions

The dilution of serum to measure the relative concentration of an antibody, including the determination of antibody titer, is a central skill employed in the diagnostic laboratory (**FIGURE 1–8**). Consisting of two components, the **solute** (material being diluted) and the **diluent** (a stable medium making up the rest of the solution), dilutions are represented as a ratio or fraction, such as 1:5, where there is 1 part solute and 4 parts diluents. Thus, a dilution is represented in the following form:

$$1/\text{Dilution (solute + diluent)} = \text{Solute}/\text{Total Volume}$$
For example, 1/5 or 1:5

Approximations of total antibody in a given serum can, therefore, be performed by creating a range of dilutions in a process called a **serial dilution**.

Titers

The **antibody titer** is not a direct detection of the concentration of an antibody, but rather the detection of the concentration of an antibody necessary to achieve an observed reaction when combined with another substance. It is often used as an indicator of the antibody's strength. The antibody titer is determined using a series of dilutions through the performance of several laboratory assays including precipitation, agglutination, coagulation, and various other immunoassays

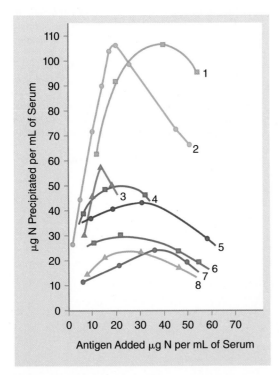

FIGURE 1–7 Example precipitin curves. These curves indicate reactions of various BSA derivatives with an anti-BSA serum.

Reprinted from *Reactions of Antibodies with Soluble Antigens: Methods in Immunology and Immunochemistry*. Vol. 3 (from prior work by Maurer 1957), Williams, C. A., & Chase, M. W., Pg. 56, copyright 1971, with permission from Elsevier.

Dilution (μL)	1:1	1:2	1:4	1:8
Saline (μL)	None	50	50	50
Serum (μL)	100	50		
Mix/transfer (50μL)				

FIGURE 1–8 Example of Serial dilution. 50 μL of serum is added to 50 μL of saline to make a 1:2 dilution, 50 μL of this solution is added to another 50 μL of saline to make a 1:4 dilution and so forth, serially.

in which a reaction product is detected. Higher antibody titers are reported as the inverse of the greatest dilution of serum in which a reaction is present, or as only the denominator of the final dilution. So, a dilution of 1:8 would be reported as a titer of 8. The greater the dilution in which a reaction is detected, the higher the concentration of the antibody in the serum when compared with the same antibody. Different antibodies may require more or less concentration for a reaction to be present. In all cases, the method of detection plays a role in the titer reported. So, comparisons between laboratories should be scrutinized as to the method employed.

Although a consensus as to the frequency of antibody titers collected from a single individual

has not been reached for all biomarkers, it has been well established that a fluctuation in the levels of patient antibody will occur after the onset of infection and during the progression of the disease, dependent on several factors including the type of immunoglobulin being detected, the type of antigen, and the rate of plasma cell production. Furthermore, the titer of an antibody has been monitored prior to and after the administration of various vaccine protective treatments, which can help to establish the need for booster shots or repeated vaccine administration. These timepoint titers are commonly referred to as acute and convalescent titers, and are important for the diagnosis and staging of disease and therapy.

▶ References

1. Mazumdar PMH, von Gruber M, Landsteiner K. *Species and specificity: an interpretation of the history of immunology.* Cambridge; New York, NY, USA: Cambridge University Press; 1995:pg. 142.
2. McCullough J. *Transfusion Medicine.* West Sussex: John Wiley & Sons, Ltd.; 2016.
3. Tas AC. The use of physiological solutions or media in calcium phosphate synthesis and processing. *Acta Biomater.* 2014;10(5):1771–1792.
4. Glick B. The bursa of Fabricius: the evolution of a discovery. *Poult Sci.* 1994;73(7):979–983.
5. Nielsen AA, Petersen PH, Green A, Christensen C, et al. Changing from glucose to HbA1c for diabetes diagnosis: predictive values of one test and importance of analytical bias and imprecision. *Clin Chem Lab Med.* 2014;52(7):1069–1077.
6. Nolan L. Pre-analytical variables: a number of factors can influence sample results in coagulation testing. *Advance for administrators of the laboratory* Vol 25: Merion Publications; 2016:14–16.
7. Riley RS, Gilbert AR, Dalton JB, et al. Widely used types and clinical applications of D-Dimer Assay. *Lab Med.* 2016;47(2):90–102.
8. Browne AS, Coffey E. Treponemal serologic tests; experiences of the Bacteriology Laboratory, California State Department of Public Health. *Calif Med.* 1958;88(4): 300–304.
9. Taylor CE. Serological techniques. *J Clin Pathol Suppl Coll Pathol.* 1969;3:14–19.

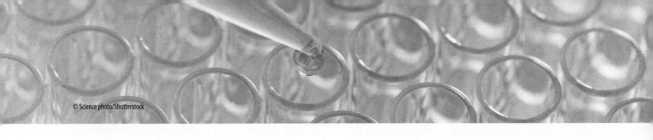

CHAPTER 2

Fundamentals of the Immune System

Barsha Dash, PhD; **Brittney Dinkel**, PhD; and **Ian Clift**, PhD, MLS(ASCP)^{CM}

KEY TERMS

Alternative pathway
Basophils
Chemokines
Classical pathway
Clonal expansion
Cytokines
Dendritic cells (DCs)
Hematopoietic stem cells (HSCs)
Histology

Immune organs
Lectin pathway
Lymphoid tissue inducer
  cells (LTi)
Macrophages
Major histocompatibility
  complex (MHC)
Mast cells
Monocytes

Neutrophils
Pattern recognition receptors
  (PRR)
Plasma cells
Primary lymphoid tissues
Secondary lymphoid tissues
Terminal pathway

LEARNING OBJECTIVES

Upon completion of this chapter, the reader should be able to:

1. Review the history of immunology up to present laboratory practices.
2. Understand and differentiate the three lines of defense that make up the immune system.
3. Specify the function of the major immune organs.
4. Outline the pathway of development for B and T cells via lineage and location.
5. Compare and contrast the pathophysiological role of the various complement pathways.
6. Identify and specify pattern recognition particles involved in innate immune response based on pathology.
7. Demonstrate understanding of the cell types, function and form of MHC molecules.

▶ Introduction

The immune system has the remarkable ability to discriminate between host and pathogens to eliminate infections and preserve organismal homeostasis. To this end, it relies on two key elements—the innate and adaptive systems—that work hand in hand to eradicate bacteria, viruses, and parasites. Innate responses are driven by encoded **pattern recognition receptors (PRR)** that detect a limited and conserved set of molecular patterns present on microbes and usually absent on mammalian cells. However, adaptive mechanisms depend on many genetic rearrangements, engendering spectacular diversity in molecules that aid in recognition of pathogen-derived substances called antigens. In addition, a salient feature of the adaptive immune system is clonal expansion whereby adaptive cells that find their cognate antigen undergo rapid expansion. These cells then partake in pathogen elimination and memory formation, which is essential for rapid elimination of pathogens upon reencounter. To summarize, collective specificities of the innate and adaptive responses allow for detection and mounting of potent defenses against invading pathogens, while minimizing harm to the host. The specificity of the adaptive cell repertoire to minimize host damage is called immune tolerance. Breakdown of tolerance can result in autoimmune diseases that entail immune-mediated destruction of organs. This chapter aims to provide an overview of immune cell development, function, and immune organs at the anatomical and molecular levels.

History

Nineteenth century paradigms created a fertile foundation for modern immunology. Louis Pasteur, a French scientist, and Robert Koch, a German scientist, put forth the "germ theory", i.e., the postulation that microorganisms cause diseases. Pasteur hypothesized that the bacterium *Bacillus anthracis* caused Anthrax disease

in cattle, and Koch experimentally demonstrated the virulence of the bacteria by first isolating it, and then injecting healthy animals with it. Injected animals developed disease, definitively demonstrating the bacteria to be the causative agent of the disease. Koch developed numerous techniques to isolate, grow, and inoculate bacteria that are still in use today. The works of Pasteur and Koch elucidated the importance of hypothesizing and developing experimental tools to demonstrate the cause of an infectious disease, enabling departure from early ideas of spontaneous generation of disease. Koch went on to demonstrate that tuberculosis was caused by a bacterium (*Mycobacterium tuberculosis*). Pasteur also discovered that long-term culturing of bacteria attenuated the bacteria or made them less virulent, generating the roots for attenuated vaccine applications, which involves administration of a weakened pathogen as vaccine to create memory. Edward Jenner, an 18th century physician from England, had already shown that inoculation with cowpox conferred protection against smallpox by immunizing a young boy with bacteria from cowpox of a dairy farmer. These observations and heroic experimental endeavors emphasized the importance of understanding biology, establishing methodologies to find disease etiology and methods to exploit immunological memory, although immunity had not yet been understood.

In the 1800s, Paul Erlich, a German physician-scientist, developed histologic methods to examine innate cells such as neutrophils, basophils, and eosinophils. **Histology** involves staining of cells with different compounds to enable visualization of cell morphology. Erlich's background in chemistry allowed him to put forth early theories of immune recognition of microbes and microbe-derived substances. He proposed that "antitoxins," produced by certain cells of the host, bind via chemically specific interactions with toxins, neutralizing their virulence. He demonstrated this by isolating serum containing "antitoxin" and inoculating animals exposed to diphtheria toxin. Animals that were given the "antitoxin" survived.

Now, it is well known that B cells, cells of adaptive immunity, produce antibodies that bind to toxins and neutralize their virulence, protecting the host. This was the first step toward understanding humoral or B-cell mediated immunity. As new methodological tools, enabling protein separation based on charge and size, enzymatic digestive methods for proteins, and protein structural analysis techniques were developed, appreciation of the structure and chemical nature of antibodies grew. In the 20th century, focus shifted to an examination of the immune cells, laying down foundations for cellular immunology.

Frank Macfarlane Burnet, an Australian immunologist, proposed the theory of clonal expansion. This theory postulated that there were many immune cells of varying specificities, and that upon exposure to a stimulant, such as a bacterium, the cell with highest recognition affinity would multiply, i.e., clonally expand. It is now known that both T and B cells of the adaptive arm of the immune system undergo clonal expansion upon antigen encounter. Australian scientists Peter Doherty and Rolf Zinkernagel discovered that T cells recognized antigens presented by molecules called **major histocompatibility complex (MHC)**. This was a seminal finding and is called MHC-restriction and the fundamental basis of T-cell immune recognition.

With the advent of cloning techniques and protein crystallization techniques, these ideas paved the way to greater structural knowledge of immune-cell receptors and proteins, ultimately leading to discovery of the T-cell surface receptor (TCR) by Mark Davis, an American immunologist; and to the structural characterization of a MHC molecule, by Pamela Bjorkman, also an American immunologist. The TCR guides T-cell functions, including direct killing of infected cells (cytolytic function) and helper T-cell functions that allow for B-cell activation. It soon became clear that innate and adaptive cells

must cooperate to mount immune responses, i.e., phagocytes express MHC molecules that display peptides derived from antigens for activation of T cells. Currently, with the help of gene sequencing and protein structure determination, it is well appreciated that MHC molecules are highly diverse (polymorphic) within the human population and govern susceptibility to infectious diseases, autoimmunity, and cancer.

Elegant experiments of the past have built the foundations of modern immunology. Our understanding of immunology has led to development of diagnostic tools, which, in turn, have led to fine-tuning of our knowledge about the immune system, giving birth to many avenues of immunology: developmental immunology, host-pathogen interaction, structural immunology, cancer immunology, and autoimmunity. These fundamental understandings underpin our clinical aptitude in immunodiagnostics and serology.

▶ Antimicrobial Small Molecules as the First Barrier of Protection

Before antigens encounter immune cells, they are confronted by barrier immunity, a combination of physical and biochemical protection[1] (**FIGURE 2–1**). Physical protection primarily consists of the skin and walls of the oral, intestinal, and respiratory systems. Biochemical protection consists of tears, mucus, antimicrobial peptides (APPs), and proteins such as defensins and cathelicidins; and proteolytic enzymes such as lysozyme secreted by specialized epithelial cells of the skin and respiratory and digestive tracts. APPs are primarily cationic molecules and prevent pathogen dissemination by disrupting anionic bacterial cell walls through electrostatic interactions. Physical mechanisms such as ciliary motions and peristalsis facilitate the expulsion of pathogens trapped in mucus. Thus,

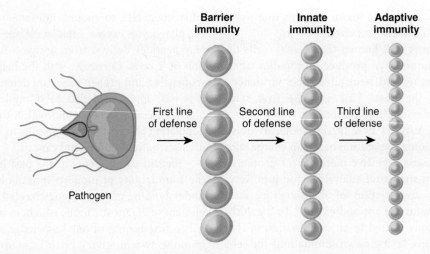

FIGURE 2-1 The three major lines of defense against pathogens. Barrier immunity including skin and intact mucous membranes, innate immunity including in inflammation and phagocytosis, and adaptive immunity or the cellular response.

Modified from Engelkirk, P., et al. Microbiology for the Health Sciences, 11e. Philadelphia, Pennsylvania: Lippincott Williams & Wilkins, 2018.

biochemical barriers aid in pathogen destruction and prevent their dissemination.

Only a few weeks before the birth of a human baby, fetal skin produces copious quantities of antimicrobial molecules in anticipation of exposure to microbes following birth, forming a thick protective layer called vernix caseosa. Immediately after birth, the skin is still vulnerable to microbial breach as its most resilient layer is still in the making. Hence, a baby born before the burst of microbial molecule secretion occurs is susceptible to fungal and gram-negative bacterial infections. With current knowledge about the importance of barrier functions and the mechanisms of APP activity, research is being geared toward treatment of infants with antimicrobial peptides that are effective in reducing incidence of severe diseases such as meningitis and sepsis caused by bacteria. An important implication of using APPs in preterm infants is the reduction of antibiotic administration to combat opportunistic infections. In recent years, numerous bacterial strains are gaining antibiotic resistance, and it is an urgent necessity to find alternative treatment options.

Pathogens that evade microbicidal activities of the skin and other barrier defenses create a

focus of infection, leading to the recruitment of innate and adaptive cells, setting off more complex molecular pathways, cellular crosstalk, and activity.

▶ Organs of the Immune System: Sites of Immune Cell Development and Activity

The immune system is highly compartmentalized. The organs of the immune system provide niches for development of immune cells and the generation of immune responses via immune cell activation[2] (**FIGURE 2-2**). Lymphocytes develop in the **primary lymphoid tissues**: bone marrow or thymus. **Secondary lymphoid tissues**, such as lymph nodes and spleen, help maintain mature lymphocytes until an infection arises.

During development, these **immune organs** (including lymphoid organs) provide optimal niches replete with necessary developmental cues

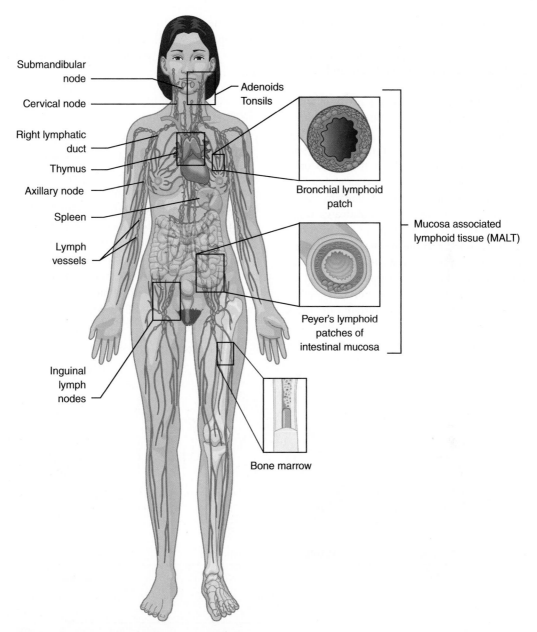

FIGURE 2–2 Lymphoid organs of the human body.

Modified from McConnell, Thomas H. The nature of Disease: Pathology for the Health Professions. Lippincott Williams & Wilkins, 2013.

such as **cytokines**; soluble messengers that bind receptors on cell surface and initiate gene expression changes, and **chemokines**; soluble and insoluble molecular cues for migration. These cues allow for cell-fate determination and maturation. During immune cell activation, they serve as foci for efficient interaction between innate and adaptive cells, allowing for the concentration of antigens and an increasing chance for antigenic encounter with T cells and B cells possessing the optimally specific receptors for the antigens. DCs initiate cell activation, functioning as a crucial link between innate and adaptive systems. Cellular interactions within lymphoid organs are mediated via receptor engagement, communication through secretion of cytokines, and chemokines.

Integrity and homeostasis of these organ systems are imperative for functional immunity and are indicators of the general health of the host. Examination of lymphoid organs may reveal vital information about the status of an individual's health during the diagnosis of the disease. For example, lymphadenopathy, or the enlargement of lymph nodes, indicates ongoing inflammation as a result of an infection. Lymphadenopathy in the absence of infection is often because of the breakdown of immune tolerance or autoimmune diseases such as Myasthenia Gravis, whereby the immune system attacks the neuromuscular system, or IPEX, (Immune dysregulation, polyendocrinopathy, enteropathy, X-linked) in which the immune system attacks many different organs in a systemic manner.[3]

Hematopoiesis

Hematopoiesis is the process of creating all of the blood cells in the body, i.e., red blood cells and immune cells (innate and adaptive).[4] Over the course of development of humans, hematopoiesis takes place at three main locations. Primitive hematopoiesis begins in the yolk sac and upon onset of blood circulation, shifts to the liver, followed by a final shift to the bone marrow, the site of definitive hematopoiesis, supporting the development of blood cells in young and adult humans (**FIGURE 2–3**).

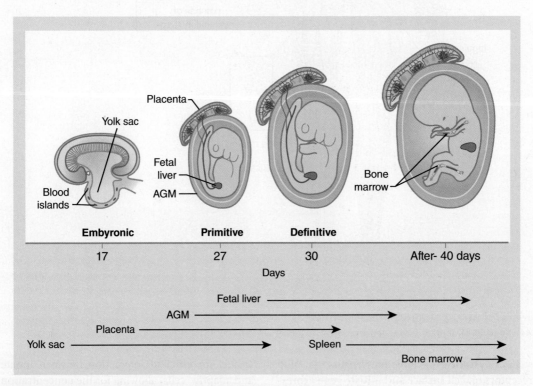

FIGURE 2–3 Sites of hematopoiesis during human development. The major sites of hematopoiesis shift during embryonic and fetal development with hematopoiesis starting in the yolk sac, then shifting to the aorta-gonado-mesonephros (AGM), then to the fetal liver, and then to the bone marrow. The arrows indicate the various sites of hematopoiesis based on the developmental stage.

Primary Lymphoid Organs: Bone Marrow

The bone marrow is a spongy tissue in the central cavity of bone.[5] It is the home to hematopoietic stem cells and their renewal, the site of generations of myeloid and lymphoid precursors (**FIGURE 2–4**), and the primary organ of B-cell development. Hematopoietic stem cells (HSCs) reside in the bone marrow. The two salient features of HSCs are self-renewal and differentiation.[4] HSCs are found along with nonhematopoietic cell types such as endothelial cells, osteoblasts, chondrocytes, and many other cells that regulate and support self-renewal of HSCs and differentiation of HSCs into myeloid and lymphoid lineages. The marrow is abundantly vascularized, allowing for influx of oxygen and nutrients via arteries, trafficking of precursors to distant locations and egress of mature cells that have completed development via venules (very small veins) called sinusoids. Migratory patterns are governed by chemokines. HSCs are found close to these sinusoids surrounded by nonhematopoietic stromal cells.

The knowledge of regenerative capacity of HSCs, i.e., self-renewal, has been critical for

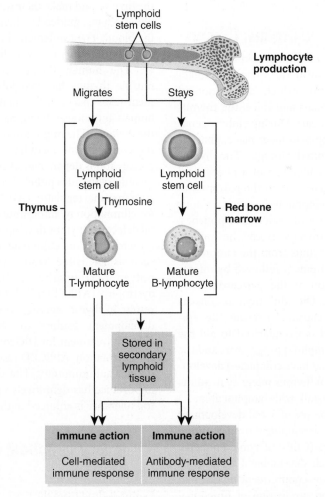

FIGURE 2–4 Lymphocytes are produced in the bone marrow. Lymphocytes emerge in the red bone marrow and either stay and mature into B lymphocytes or migrate to the thymus to become T lymphocytes.

Modified from Archer, Pat, and Lisa A. Nelson. Applied Anatomy & Physiology for Manual Therapists. Lippincott Williams & Wilkins, 2012.

modern medicine regenerative therapies such as bone marrow transplantation.[6] In addition, greater understanding of step-by-step hematopoiesis and markers to identify precursor cells and terminally differentiated cells have been instrumental in characterizing hematopoietic failures in aplastic anemia, whereby Th1 cells mediate destruction of HSCs and chronic myeloid leukemia (CML) characterized by malignant transformation of an HSC that gives rise to myeloid progenitors with self-renewal capacity and superior proliferative capacity. Treatments for both of these conditions include bone marrow transplantation in combination with other treatments.

Primary Lymphoid Organs: Thymus

The thymus consists of two main kinds of cells: epithelial cells that form the thymic architecture, and thymocytes, which are lymphoid cells.[7,13] In adult humans and mice, the thymus is located above the heart. During embryogenesis, as foregut development takes place, pharyngeal pouches arise from the foregut. The thymus originates from the endoderm of a pharyngeal pouch, which also gives rise to the parathyroid gland. Thymus development happens in four major steps: formation of pharyngeal pouches, formation of the thymus from the pouch, detachment of the thymus from the endoderm, and continued development followed by migration to final location at the pericardium by 9 weeks of gestation. The adult thymus consists of a mesenchymal capsule covering the epithelial framework. It is vascularized to aid the influx of common lymphoid progenitors and the exit of thymocytes that have completed development. Maintenance of thymus integrity in adults is dependent on crosstalk with lymphocytes.

The thymus is the site of T-cell development from the site of T-cell development from common lymphoid progenitors (CLPs). Thymic epithelial cells orchestrate T-cell development by providing molecular cues for commitment of CLPs to the T-cell lineage and production of functional T cells. Development of T cells involves genetic rearrangement at the T-cell receptor gene loci,

culminating in a large repertoire of cells with novel specificities, which may include potentially autoreactive TCRs, and nonfunctional receptors. Thymic epithelial cells not only support the development of cells but also aid in the selection of cells that are functional and nonautoreactive. In addition, the thymus harbors DCs, macrophages, and B cells that facilitate T-cell selection. Two major kinds of T cells develop in the thymus, CD4 T cells and CD8 T cells.[8] As mentioned earlier, CD4 T cells, when activated, differentiate into helper T cells, activating B cells and CD8 T cells; and CD8 T cells mediate direct killing of infected cells. Following development, T cells egress from the thymus and make their way to secondary lymphoid organs, guided by chemokine molecules in the blood. The fundamental role that the thymus plays in immunity is now well appreciated.

The human thymus is multilobed while murine thymus has two lobes. T-cell development takes places in two main locations in both human and mouse thymi, namely, the cortex and the medulla. The migration of T cells occurs from the cortex to the medulla as development progresses and is dependent on chemokine cues. The medullary thymic epithelial cell is a gene called an autoimmune regulator (AIRE), which is critical for elimination of autoimmune T cells.[9] Congenital defects in thymus development or loss of AIRE protein function culminate in severe disorders such as DiGeorge Syndrome and autoimmune polyendocrinopathy-candidiasis-ectodermal dystrophy (APECED).[10–13] DiGeorge syndrome results in thymic aplasia, creating reduced T-cell development leading to recurrent infections. Current treatment for DiGeorge includes thymus transplantation. APECED results in a severe multiorgan autoimmunity. The discovery of AIRE's importance has definitively established that central tolerance is enforced in the thymus.

Secondary Lymphoid Organs: Lymph Nodes

Lymph is fluid from the tissue that is drained away from tissues into lymph nodes (LN) (**FIGURE 2–5**) for filtration and supplied back to the blood.[14]

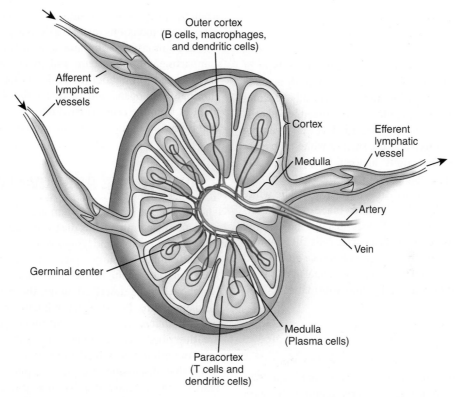

FIGURE 2–5 Anatomy of a Lymph Node.

Data from Reisner, H. (2017). Crowley's an introduction to human disease, 10e. Jones & Bartlett Learning.

Lymph nodes develop from **lymphoid tissue inducer cells (LTi)**.[15–17] LTi cells arise at around 8 weeks of gestation from the fetal liver. Lymph nodes form when LTi cells interact with mesenchymal cells required for organization of lymph nodes in the presence of appropriate molecular signals. These signals have not been fully dissected in humans. During inflammatory responses, tertiary lymph nodes may arise from cells that resemble LTi cells in their molecular signature. LNs are hubs of interaction for innate cells and adaptive cells and for the concentration of antigens for immune cell activation.

LNs are scattered throughout the body and capture pathogens that are not eliminated by initial innate responses by filtering lymph- and chemokine-mediated recruitment of activated DCs carrying antigens. Afferent lymphatic vessels drain lymph into subcapsular sinuses (SCS). The subcapsular sinuses within the LN are lined by macrophages, awaiting antigen entry, and poised to capture and present to B cells and T cells to trigger adaptive responses. Chemokines produced by LN attract lymphocytes to enter the LN via the high endothelial venules. B cells entering the LNs are confined to follicles called the B-cell zone, while T cells are found in paracortical areas called T-cell zones where DCs are positioned to stimulate T cells. The positioning of these cells is dependent on chemokine gradients within the LN. The encountering of B cells and T cells with antigens begins a cascade of events that include interaction of B cells with T cells, clonal expansion to create effector cells that will actively fight infections, and long-lived memory cells for future responses. In addition, LNs are important sites for tolerance enforcement. DCs from tissues continually present self-derived peptides to T cells that may be potentially autoreactive, rendering them anergic or in a state of inactivity, a form of peripheral tolerance.

Secondary Lymphoid Organs: Spleen

The spleen arises from the mesenchymal layer of tissue during embryonic development. It is made of two functionally and anatomically distinct regions: a large red pulp area where red blood cells are broken down and discarded as well as acting in iron turnover, and the smaller white pulp area. Immune interactions happen primarily in the white pulp. Lymphocytes enter the white pulp via the highly branched trabecular artery. The white pulp is organized similarly to that in LN, consisting of B-cell and T-cell zones. Just like the LNs, the spleen has resident phagocytic cells that capture antigens to aid in pathogen clearance and T- and B-cell activation essential for clonal expansion, effector functions, and memory formation.

Secondary Lymphoid Organs: Mucosa-Associated Lymphoid Organs

Ingestion of food and colonization of the gut with friendly but foreign bacteria requires constant immune modulation at the interface of mucosal surfaces that like the gut.[17,18] Additionally, the air that we breathe via the nose contains foreign particles and pathogens, which must be tackled by the mucosa lining the nose and respiratory tract. The mucosal tissues that line these surfaces have many lymphoid structures specialized in antigen capture and clearance. The fundamental architecture of these structures is akin to that of the LN and spleen, consisting of demarcated areas for B cells and T cells and the presence of phagocytic cells for antigen capture and display. These tissues are called Nasal Associated Lymphoid Tissue (NALTS), Bronchus Associated Lymphoid Tissue (BALTS) and Gut Associated Lymphoid Tissue (GALTS).[19] These surfaces are colonized by commensal bacteria, which are critical for overall immune system maturation. Epidemiological studies suggest an increased association of aberrant immune function, such as allergies to innocuous substances because of lack of exposure to commensal as well as infectious microbes. This observation has led to the hygiene hypothesis, whereby allergies and autoimmunity increase as exposure to infectious microbes decrease.[20]

In summary, the immune system is a highly compartmentalized system, and its components are scattered throughout the body to capture and eliminate pathogens and to direct the development of immune cells. This widespread distribution is important for local tissue surveillance.[16]

▶ Innate and Adaptive Cells

The cells of the immune system are what we are most familiar with in the diagnostic laboratory. The various myeloid and lymphoid cells that make up the cellular immune system are a common source of information in the clinic. Along with the lymphoid organs described above, these cells are fundamental to the processes of innate and adaptive immunity. The myeloid and monocytic cells are described below, which have fundamental roles in both innate and adaptive systems. Absent from this discussion are the lymphocytes, in which a more robust discussion is provide in a subsequent chapter.

Myeloid Cells: Granulocytes: Neutrophils, Basophils, Eosinophils, and Mast Cells

Neutrophils are polymorphonuclear leukocytes with lobulated nuclei[21] (**FIGURE 2–6**). Their cytoplasms are rich in granulocytic factors that develop in the bone marrow. During infections, neutrophil production increases and neutrophils migrate to tissues for pathogen clearance. Neutrophils kill pathogens by phagocytosis followed by killing with the help of reactive oxygen species (ROS), degranulation of proteolytic enzymes, or NET (Neutrophils Extracellular Traps) formation. NETs consist of DNA and protein traps to prevent dissemination of pathogens. These are short-lived cells with a half-life of 1.5 hours in mice and 8 hours in humans.

Basophils are also granulocytes that develop in the bone marrow.[22] They harbor granules containing histamines, proteoglycans, granzyme B, as

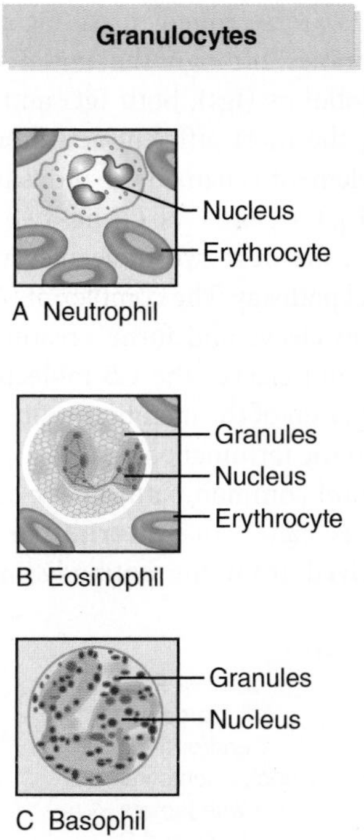

Granulocytes

Nucleus
Erythrocyte

A Neutrophil

Granules
Nucleus
Erythrocyte

B Eosinophil

Granules
Nucleus

C Basophil

FIGURE 2–6 Granulocytes images of N, E, B.

Modified from Ruth McCall, Phlebotomy Exam Review, Jones & Bartlett Learning, 2015.

well as growth factors (Figure 2–6). Upon activation, basophils degranulate. Like neutrophils, they also have a short lifespan. Eosinophils are granulocytes with bi-lobed nuclei and which contain secretory granules.[23] They leave the bone marrow fully mature and circulate in the blood. Eosinophils are known to modulate functions of other immune cells by secretion of growth factors and molecular cues known as chemokines. Similarly, mast cells are granulated leukocytes that originate in the bone marrow.[24] They circulate in the blood and take up residence in tissues where they mature further. Engagement of receptors on **mast cells** leads to degranulation, causing the release of histamines, proteases, and other molecules that aid in pathogen clearance.

Mononuclear Phagocytes: Monocytes, Macrophages, and DCs

Monocytes are mononuclear leukocytes that circulate in the blood and differentiate into macrophages and DCs (dendritic cells).[25,26] Macrophages and DCs are phagocytic professional antigen-presenting cells (pAPCs). **Macrophages** are large mononuclear leukocytes that inhabit lymphoid and nonlymphoid organs. They are important sentinels of immune surveillance because of their superior phagocytic capacity. Phagocytosis allows them to sample their environment for potential tissue damage or infection, leading to initiation of mechanisms to kill pathogens, mitigate damage, and reestablish tissue homeostasis. Macrophages are a heterogeneous population of cells and are highly plastic; their immediate environments shape their properties. The different kind of macrophages are Kupffer cells in the spleen, Langerhans cells in the skin, and microglia in the brain.

Dendritic cells (DCs) are phagocytic leukocytes that circulate in the blood or take up residence in peripheral tissues.[25,27,28] They are essential for immune surveillance and activation of adaptive immune cells. While there are subcategories of DCs, all DCs are derived from common DC progenitors (cDCPs).[29] In the bone marrow, cDCPs differentiate into pre-DCs that migrate via blood to tissues to complete differentiation in lymphoid and nonlymphoid organs. cDCPs are also precursors to plasmacytoid DCs that aid in virus clearance. DCs sample the environment for pathogens using their PRRs and, upon antigen encounter, they mature and migrate to lymph nodes to activate T cells and secrete chemokines to shape the course of the adaptive immune responses.

DC macrophages are professional antigen-presenting cells.[26] They engulf antigens and display them as small peptide fragments on their cell surface to activate T cells, setting off the adaptive responses in motion. Fragmented peptides are displayed on protein molecules called major histocompatibility complex (MHC). T cells recognize peptide-MHC complexes; this recognition is a prerequisite for T-cell priming and activation for their adaptive immune functions.

▶ Complement Cascade

In the late 19th century, Hans Buchner, a German bacteriologist, is credited with describing, for the first time, protective substances, which he called alexins; alexins were capable of killing micro-organisms. These humoral molecules were later called "complement" by Paul Ehrlich, when they were found to be important in both cellular and humoral responses. Unlike the antibody system, also described by Ehrlich, the complement system is considered a nonadaptive piece of the humoral response. Currently, the term "complement" describes 35 proteins found in plasma or on the cell surface.

The complement cascade may be mediated by both innate and adaptive immune mechanisms (**FIGURE 2–7**). Specifically, the **classical pathway** of complement activation is through an antibody-dependent trigger. The first complement components are recruited to pathogens or host-cell membranes through the initial binding of immunoglobulins (Igs), both IgG and IgM, with IgM being the most efficient activator. The first recruited element is named C1 and is broken into subunit C1q, C1r, and C1s. C1 has two substrates, C4 and C2, the next two molecules activated in the classical pathway. The complex of C4b2a stimulates C3 to cleave and form, creating C4b2a3b that binds and cleaves the C5 molecule, leading to the formation of the membrane attack complex (MAC) and the terminal pathway.

A second common pathway for complement activation is called the **alternative pathway**, which derived from the antibody independent

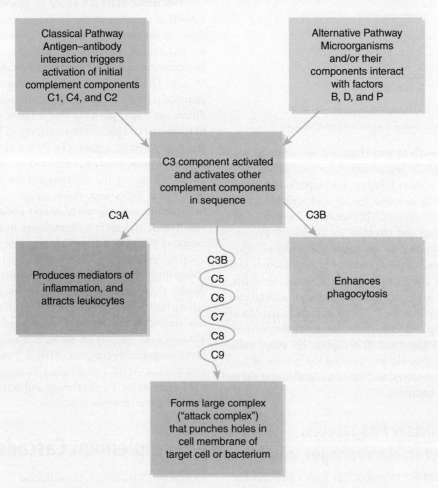

FIGURE 2–7 Complement Pathways.

Data from Reisner, H. (2017). Crowley's an introduction to human disease, 10e. Jones & Bartlett Learning.

activation of complement from certain pathogens. Current speculation exists as to whether this pathway is completely independent of the classical pathway, or if it simply acts as an amplification to that pathway. Nonetheless, it does require the recruitment of several components not found in the classical pathway, namely Factors B, D, and P, which can bind the C3 component and converge with the classical pathway through the stimulation of C5b and the formation of the MAC.

A third complement pathway, known as the **lectin pathway** is also antibody independent and has similar conversion points to the prior two, but is distinctive in its initiation through the mannan-binding lectin (MBL), a lectin that shares structural similarities with the C1 complex found in the classical pathway. Beyond this point, the pathway converges with the stimulation of C4 and C2 as before, and leads to the formation of the MAC and the terminal pathway.

The **terminal pathway**, also referred to as the membrane attack pathway, begins with the cleavage of the molecular C5 on the surface of the target cell. The C5b component is joined by molecules C6, C7, and C8, which, together, can cause membrane disruptions. However, the MAC is completed by the recruitment of multiple copies (estimated at 10) of complement molecular C9, which forms a 10 nm pore in the surface of the cell, releasing water and ions from the cell.

The complement cascade and MAC are highly effective at destroying and inactivating many bacterial pathogens, including *Neisseria meningitides*, *Streptococcus pneumonia*, and *Haemophilus influenzae*. Complement is also consumed at a higher rate during certain autoimmune diseases such as systemic lupus erythematosus (SLE). Serum is collected for detection of the C3 and C4 components via the immunoturbidometic method in many labs as an assessment of a number of pathophysiologic conditions.

▶ Pattern Recognition Receptors

Pattern recognition receptors (PRRs) allow detection of pathogens by innate immune cells outside of the cell and within different cellular compartments[27,30] (**TABLE 2–1**). They recognize common pathogen-associated molecular patterns, such as bacterial cell-wall molecules and viral RNA. Macrophages and DCs use PRRs to sense antigens in secondary lymphoid organs and within tissues. PRR sensing of pathogens activates macrophages and DCs, promoting their ability to

TABLE 2–1 Pattern Recognition Receptor			
Pattern Recognition Receptor	**Ligand**	**Location**	**Primary Outcome**
Toll-like receptors (TLRs)	Viral RNA, bacterial flagellin, bacterial LPS	Cell surface and luminal space	Modulation of immune response
RIG-I like receptors (RLRs)	Microbial nucleic acids	Cytosol	Modulation of immune response
Dectins	Microbial carbohydrates	Cell surface	Internalization of pathogen
LPS receptor	Bind to bacterial Lipopolysaccharide walls	Cell surface	Internalization of pathogen

(continues)

TABLE 2–1 Pattern Recognition Receptor			*(Continued)*
Pattern Recognition Receptor	**Ligand**	**Location**	**Primary Outcome**
Mannose receptors	Mannose residues on bacterial and viral proteins	Cell surface	Internalization of pathogen
Complement receptors	Bind to pathogens opsonized by complement	Cell surface	Internalization of pathogen
Fc receptors	Bind to Fc portions of antibodies that bind pathogens	Cell surface	Internalization of pathogen

create an inflammatory milieu and to modulate immune responses by interaction with innate and adaptive cells. Engagement of pathogens with PRRs initiates signaling cascades that aid in the production of inflammatory chemokines and enhance internalization of pathogen.

The production of various chemokines leads to recruitment of neutrophils, basophils, and eosinophils to the area of inflammation. In addition, macrophages and DCs produce cytokines to enhance activation of innate and adaptive cells. PRRs are strategically positioned in different subcellular compartments to maximize the chances of detecting a pathogen that is present extracellularly or is phagocytosed and is located within phagosomes or the cytosol. For example, toll-like receptors (TLRs) are found on the cell surface and cell vacuoles, while nod-like receptors (NLRs), are found in the cytosol.

▶ Mechanism of Internalization of Pathogens: Endocytosis

Endocytosis or internalization of extracellular particles can occur in two main ways: Phagocytosis and pinocytosis.[16,27,28,31–33] Phagocytosis refers to uptake of extracellular particles, which includes

both foreign antigen and self. For efficient phagocytosis, particles derived from foreign antigens are coated by small molecules present in the blood called opsonins, such as complement proteins or lectins that facilitate uptake of these particles by phagocytic cells. Receptors such as dectins, Fc receptors, complement receptors, scavenger receptors, and many others on phagocytic cells bind to opsonized fragments and internalize them. Bound antigens are taken up into phagosomes, which undergo acidification and subsequent fusion with lysosomes that contain digestive enzymes. Low pH of the acidified phagosome activates proteolytic enzymes allowing for enzymatic degradation of antigens. Pinocytosis refers to fluid-phase engulfment of pathogens. Macrophages are more phagocytic and DCs are less phagocytic, but are superior at pinocytosis and are thought to be better T-cell activators.

Phagocytosis of antigens has a two-pronged effect: it results in activation and maturation of the phagocytic cells, which allows them to migrate to the LN in search of the right T-cell clone and enhances their ability to activate T cells by upregulation of MHC molecules and cytokine expression.

The response of the innate immune system provides mechanisms to keep an infection under control, such as pathogen recognition via various pathogen-associated molecular patterns (PAMPS), while the adaptive response has time to form. The innate immune response also works to prime the adaptive immune response by processing the antigen for presentation to T cells and releasing proinflammatory cytokines. The adaptive immune response, which is composed of T and B cells, provides a specific targeted response to antigens associated with the pathogens while also forming a memory response to provide protection against re-exposures to the same pathogen. It is the adaptive response to disease that has been exploited by immunodiagnostic manufacturers for the production of commercially available antibodies with specific targets.

The adaptive immune system has several unique features that are not shared with the innate immune system. The cells of the innate immune system have receptors on their surface that recognize pathogens that are coded for by germline genes, i.e., genes that are found in all cells of the organism. The adaptive immune system requires receptor assembly through gene rearrangement, i.e., genes that are specific to the cells. Adaptive immune cells undergo a process of gene rearrangement that combines gene segments to produce their receptors. This receptor assembly provides a unique ability to express more than 10^{11} unique receptors. The ability of the adaptive immune system to create the large repertoire of unique receptors allows for greater protection against more pathogens than a static germline system would allow. Another unique feature to the adaptive immune system is memory. Once there has been an adaptive immune response to the pathogen, memory toward that pathogen is generated, protecting against future infections. This memory allows a quicker and more robust response to the pathogen upon re-exposure.

The adaptive immune system is composed of lymphocytes. Lymphocytes are composed of two specific cell types: B cells and T cells. B cells, originally isolated and named for the bursa of chickens, have a unique B-cell receptor (BCR) expressed on the cell surface and develop in the bone marrow. Each B-cell clone expresses a unique BCR that recognizes a specific antigen. Once the BCR binds to its antigen, it activates the B-cell to proliferate and differentiate into plasma cells. **Plasma cells** secrete their BCRs as immunoglobulin, also known as antibodies. T cells develop in the thymus and express a T-cell receptor (TCR) that recognizes antigen in the context of peptide bound to the Major Histocompatibility Complex (MHC).[34] T cells play a key role in the immune response by directing the response of other immune cells through cytokines or by killing infected cells.

Each B-cell and T-cell has a unique BCR or TCR that allows it to recognize a specific pathogen. When a B or T-cell recognizes its antigen through the binding of its receptor, it undergoes **clonal expansion** where every cell that is generated from that activated cell expresses the same clone of the receptor.

Broadly, two lineages of cells carry out immune functions: the myeloid and the lymphoid lineages.[4] Myeloid cells are innate cells, composed of dendritic cells (DCs), macrophages, neutrophils, eosinophils, and basophils. The lymphoid lineage consists of T cells and B cells, which are adaptive cells, and NK cells, which harbor both innate and adaptive features. A more extensive examination of these two systems can be found in Chapter 5: Innate Immunity, and Chapter 6: Adaptive Immunity.

Immune cells develop in primary lymphoid organs, namely, the bone marrow and the thymus, and undergo activation in secondary lymphoid organs such as the spleen and the lymph nodes. All immune cells develop from bone marrow residing pluripotent **hematopoietic stem cells (HSCs)**.[4] The two defining features of HSCs are the ability to self-renew and to differentiate into precursors of immune cells. HSCs differentiate into CLP, which give rise to the lymphoid lineages and the common myeloid progenitors (CMP), which differentiate into the myeloid lineages.

Major Histocompatibility Complex

Major histocompatibility complex consists of a class of heterodimeric glycoprotein molecules, mainly important for antigen presentation to T cells and for directing NK cell function.[35,36] The two main classes of MHC proteins responsible for peptide presentation to T cells are MHC-I and MHC-II.

Central to understanding the role of MHC in immunity is the appreciation of structures of these molecules as well as the genetics that drive their expression.[37] MHC molecules are polygenic, i.e., within one individual, multiple genes will encode MHC-I and II. In addition, MHC molecules are highly polymorphic, which means that many variants of a single gene exist in a population. MHC-I molecules consist of two chains, the α and β domains. α chain comprises the larger part of the molecule, folding into three domains α1, α2, and α3. Folding of the α1 and α2 domains into anti-parallel, β-pleated sheets gives rise to the peptide-binding groove, while α3 is transmembrane and pairs with β2-microglobulin for structural stability. Amino acids that form the groove are areas of a high degree of polymorphism, allowing MHC proteins to display a wide variety of peptides.

Amino-acid residues of the peptide that facilitate its binding to the MHC groove are called anchor residues and are generally aromatic residues with the ability to have ionic interactions as well as the ability to form hydrogen bonds (**BOX 2–1**). MHC-II molecules have two chains, α and β, which pair and contribute to the peptide-binding groove that is structurally similar to MHC-I's peptide binding groove (**FIGURE 2–8**, **BOX 2–2**). Peptides that bind MHC-II are longer and more variable than those

that bind MHC-I. Structural stability of MHC molecules is determined by the peptides loaded onto these molecules. Peptides ensure appropriate folding of MHC molecules and their stability on the cell's surface.

Peptide-MHC complexes serve as signals of cellular health. While MHC-I genes are expressed on all nucleated somatic cells, MHC-II is expressed only on DCs, macrophages, and thymic epithelial cells. MHC molecules present on thymic epithelial cells are critical for instructing developing T cells to recognize peptides in the context of MHC. This is called MHC restriction and allows CD4+ T cells to recognize peptides in the context of MHC-II and CD8+ T cells to recognize peptides in the context of MHC-I. Stimulation of CD4+ T cells by antigenic peptides causes them to differentiate into various helper lineages that facilitate CD8+ T-cell and B-cell activation. CD8+ T cells are direct killers of infected cells.

In addition to classical MHC molecules that present peptides to T cells, nonclassical MHC-like molecules (structurally similar to classical MHC) play important roles in the modulation of immune responses. MHC studies have been pivotal in understanding the self-vs-nonself

A DEEPER LOOK BOX 2–1

Bonds are chemical interactions between atoms to create molecules (intramolecular) or an interaction between molecules (intermolecular) to create macromolecular networks and structure.

Intramolecular forces are ionic or covalent bonds. Ionic bonds are electrostatic interactions between atoms of opposite charges that occur as a result of donation and acceptance of electrons. For example, sodium (Na) donates an electron to chlorine (Cl) to form sodium chloride (NaCl). In the process, Na becomes positively charged and Cl becomes negatively charged. Covalent bonds involve the sharing of electrons between atoms. Carbon (C) bonding is covalent and is abundant in biological molecules. Carbon can make single, double, and triple bonds, allowing it to create a multitude of interactions. In a single water molecule, the interaction between one oxygen (O) molecule and two hydrogen (H) molecules is a covalent bonds.

Intermolecular forces are weak bonds. These include Van der Waals forces and hydrogen bonds. Van der Waals forces are distance dependent and exist between temporary dipoles. Hydrogen bonds are electrostatic interactions between electronegative (electron pulling) atoms. Although water molecules are a result of electron sharing, the sharing is unequal between O and H. O is electronegative and pulls electrons toward itself in a H–O–H molecule, becoming slightly negatively charged, and H atoms adopt a slightly positive charge (dipole formation). The slightly negative charge on O in a water molecule can attract a slightly positive charge on H on a neighboring water molecule. Hydrogen bonding confers high surface tension to water. Such interactions can lend stability to a molecule. For example, DNA consists of two strands held together by stacking hydrogen bond interactions.

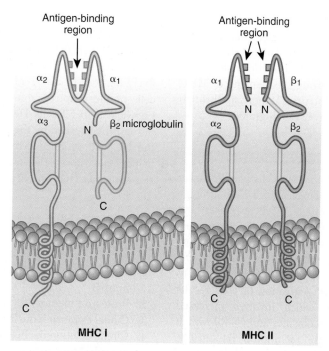

FIGURE 2–8 MHC I and MHC II. The major histocompatibility complex (MHC) I and II (also called Human Leukocyte Antigens; HLA in humans) are glycoproteins expressed on the surface of cells. MHC I is expressed in a variety of nucleated cells and is recognized by cytotoxic T cells prior to targeted destruction of the cell. MHC II, by contrast, is found only on specific antigen-presenting cells (APCs) and when bound with antigen, is recognized by helper T cells.

Modified from Michael H Ross, Wojciech Pawlina. Histology: A Text and Atlas: With Correlated Cell and Molecular Biology, Lippincott Williams & Wilkins, 2015.

recognition capacity of the immune system. This understanding has been critical for appreciating the role of MHC in transplantation of organs. During T-cell development, T-cell repertoire of an individual is instructed to recognize peptides in the context of self-MHC. If a T-cell encounters a foreign MHC, it will perceive the MHC as "nonself." Hence, the MHC match between organ donors and recipients is critical to prevent immune-mediated rejection of grafts after

---

A DEEPER LOOK BOX 2–2   The Major Histocompatibility Complex (MHC)

The two classes of MHC molecules, class I and class II, are a reflection of the health of the cell that synthesized them (class I) or the local cellular environment (class II). In humans, the MHCs are typically referred to as HLA (for human leukocyte antigen), but have been named variously in other organisms. Nomenclature for newly found HLA antigens are governed by the World Health Organization (WHO).

In general, the class of glycoproteins called MHC are recognized to perform a range of immunological functions on the surface of somatic cells. In their prototypical form, they are known for presenting foreign and self-antigens to the surface of the cell, whereby they can be detected by the TCR on T cells or the NK cell receptors on NK cells. These antigens can be the debris from a pathophysiological condition underway within the cell, such as a viral infection, or as a result of a cellular dysregulation as may occur in certain cancers or autoimmune diseases. HLA matching is crucially important for determining transplantation acceptance or rejections. Furthermore, a large number of human diseases are affected by expression or polymorphisms of this molecule. Therefore, it is an important antigenic target in immunodiagnostic analysis.

transplantation. MHC-related studies within human populations have revealed that these are important determinants of cancer, autoimmunity, and susceptibility to infections. Diversity of MHC is studied through sequencing of MHC encoding genes and structural analysis through methods such as X-ray crystallography.

The Adaptive Immune Response

Both the innate and adaptive cells play key roles in determining pathogen clearance. DCs have the unique capacity to initiate T-cell responses, and macrophages synergize and amplify the process of activation of T and B cells by capturing antigens. Pathogens can either be transported by DC cells to the LN, or free pathogens can migrate to SLOs activating DCs. Activation of DCs results in DC maturation, which involves increased expression of MHC molecules and CCR7, which results in migration and retention of DCs in LN. Pathogen proteolytic degradation leads to peptide presentation and T-cell activation. Activated CD4 T cells facilitate the activation of B cells, CD8 T cells, (which deliver humoral immunity) and targeted cellular killing of infected cells, respectively. Because T cells offer help in activating other cells of the adaptive immune system, they are known as helper T cells. Depending on the nature of the PRR engaged by the pathogen on the DC, the DC will produce cytokines to differentiate helper cells into specific fates, which need superior capacity to fight specific pathogens.

Key Tenets of Adaptive Immune Response

1. The ability to discriminate between self and nonself
2. Protective memory formation
3. Clonal expansion during activation
4. Clonal deletion during development as basis of central tolerance

CASE STUDY

Three Immune System Disorders
Case Study 1
This case has been adapted from Markert et al, *N Engl J Med*, 1999.[38]

The DiGeorge syndrome is a heritable disorder that prevents normal thymus development leading to a reduction of T-cell function. Five infants, from age 1 to 4 months with profound DiGeorge syndrome were treated with transplantation of postnatal thymus tissue. Follow-up tests involved immune phenotyping, proliferation assays of peripheral-blood mononuclear cells. Thymic production of new T cells was assessed in peripheral blood. Following transplantation, T-cell proliferative responses developed in four infants. Two patients survived and attained immune function. The remaining three patients died from infections or anomalies independent of transplantation. Biopsies of grafted thymus in the surviving patients showed normal morphologic features and active T-cell production. In one surviving patient, T-cell development occurred within the graft, leading to accumulation of recently developed T cells in the periphery and acquisition of normal T-cell function. In the second patient, thymus function and T-cell development was observed for more than 5 years after transplantation. This study led to the conclusion that in some infants with severe DiGeorge syndrome, transplantation of the thymus can lead to restoration of the T-cell compartment and function. However, it is likely that early thymus transplantation is essential, prior to any infections, to increase chances of survival.

Critical Thinking Question
With crucial knowledge about DiGeorge syndrome in hand, you diagnose it in a newborn. Suppose you are a physician. What treatment would you administer to restore T-cell function in the infant?

Case Study 2

This case was adapted from Gottleib et al., *N Engl J Med*, 1981.[39]

In 1981, the first cases of Acquired Immunodeficiency Syndrome (AIDS) arose around the world. The following is an (edited) abstract from a case study from 1981 published in the *New England Journal of Medicine* documenting initial observations of AIDS-positive patients. Four homosexual patients displayed opportunistic infections, loss of CD4 helper T cells, and telltale signs of inflammation such as lymphadenopathy.

Soon a virus, Human Immunodeficiency Virus 1 (HIV1), was cloned and described as the causative agent of AIDS. The key observation of depletion of helper CD4 T cells led to the discovery of CD4 as a key receptor that HIV1 used to bind to CD4 T cells and initiate its replication cycle within CD4+ T cells that caused T-cell death. CD4 T-cell count is now an important criterion to monitor HIV status of patients. HIV struck at a time when clinicians and scientists were armed with tools such as monoclonal antibodies to immune phenotype cells, sequencing techniques to isolate the virus and monitor its evolution. Furthermore, general knowledge of the immune system, coupled with ideas about viral, bacterial, and fungal infections, were already in place to recognize that patients were susceptible to opportunistic infections that an immune-competent person could easily thwart. Although HIV remains a global infectious disease challenge with no effective vaccine in place, powerful antiviral drugs that halt viral replication and allow for CD4 T-cell persistence have enabled patients to lead longer and healthier lives. The case of HIV demonstrates an ongoing global collaboration between clinicians and scientists to overcome an enormous public health challenge with many successes and many failures and along the way. The following study was adapted from "Pneumocystis Carinii Pneumonia and Mucosal Candidiasis in Previously Healthy Homosexual Men.

Evidence of a New Acquired Cellular Immunodeficiency

Four previously healthy patients were hospitalized with fever, lethargy and lymphadenopathy, candidiasis infection, and respiratory infections. All patients had reduced T-cell numbers, as determined by monoclonal antibody function and virtual absence of T-cell proliferative response. Cytomegalovirus infection was determined by viral cultures performed in human-embryonic-lung fibroblasts. Antibodies to cytomegalovirus, adenovirus, and herpes simplex were found in the sera of the patients. Bronchial brushings showed evidence of Pneumocystis carinii in all patients. One patient died, two patients recovered, and Kaposi's sarcoma developed in the remaining patient. These manifestations suggest severe immunosuppression.

Critical Thinking Question

Confronted with a conglomeration of symptoms that you have never seen before, how do you go about characterizing a disease?

Case Study 3: RAG Deficiency Leading to Impaired Antibody Production

This case has been adapted from Geier et al, *PLoS One*, 2015.[40]

Patient A, a 27-year-old woman, was tested for a primary immunodeficiency. The woman's family had no history of immunological defects. The woman suffered from reoccurring bacterial infections of the upper respiratory system starting at age 7. At the age of 8, she was hospitalized due to inflammation of the blood vessels of the skin of both legs, which reoccurred at age 13. When she was 10 years old, she was diagnosed with chronic interstitial pneumonia. The chronic bacterial infections of the lungs led to chronic obstructive airway disease. At age 13, she was diagnosed with hypogammaglobulinemia, the lack of antibodies. She started intravenous (IV) IgG (IVIG) infusions at the age of 20. Prior to IgG infusions, she had a serum IgG level of 393 mg/dL and normal levels of IgA and IgM. Despite recurrent *Streptococcus pneumoniae* infections, the patient had very low levels of S. pneumoniae-specific IgG antibodies but high levels of pathogen-specific IgM antibodies. Continued susceptibility to pulmonary and middle ear infections required regular IVIG substitution therapy. Unfortunately, the chronic lung infections led to decreasing lung function, resulting in the patient's death at age 48.

(continues)

CASE STUDY   (Continued)

Patient B is a 41-year-old woman who was tested for a primary immunodeficiency at the age of 35. The patient has two healthy children. She has a history of pneumonia and recurrent bacterial bronchitis. She presented with low levels of IgM, IgA, and IgG. She also lacked antibodies against common bacterial polysaccharides. The patient was successfully treated with IV infusions of IgG and sinus surgery.

Laboratory Diagnostics

The patients' blood samples were evaluated for serum antibodies against common bacterial and viral antigens. The first laboratory test was to determine the serum concentrations of the various antibody isotypes. Serum antibody concentrations are calculated by nephelometry. Nephelometry (discussed in more detail in Chapter 2: The Serological Specimen) measures the concentration of the antibodies in suspension via laser light. The more the light that is scattered, the higher the concentration of antibodies present. The antibody specificity is determined by ELISA. ELISA plates are coated with the antigens of interest (tetanus, diphtheria toxin, *Haemophilus influenzae* type b, or pneumococcal capsular polysaccharide). The patient's serum is added to the wells and any antibodies specific to those antigens will bind. Noncognate antigens will be washed away. A secondary antibody that recognizes human IgG or IgM linked to an enzyme will be added to the wells to detect the antigen-specific antibodies. The enzymes linked to the end of the secondary antibody will interact with its substrate to produce fluorescence that can be quantified. These laboratory diagnostic tests revealed that the two patients had low antibody concentrations and lacked antigen-specific antibodies.

Diagnostic tests were also performed to look at B-cell antibody secretion and proliferation. The patient PBMCs and control cells were stimulated with Epstein-Barr virus (EBV) and cultured for 8 days. The antibody secretion was measured by nephelometry. Proliferation of the B cells was measured by ^{3}H-Thymidin incorporation, which incorporates as the cells grow and divide. The patients' B cells had decreased IgG production and proliferation. B-cell differentiation was also tested by flow cytometry. Patient A had normal levels of B cells in the periphery (CD19+ and CD20+) while patient B had decreased numbers. A decrease was detected in class-switched B cells and memory B cells. The patients also had increased CD21^{low} B cells, which are characterized by an exhausted phenotype. Overall, the diagnostic tests revealed a defect in B cells.

The patients also had their T cells tested. The patients had decreased CD3+, CD4+, and CD56+ lymphocytes and decreased Tregs. Further testing revealed decreased levels of naïve CD4+ T cells but normal levels of memory and effector cells. The CD8+ population was normal. A spectratyping analysis was done to examine the TCR Vβ repertoire of CD3+ T cells. Spectratyping analysis purifies RNA from the T cells and it is converted into cDNA. Polymerase chain reaction (PCR) amplifies the cDNA. During PCR, the complementary-determining region-3 (CDR3) is fluorescently labeled with various primers. The cDNA is passed through a laser that measures the frequency of the different Vβ chains. The spectratyping of the patient samples revealed normal diversity of the TCR Vβ chains. These tests revealed a defect in T cells as well as the B cells.

The defect in T and B cells suggested a possible role for the endonucleases RAG1 and RAG2. RAG1 and RAG2 are required for T-cell receptor and B-cell receptor generation. DNA sequencing revealed mutations in the RAG1 and RAG2 loci. Patient A was heterozygous for a RAG1 mutation. Patient B was heterozygous for a RAG2 mutation. Molecular characterization of RAG expression by Western Blot showed significantly decreased levels of RAG in these patients. The mutation did not completely delete RAG, resulting in an intermediate phenotype instead of severe combined immunodeficiency (SCID). The lower levels of RAG allowed some B cells and T cells to rearrange their receptors and successfully mature. The RAG defect did, however, decrease the number of T and B cells able to develop. The decrease in the number of CD4+ T cells would result in less T-cell help for the B cells, resulting in decreased class switching and affinity maturation.

Critical Thinking Questions

1. Which immunodiagnostic tests were incorporated into this diagnosis?
2. How did the RAG1 and RAG2 deficiencies affect the patients' antibody production?

▶ References

1. Kollmann TR, Kampmann B, Mazmanian SK, et al. Protecting the newborn and young infant from infectious diseases: lessons from immune ontogeny. *Immunity.* 2017;46(3):350–363.

2. Cyster JG. Lymphoid organ development and cell migration. *Immunol Rev.* 2003;195:5–14.

3. Leite MI, Jones M, Ströbel P, et al. Myasthenia gravis thymus: complement vulnerability of epithelial and myoid cell, complement attack on them, and correlations with autoantibody status. *Am J Pathol.* 2007;171(3): 893–905.

4. Orkin SH, Zon LI. Hematopoiesis: an evolving paradigm for stem cell biology. *Cell.* 2008;132(4):631–644.

5. Morrison SJ, Scadden DT. The bone marrow niche for haematopoietic stem cells. *Nature.* 2014;505(7483): 327–334.

6. Gratwohl A, Baldomero H, Aljurf M, et al. Hematopoietic stem cell transplantation: a global perspective. *JAMA.* 2010;303(16):1617–1624.

7. Rodewald HR. Thymus organogenesis. *Annu Rev Immunol.* 2008;26:355–388.

8. Hogquist KA, Jameson SC. The self-obsession of T cells: how TCR signaling thresholds affect fate 'decisions' and effector function. *Nat Immunol.* 2014;15(9):815–823.

9. Bansal K, Yoshida H, Benoist C, et al. The transcriptional regulator Aire binds to and activates super-enhancers. *Nat Immunol.* 2017;18(3):263–273.

10. Baldini A. Dissecting contiguous gene defects: TBX1. *Curr Opin Genet Dev.* 2005;15(3):279–284.

11. Davies EG. Immunodeficiency in DiGeorge syndrome and options for treating cases with complete athymia. *Front Immunol.* 2013;4:322.

12. Malchow S, Leventhal DS, Lee V, et al. Aire enforces immune tolerance by directing autoreactive T cells into the regulatory T-cell lineage. *Immunity.* 2016;44(5):1102–1113.

13. Pitkänen J, Peterson P. Autoimmune regulator: from loss of function to autoimmunity. *Genes Immun.* 2003;4(1):12–21.

14. Ruddle NH, Akirav EM. Secondary lymphoid organs: responding to genetic and environmental cues in ontogeny and the immune response. *J Immunol.* 2009;183(4): 2205–2212.

15. Cupedo T. Human lymph node development: an inflammatory interaction. *Immunol Lett.* 2011;138:4–6.

16. Delves PJ, Roitt IM. The Immune system: first of two parts. *N Engl J Med.* 2000;343(1):37–49.

17. van de Pavert SA, Mebius RE. New insights into the development of lymphoid tissues. *Nat Rev Immunol.* 2010;10(9):664–674.

18. Randall TD, Mebius RE. The development and function of mucosal lymphoid tissues: a balancing act with micro-organisms. *Mucosal Immunol.* 2014;7(3):455–466.

19. Elmore SA. Enhanced histopathology of mucosa-associated lymphoid tissue. *Toxicol Pathol.* 2006;34(5):687–696.

20. Okada H, Kuhn C, Feillet H, et al. The 'hygiene hypothesis' for autoimmune and allergic diseases: an update. *Clin Exp Immunol* 2010;160(1):1–9.

21. Kolaczkowska E, Kubes P. Neutrophil recruitment and function in health and inflammation. *Nat Rev Immunol.* 2013;13(3):159–175.

22. Chirumbolo S. State-of-the-art review about basophil research in immunology and allergy: is the time right to treat these cells with the respect they deserve? *Blood Transfus.* 2012;10(2):148–164.

23. Rosenberg HF, Dyer KD, Foster PS. Eosinophils: changing perspectives in health and disease. *Nat Rev Immunol.* 2013;13(1):9–22.

24. Wernersson S, Pejler G. Mast cell secretory granules: armed for battle. *Nat Rev Immunol.* 2014;14(7):478–494.

25. Auffray C, Sieweke MH, Geissmann F. Blood monocytes: development, heterogeneity, and relationship with dendritic cells. *Annu Rev Immunol.* 2009;27(1):669–692.

26. Guilliams M, Ginhoux F, Jakubzick C, et al. Dendritic cells, monocytes and macrophages: a unified nomenclature based on ontogeny. *Nat Rev Immunol.* 2014;14(8):571–578.

27. Pauwels AM, Trost M, Beyaert R, et al. Patterns, receptors, and signals: regulation of phagosome maturation. *Trends Immunol.* 2017;38(6):407–422.

28. Savina A, Amigorena S. Phagocytosis and antigen presentation in dendritic cells. *Immunol Rev.* 2007; 219:143–156.

29. Mildner A, Jung S. Development and function of dendritic cell subsets. *Immunity.* 2014;40(5):642–656.

30. Takeuchi O, Akira S. Pattern recognition receptors and inflammation. *Cell.* 2010;140(6):805–820.

31. Henneke P, Golenbock DT. Phagocytosis, innate immunity, and host-pathogen specificity. *J Exp Med.* 2004;199(1):1–4.

32. Iadecola C, Anrather J, Nat, et al. Mannose-binding lectin—the forgotten molecule? *Nature Medicine.* 2011; 17(26):796–808.

33. Jin J, He S. The complement system is also important in immunogenic cell death. *Nat Rev Immunol.* 2017; 17(2):143.

34. De Silva NS, Klein U. Dynamics of B cells in germinal centres. *Nat Rev Immunol.* 2015;15(3):137–148.

35. Wieczorek M, Abualrous ET, Sticht J, et al. Major histocompatibility complex (MHC) class I and MHC class II proteins: conformational plasticity in antigen presentation. *Frontiers Immunol.* 2017;8:292.

36. Bjorkman PJ, Parham P. Structure, function, and diversity of class I major histocompatibility complex molecules. 1990;59:253–288.

37. Trowsdale J, Knight JC. Major histocompatibility complex genomics and human disease. *Annu Rev Genomics Hum Genetics.* 2013;14(1):301–323.

38. Markert ML, Boeck A, Hale LP, et al. Transplantation of thymus tissue in complete DiGeorge syndrome. *N Engl J Med*. 1999;341(16):1180–1189.

39. Gottlieb MS, Schroff R, Schanker HM, et al. Pneumocystis carinii pneumonia and mucosal candidiasis in previously healthy homosexual men: evidence of a new acquired cellular immunodeficiency. *N Engl J Med*. 1981;305(24): 1425–1431.

40. Geier CB, Piller A, Linder A, et al. Leaky RAG deficiency in adult patients with impaired antibody production against bacterial polysaccharide antigens. *PLoS One*. 2015;10(7):e0133220.

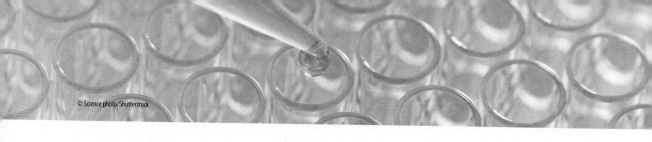

CHAPTER 3

Lymphocytes in Adaptive Immunity

Barsha Dash, PhD; **Brittney Dinkel**, PhD; and **Ian Clift**, PhD, MLS(ASCP)^{CM}

KEY TERMS

12/23 rule
Activation Induced Cytidine Deaminase (AID)
Affinity
Affinity maturation
Antibodies
Apurinic/apyrimidinic endonuclease (APE1)
Autoimmune regulator (AIRE)
Avidity
calcium release-activated channels (CRAC)
CD4
CD8
Centroblasts
Centrocytes
Class switching
Class switch recombination (CSR)
Cluster of differentiation 3 (CD3)

Common lymphoid progenitors (CLPs)
Constant region
Cytotoxic T cells
Double negative (DN)
Double positive (DP)
Early thymic progenitors (ETP)
ERK
Follicular T cells (Tfh)
Germinal center
Hematopoietic stem cells (HSCs)
IκB
Immune complexes
Kinases
LAT
LCK (lymphocyte-specific protein tyrosine kinase)
Linked recognition
Phosphatases

PKCθ
Plasmablasts
PLCγ
RAG genes
Recombination Activating Gene (RAG-1 and RAG-2)
Recombination signal sequences (RSSs)
Secondary lymphoid organs
SLP76
Switch regions (S regions)
Th1
Th2
Th17
T helper cells (T$_H$)
Tregs
Uracil DNA glycosylase (UNG)
Variable region
ZAP70 (zeta-chain-associated protein kinase 70)

▶ Lymphocytes

While both T- and B-cell mediated immunity require antigen recognition in some form, only B cells produce and release antibodies into circulation. T cells rely on detection of antigens associated with MHC complexes that reside within a number of antigen-presenting cells (APCs) and lead to the direct destruction of cells that are pathogen infected. B cells, on the other hand, rely on what is known as humoral immunity, or the release of macromolecules such as antibodies and complement proteins. Humoral immunity depends on these macromolecules in the body fluid and blood, as well as the cellular mediators of pathogen detection and destruction. Clinical immunodiagnostics is underpinned by the actions of both T and B cells for the production of antibodies (**FIGURE 3–1**) in vivo; therefore, an in-depth understanding of their function and development is crucially important in the diagnosis of diseases in the clinical setting.

This chapter primarily focuses on the B and T lymphocytes (B and T cells) that mediate humoral or adaptive immunity.

▶ B Cells

B cells are lymphocytes that develop in the bone marrow. After B cells have matured, they can migrate through the blood stream as naïve B cells.[1,2] Naïve B cells also enter the lymphoid tissues or lymphoid organs, lymph nodes, spleen, and mucosal lymphoid tissues. When a B-cell binds its cognate antigen through the B-cell receptor (BCR), the BCR internalizes the antigen and possibly the entire pathogen. This allows the B-cell to process that captured antibody and present it on MHC to activate T cells. A signaling cascade between these cells determines the

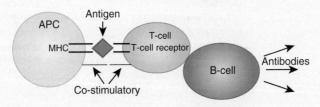

FIGURE 3–1 Antigen presentation to T and B cells in the production of antibodies.

Data from Reisner, H. (2017). Crowley's an introduction to human disease, 10e. Jones & Bartlett Learning.

pathogenicity of the antigen. After a B-cell has been activated through its BCR, it can differentiate into a plasma cell and secrete its BCR in the form of antibodies.

B-cell development is centered around creating functional BCRs that can recognize a broad variety of antigen.[3] BCR expression involves V(D)J recombination mediated by RAG enzymes. Functional B cells that become activated can differentiate into plasma cells in B-cell zones of secondary lymphoid organs and home back to the bone marrow. Plasma cells produce copious quantities of a secreted version of BCRs called antibodies. Antibodies are essential for humoral immunity for B-cell mediated immunity, providing protection against pathogens by neutralizing toxins and pathogens, and mediating their phagocytosis by macrophages and DCs. Antibodies and BCRs are Y-shaped molecules composed of two heavy chains and two light chains (**FIGURE 3–2**). The light regions pair with the heavy chains via disulfide bridges, and the two heavy chains pair via disulfide bridges. The "arms" of the Y are called the Fab fragments and the stalk is the Fc region. Arms engage in interactions with antigens. DCs have receptors that recognize the Fc region, and any antibody bound to an antigen can undergo receptor-mediated endocytosis for antigen processing. In this way, B-cell and T-cell immunity is intricately linked. Subsequent sections will introduce more concepts of B-cell and T-cell collaboration in immune responses. The Fab fragments resemble the TCR variable and constant regions and are attached to the Fc region, which is composed of constant regions via a flexible linker called the hinge region. Thus, the antibody has regions that are variable and that are highly conserved, depending on the roles that these regions play.

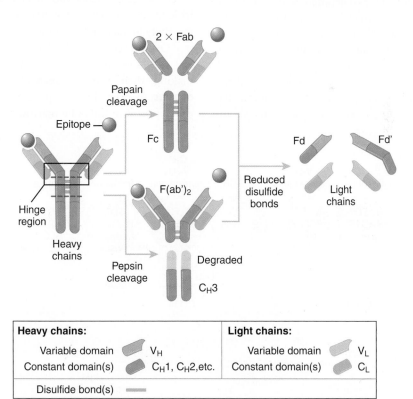

FIGURE 3–2 Antibody structure and fragmentation.

Modified from Thao Doan, et al. Lippincott Illustrated Reviews: Immunology, Lippincott Williams & Wilkins, 2012.

B-Cell Development

Following birth, B-cell development occurs in the bone marrow in humans and mice (**FIGURE 3–3**). Simply put, **hematopoietic stem cells (HSCs)** differentiate into the **common lymphoid progenitors (CLPs)**,[4–8] which develop into B cells. Molecular networks orchestrate the commitment of CLPs to the B-cell lineage and subsequent stages of development and selection. CLPs differentiate into Pro-B cells. At this stage, genes encoding the heavy chain begin to rearrange, catalyzed by **RAG genes**. The D and J regions are joined first, followed by recombination of the V region to the already-assembled D-J regions. When the heavy chain is completely assembled, it is expressed on the cell surface and paired with a surrogate light chain called the VpreB, and the B-cell is called the pre-B cell. Together they signal for the pre-B cells to proliferate. Proliferation results in many daughter cells carrying a heavy chain that is properly folded; each cell can then start rearranging its light chain loci. Assembly of the light chain involves joining of V to J regions. Together, the light and heavy chains make up the B-cell receptor (BCR).

Just like random gene rearrangement can give rise to autoreactive T cells, autoreactive B cells are also generated. An autoreactive B-cell can undergo one of several fates. If it encounters a self-ligand in the bone marrow, it undergoes clonal deletion, just as T cells undergo negative selection. It may also undergo receptor editing whereby the existing light chain can be replaced by further rearrangement at the light chain loci. The combination of the new light chain with the previous heavy chain can yield a novel BCR that is no longer self-reactive. If B cells are not self-reactive, they migrate to secondary lymphoid organs where they complete B-cell maturation. Loss of B-cell tolerance can cause autoimmunity such as systemic lupus erythematosus (SLE).[9] B-cell tolerance breakdown can be determined by detection of antibodies against mammalian, double-stranded DNA and histones (antinuclear antibodies, or ANA). Serum-containing antibodies can be isolated from the blood of SLE patients and incubated with fixed irradiated cells such as hepatocytes to determine reactivity to nuclear proteins and DNA.

Over the course of B-cell development, B cells exit the bone marrow via the central arteriole, making their way to **secondary lymphoid organs**. B cells that complete initial stages of development in the bone marrow, migrate to the

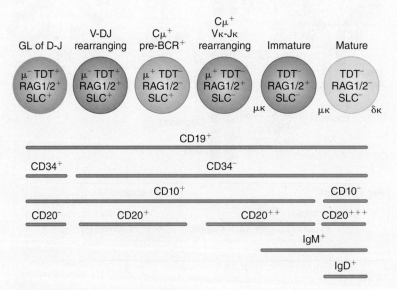

FIGURE 3–3 B-cell development summary.

Modified from William E Paul. Fundamental Immunology, Lippincott Williams & Wilkins, 2012.

spleen to complete additional stages of maturation to achieve functional competency. Maturing B cells go through three transitional stages, namely, T1, T2, and T3 populations. B-cell maturation is also a mechanism to ensure B-cell tolerance or to prevent B-cell activation against self, driven by the nature of BCR signals.

Cytokine signaling and transcription factors direct B-cell development. Pax5, a key transcription factor in B cells, drives CD19 (B-cell coreceptor) expression. CD19 expression is a marker of Pro-B cells. Pro-B cells start their IgH (heavy chain) rearrangement. Once an IgH chain is rearranged, it is expressed on the surface of the B-cell with a surrogate light chain to form the Pre-BCR. Signaling through the pre-BCR drives clonal proliferation and allelic exclusion. Allelic exclusion occurs when the B-cell stops rearranging the IgH and shuts down rearrangement of the other allele for the heavy chain. Allelic exclusion occurs by downregulating RAG1/2 gene, phosphorylating RAG2 causing its degradation, and epigenetic modifications of the heavy chain locus. The pre-BCR is expressed during the pre-B-cell stage of development. Signaling through the pre-BCR also starts the rearrangement of the IgL (light chain). After rearrangement of the IgL chain, the BCR is expressed on the cell surface and tested for self-reactivity. Immature B cells will test their BCR in the bone marrow first. B cells that recognize self-antigen in the bone marrow have four possible fates: death by apoptosis (clonal deletion), light chain replacement by receptor editing, induction of anergy (absence of immune response), or induction of ignorance (production below the threshold of immune responsiveness). High-affinity, self-antigen binding that crosslinks the BCRs in the bone marrow, results in clonal deletion of the B cells. Another possible fate that can occur with the high-affinity, self-reactive antibody is receptor editing. B cells have two kappa light chain alleles and two lambda light chain alleles. The self-reactive B-cell can turn on RAG1 and RAG2 expression again and rearrange the remaining light chain loci. Once a new light chain is rearranged, it will be tested by the same mechanism. The third possible fate, anergy, occurs when the B-cell binds weakly, cross-linking antigen-like soluble proteins. Anergic B cells express low levels of IgM on the cell surface and are in a state of unresponsiveness. Stimulation with antigen and T-cell help cannot overcome the anergic state. The final possible fate, ignorance, is induced by weak affinity for self-antigen. Ignorant B cells mature and migrate through the periphery and can become activated under the right circumstances. Immunologically ignorant B cells are kept under control by lack of appropriate T-cell help (autoreactive T cells are deleted from the periphery), inaccessibility to antigen, and peripheral tolerance. Immature IgM+ B cells exit the bone marrow and enter the spleen for antigen-dependent B-cell development.

Generation of the BCR

B cells can recognize very large number of different antigens or epitopes. The antibody repertoire, or the total number of different antibodies possible for humans, is greater than 10^{11}. Through the Human Genome project, it is estimated that humans have about 20,000 to 25,000 protein-coding genes. If we have only approximately 20,000 genes, how can we generate so many different BCRs? B cells and T cells undergo a process called somatic recombination that combines germline gene segments to produce their receptors. It is important to note here that the BCR generation and gene rearrangement are random processes that occur during B-cell development in the absence of antigen.

BCRs contain two polypeptides, the light chain and the heavy chain. Both the light and heavy chains are made by combining gene segments to produce a single polypeptide.[10–13] The light chain is made up of a **variable region** and a **constant region**. The variable region is made up of a variable or V gene and a joining or J gene segment. There are two genetic loci (κ and λ) that can be used to generate the variable region of the light chain. Generally, healthy individuals have a κ:λ ratio of 3:1. The heavy chain is also made up of a variable region and a constant region. The variable region of the heavy chain can be divided into three gene segments: V_H gene, J_H gene, and diversity or D_H gene. The heavy chain has only one genetic locus that can be used to generate the variable region. Each of the genes has multiple, different functional gene segments that can be used to generate the receptor. The different combinations of V (variable segment) and J (joining segment) for the light chain, and V, D (diverse segment), and J for the heavy chain, creates combinatorial diversity (**FIGURE 3-4**). For example, light chain λ has 30 different V genes and 4 different J genes resulting in approximately 120 different λ light chains. The diversity of the antibody does not only come from the different combination of gene segments in the light or heavy chain, but also from all of the different combinations of different heavy and light chains. There are approximately 200 different κ light chains and 120 different λ light chains that could be combined with approximately 18,000 different heavy chains resulting in 5,760,000 different antibodies that can be produced. However, that represents only the magnitude of 10^6 for diversity, whereas it has been estimated that there are approximately 10^{11} different antibodies possible. So where does the rest of the diversity come from? The process of gene recombination also creates junctional diversity.

Antibodies are secreted BCRs that are crucial to the immune response **BOX 3-1**. Antibodies are produced from the same gene rearrangement that created the surface BCR, but they are slice variants that no longer have the transmembrane domain linking them to the cell

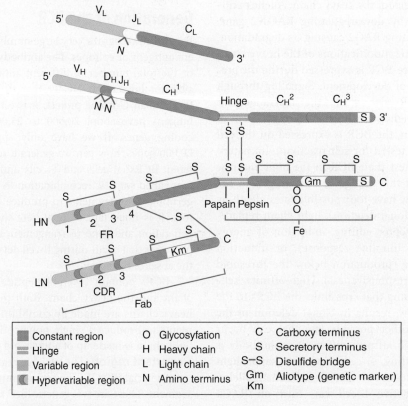

FIGURE 3-4 Detailed antibody structure.

Modified from William E Paul. Fundamental Immunology, Lippincott Williams & Wilkins, 2012.

Antibodies are made up of two different polypeptide chains.[14] The larger polypeptide chain that is approximately 50 kDa is the heavy chain. The smaller polypeptide is the light chain and is about 25 kDa. Each antibody is composed of two heavy and two light chains linked by disulfide bonds. The heavy chains contain a variable region that recognizes the antigen, and a constant region that makes up the stem or the Fc portion of the antibody. The light chains contain variable and constant regions that are part of the arms of the Y. The Y shape of antibodies allows them to have two binding sites that recognize the same antigen on each molecule. The strength of the interaction of a single binding site on the antibody to the antigen is its **affinity**. Combining the affinities of the binding sites on the antibody is the **avidity** of the molecule.

The heavy chain of the antibody defines the class and effector function of the antibody. The heavy chains have five classes or isotypes that control the function of the antibody. The five isotypes are immunoglobulin M (IgM), IgD, IgG, IgA, and IgE. The heavy chains that make up each isotype are designated by lowercase Greek letters (μ, δ, γ, α, or ε).

surface; therefore, they are released to circulate in the tissue and bloodstream. BCRs and antibodies are Y-shaped molecules where the two arms recognize and bind to the pathogen, and the stem interacts with effector cells and molecules (Figure 3–2 and Figure 3–4). If we break down the structure of the antibodies further, the arms contain a variable region that recognizes and binds to the antigen, and a constant region that provides the structure of the antibody. The stem of the Y is the Fc portion or a constant region that effector cells or complement can recognize and bind to in order to carry out their effector functions.

The BCR itself does not actually contain any signaling domains that result in downstream activation of the B-cell. The BCR forms a complex with Igβ and Igα. Igβ and Igα form a complex that is linked through a disulfide bond and contains immuno-receptor tyrosine-based activation motifs (**ITAMS**) that are responsible for downstream signaling and activation. Igβ and Igα are also required for the BCR to be transported to the cell surface and expressed. Igα:Igβ complexes with the BCR through hydrophilic interactions between transmembrane domains. Later in the chapter, we will cover BCR and TCR signaling and activation more thoroughly.

Recombination Activation Genes (RAGs)

During genetic recombination to produce the BCR, **recombination signal sequences (RSSs)** guide the recombination machinery to insure the proper recombination of V to J for the light chain, and V to D to J for the heavy chain.[15] The RSS is a heptamer of seven conserved nucleic acids followed by a spacer that is 12 or 23 base pairs long followed by a nonamer. During V-region rearrangement or V(D)J recombination, genes are recombined following the **12/23 rule**: Genes with a 12 nucleotide spacer can be combined only with genes that have a 23 nucleotide spacer (**FIGURE 3–5**). This means, for example, if the V_λ gene segment has a 12 nucleotide spacer, the J_λ must have a 23 nucleotide spacer. With the heavy chain, which combines a V, D, and J segment, the V_H and J_H gene segments both have a 23 nucleotide spacer, and the D_H segment has a 12 nucleotide spacer on both ends of the gene, allowing it to be sandwiched between the V_H and J_H segments. This pattern recognition provides a way to regulate gene rearrangement and prevent random genes from being combined, possibly resulting in dangerous mutations that could lead to cancer.

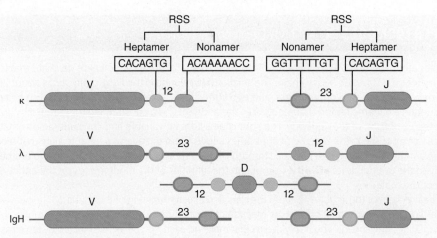

FIGURE 3-5 The 12/23 Rule. The 12/23 rule describes the structure of the recombination signal sequences, which contain a conserved nonamer and heptamer, flanking either a 12 bp (basepair) or 23 bp spacer region. V or J regions may be flanked by either the 12 bp or 23 bp; however, one of each must be present for recombination to occur.

Modified from William E Paul. Fundamental Immunology, Lippincott Williams & Wilkins, 2012.

The RSSs not only provide some regulation as to how the genes rearrange but also serve as binding sites of the recombination machinery[16] (**FIGURE 3-6**). **Recombination Activating Gene (RAG-1 and RAG-2)** are two proteins that act in synergy to carry out V(D)J recombination. The RAG proteins are expressed at high levels only in B and T cells. RAG-1 and RAG-2 recognize the RSSs and form a dimer, bringing the two genes into close proximity. RAG then acts as an endonuclease that makes two single-stranded DNA breaks just 5' of each of the RSS, leaving a free 3'-OH group at the ends. After RAG breaks the DNA, the free 3'-OH group reacts with the phosphodiester bond on the other DNA strand to form a hairpin. This hairpin results in the formation of a blunt double stranded break (DSB) in the DNA.

The double stranded breaks in the DNA are ligated together using nonhomologous end joining (NHEJ) mechanisms used in all cell types, not just B and T cells.[17,18] The first proteins of NHEJ recruited to the DSB are a heterodimer of DNA-modifying proteins Ku70 and Ku80. Ku70:Ku80 forms rings around the breaks, allowing DNA-dependent protein kinase (DNA-PK) to bind and recruit the nuclease Artemis. The PK:Artemis complex opens the hairpin by cleaving the DNA, producing two free ends of DNA. PK:Artemis can induce breaks anywhere in the hairpin that result in even-ended, double-stranded DNA, or alternatively, an uneven-ended DNA with a single strand hanging out further than the other.

The endonuclease activity of PK: Artemis can cause the removal of nucleotides, resulting in imprecise joining. This imprecise cutting adds another level of diversity called junctional diversity. For example, the endonuclease activity can result in three nucleotides being removed from the sequence, creating a simple deletion of a single amino acid; however if only one or two nucleotides are excised, it will result in a frameshift mutation altering the amino acids after the deletion and potentially having a larger change in the structure. Because of the random nature of this process, nonproductive rearrangements can occur from a frameshift mutation, which results in a premature stop codon.

While the DNA repair enzymes can be removing nucleotides, another protein in the recombinase complex, terminal deoxynucleotidyl transferase (TdT), which is expressed only in B and T cells, can randomly add nucleotides to the single-stranded DNA.[2,19] Eventually, DNA ligase IV joins the two strands together to combine the gene segments. This variable addition and deletion of nucleotides provides

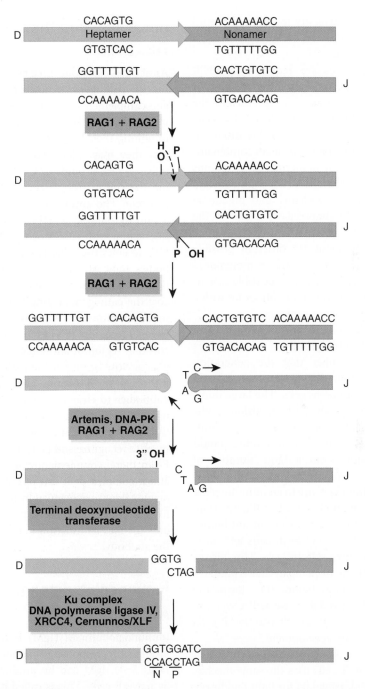

FIGURE 3–6 General Mechanism for immunoglobulin gene recombination assembly. Illustrated here is the D-J recombination, which represents a potentially common mechanism for all V-recombination reactions. The RSS appears in triangles, per convention. Two Recombination Activating Genes: RAG1 and RAG2, initiate a hairpin loop and lead to the recruitment of exonucleases, which expose the joining regions. Ligation via the Ku complex DNA polymerase ligase completes the process.

Modified from William E Paul. Fundamental Immunology, Lippincott Williams & Wilkins, 2012.

the majority of the diversity found in the third hypervariable regions (genetic regions with repeating base pairs).

Since RAG genes are required for BCR recombination, they are also responsible for antibody development as well. Specifically, the diversity of antibodies is produced by gene rearrangement as described above. We discussed two ways that the diversity is created: combinatorial diversity created by numerous combinations possible by joining various V(D)J segments and various light and heavy chains, and junctional diversity created by imprecise joining of the gene segments. Combinatorial diversity alone accounts for only about 10^6 different possible antibodies, but the combination of combinatorial and junctional diversity makes it possible to generate greater than 10^{11} different antibodies with a relatively small number of genes.

Antibodies and BCRs are a biological tool kit for binding peptides, built in advance. It is important to remember that the generation of antibodies is done during development and without exposure to pathogens. The large numbers of antibodies produced have unique abilities to recognize and bind to peptides or lipids. The large number of different antibodies should provide protection from a large number of pathogens. Only proliferation of specific antibodies occurs after exposure to an immunogenic antigen, during the process of B-cell activation. However, the random generation of antibodies also means that there will be B cells and antibodies that recognize self-antigen. This means that there must be a mechanism that eliminates self-reactive antibodies before they harm the host or cause disease. Later, we will cover the mechanisms of eliminating self-reactive B cells (or tolerance) during development.

Of importance, the generation of the T-cell receptor (TCR) in T cells uses the same mechanisms.[20] Instead of using loci for light and heavy chains, the TCR uses loci for the α and β chains. The α chain consists of a V_α and J_α similar to the light chain of an antibody. The β chain has a V_β, D_β, and J_β, as does the heavy chain of an antibody.

Antibodies and Their Effector Functions

Antibodies carry out three key functions in fighting off pathogens: neutralization, opsonization, and complement activation.[21] Antibodies neutralize pathogens by binding to them and blocking or inhibiting their binding or interaction with cells that they may infect. For example, when HIV infects a cell, it binds to CCR5 or CXCR4, causing the cell to internalize it, allowing infection to occur. The antibodies can prevent this interaction by binding to HIV, thereby blocking the interaction with CCR5 or CXCR4, which allows HIV to enter the cells. The second way that antibodies fight off infection is through opsonization. Opsonization occurs when the antibodies coat the pathogen, tagging it for phagocytosis by innate immune cells. Various innate immune cells have Fc receptors (**FIGURE 3–7**) that recognize the constant region of antibodies that allow them to phagocytose or engulf the pathogen and destroy it through the lysosome. The final mechanism of antibodies to clear infection is through complement activation. Antibodies activate complement through the classical pathway and allow complement to recognize and be recruited to a pathogen. From there, complement can form a membrane attack complex or it can opsonize the pathogen, tagging it for phagocytosis by innate immune cells like macrophages. The isotype of the antibody not only dictates its function but also the location of the antibody.

Immunoglobulins and Their Associations

Immunoglobulin M (IgM) is the first antibody produced in response to pathogens (**FIGURE 3–8**, **TABLE 3–1**). IgM can be produced and secreted by naïve B cells. This is called natural IgM. Natural IgM serves more of an innate-like role in the immune response. Natural IgM antibodies have very little diversity and low affinity. IgM antibodies are produced early in the immune response because they do not need to undergo

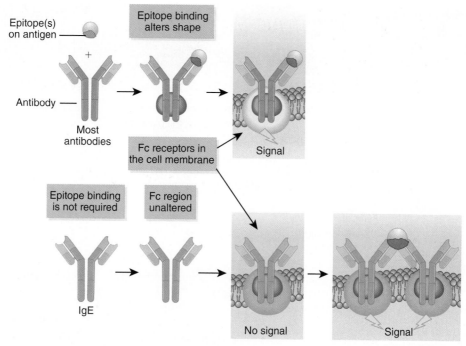

FIGURE 3–7 Fc receptors on the surface of cells can also lead to downstream signaling events when antigen is present. The Fc receptors permit phagocytic cells to ingest microbes and debris previously tagged by antibodies for destruction.

Modified from Doan, T., Melvold, R., Viselli, S., & Valtenbaugh, C. Lippincott Illustrated Reviews: Immunology, Lippincott Williams & Wilkins, 2012.

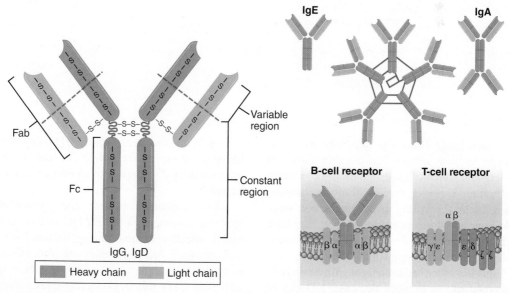

FIGURE 3–8 Antigenic receptors. While the most well-established set of antigenic receptors are the antibodies (IgG, IgM, IgA, IgD, and IgE), the two antigenic receptors of the adaptive immune system, the B-cell receptor and T-cell receptor, are extremely important for human defense and for the creation of new antibodies.

Modified from Rhoades, Rodney A., and David R. Bell, eds. Medical phisiology: Principles for clinical medicine. Lippincott Williams & Wilkins, 2017.

TABLE 3–1 Immunoglobulin (antibody) Functional Summary

Immunoglobulin Type	Function	Locations	Concentration in Normal Serum
IgG	Produced in response to a previously encountered pathogen	Most predominant in serum, able to cross the placenta	800–1,800 mg/dL
IgM	Produced first against immunogen/pathogen	Serum, plasma, upregulated after first infection/inoculation	60–250 mg/dL
IgA	Associated with the immune function of mucous membranes	Secretory in mucous membranes	150–400 mg/dL
IgD	Simulate B cells to be activated/transition from immature to mature	Low concentration, found on B cells	1.5–40 mg/dL
IgE	Associated with detection of specific allergens	Fc region binds to mast cells to exhibit an allergic response	0.002–0.05 mg/dL
B-cell receptor (BCR)	Recognizes antigen and communicates a signal to cell nucleus	Surface of B lymphocytes	Associated with cellular concentrations
T-cell receptor (TCR)	Recognizes antigen and communicates a signal to cell nucleus	Surface of T lymphocytes	Associated with cellular concentrations

class switching. They also generally have low affinity to their antigen because they have not undergone somatic hypermutation or affinity maturation. However, the low affinity is compensated for by the avidity of the interaction since IgM molecules form pentamers so that they have 10 binding sites instead of just two. IgM is responsible for most of the complement activation.

IgD is a splice variant of IgM with a relatively unknown role in immune response. IgD can be co-expressed with IgM on B cells. IgD can be found circulating in the blood but is mostly found in mucosal tissues of the upper respiratory system. While the precise role of IgD is unknown, unregulated expression of IgD can lead to auto-inflammatory disorders through overactivation of basophils.

IgG antibodies protect the extracellular spaces in tissues. High-affinity IgG antibodies are highly effective at neutralizing bacterial toxins and viruses.[22] IgG antibodies are also effective at activating complement and opsonization. IgG also plays a key role in protecting fetuses during pregnancy and newborns from infection. Because of IgG's function in protection of extracellular spaces, it is transferred through the placenta by the neonatal Fc receptor (FcRn) into fetuses, and provides protection against infection until the immune response in the infant is developed. This transfer of IgG from the mother to the fetus allows levels and antigen specificity in the newborn comparable to the mother's. The IgG isotype can be broken down further into four main subclasses: IgG1, IgG2, IgG3, and IgG4. While these subclasses have many highly conserved regions, they all vary slightly in their constant region allowing them to have different effector functions. IgG1 and IgG3 are able to activate complement much more effectively than that of IgG2 or IgG4. IgG1 and IgG3 are also able to bind to the FcγR on NK cells with high affinity, resulting in greater sensitization for killing than IgG2 or IgG4. IgG1 and IgG3 to they play a larger role in fighting viral infections than bacterial or extracellular infections. IgG2 and IgG4 are less proinflammatory than IgG1 and IgG3 and play a major role in neutralization of toxins and pathogens.

IgA is very similar to IgG in its functions but instead of being found in the extracellular fluids like IgG, IgA is located in mucosal tissues of the respiratory tract and digestive system.[23] IgA is also found in breast milk and can be transferred to a newborn's gut through ingestion, providing a first line of defense against pathogens. IgA is mostly responsible for neutralizing pathogens and toxins before they are able to infect or kill the host cells. IgA exists primarily as dimers linked together by a single J chain. This J chain plays a key role in the transport of IgA into mucosal surfaces by transcytosis (crossing through cells). The plasma cells that produce the IgA are primarily found in the lamina propria, the space below the epithelial cells of the gut. In order for the IgA to protect the epithelial cells of the gut from infection, IgA needs to be transported to the lumen of the gut. IgA then needs to be transported across the epithelial cells to bind to the polymeric immunoglobulin receptor (pIgR) on the basolateral surface of epithelial cells through the J chain. Once the IgA binds to the pIgR, it triggers endocytosis of the pIgR and its transport to the luminal surface of the epithelial cell.

IgE is the final isotype of immunoglobulin. IgE has one main function: to sensitize mast cells for activation.[24,25] Mast cells are innate immune cells that contain large granules of chemical mediators like histamine. Mast cells play a key role in fighting off parasitic infections with the help of IgE. Mast cells have specific, high-affinity Fc receptors (FcεRI) that bind to IgE, even when IgE is not bound to its antigen. When IgE binds to its target antigen, it causes crosslinking of the FcεRI, resulting in an activation signal and the release of the mast cell's granules. Without the crosslinking of the IgE bound to the Fc receptors, the masts cells will not release their granules. IgE antibodies play a key role in allergies. Patients who experience anaphylaxis with exposure to certain allergens often have IgE that recognizes the allergen and results in degranularization by mast cells and eosinophils resulting in permeabilization of blood vessels and constriction of airways.

Class Switching

Each BCR can use the different isotypes of antibodies. Depending on the signals present, the B-cell will undergo **class switching** to produce the isotype most capable of responding to the infection or pathogen[26–28] (**FIGURE 3–9**). When the BCR is first produced, it expresses the receptor with the IgM constant region (C region). The μ C region lies directly 3' of the J region for the heavy chain. When the heavy chain undergoes transcription, the μ chain is transcribed as part of the heavy chain. Class switching from IgM to another isotype occurs by excising DNA between the J region and the isotype gene. The C regions lie 3' of the J region in the following order: μ, δ, γ, ε, and α. In order for a different isotype to be expressed, the other genes must be excised from the DNA, thereby linking the desired constant region to the V region. For example, if the antibody class switches to IgE, it must excise out the μ, δ, and γ to do so. Since this is a DNA excision, it is permanent: IgE can never go back to IgM, IgD, or IgG. However, an IgE antibody can, in theory, class switch to IgA, since the IgA locus has not been excised.

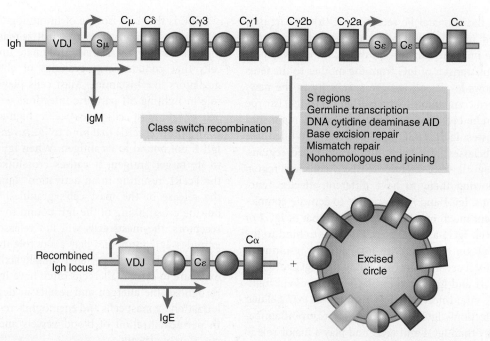

FIGURE 3-9 Mature B cells undergo class switch recombination. Class Switch Recombination is initiated through transcription events (gray arrows) utilizing the Switch regions (S) and C region. During this process, an excised circle is formed and a new constant region gene is juxtaposed downstream of the variable region exons.

Modified from Matthews AJ et al., *Adv Immunol. 2014.*

The one exception is IgD. IgD is unique in that it can be coexpressed with IgM. IgD is expressed as an mRNA transcript variant. The V_H promoter that drives transcription of the variable region also extends through both C_μ and C_δ. Alternative splicing of the mRNA transcript, therefore, determines whether the antibody expresses the μ or δ constant chain.

Class switching occurs in mature B cells that have recognized their antigen and become activated. The costimulatory signals such as cytokines and T-cell help at the time of activation decide to which isotype the B-cell will class switch. CD40 stimulation on the B-cell by CD40L on T cells or TLR-4 signaling provide the necessary signals along with antigenic stimulation to express the **class switch recombination (CSR)** machinery. Cytokines help direct the CSR machinery to the desired gene locus. Cytokines result in the opening of the DNA at **switch regions (S regions)** directing the excision events. The promoters of the

S regions have cytokine-responsive elements. The promoters for λ1 and ε have IL-4 responsive elements that drive class switching to those isotypes when IL-4 is present. IL-4 can also inhibit the production of IgM, IgG3, and IgG2a. IL-5 enhances IgA production but is not enough to induce class switching to IgA alone. Class switching to λ2b and α is regulated by the transcription factors Smad and Runx, which are activated by TGF-β. TGF-β inhibits production of IgM and IgG3. IFN-λ drives IgG2a and IgG3 class switching while inhibiting IgM, IgG1, and IgE class switching.

Class switching occurs when the DNA between two S regions is excised and the VDJ is recombined with the C region. Class switching is guided by the S regions, highly conserved G-rich regions. Class switch recombination occurs between the S_μ and the S region right before the constant region for the desired isotype. Transcriptional activity at the switch regions opens the DNA, creating areas of single-stranded

DNA. Once a B-cell is activated, it expresses **Activation Induced Cytidine Deaminase (AID)**, which converts cytidine (C) residues in DNA into uridine (U) in single-stranded DNA. AID can bind only to single-stranded DNA, which is a mechanism that acts to guide the class-switching process. Since uridine is typically not associated with DNA, it will generally be excised by nucleotide excision repair machinery. **Uracil DNA glycosylase (UNG)** removes the uracil and leaves an empty ribose backbone. The **apurinic/apyrimidinic endonuclease (APE1)** will cleave out the ribose backbone, resulting in a single-stranded break. During class switching recombination, this process will result in numerous single-stranded breaks in clusters around the S region of the DNA, resulting in a staggered, double-stranded break. The double-stranded break is then repaired by the same machinery used during generation of the BCR. The two switch regions are brought together by the DNA repair machinery including DNA-PKcs and Artemis and joined together.

Affinity Maturation

In 1984, Dr. David McKean showed that multiple, different antibodies with the same Vκ-Jκ junction arose when he immunized a mouse with Influenza HA protein.[29] The common Vκ-Jκ junction showed that these antibodies all likely arose from a single original clone. Further studies showed a genealogical relationship consisting of a sequential accumulation of mutations. This provided evidence for affinity maturation. Activated B cells can undergo **affinity maturation** or a series of random mutations in the variable regions of the antibody that can result in higher affinity interactions with antigen. Affinity maturation occurs by the same mechanisms used during class switching.[30]

The process of affinity maturation results in random mutations. This means that an antibody may be generated with higher affinity to the antigen, lower affinity, or even with new specificity for another antigen. Selecting the higher affinity antibodies occurs through better activation of the B cells when a low concentration of the antigen is present. When the antigen is present at a high concentration, all of the antibodies with specificity toward that antigen will bind. As an infection is cleared and the concentration of the antigen decreases, there is more and more competition for binding and the B cells that express higher affinity antibodies will bind more of the antigen and continue to be stimulated, allowing clonal expansion.

The mechanism of action is as follows. Transcriptional activity opens the DNA-producing areas of single-stranded DNA. AID converts cytidines to uridines in the DNA. If the DNA repair mechanisms do not see the error, a transition mutation occurs and the cytidine is replaced by a thymine in the genomic sequence. If the DNA repair mechanisms catch the error, UNG will remove the uracil, leaving the ribose backbone. If DNA replication occurs at this point, the gap will be filled using a random mutation, resulting in transition mutation (purine to purine or pyrimidine to pyrimidine) or transversion mutation (purine to pyrimidine or pyrimidine to purine) mutations. After UNG removes the uracil, the gap is fixed by APE1 excising the ribose and causing a single-stranded nick in the DNA. The DNA repair machinery will try to pair the gap with a homologous sequence that can cause a partial gene conversion to repair the break.

The goal of affinity maturation is to improve the binding of antibodies to the pathogen. Because this is a random process, new antibodies that can recognize other epitopes may be generated through this process. These new antibodies may even recognize self-antigen now. To prevent the generation of self-reactive antibodies, the B cells go through a selection process that ensures that the self-reactive antibodies do not make it into circulation.

B Cells Response to Pathogens

Naïve B cells enter the circulation after development and migrate to the secondary lymphoid organs—the lymph nodes and spleen. In the secondary lymphoid organs (SLO), B cells constantly test their surroundings for antigen brought in through the lymph.[31,32] The antigen can enter the B-cell zone of the SLO by three mechanisms, depending on the size of the antigen. Large, opsonized antigen-like viruses will be carried into the B-cell zone by macrophages. The large opsonized antigen will localize to the subcapsular sinus of the lymphoid organ where macrophages can pick up the antigen by binding to the complement through complement receptors. The macrophages can present the antigen to B cells. Small, soluble antigens can rapidly and freely flow in the B-cell zone through the conduit system, allowing B cells to bind to their antigen. The third mechanism occurs when noncognate B cells mediate complement-dependent transfer of antigen to follicular DCs that will present the antigen for long periods of time. **Immune complexes** consisting of antibody, antigen, and complement play a key role in the transport of antigen.[33] Immune cells (B cells in particular) can take up immune complex found in the blood or lymph through their complement receptors or FcRs (Fc Receptors).

B-Cell Activation

Activation of B cells involves binding of BCR to antigens and internalization of BCR-antigen complex. This is followed by presentation of internalized antigens in the form of peptides on MHC molecules on the B-cell surface to engage antigen-specific T cells. B cells find their antigens and migrate to the T-cell area in search for a cognate T-cell. The engagement between B cells and T cells is called linked recognition and occurs in the T-cell area. This is an effective mechanism of mobilizing B-cell or humoral immunity against a pathogen detected by the T-cell. Recognition by T cells leads to cytokine production, which induces B-cell proliferation and differentiation into antibody-secreting plasma cells. Cytokine production also includes the switching of antibody isotypes to IgG, IgE, and IgA. In addition, activated B cells undergo somatic hypermutation, which involves alteration of the specificity at the V region of antibody to create antibodies of higher affinity for the pathogen. This results in selection of high-affinity

B cells to differentiate into plasma cells whereas low affinity cells undergo death.

When a B-cell recognizes its specific antigen, also called cognate antigen, a series of events occurs that allow B cells to interact with T cells for costimulation. When a BCR binds to its antigen, it results in crosslinking and actin rearrangement to form an immune synapse. The B-cell will start to endocytose its receptors along with whatever is bound through a clathrin-dependent mechanism.[31,34,35] It will then process the antigen through antigen processing and present antigens on their MHC class II. The B-cell will also migrate to the B-T-cell zones to find its cognate T-cell. The B-cell will look for T cells that recognize part of the antigen or pathogen that was internalized and processed by the B-cell. The cognate T-cell does not have to recognize the exact same epitope or even the same protein, but it will recognize a small part of what was internalized by BCR stimulation. This is called **linked recognition**.[36,37] When it is activated, the T-cell will upregulate CD40L, which will bind to CD40 on the B-cell and provide costimulation. The T-cell will also secrete cytokines like IL-4 and IFN-γ, which will induce class switching. T-cell help is critical to promote a B-cell response.

After a B-cell has encountered its antigen, it will migrate out of the lymph node and form a **germinal center**, an area of massive proliferation.[38] The germinal center is where B cells undergo affinity maturation and class switching. The germinal center has two zones: the dark zone, in which there is rapid proliferation and affinity maturation and in which class-switching occurs, and the light zone, in which the B cells test their new BCRs.[39,40] B cells in the dark zone of the germinal center are called **centroblasts**. The centroblasts will proliferate and undergo somatic hypermutation and class switching. They will then differentiate into nondividing **centrocytes**. The centrocytes will test their BCRs through interactions with follicular dendritic cells and T follicular helper cells. B cells with low affinities or that are self-reactive will undergo apoptosis and be removed from the repertoire. Centrocytes with high affinity BCRs can differentiate back into centroblasts to proliferate and undergo another round of affinity maturation, or they can differentiate into long-lived plasma cells or memory B cells and migrate out of the germinal center.

T-dependent antibody responses occur in two waves: primary and secondary.[41] The primary antibody response is the secretion of low-affinity IgM or IgG1 that has not undergone affinity maturation. The primary antibody response is essentially the production of the original clone of the BCR or antibody. The first wave of antibodies is produced by the activated B cells that differentiate into short-lived **plasmablasts** that migrate to sites of infection and secrete their antibodies. This provides a rapid response that provides time for a secondary response to be built up. The secondary response will produce high-affinity class switched antibodies. The secondary antibody production includes the antibodies produced by class switching and affinity maturation. The secondary responders will proliferate and differentiate into long-lived plasma cells that secrete high-affinity antibodies from the bone marrow and long-lived memory B cells that recirculate for years. The plasma cells secrete antibodies and do not express a membrane bound BCR. Memory B cells express their BCR on their membrane and are able to respond much more quickly and robustly if they encounter their antigen again, even years later.

Formation of Memory

Mounting an adaptive immune response results not just in effector cells but also gives rise to a small population of memory cells that are long-lived and persist after infection resolution.[42] These can respond to the same infection more rapidly and more effectively when the pathogen invades the host again. Activation of T and B cells, through exposure to antigens, leads to the production of long-lived cells that are antigen specific and are poised to act in response to re-exposure to antigen, a process called clonal selection (**FIGURE 3–10**). Memory is maintained independently of antigenic stimulation, and, upon re-exposure to pathogen, a rapid response is mounted. Memory T cells are found in lymph nodes (central memory T cells)

and patrol tissues (effector memory T cells). Memory B cells and long-lived plasma B cells that secrete antibodies are immunologic memory following B-cell activation. It is this ability of the immune cells to bifurcate into memory and effector cells that immunologists can exploit for vaccination. Vaccination has played important roles in eradication of infectious diseases such as polio in many countries. However, currently, no effective vaccines exist for two dangerous infectious diseases that afflict a large number of people around the world: HIV and tuberculosis (TB).

Laboratory Roles for Antibodies

Antibodies are important for fighting infections in vivo, but they have also become important tools in the laboratory and in the clinic. In this section, we will cover some of the common uses of antibodies in research and some that are being used in clinical trials.

Antibodies for laboratory use are generated by immunizing lab animals such as mice, rats, rabbits, and goats with a peptide of interest or a specific epitope of a peptide that is targeted for the antibody response. After the immune response and the antibodies have been generated, antibodies specific for the peptide of interest can be purified using column purification. There are two types of antibodies commonly used in the laboratory: monoclonal and polyclonal. Monoclonal antibodies are produced from a single B-cell clone and all of the antibodies are identical. Production of monoclonal antibodies is a more complicated process. After the immunization and generation of the high-affinity B cells, the spleen is harvested and the B cells are fused with a multiple myeloma cell line to produce a hybridoma. These hybridomas grow up rapidly in culture and can produce large amounts of a single clone of antibody. Monoclonal antibodies are useful because every batch will be the same and will not have variability. Polyclonal antibodies are a combination of multiple, different antibodies that recognize a single antigen. Polyclonal antibodies are more representative of an immune response. There will be diversity in the affinities of the antibodies and what epitopes

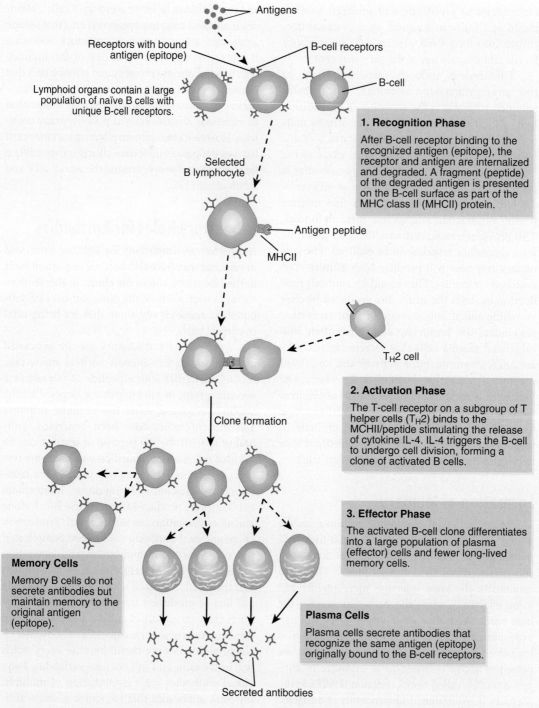

Antigens

Receptors with bound antigen (epitope)

B-cell receptors

B-cell

Lymphoid organs contain a large population of naïve B cells with unique B-cell receptors.

Selected B lymphocyte

Antigen peptide

MHCII

T_H2 cell

Clone formation

Memory Cells

Plasma Cells

Secreted antibodies

1. Recognition Phase

After B-cell receptor binding to the recognized antigen (epitope), the receptor and antigen are internalized and degraded. A fragment (peptide) of the degraded antigen is presented on the B-cell surface as part of the MHC class II (MHCII) protein.

2. Activation Phase

The T-cell receptor on a subgroup of T helper cells (T_H2) binds to the MCHII/peptide stimulating the release of cytokine IL-4. IL-4 triggers the B-cell to undergo cell division, forming a clone of activated B cells.

3. Effector Phase

The activated B-cell clone differentiates into a large population of plasma (effector) cells and fewer long-lived memory cells.

Memory Cells

Memory B cells do not secrete antibodies but maintain memory to the original antigen (epitope).

Plasma Cells

Plasma cells secrete antibodies that recognize the same antigen (epitope) originally bound to the B-cell receptors.

FIGURE 3–10 Clonal selection of B cells.

Data from Pommerville, J. C. (2017). Fundamentals of Microbiology, 11e. Jones & Bartlett Learning.

of the antigen they bind. Polyclonal antibodies are more easily produced, but will vary from batch to batch, and are harder to control cross-reactivity of the antibodies to other peptides.

Antibodies have many uses in the research lab or as clinical diagnostic tools. For example, antibodies can be used for classical and labeled immunoassays, such as ELISA, as well as flow cytometry, immunohistochemistry (IHC), Western blotting, and immunoprecipitations.

Antibodies in the Clinic

Antibodies are also useful for therapeutic treatments. In this section, we will cover three common clinical uses for antibodies: neutralization of a toxin, passive immunity, and cancer therapies. Antibodies are often used to neutralize toxins, for example, snake venom.[43,44] Antibodies to snake venom are generated by immunizing horses with sublethal doses of the venom. The antibodies generated can then be injected into a patient with a snake bite by IV and they will neutralize the venom. Another common use of antibodies is passive immunity.[45,46] For patients who have immunodeficiencies, where they lack B cells or are unable to produce antibodies, they often experience reoccurring bacterial infections that can lead to pneumonia. To help treat these patients, they receive IV infusions of IgG to provide a source of antibodies to prevent infection. However, because of the short half-life of the antibodies, patients need to have regular infusions. A relatively new use of antibodies in the clinic that is rapidly growing is for cancer therapies.[47] Recently, monoclonal antibody therapy targeting, and immune checkpoint receptor PD1 that is expressed on exhausted T cells, and its ligand PD-L1, were approved for treatment of melanoma and renal cancer. The antibody works to prevent the immune checkpoint inhibitor and reinvigorates the ability of anti-tumor T cells to target and lyse tumor cells. Monoclonal antibodies can also be used to target tumor cells directly through inhibiting signaling, by binding specific markers, or by targeting them for killing by immune cells.

▶ T Cells

T cells, lymphocytes that develop in the thymus and are characterized by the presence of a T-cell receptor (TCR), play a key role in directing the overall immune response. T cells are key players in cell-mediated immunity. The majority of T cells have a TCR that is composed of an alpha chain with a beta chain.[48] However, there is a subset of T cells called γδ T cells that have a TCR composed of delta and gamma chains.[49–53] The alpha and beta chains of the TCR provide the specificity of the T-cell to recognize their specific or cognate peptide presented by the MHC. The TCR alpha and beta chains heterodimerize (come together) and are each composed of a transmembrane region that allows surface expression, a constant region that is conserved across TCRs, and the variable region of the TCR that provides the specificity of the TCR. The TCR is also composed of **cluster of differentiation 3 (CD3)** subunits that provide the signaling motifs. The TCR is composed of 2 CD3ε, 1 CD3δ, 1 CD3γ, and 2 CD3ζ subunits (**FIGURE 3–11**). Each of the CD3 subunits contains transmembrane domains, and an intracellular domain that has immunoreceptor tyrosine-based activation motifs (ITAMs) that are the signaling domains. ITAMs are sites of tyrosine phosphorylation that serve as binding sites for downstream signaling molecules.

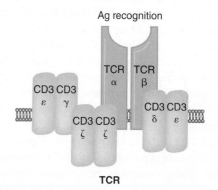

FIGURE 3–11 T-Cell Receptor with CD3 subunits. The TCR is expressed as two polypeptide chains (a and b) with a variety of associated CD3 subunits that link to signaling domains.

Adapted from Tan, D.S., & Lynch, H.T. (2012). Principles of molecular diagnostics and personalized cancer medicine, LWW Wolters Kluwer.

The T-cell surface receptor (TCR) is a glycosylated heterodimer composed of two chains, and is anchored to the cell surface with a transmembrane.[54] Predominantly, T cells bear TCR composed of two chains, α and β, while a small fraction of T cells carry a TCR made of γ and δ chains. αβ and γδ pair with covalent disulfide bridges. Together, the two chains make the variable and constant domains; the variable domain is farther away from the transmembrane domain while the constant is closer to the transmembrane domain. Variable domains contain complementarity-determining regions (CDRs), which arise as a result of recombination of gene segments at the TCR chain encoding loci. CDRs are highly diverse in nature and are primarily responsible for binding peptide-MHC complexes.

T-Cell Development

At the heart of adaptive immunity lies the ability to create an enormous diversity of receptors for recognition of pathogens. These receptors are made during the development of T and B cells and are screened for quality via several selection checkpoints.

The generation of the TCR or the BCR occurs via a step-by-step process as well as cell-fate decisions relying on signaling molecules that direct gene expression changes.[55,56] During T-cell development, CLPs migrate from the bone marrow to the thymus via blood, entering the thymus through the cortico-medullary junction to begin the process of development; CLPs commit to the T-cell lineage by differentiating into **early thymic progenitors (ETP)**. From the ETP stage onward, development requires assembly of the T-cell receptor (TCR). Diversity of TCRs is guided by sequential gene rearrangements of genes encoding the TCR subunits. These genes constitute many gene segments that can be broadly categorized into variable regions (V), diversity regions (D), and joining (J) regions. The process of TCR creation is called VDJ recombination whereby randomly selected V regions combine with randomly selected D and randomly selected J regions.[57] It is random joining of these regions that gives rise to various permutations of the TCR, allowing for large repertoire of T cells. Recombinases RAG1 and RAG2 catalyze the recombination process that broadly encompasses two key steps: DNA cleavage and DNA joining.

Individuals lacking functional RAG proteins develop primary immunodeficiency as they lack functional T and B cells (BCR generation is also dependent on RAG catalytic activity).[58,59] Diagnosis of RAG functional deficiency as a result of missense mutations entails quantification of T- and B-cell frequency. However, to definitely associate RAG mutations with loss of its function, RAG encoding genes are sequenced, cloned, and introduced into human dermal fibroblasts along with substrate vectors to determine whether the protein can allow V(D)J recombination. The aforementioned scenario is an example of diagnosis of disease at the molecular level.

T cells generate their TCR by the same mechanism that B cells use. T cells develop in the thymus and undergo a selection mechanism that prevents autoreactive T cells from escaping into the periphery.[60,61] In general, T cells that have successfully rearranged their receptors, test their receptors by binding to peptide:MHC complexes (pMHC) in the thymus presented by dendritic cells. T cells that weakly interact with pMHC are positively selected, while T cells that strongly bind pMHC in the thymus are negatively selected and deleted from the repertoire.[62]

Naïve, Effector, and Memory T Cells

Naïve T cells are CD4+ or CD8+ T cells that have successfully passed through positive and negative selection and development in the thymus.[63,64] After development, naïve T cells leave the thymus and circulate through the periphery. When naïve T cells initially leave the thymus, they express low levels of the coreceptor CD28 and IL-7 receptor (IL-7R). The T cells continue their maturation process in the secondary lymphoid organs to insure that they do not react with self-antigens. If after the course of the first 2 weeks, the immature naïve T cells do not encounter their cognate peptide:MHC, they finish their maturation process and are now ready to respond to antigenic stimulation. Naïve T cells spend the majority of their lifespan recirculating through the secondary lymphoid organs probing for their cognate antigens. The naïve T cell's survival requires IL-7 and weak TCR signals from recognizing MHC.

If a naïve T-cell encounters its cognate antigen, it begins to produce lymphokines, proliferate, and differentiate into effector T cells.[2,65] Effector T cells differentiate to help eliminate infection. Effector CD4+ T cells produce large amounts of proinflammatory cytokines that direct the immune response of other cells such as macrophages, neutrophils, or eosinophils or CD8+ T cells. Effector CD8+ T cells are cytotoxic T cells that eliminate virally infected cells or mutated self through a perforin/granzyme B mechanism. Effector memory cells can also differentiate into memory T cells.

During an infection, effector T cells rapidly proliferate. The proliferation reaches a peak roughly a week after infection. After the infection is cleared, effector T-cell numbers rapidly decrease to about 10% of the peak after about 2 weeks. The T cells that remain after this contraction period are long-lived memory T cells that circulate and respond to the antigen for the remainder of the host's life. Memory T cells contain high levels of IL-7R and IL-15R that allow them to survive. These memory cells require lower threshold of stimulation to respond to antigen and provide protection from infection for life.

T-Cell Response to Pathogens

Naïve T cells are constantly circulating through the lymph nodes searching for their cognate antigen. At the same time, tissue resident dendritic cells (DCs) are always sampling their surroundings and taking antigen back to the lymph node to present to T cells.

There are three main kinds of antigens: extracellular, cytoplasmic, and phagolysosomal. Professional antigen-presenting cells are DCs, macrophages, and B cells.[66] Of the three kinds of cells, DCs and macrophages have superior capacity to present antigens. Activation of DCs and macrophages enhances their ability to present antigens. They take up pathogens and relay information to T cells about an infection by breaking up pathogen-derived proteins into smaller peptides and displaying them on their cell surface to activate T cells. Presentation of peptides occurs on MHC molecules. There are two main classes of MHC molecules: MHC-I and MHC-II. MHC-I is expressed by all nucleated cells and MHC-II is expressed exclusively by professional antigen-presenting cells.

CD4 T cells recognize peptides in the context of MHC-II while CD8 T cells recognize peptides in the context of MHC-I.[66,67] Hence, all infected cells can process antigens and display on MHC-I, allowing self-killing by CD8 T cells before they can be propagated. Hence, peptides made in acidified endocytic vesicles following phagocytosis are loaded onto MHC-II molecules. This occurs when vesicles containing peptides fuse with vesicles containing MHC-II molecules. Some proteins can be translocated from endocytic vesicles to the cytosol where they can undergo degradation by the proteasomes, a multiunit catalytic protein complex. Peptides derived from this process are loaded onto MHC-I. This mechanism of "crosspresentation" is effective for priming CD8 T cells by DCs that do not naturally get infected by the pathogen. Further, DCs are better at crosspresentation than macrophages due to their phagocytic and pinocytic abilities.

B cells can take up antigens via their BCR-mediated endocytosis and this is important for engagement between B and T cells in a process called linked-recognition, critical for B-cell activation and expansion.[68] In addition, presentation of peptides is not just critical for T-cell activation but also for T-cell development. Normal catabolism of cytosolic and nuclear products results in peptides that are also presented. However, these products do not elicit immune responses as they are derived from self-proteins.

During an infection or tissue damage, signals such as cytokines or TLR signaling activate the DCs to express the cell-surface marker B7. The expression of B7 of the DCs acts as a costimulatory signal to T cells. T cells require three signals to be activated and to respond to pathogens: TCR stimulation, costimulation through CD28 on the T-cell binding B7 on the APC, and cytokine signaling.[69] Signal one (TCR stimulation) without signal two (CD28:B7) will result in the T-cell becoming anergic. Four to 5 days after the T-cell has recognized its cognate antigen, it will have differentiated and proliferated into an effector T-cell. CD8+ T cells are now cytotoxic T cells and will kill any cell that presents the antigen, while CD4+ will have differentiated into T_H1, T_H2, T_H17, or Tregs, depending on the cytokine signals.

T-Cell Selection: Positive and Negative Selection

T-cell development begins with bone marrow progenitors that are **double negative (DN)** for CD4 and CD8 coreceptors, which are maintained through several rounds of development. First, these bone marrow progenitor cells exit the bone marrow and enter the thymus. T cells at this point are in the DN1 phase of development. T cells now have to make the T-cell fate decision of becoming γδ T cells or conventional αβ T cells. The current theory is that there is a race that decides the cell fate. At the double negative (DN2, CD4-CD8-, TCR-) stage, the T cells begin to rearrange their γ, δ, and β chains. If the γδ receptor is rearranged first, it will signal and shut down β chain rearrangement. If the β chain is rearranged first, it will associate with a surrogate α chain and be expressed on the surface, which signals to shut down γδ rearrangement.

We will focus on αβ T-cell development as it makes up the majority of T cells. Similar to the B-cell receptor development mechanism, the β chain is rearranged before the α chain. Once a β chain has been successfully rearranged, the β chain forms a pre-TCR that signals to promote proliferation and stops further β chain rearrangement. Signaling through the pre-TCR also induces rearrangements of the α chain. Once the α chain is finished being rearranged, it will be expressed on the cell surface for selection. At this point, the T-cell also begins to express both CD4 and CD8 and is

now in the **double positive (DP)** stage of development. This stage of development decides whether the T-cell becomes CD4 single positive (SP) or CD8 single positive. T cells in the DP stage test their new TCR for interactions with pMHC complexes. If the TCR weakly interacts with MHC I, it will develop into a CD8+ T-cell. If it interacts weakly with an MHC II molecule, it will become a CD4+ T-cell.

After the TCR is made, T cells express the coreceptors CD4 and CD8.[67] At this stage, they are called CD4 CD8 double positive (DP) cells. Coreceptors facilitate the engagement of newly produced TCRs with MHC molecules. At the DP stage, T cells that have made properly folded and functional TCRs and can recognize peptide-MHC are selected to enter the next developmental stage. This interaction ensures that the T-cell can recognize foreign peptides in the context of MHC in the future. Following positive selection, T cells make a lineage choice by becoming either CD4 or CD8 single positive (SP), thus, coreceptor expression becomes mutually exclusive following positive selection. While CD4 T cells are MHC-II restricted, CD8 T cells are MHC-I restricted. CD4 or CD8 lineage commitment of T cells is dependent on cytokine signaling, TCR signaling that regulates transcriptional changes associated with CD4 or CD8 fate adoption by T cells.

The random nature of the process comes at the cost of generating TCRs that can recognize host antigens, giving rise to T-cell-mediated autoimmunity.[70] Following the arrangement of the TCR and positive selection comes negative selection that involves the weeding out of T cells that are potentially autoreactive, i.e., can cause autoimmunity. The physical elimination of T-cell clones that have the potential to attack host tissues and organs is called central tolerance and is the fundamental basis of discrimination between host and pathogens by the immune system.

Central tolerance is mediated by the **autoimmune regulator (AIRE)** protein. AIRE is a transcription factor that is expressed in the thymus.[71] AIRE drives transcription of tissue-specific genes so that more diversity of self-antigen is present in the thymus for negative selection. AIRE enables promiscuous expression of tissue-restricted antigens by medullary thymic epithelial cells, which process and present the proteins on MHC molecules, enabling negative selection of autoreactive T cells.[72] Loss of AIRE function results in multiorgan autoimmunity called APECED. The underlying explanation of APECED is the escape of auto-reactive T cells into the peripheral lymphoid organs where they initiate immune responses against the host.

The outcome of random generation of the TCR is that a very diverse repertoire of T cells is constructed and carefully curated to keep those that are useful and get rid of those that may unleash autoimmunity or are nonfunctional by failing to fold properly.

T-Cell Maturation

Development of T cells does not cease postpositive selection. Additional steps of maturation are required for T cells to undergo to acquire a number of phenotypic and functional competencies.[73,74] Some of these include the ability to egress, the ability to proliferate and produce cytokines upon TCR stimulation, and the ability to persist long term in the mature T-cell pool. Therefore, to mount a functional T-cell response, T-cell maturation is critical. Finer knowledge about the various steps needed to equip T cells with functional capacity will allow investigators and clinicians to manipulate maturation status of T cells in treatments such as transplantation which require immune suppression to prevent graft rejection.

Other T-Cell Lineages That Arise in the Thymus

Negative selection is not the only fate of a potentially autoreactive T-cell. In the presence of additional cellular and molecular cues, T cells can commit to the regulatory T (Tregs) cell lineage.[75,76] Tregs play the critical role of dampening immune responses, maintaining tissue homeostasis, and

TABLE 3–2 Summary of Types of T Cells

Type of T-Cell	Function
αβ Conventional T-cell	Adaptive immunity
αβ Regulatory T cells	Regulation of immune response
γδ T cells	Innate
iNKT cells	Innate
αα CD8 iELs	Innate

preventing autoimmunity. Loss of Treg function or development causes severe autoimmunity in humans known as immunodysregulation polyendocrinopathy enteropathy X-linked syndrome (IPEX) in humans.[77] In addition, γδ and iNKT cells, which are innate-like in nature, can also arise in the thymus (**TABLE 3–2**). These cells recognize a limited set of molecular patterns and are initial responders in an infection.

It is well established that Tregs function through the suppression of the proliferation of autoreactive T cells. In vitro proliferation assays can be used to determine Treg functional deficits in humans. These assays involve stimulation of T cells in the presence or absence of patient's Tregs (negative control) in comparison to normal Tregs (positive control). It is also known that the transcriptional regulator Foxp3 is critical for Treg development and function. Gene sequencing techniques can be used to determine loss of Foxp3 function mutations. IPEX is almost always fatal but bone marrow transfer may prolong life.

CD4+ vs CD8+ T Cells

T cells can be divided initially into two subgroups, depending on the coreceptor that they express. T cells express either the coreceptor

CD4 or CD8. **CD4** is a glycoprotein that has a single transmembrane domain and recognizes MHC class II.[78] **CD8** is another glycoprotein that consists of a heterodimer of αβ subunits with two transmembrane domains and recognizes MHC class I. CD4 and CD8 contribute to the T-cell response by enhancing the binding of the TCR to MHC (**FIGURE 3-12**) to stabilize weak interactions between the TCR and peptide:MHC and recruit signaling molecules such as LCK to the TCR complex.[79]

The expression of CD4 or CD8 determines the function of the T-cell. CD4+ T cells are classified as **T helper cells (T$_H$)** and influence the immune response through their production of cytokines that direct the immune response toward a viral or intracellular response (T$_H$1), extracellular response (T$_H$2), or a fungal/parasitic response (T$_H$17)[80] (**FIGURE 3-13**). CD8+ T cells are **cytotoxic T cells** that recognize mutated self or

virally infected cells. CD8+ T cells clear infected or mutated cells through a perforin/granzyme B killing mechanism.

To ensure that a self-reactive T-cell does not escape into the periphery, there needs to be a mechanism that allows expression of tissue-specific antigens in the thymus.

T Helper Subsets

Naïve CD4+ T cells differentiate into different helper subtypes (**TABLE 3-3**), depending on the cytokine signal they receive when they recognize their cognate antigen. CD4+ T cells can be differentiated into five different, well-characterized subsets: T$_H$1, T$_H$2, T$_H$17, Treg (regulatory T cells), and T$_{FH}$ (follicular helper T cells).[81,82]

Th1 cells are differentiated from naïve CD4+ T cells by the cytokines interleukin-12 (IL-12) and interferon gamma (IFN-γ). Th1 expresses

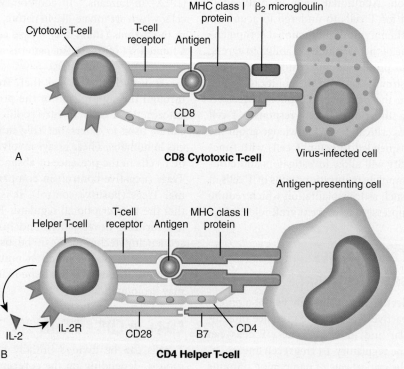

FIGURE 3-12 Interaction of CD8+ and CD4+ T cells with MHC. **(A)** CD8 (or cytotoxic) T cells interact with MHC class I. **(B)** CD4 (or helper) T cells interact with MHC class II.

Modified from Golan, D. E., Tashjian, A. H., & Armstrong, E. J. (Eds.). Principles of Pharmacology: The Pathophysiologic Basis of Drug Therapy, Lippincott Williams & Wilkins, 2011.

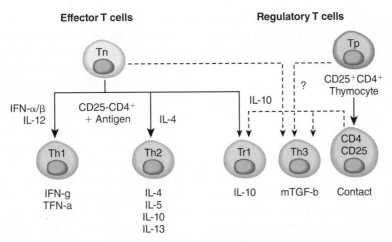

FIGURE 3–13 T-cells found in peripheral blood are differentiated into two distinct lineages: Effector or regulatory cells. They are characterized by surface antigen profiles and soluble factors such as the interleukins (ILs).

Modified from William J Koopman; Larry W Moreland. Arthritis and Allied Conditions: A Textbook of Rheumatology, Lippincott Williams & Wilkins, 2004.

TABLE 3–3 T Effector Fates

Type	Nature of Pathogen	Outcome
CD4 Th1	Intracellular bacteria	Helper
CD4 Th2	Parasitic	Helper
CD4 Th17	Fungal	Helper
CD8 cytotoxic T-cell	Virus and intracellular bacteria	Killer

the transcription factor Tbet and secretes proinflammatory cytokines IFN-γ and tumor necrosis factor (TNF). These proinflammatory cytokines enhance the functions of NK cells, macrophages, and CD8+ T cells to clear intracellular pathogens.

Th2 cells differentiate from naïve CD4+ T cells in the presence of IL-4. Th2 cells express the transcription factor GATA3 and produce IL-4, IL-5, and IL-13, which play a role in directing B cells, mast cells, and eosinophils to respond against extracellular pathogens. While a Th2 response is important for clearing pathogens, an aberrant Th2 response can lead to allergies or asthma.

A combination of transforming growth factor β (TGF-β) and IL-6 results in the differentiation of **Th17** cells from naïve CD4+ cells. Th17 cells express the transcription factor RORγt and produce the proinflammatory cytokines IL-23 and IL-17. The Th17 immune response is targeted against parasitic and fungal infections. A deregulated Th17 immune response has been implicated in playing a role in tumor genesis and cancer.

CD4+ T cells differentiate into Tregs in the presence of high levels of IL-2 and TGF-β. **Tregs** express the transcription factor FOXP3 and produce IL-10, an immune-suppressive cytokine. Tregs promote tolerance against self-antigen, the microbiota, and can provide protection for tumors.

The final T helper subset is **follicular T cells (Tfh)**. IL-6 and IL-21 drive differentiation of Tfh cells. Tfh cells express the BCL-6 and produce IL-21. Tfh cells provide essential help to germinal center B cells, driving germinal center formation, affinity maturation, and B-cell memory formation. Tfh cells have also been implicated in playing a role in driving autoimmune diseases.

The regulation of the T helper cell differentiation provides important regulation of the immune response. Aberrant or deregulated differentiation of T cells can result in a variety of diseases including autoimmune, allergy, and cancer.

T-Cell Receptor Signaling

Activation of the T-cell through its TCR activates three main signaling pathways that regulate the T cell's effector function: NFAT, AP-1, and NFκB.[2,83] In this section, we will cover these three main pathways, but first, it is important to understand how signaling proteins can interact with each other to pass the message forward. Signal transduction uses posttranslational modifications of signaling proteins to activate the signaling molecules. Alterations in the signal transduction cascade have been linked to changes in T-cell function, immunity, rates of cancer, and other disease. The most common posttranslational modification involved in signal transduction is phosphorylation of amino acids with a hydroxyl group like tyrosine or serine by kinases. Often, phosphorylation of proteins by **kinases** activates the enzymatic activity of signaling protein. Activated signaling molecules can be turned off by **phosphatases** that shut down enzymatic activity. Protein phosphorylations can serve to activate proteins by changing the conformation of the protein to open binding sites or phosphorylation sites can act as binding motifs to recruit other proteins into the complex. Signaling proteins with an SH2 domain bind to phosphorylated tyrosine residues.

NFAT, AP-1, and NFκB signaling all share early TCR signaling. When the TCR binds its cognate peptide:MHC complex, it has to somehow transmit that signal across the plasma membrane to the signaling domains on the CD3 subunits. Currently, there are three hypotheses about how the TCR transmits this message. The first hypothesis is aggregation. When the TCR binds to the peptide:MHC, CD4 or CD8 also binds to the MHC complex, thereby bringing CD4 or CD8 into close proximity to the TCR. The tyrosine kinase **LCK (lymphocyte-specific protein tyrosine kinase)** that phosphorylates

the ITAMS on the CD3 is associated with CD4 in resting T cells. By bringing CD4 into close proximity with the TCR complex, LCK is also brought in and this is thought to allow the signal from the TCR to be transmitted across the plasma membrane. The second hypothesis is that the TCR undergoes a conformational change that allows the transfer of the signal. The third mechanism is similar to the first: segregation. When the TCR binds and forms the immune synapse, inhibitory signaling receptors are pushed away from the TCR-removing phosphatases that inhibit TCR signaling. These hypotheses are not mutually exclusive: All three of these mechanisms could be playing a role.

When the TCR transmits its signal across the membrane, LCK phosphorylates the ITAMS of the CD3 subunits. **ZAP70 (zeta-chain-associated protein kinase 70)** is recruited to the phosphorylated CD3 subunits and is activated by LCK. ZAP70 then associates with **LAT** (Linker for Activation of T cells). ZAP70 phosphorylates LAT at several tyrosine residues. LAT serves as a common binding site for several different proteins and adaptor molecules. LAT does not have any enzymatic abilities but recruits proteins into a central location. ZAP70 also phosphorylates **SLP76** (SH2 domain containing leukocyte protein of 76 kDa) and GADS. GADS binds to the phosphorylated tyrosine residues on LAT and recruits phosphorylated SLP76 to LAT. SLP-76 serves as another adaptor molecule and recruits VAV1 and PLCγ. The phospholipase **PLCγ** cleaves the phospholipid PIP2 into IP3 and DAG. From here, the pathways leading to NFAT, AP-1, and NFκB start to diverge.

The NFAT pathway uses the IP3 from the PIP2 cleavage. IP3 acts as a signal by binding the IP3 receptor (IP3R) on the endoplasmic reticulum (ER), causing the ER to release its intracellular calcium storage. The release of the calcium from the ER opens the **calcium release-activated channels (CRAC)**. CRAC lets extracellular calcium enter the cell. The high levels of intracellular calcium cause calmodulin to release calcineurin. Calcineurin is a phosphatase that dephosphorylates cytoplasmic NFAT and allows it to translocate to the nucleus and bind to DNA.

The AP-1 pathway uses the other product of the PIP2 cleavage: DAG. DAG recruits the guanine exchange factor (GEF) RasGRP to the membrane where it activates Ras by exchange of GDP for GTP on Ras. Ras then activates the mitogen-activated kinase (MAPK) **ERK** by phosphorylation. Phosphorylated ERK then phosphorylates c-Fos, one subunit of the AP-1 transcription factor. AP-1 activation also relies on a second pathway downstream of VAV. VAV is a RacGEF that activates Rac1. Rac1 signals downstream by phosphorylating the MAPK JNK. JNK phosphorylates and activates c-JUN, the second subunit of AP-1. Activated c-Fos and c-JUN translocate from the cytoplasm to the nucleus and bind to the DNA.

The final pathway NFκB also relies on the secondary messenger DAG. DAG signaling activates PKCθ. **PKCθ** phosphorylates Carma1, causing it to complex with MALT1 and BCL-10. This complex activates the E3 ligase TRAF6. TRAF6 ubiquitinates IκB and targets it for degradation. **IκB** inhibits NFκB signaling by preventing NFκB from localizing to the nucleus. The degradation of IκB allows NFκB to translocate into the nucleus and bind to the DNA.

The combination of NFAT, AP-1, and NFκB signaling results in transcription of cytokines and other genes that regulate survival and proliferation of the T cells. B cells signal through the same pathways although some of the signaling molecules are a little different.

T-Cell Activation and Clonal Expansion

DC activation leads to increased expression of MHC-II and adhesive molecules, allowing prolonged contacts with T cells. T-cell activation involves three main signals: TCR-MHC-II interaction (signal 1); costimulation (signal 2) and cytokine signaling (signal 3) to mediate activation, survival, differentiation, and proliferation, respectively **BOX 3–2**. Signal 2 by T cells allows for their proliferation via a called clonal expansion. The making of multiple cells of the same specificity that allows for faster eradication of the infection, is a

A DEEPER LOOK BOX 3–2 Immune Cell Migration Into Tissues

During an infection, the immune cells need to be able to migrate out of the circulation and into the tissues where the pathogens are located.[2,64] Cells at the site of infection will release a chemo-attractant called a chemokine. The chemokines will form a gradient: Chemokines will be most concentrated at sites of infection and diffuse out to lower concentrations. The immune cells will recognize the chemokine gradient and follow it to the sites of infection. The immune cells (T cells, B cells, neutrophils, etc.) traveling through the blood vessels will sense the gradient and upregulate L-selectin. L-selectin is an adhesion molecule on immune cells that will transiently bind to CD34 on the endothelial cells of the blood vessel. This binding between L-selectin and CD34 will slow the immune cell down so that it is rolling along the endothelial cells. Next, the immune cells will upregulate an integrin such as LFA-1 that binds tightly to ICAM-1 on the endothelial cells, causing the immune cell to stop rolling. The immune cell can then exit the vessel by diapedesis and enter the tissues.

central tenet of adaptive immune response. Lack of signal 2 leads to anergy or a state of unresponsiveness whereby the T-cell cannot undergo further activation. This is a process that checks activation of autoreactive T cells, which may engage with self-peptides displayed on MHC. Activation of T cells in specific cytokine milieu guides them to adopt different cell fates. CD8 T cells mitigate infections by direct killing of infected cells.

Methods to Detect Immune Cells' Development, Activation

The process of cellular identification is an important experimental tool of modern immunology to ascertain numbers and ratios of different cell types. Combinations of molecules called "cell markers" can be reliably used to demarcate stages of cell development and status of activation of cells. An example of a cell-surface maker is the T-cell surface receptor (TCR), which is exclusively present on T cells. Within the T-cell lineage, further characterization of cells can be accomplished using other markers such as CD4 and CD8; the former is present on helper T cells that potentiate other members of the immune system and later identifies cytotoxic T cells that carry out direct killing of infected cells to eliminate pathogen and prevent its spread. Immune phenotyping is also a critical tool for disease diagnosis. In the 1980s, it was used to determine the loss of CD4 T-cell in human immunodeficiency virus- (HIV) infected patients. This observation incited experimental studies that subsequently demonstrated that HIV multiplied within CD4 T cells, causing their death and rendering the host immune deficient.

How is immune phenotyping conducted? One method of marker detection is to use antibodies with reactivity against certain markers. These antibodies are conjugated with different fluorescent compounds called fluorochromes. Using flow cytometry, a system consisting of lasers to excite fluorochromes and detectors to read out emissions from fluorochromes, can be used to detect the binding of fluorochrome-conjugated antibodies to a cell. Sample preparation for flow cytometry involves crushing an organ such as the spleen to release cells, incubating harvested cells with fluorochrome-conjugated antibodies and finally, detection with flow cytometry. "Cell markers" can be reliably used to demarcate stages of cell development, i.e., tell apart the various precursors and the terminally differentiated cell and activation status of cells.

Astute understanding of development or cellular activation is also dependent on understanding the relationship between cell signaling and gene expression changes. Cell signaling involves binding of soluble molecules, such as cytokines, in the environment that trigger molecular signaling cascades within the cell, leading to alterations in genetic expression in the nucleus, thus orchestrating the future course of development. Cytokine presence in the serum can be detected using enzyme-linked immunosorbent assay (ELISA). The sample is first immobilized to a solid surface and detection antibodies are used to quantify the presence of cytokines. Many variants of the technique have been developed for several purposes, which will be discussed elsewhere in the book.

Cytokine signaling leads to activation of transcription factors, which bind DNA and recruit other transcriptional machinery to allow for gene expression.[84] For example, during T-cell development, CD4 T cells and CD8 T cells develop from CD4 CD8 double positive (DP) immature precursors. These precursors frequently bifurcate into either the CD8 lineage of T cells or CD4 lineage of T cells. Cytokine signaling leads to expression of Runx3 of the master transcriptional regulator of CD8 T cells, while prolonging signaling through the T-cell surface receptor (TCR) leads to a commitment to the CD4 lineage by expression of ThPOK, the CD4 master transcriptional regulator. Additionally, cytokine signaling can lead to chromatic alterations. Chromatin consists of DNA and DNA-associated proteins such as histones. Alteration of chemical properties of histones and repositioning of histones can lead to increased accessibility of DNA to transcriptional regulators, resulting in gene-expression changes.

How is transcriptional regulation studied? Several methods can be used to ascertain the transcriptional regulation, and these methods are based on fundamental principles of immune-precipitation. Immune precipitation involves the use of antibodies to precipitate out a protein of interest that is bound to another protein or DNA from cell lysates. For instance, an antibody that specifically binds to Runx3 can be used to precipitate Runx3 while it is bound to DNA. The methodology involves using a crosslinker such as formalin to stably cross-link protein and DNA, using the antibody to precipitate the protein and uncross-linking protein and DNA to recover DNA targeted by protein of interest (e.g., Runx3). Precipitated DNA can then be sequenced to determine the regions of the genome Runx3 localized to drive a developmental fate such as CD8 T-cell lineage commitment. This method is called ChipSeq (chromatin immunoprecipitation).

Additionally, to assess the nature of gene expression of a cell at a specific stage in development, RNA can be profiled using various methods. One

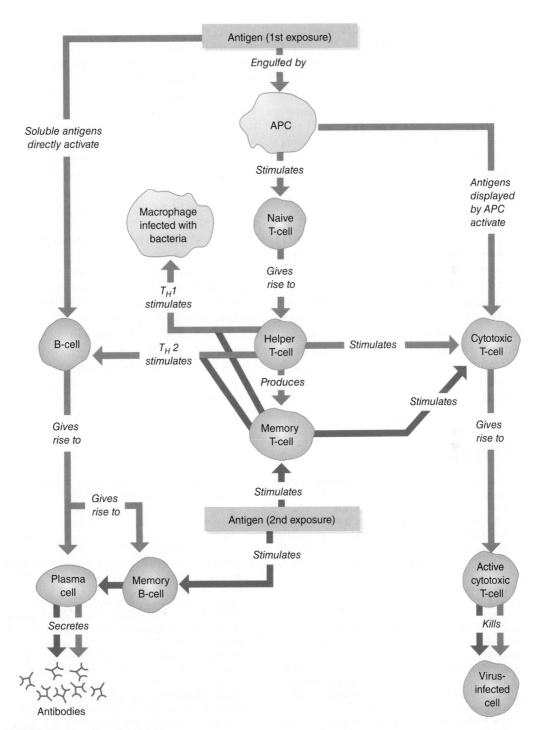

FIGURE 3–14 B- and T-cell activation.

Data from Reisner, H. (2017). Crowley's an introduction to human disease, 10e. Jones & Bartlett Learning.

such method is RNA-seq, which entails extraction of RNA from cells purified based on cell marker expression, followed by the sequencing of extracted RNA to determine identity and levels of transcripts present at a specific stage of development. Hence, cell markers and gene expression profiles of cells can be harnessed to understand development of cells and how the immediate environment of precursors instructs their development. Some other methods to ascertain mRNA levels are real-time PCR and microarrays.

Conclusion

The adaptive immune system provides a unique mechanism for fighting off pathogens. B cells and T cells both express receptors that have undergone gene rearrangement. The generation of BCRs and TCRs is a random process that occurs without antigens and therefore, self-reactive receptors can be generated. To prevent self-reactive B cells and T cells from entering the periphery, B cells and T cells undergo an extensive development process that negatively selects auto-reactive cells. B cells,

after an encounter with their antigen, can continue to alter their receptors by affinity maturation to produce high affinity antibodies against pathogens. B cells can differentiate into plasma cells that secrete their BCRs as antibodies. Antibodies have three main effector functions: neutralize, opsonize, and activate complement.

T cells recognize their antigens in the context of peptides present on MHC molecules. CD4+ T cells recognize MHC II and differentiate into T helper subsets that help direct the immune response against pathogens. CD8+ T cells recognize MHC I and develop into cytotoxic T cells that lyse infected cells through a perforin/granzyme B mechanism.

Both B and T cells can produce long lasting memory cells. In general, first exposure to an antigen can engage either a B-cell directly or an APC, which activates the naïve T-cell leading to the production of longer lasting memory B and T cells (**FIGURE 3–14**). The memory cells require lower thresholds for activation, allowing a quicker, more robust response following re-exposure to a pathogen.

▸ References

1. Granato A, Chen Y, Wesemann DR. Primary immunoglobulin repertoire development: time and space matter. *Curr Opin Immunol*. 2015;33:126–131.
2. Gottlieb MS, Schroff R, Schanker HM, et al. Pneumocystis carinii pneumonia and mucosal candidiasis in previously healthy homosexual men: evidence of a new acquired cellular immunodeficiency. *The New England journal of medicine*. 1981;305(24):1425–1431.
3. Hardy RR, Hayakawa K. B-Cell Development Pathways. *Annu Rev Immunol*. 2001;19:595–621.
4. Melchers F, Strasser A, Bauer SR, et al. Cellular stages and molecular steps of murine B-cell development. *Cold Spring Harb Symp Quant Biol*. 1989;54 Pt 1:183–189.
5. Melchers F, ten Boekel E, Seidl T, et al. Repertoire selection by pre-B-cell receptors and B-cell receptors, and genetic control of B-cell development from immature to mature B cells. *Immunol Rev*. 2000;175:33–46.
6. Rolink AG, Schaniel C, Andersson J, et al. Selection events operating at various stages in B-cell development. *Curr Opin Immunol*. 2001;13(2):202–207.
7. Melchers F. Checkpoints that control B-cell development. *J Clin Invest*. 2015;125(6):2203–2210.
8. Pitkänen J, Peterson P. Autoimmune regulator: from loss of function to autoimmunity. *Genes and immunity*. 2003;4(1):12–21.
9. Brooks WH, Renaudineau Y. Epigenetics and autoimmune diseases: the X chromosome-nucleolus nexus. *Frontiers in genetics*. 2015;6:22–22.
10. Brandtzaeg P. Structure, synthesis and external transfer of mucosal immunoglobulins. *Ann Immunol (Paris)*. 1973;124(3):417–438.
11. Early PH, H. Davis, M. Calame, K., and Hood, L. An immunoglobulin heavy chain variable region gene is generated from three segments of DNA: V_H, D and J_H. *Cell*. 1980(19):981–992.
12. Hozumi N, Tonegawa S. Evidence for somatic rearrangement of immunoglobulin genes coding for variable and constant regions. 1976 [classical article]. *Journal of immunology*. 2004;173(7):4260–4264.
13. Merler E, Rosen FS. The gamma globulins. I. The structure and synthesis of the immunoglobulins. *The New England journal of medicine*. 1966;275(10):526–542 concl.
14. Ballieux RE. Immunoglobulins: an introduction to the structure, synthesis and pathology. *Vox Sang*. 1969;16(4):279–285.

15. Sakano H, Huppi K, Heinrich G, Tonegawa S. Sequences at the somatic recombination sites of immunoglobulin light-chain genes. *Nature.* 1979;280(5720):288–294.

16. Agrawal A, Schatz DG. RAG1 and RAG2 form a stable postcleavage synaptic complex with DNA containing signal ends in V(D)J recombination. *Cell.* 1997;89(1):43–53.

17. Lieber MR. The mechanism of human nonhomologous DNA end joining. *The Journal of biological chemistry.* 2008;283(1):1–5.

18. Ma Y, Pannicke U, Schwarz K, Lieber MR. Hairpin opening and overhang processing by an Artemis/DNA-dependent protein kinase complex in nonhomologous end joining and V(D)J recombination. *Cell.* 2002;108(6):781–794.

19. Komori T, Okada A, Stewart V, Alt FW. Lack of N regions in antigen receptor variable region genes of TdT-deficient lymphocytes. *Science.* 1993;261(5125):1171–1175.

20. Schatz DG. V(D)J recombination. *Immunol Rev.* 2004;200:5–11.

21. Low TL, Liu YS, Putnam FW. Structure, function, and evolutionary relationships of Fc domains of human immunoglobulins A, G, M, and E. *Science.* 1976;191(4225):390–392.

22. Clark MR. IgG effector mechanisms. *Chem Immunol.* 1997;65:88–110.

23. Corthesy B, Kraehenbuhl JP. Antibody-mediated protection of mucosal surfaces. *Current topics in microbiology and immunology.* 1999;236:93–111.

24. Sutton BJ, Gould HJ. The human IgE network. *Nature.* 1993;366(6454):421–428.

25. Kawabe T, Maeda Y, Takami M, et al. Human Fc epsilon RII and IgE-binding factor; triangular network with IL-2 and IL-4. *Res Immunol.* 1990;141(1):82–85; discussion 105–108.

26. Bransteitter R, Pham P, Scharff MD, et al. Activation-induced cytidine deaminase deaminates deoxycytidine on single-stranded DNA but requires the action of RNase. *Proc Natl Acad Sci U S A.* 2003;100(7):4102–4107.

27. Corcoran LM, Tarlinton DM. Regulation of germinal center responses, memory B cells and plasma cell formation-an update. *Curr Opin Immunol.* 2016;39:59–67.

28. Rush JS, Fugmann SD, Schatz DG. Staggered AID-dependent DNA double strand breaks are the predominant DNA lesions targeted to S mu in Ig class switch recombination. *Int Immunol.* 2004;16(4):549–557.

29. McKean D, Huppi K, Bell M, et al. Generation of antibody diversity in the immune response of BALB/c mice to influenza virus hemagglutinin. *Proc Natl Acad Sci U S A.* 1984;81(10):3180–3184.

30. Muramatsu M, Kinoshita K, Fagarasan S, et al. Class switch recombination and hypermutation require activation-induced cytidine deaminase (AID), a potential RNA editing enzyme. *Cell.* 2000;102(5):553–563.

31. Hoogeboom R, Tolar P. Molecular Mechanisms of B-Cell Antigen Gathering and Endocytosis. *Current topics in microbiology and immunology.* 2016;393:45–63.

32. Phan TG, Gray EE, Cyster JG. The microanatomy of B-cell activation. *Curr Opin Immunol.* 2009;21(3):258–265.

33. Heesters BA, Chatterjee P, Kim YA, et al. Endocytosis and recycling of immune complexes by follicular dendritic cells enhances B-cell antigen binding and activation. *Immunity.* 2013;38(6):1164–1175.

34. Clark MR, Massenburg D, Zhang M, et al. Molecular mechanisms of B-cell antigen receptor trafficking. *Annals of the New York Academy of Sciences.* 2003;987:26–37.

35. Kurosaki T. Molecular mechanisms in B-cell antigen receptor signaling. *Curr Opin Immunol.* 1997;9(3):309–318.

36. Gong YF, Xiang LX, Shao JZ. CD154-CD40 interactions are essential for thymus-dependent antibody production in zebrafish: insights into the origin of costimulatory pathway in helper T-cell-regulated adaptive immunity in early vertebrates. *Journal of immunology.* 2009;182(12):7749–7762.

37. McHeyzer-Williams LJ, Malherbe LP, McHeyzer-Williams MG. Helper T-cell-regulated B-cell immunity. *Current topics in microbiology and immunology.* 2006;311:59–83.

38. Allen CD, Okada T, Cyster JG. Germinal-center organization and cellular dynamics. *Immunity.* 2007;27(2):190–202.

39. Allen CD, Ansel KM, Low C, et al. Germinal center dark and light zone organization is mediated by CXCR4 and CXCR5. *Nat Immunol.* 2004;5(9):943–952.

40. Kelsoe G. The germinal center: a crucible for lymphocyte selection. *Semin Immunol.* 1996;8(3):179–184.

41. Liu YJ, Zhang J, Lane PJ, et al. Sites of specific B-cell activation in primary and secondary responses to T-cell-dependent and T-cell-independent antigens. *Eur J Immunol.* 1991;21(12):2951–2962.

42. Farber DL, MG N, A R, K R, RM Z. Immunological memory: lessons from the past and a look to the future. *Nat Rev Immunol* 2016;16(2):124–128.

43. Selvanayagam ZE, Gopalakrishnakone P. Tests for detection of snake venoms, toxins and venom antibodies: review on recent trends (1987–1997). *Toxicon.* 1999;37(4):565–586.

44. Theakston RD, Pugh RN, Reid HA. Enzyme-linked immunosorbent assay of venom-antibodies in human victims of snake bite. *J Trop Med Hyg.* 1981;84(3):109–112.

45. Filipovich AH, Peltier MH, Bechtel MK, et al. Circulating cytomegalovirus (CMV) neutralizing activity in bone marrow transplant recipients: comparison of passive immunity in a randomized study of four intravenous IgG products administered to CMV-seronegative patients. *Blood.* 1992;80(10):2656–2660.

46. Pierce NF, Reynolds HY. Immunity to experimental cholera. I. Protective effect of humoral IgG antitoxin demonstrated by passive immunization. *Journal of immunology.* 1974;113(3):1017–1023.

47. Hatae R, Chamoto K. Immune checkpoint inhibitors targeting programmed cell death-1 (PD-1) in cancer therapy. *Rinsho Ketsueki.* 2016;57(10):2224–2231.

48. Rudolph MG, Stanfield RL, Wilson IA. How TCRs bind MHCs, peptides, and coreceptors. *Annu Rev Immunol.* 2006;24:419–466.

49. Allison TJ, Garboczi DN. Structure of gammadelta T-cell receptors and their recognition of non-peptide antigens. *Mol Immunol.* 2002;38(14):1051–1061.

50. Rubin B, Knibiehler M, Gairin JE. Allosteric changes in the TCR/CD3 structure upon interaction with extra- or intra-cellular ligands. *Scand J Immunol.* 2007;66(2–3): 228–237.

51. Wang L, Zhao Y, Li Z, et al. Crystal structure of a complete ternary complex of TCR, superantigen and peptide-MHC. *Nat Struct Mol Biol.* 2007;14(2):169–171.

52. Feito MJ, Jimenez-Perianez A, Ojeda G, et al. The TCR/CD3 complex: molecular interactions in a changing structure. *Arch Immunol Ther Exp (Warsz).* 2002;50(4):263–272.

53. de la Hera A, Muller U, Olsson C, et al. Structure of the T-cell antigen receptor (TCR): two CD3 epsilon subunits in a functional TCR/CD3 complex. *J Exp Med.* 1991;173(1):7–17.

54. Wucherpfennig KW, Gagnon E, Call MJ, et al. Structural Biology of the T-cell Receptor: Insights into Receptor Assembly, Ligand Recognition, and Initiation of Signaling. *Cold Spring Harb Perspect Biol* 2010 2(4).

55. Koch U, Radtke F. Mechanisms of T-Cell Development and Transformation. *Annual Review of Cell and Developmental Biology.* 2011;27(1):539–562.

56. Krueger A, Ziętara N, Łyszkiewicz M. T-Cell Development by the Numbers. *Trends in Immunology.* 2016;xx(2):1–12.

57. Bassing CH, Swat W, Alt FW. The mechanism and regulation of chromosomal V(D)J recombination. *Cell.* 2002;109:Supp: 45–55.

58. Schuetz C, Huck K, Gudowius S, et al. An Immunodeficiency Disease with RAG Mutations and Granulomas. *The New England journal of medicine.* 2008;19358(8):2030–2038.

59. Nathan C. Fundamental immunodeficiency and its correction. *J Exp Med.* 2017;214(8):2175–2191.

60. Mechanisms of lymphocyte activation and immune regulation III. Developmental biology of lymphocytes. Proceedings ot the Third International Conference on Lymphocyte Activation and Immune Regulations, February 16–18, 1990, Newport Beach, California. *Adv Exp Med Biol.* 1991;292:1–258.

61. von Boehmer H, Bluethmann H, Staerz U, et al. Developmental biology of T lymphocytes. Deletion of autoreactive T cells and impact of the alpha, beta receptor on the CD4/CD8 phenotype. *Annals of the New York Academy of Sciences.* 1988;546:104–108.

62. Starr TK, Jameson SC, Hogquist KA. Positive and negative selection of T cells. *Annu Rev Immunol.* 2003;21:139–176.

63. Itano AA, Jenkins MK. Antigen presentation to naive CD4 T cells in the lymph node. *Nat Immunol.* 2003;4(8): 733–739.

64. Picker LJ, Butcher EC. Physiological and molecular mechanisms of lymphocyte homing. *Annu Rev Immunol.* 1992;10:561–591.

65. Gudmundsdottir H, Wells AD, Turka LA. Dynamics and requirements of T-cell clonal expansion in vivo at the single-cell level: effector function is linked to proliferative capacity. *Journal of immunology.* 1999;162(9):5212–5223.

66. Blum JS, Wearsch PA, Cresswell P. *Pathways of Antigen Processing.* Vol 312013.

67. Klein L, Kyewski B, Allen PM, et al. Positive and negative selection of the T-cell repertoire: what thymocytes see (and don't see). *Nature Reviews Immunology.* 2014;14(6):377–391.

68. Yuseff M-I, Pierobon P, Reversat A, et al. How B cells capture, process and present antigens: a crucial role for cell polarity. *Nature Reviews Immunology.* 2013;13(7):475–486.

69. Greenwald RJ, Freeman GJ, Sharpe AH. The B7 family revisited. *Annu Rev Immunol.* 2005;23:515–548.

70. Gray D. The thymic medulla: who needs it? *Immunology and Cell Biology.* 2013;91(10):541–542.

71. Anderson MS, Su MA. Aire and T-cell development. *Curr Opin Immunol.* 2011;23(2):198–206.

72. Malchow S, Leventhal DS, Lee V, et al. Aire Enforces Immune Tolerance by Directing Autoreactive T Cells into the Regulatory T-Cell Lineage. *Immunity.* 2016;44:1102–1113.

73. Hogquist KA, Xing Y, Hsu F-C, et al. T-Cell Adolescence: Maturation Events Beyond Positive Selection. *The Journal of Immunology.* 2015;195(195):1351–1357.

74. Fink PJ, Hendricks DW. Post-thymic maturation: young T cells assert their individuality. *Nature.* 2011;11:544–549.

75. Moran AE, Holzapfel KL, Xing Y, et al. T-cell receptor signal strength in Treg and iNKT cell development demonstrated by a novel fluorescent reporter mouse. *J Exp Med.* 2011;208(6):1279–1289.

76. Lio CWJ, Hsieh CS. A Two-Step Process for Thymic Regulatory T-Cell Development. *Immunity.* 2008;28(1): 100–111.

77. Wildin RS, Freitas A. IPEX and FOXP3: Clinical and research perspectives. Vol 252005:56–62.

78. Zamoyska R. CD4 and CD8: modulators of T-cell receptor recognition of antigen and of immune responses? *Curr Opin Immunol.* 1998;10(1):82–87.

79. van der Merwe PA, Dushek O. Mechanisms for T-cell receptor triggering. *Nature reviews Immunology.* 2011; 11(1):47–55.

80. Murphy KM, Reiner SL. The lineage decisions of helper T cells. *Nature reviews Immunology.* 2002;2(12):933–944.

81. O'Shea JJ, Paul WE. Mechanisms underlying lineage commitment and plasticity of helper CD4+ T cells. *Science.* 2010;327(5969):1098–1102.

82. Geier CB, Piller A, Linder A, et al. Leaky RAG Deficiency in Adult Patients with Impaired Antibody Production against Bacterial Polysaccharide Antigens. *PLoS One.* 2015;10(7):e0133220.

83. Lin J, Weiss A. T-cell receptor signalling. *J Cell Sci.* 2001;114(Pt 2):243–244.

84. Singer A, Adoro S, Park J-H. Lineage fate and intense debate: myths, models and mechanisms of CD4- versus CD8-lineage choice. *Nature Reviews Immunology.* 2008;8(10):788–801.

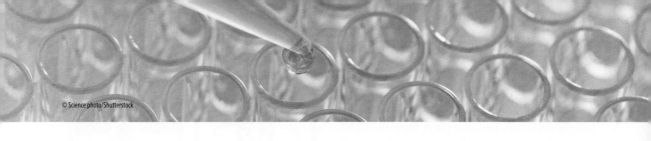

CHAPTER 4

Safety and Standards

Ian Clift, PhD, MLS(ASCP)^{CM}

KEY TERMS

Aliquots
Biohazardous
Continuing education
Material Safety Data Sheet (MSDS)
Method validation

Personal protective equipment
 (PPE)
Proficiency testing
Quality assurance (QA)
Quality controls

Quality indicators (QI)
Sharps
Standard operating procedures
 (SOPs)

LEARNING OBJECTIVES

Upon completion of this chapter, the reader should be able to:

1. Define governing and regulatory bodies with oversight in the laboratory.
2. Explain the types of error encountered in the lab and how to control for each.
3. Name four safety measures used to prevent disease spread and infection risk in the laboratory.
4. Compare and contrast quality assurance and quality control.

▶ Fundamentals

Safe handling of body fluids and reagents as well as proper laboratory practices are everybody's business. All biosafety and clinical diagnostic laboratories must ensure safety conditions to avoid the hazards associated with biological materials but are also responsible for protecting the public from these potential hazards through risk-management measures. Despite the common myth that laboratory teachers and training coordinators have gone to school for a long time and, therefore, know everything about safety in the lab, both teachers and students need to keep informed on safety practices, and reacquaint themselves periodically to maintain the level of excellence that is required of laboratory professionals. Laboratory-acquired infections (LAI) have always been reported in the literature, but in the 1970s they were quantitatively evaluated. Recent reports from the CDC suggest that >40% of infections are of bacterial origin; however, the virus hepatitis B remains the most frequent LAI viral infection.[1] Both employers and employees have specific responsibilities when it comes to preventing infections, injuries, and contamination-related risks. Therefore, this chapter is an essential component of every laboratory-based curriculum. Provided here are the fundamental standards and practices established to facilitate laboratory safety; however, most organizations require some sort of continuing, typically annual, review of safety protocols, which should be consulted for updates and site-specific examinations.

Biosafety Oversight

Jurisdiction and institution-specific biosafety oversight should be considered when developing a laboratory safety program. The organizational oversights presented here are based on current United States (US) standards; however, several of these organizations also provide oversight at the international level and may be a practical resource in other jurisdictions.

OSHA

The US Occupational Safety and Health Act (OSHA) was established in 1970 with the goal of providing employees with a safe work environment based on a federal regulatory standard. Included in this broad set of workplace regulations are standards that are associated with safety in clinical and diagnostic laboratories. These standards include those for Bloodborne Pathogens, Hazard Communication, and Occupational Exposure to Hazardous Chemicals in the Laboratory standards. The OSHA standards apply to all businesses in the United States with one or more employees and are administered through the U.S. Department of Labor.

In general, OSHA programs apply to many aspects of safety and health protection that are reflected in organizational policies and procedures including system administration and operation,

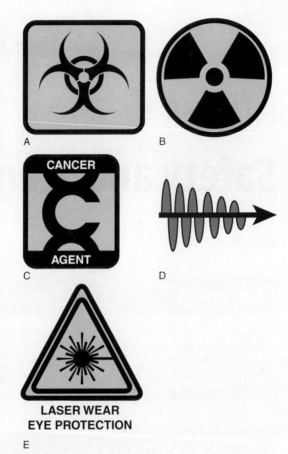

FIGURE 4–1 Common Hazard Symbols Seen in the Laboratory. **(A)** Biohazard. **(B)** Radioactive. **(C)** Cancer Agent. **(D)** Ultraviolet Rays, **(E)** Laser in use.

inspection procedures, compliance arrangements, complaint procedures, and duties and responsibilities for specific laboratory personnel. They include provisions for proper warning signs (**FIGURE 4–1**), e.g., reagent labels, and also mandate that laboratories implement an exposure control plan, a chemical hygiene plan, and provide guidelines on bloodborne pathogens through standard 1910.1030. For example, the Safety Data Sheets (SDSs) (**TABLE 4–1**), formerly known as Material Safety Data Sheets (MSDS), are required to be provided by manufacturers and be readily available within all laboratories for assurance of safe product use.

State organizations have policies that are at least as stringent as the federal policies and, in many cases, duplicate the OSHA terminology exactly.

TABLE 4–1 Inclusions within Safety Data Sheets

Hazard Communications Safety Data Sheet Sections*

Section 1, Identification	Includes product identifier; manufacturer or distributor name, address, phone number; emergency phone number; recommended use; restrictions on use.
Section 2, Hazard(s) identification	Includes all hazards regarding the chemical; required label elements.
Section 3, Composition/information on ingredients	Includes information on chemical ingredients; trade secret claims.
Section 4, First Aid measures	Includes important symptoms/effects, acute, delayed; required treatment.
Section 5, Fire-fighting measures	Lists suitable extinguishing techniques, equipment; chemical hazards from fire.
Section 6, Accidental release measures	Lists emergency procedures; protective equipment; proper methods of containment and cleanup.
Section 7, Handling and storage	Lists precautions for safe handling and storage, including incompatibilities.
Section 8, Exposure controls/ personal protection	Lists OSHA's Permissible Exposure Limits (PELs); ACGIH Threshold Limit Values (TLVs); and any other exposure limit used or recommended by the chemical manufacturer, importer, or employer preparing the SDS where available as well as appropriate engineering controls; personal protective equipment (PPE).
Section 9, Physical and chemical properties	Lists the chemical's characteristics.
Section 10, Stability and reactivity	Lists chemical stability and possibility of hazardous reactions.
Section 11, Toxicological information	Includes routes of exposure; related symptoms, acute and chronic effects; numerical measures of toxicity.
Section 12, Ecological information	Mandated by other agencies (not OSHA)
Section 13, Disposal considerations	Mandated by other agencies (not OSHA)
Section 14, Transport information	Mandated by other agencies (not OSHA)

(continues)

TABLE 4–1 Inclusions within Safety Data Sheets	*(Continued)*
Hazard Communications Safety Data Sheet Sections*	
Section 15, Regulatory information	Mandated by other agencies
Section 16, Other information	Includes the date of preparation or last revision.

*Hazard Communication Safety Data Sheets, Occupational Safety and Health Administration, Retrieved from https://www.osha.gov/Publications/HazComm_QuickCard_SafetyData.html

CAP

The College of American Pathology (CAP) is an accrediting organization for clinical laboratories in the United States. It has counterparts in other countries as well, such as Clinical Pathology Accreditation (CPA) in the United Kingdom. CAP provides inspectors who perform site visits and provides resources for in-house proficiency testing. Inspectors, including pathologists, lab managers and technologists, perform on-site inspections in which the laboratories record of quality control and procedures for the past 2 years are assessed. Laboratories that subscribe to CAP proficiency testing programs receive periodic samples for analysis and then return the results to CAP. This testing helps to ensure high levels of quality.

TJC

The Joint Commission (TJC), also known as the Joint Commission on Accreditation of Healthcare Organizations (JCAHO), mandates that all healthcare organizations, including those associated with clinical and diagnostic laboratory testing, have a hospital preparedness plan for disaster management, which includes responses to tornados, earthquakes, and other natural or unintentional manmade mass casualty events.[2]

In response to this mandate, many organizations developed their own specific plans for managing emergency situations and external disasters. In 2008, the Mayo Clinic began developing a standardized internal approach to handling TJC's mandate through the development of their Mayo Emergency Incident Command System (MEICS) (**FIGURE 4–2**).[3]

Specific laboratory units have also developed disaster management plans. These plans establish a chain of command and a procedure for communicating and recruiting supporting units to handle the disaster. In specific areas, such as transfusion medicine, actions such as notification of outside blood donation testing laboratories and transportation providers, as well as evaluation of the blood supply needs should be considered.[3] In such an emergency, laboratory personnel may be recruited for additional shifts, asked to relocate for safety, or tasked with a very specific workload. The depth of such a plan will be dependent upon the type of facility and type of testing performed.

CDC

Another important partner in disaster planning is the Centers for Disease Control and Prevention (CDC). The primary role of the CDC is to assess infectious disease risks that pose a risk to public health. In support of this role, they provide guidelines and regulatory mandates to clinical laboratory organizations. In 2008, the CDC gathered a panel to address the issues of clinical laboratory safety and incidence of laboratory-acquired infection. This was part of a larger federal effort to assess the role of laboratory biosafety on biosecurity and threats to public health.[4] The result of this effort was a modification and increased regulation of the competencies required of laboratory personnel in the areas of safety and risk management in order to establish a culture of safety (**FIGURE 4–3**).

In addition to developing guidelines for laboratory practice, the CDC collects data on the rates of LAIs caused by microorganisms, most of which

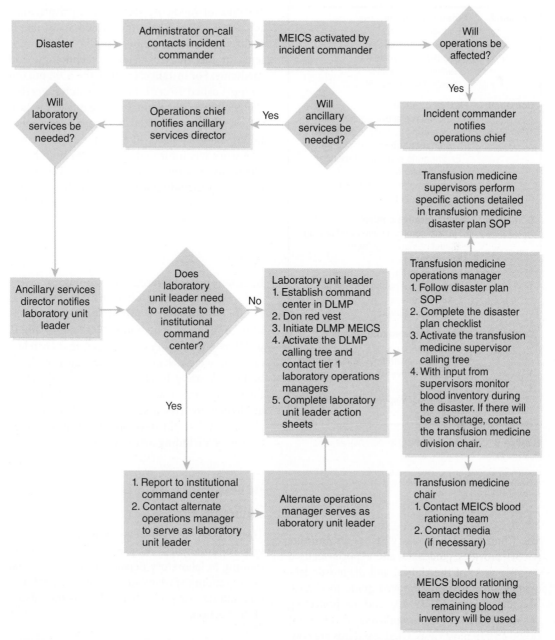

FIGURE 4–2 A high-level summary diagram disaster response plan from the Mayo Clinic. The Mayo Emergency Incident Command System (MEICS) is an example of an institutional disaster response system.

Bundy KL, Foss ML, Stubbs JR. Transfusion service disaster planning. *Immunohematology*. 2008;24(3):93–101. Used with permission from American Red Cross.

result from improper handling of blood and body fluid specimens or inadequate/improper usage of laboratory safeguards. Specifically, the CDC has indicated that needle punctures, glass cuts, bruises, cuts, and splashes in the eye account for the majority of LAIs.[1]

Domain I: **Potential hazards**
              Biologic materials
              Research animals
              Chemical materials
              Radiologic materials
              Physical environment

Domain II: **Hazard controls**
              Personal protective equipment
              Engineering controls – equipment
                (primary barriers)
              Engineering controls – facility
                (secondary barriers)
              Decontamination and waste control
                management

Domain III: **Administrative controls**
              Hazard communication and signage
              Guidelines and regulatory
                compliance
              Safety program management
              Occupational health – medical
                surveillance
              Risk management

Domain IV: **Emergency preparedness and
              response**
              Emergencies and incident response
              Exposure prevention and hazard
                mitigation
              Emergency response – exercises
                and drills

FIGURE 4–3 Domains of Safety Competency Established by the CDC.

Delany JR, Pentella MA, Rodriguez JA, et al. Guidelines for biosafety laboratory competency: CDC and the Association of Public Health Laboratories. *MMWR Suppl*. 2011;60(2):1–23. Retrieved from https://www.cdc.gov/mmwr/preview/mmwrhtml/su6002a1.htm

CLSI

The Clinical and Laboratory Standards Institute (CLSI) provides guidelines and reports focused on all aspects of the clinical and diagnostic laboratory, including an approved guide to clinical laboratory safety (GP17-A3) and to protecting laboratory workers from work-related infections (M29-A4). In most cases, CLSI standards are considered the standard of care that a laboratory must meet and are often referred to in legal proceedings.

HMD

The Health and Medicine Division (HMD) of the National Academies of Sciences, Engineering, and Medicine, formerly known as the Institute of Medicine (IOM), is a private, not-for-profit institution in the United States that is focused on solving complex public policy problems in the areas of science, technology, and medicine. For instance, in 1999, the IOM put out a report called *To err is human*, which suggested that 98,000 deaths annually were due to medical errors, underscoring the importance of quality practices in all parts of the medical system.[5,6] The work has informed policy reform and provided insights into improving practices in the laboratory including aspects of public concern. The website is a valuable resource for health-related information.

WHO

International standards for laboratory safety and quality have been established by the World Health Organization (WHO). The WHO periodically updates its *Laboratory Biosafety Manual*, which contains general guidelines that correlate infective agent risk groups (1 through 4) with the biological safety levels (BSL) examined below. Like other organizations on this list, it provides guidelines for risk assessment, and serves as a global standard for developing healthcare organizations, including laboratory facilities.

Developing a Safe Laboratory Environment

The primary step in developing a safe laboratory environment is to provide the appropriate training to laboratory personnel. A fundamental understanding of what causes errors in the laboratory and the ways to mitigate them is the subject of this section.

Types of Error

In the clinical diagnostic laboratory, the technologist must confront both analytical and procedural errors. In both cases, there may be a risk either to the patient, the practitioner, the institution, or all of the above. Managing these risks is helped by understanding whether an error is systematic (within a procedure or process) or random. Clinical laboratory systems aim to reduce all forms of random error by establishing strict processes to be followed at all times: i.e., Standard Operating Procedures (SOPs).

Systematic Errors. A systematic error is part of a procedure or process that is both reproducible and discoverable and can, therefore, be eliminated. These are also known as determinate errors. Most errors have a cause that can be detected and eliminated. Instrument errors, method errors, and training errors are all systematic and can be mitigated or eliminated by modifications to the protocol design or through retraining. A focus on quality and safety is established to reduce the number of systematic errors.

Random Errors. In contrast to determinate errors, random errors are considered indeterminate and are caused by unknown variables that and therefore cannot be defined or eliminated. These may be caused by imprecision in an instrument or unknown variables in the sample, but are often human in nature. Even when a laboratory is focused on quality and safety, unknown factors remain. Therefore, no laboratory procedure or activity is without risk. Carelessness and imprecise techniques in the laboratory increase the potential for random error. Even subtle changes in a procedure may lead to changes in assay results, for example. Following strict procedures in the laboratory is one way to reduce the rate of random error.

Lab Setup

The best time to implement lab safety systems is during the design and setup of the clinical diagnostic laboratory. These general precautionary measures should include the installation of appropriate safety equipment, i.e., fire extinguishers, safety showers, and nonslip flooring for the laboratory. It is also during the design phase redundant that a specific chemical hygiene plan and hazard-tracking system can be best implemented. While OSHA standards provide a sensible starting point, they are generic in nature; and lab-specific

considerations should also be examined. Furthermore, laboratories within an institutional system should examine internal institutional guidelines for laboratory set-up and safe operation. Many institutions may have a group called a biosafety committee that performs periodic inspections and defines deficiencies needing correction. These inspections provide documentation to internal and external stakeholders to demonstrate operations are performed in a safe manner throughout the institution.

Unlike research laboratories, clinical laboratories are more process-oriented; focus on both accuracy and efficiency of test results, therefore, requires, process-engineering steps to be included in the lab design phase. Specifically, three aspects of lab design can facilitate increased safety and productivity in the lab: the physical layout of the lab, the heating ventilation and air conditioning (HVAC) systems, and the installation of emergency-response equipment[7] (**TABLE 4–2**). For instance, the location of benches and other obstacles should be situated to avoid collision and to accommodate traffic. Biological safety cabinets

TABLE 4–2 Common Built-in Laboratory Safety Features
Handwashing stations
Eye washing stations
Process alarm systems
Flammable liquid storage
Special hazardous chemical storage
Durable/cleanable work surfaces, flooring, and walls
Fire and gas detection systems
Biological safety cabinets
Chemical fume hoods

TABLE 4–3 Common Hazard Sources in the Clinical Laboratory
Chemicals
Biological Agents
Radiation-producing Agents
Electrical
Physical
Mechanical
Noise
Heat

should be installed to circulate pathogens away from workers and to filter toxic fumes. Toxic chemicals should be separated and contained securely. Fire suppression and detection systems should be installed (**TABLE 4–3**).

Revisions and updates to safety protocols should be performed periodically during the normal operation of the laboratory, and specifically conducted during the development of new test or assay implementations.

Biosafety Levels. Laboratories are designated by a common nomenclature regarding biomedical safety. These biosafety levels are used to inform and establish appropriate containment and procedures for infectious agents used in the specified laboratory. The BSL numbers have been correlated to the WHO Risk Group classifications (1 through 4).[8]

BSL-1 Laboratories do not work with agents that consistently cause disease in healthy humans.

BSL-2 Laboratories work with agents that can cause infections if ingested, percutaneously passed, or through mucous membrane exposure.

BSL-3 Laboratories work with exotic agents with potential for aerosol transmission that may have serious or lethal consequences.

BSL-4 Laboratories are designated to work with exotic agents that cause known life-threatening diseases, such as Ebola and Marburg viruses, in which no known treatment is available.

Biological Safety Cabinets. The biological safety cabinet (BSC) is designed to provide a protective barrier for laboratory personnel to prevent exposure to infections from splashes and aerosols (**FIGURE 4–4**). If work with bacteria, viruses, or

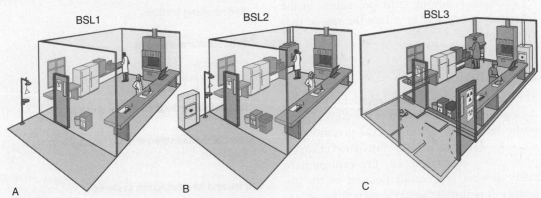

FIGURE 4–4 Biosafety level lab design examples. **(A)** Biosafety level 1—minimum level of controls, lowest risk organisms examined. **(B)** Biosafety level 2—moderate level of controls, moderate risk organisms examined. **(C)** Biosafety level 3—high level of controls, extreme risk organisms examined.

Adapted from Biosafety level lab design examples, Architects USA, Retrieved from http://architectsusa.com/

potentially infected cells to be conducted in the laboratory, a BSC should be installed during laboratory setup. Activities such as shaking, pouring, mixing, and dispensing liquids can lead to aerosolized particles. These particles, sometimes as small as 5 μm, are undetectable by the naked eye and are, therefore, commonly inhaled or spread to other work surfaces without notice. BSCs help to mitigate this risk. Three classes: class I, class II, and class III of BSCs have been designed to account for different types of protection. In most laboratories, any class of BSC will protect against microorganisms encountered; however, only class II and higher BSCs will provide protection for the products being examined. Specifically, when working with viruses or cell cultures, air from a HEPA-filtered (sterile) source flows over the work surface, preventing contamination of the cultures from outside air. Class II BSCs can be used with the highest risk organisms (WHO group 4) when positive pressure suits are worn, and Class III BSCs, also known as "glove boxes", can be used with this highest-risk group and is sometimes connected with a double-door autoclave to decontaminate and sterilize all entering and exiting materials.[8]

The selection of a BSC should be part of the initial lab design or revised lab design, depending on the types of pathogenic organisms to be considered and the level of sterility needed for conducting common procedures. Operators of BSCs should be appropriately trained to avoid misuse, which can diminish the protective benefit of the cabinet.

Essential Safety Guidelines

In addition to environmental protections, a laboratory safety program also includes elements focused on hazard recognition, risk assessment, and risk/hazard mitigation. Through the process of training, individuals in the laboratory should reduce the overall risk to themselves and others from exposures to toxic and infectious materials, as well as the unintended release of toxins or infectious agents.

The CDC found that the predominant routes to laboratory-associated infections (LAI) are from needle sticks, splashes/spills, ingestion through mouth pipetting/transfer from infected objects, animal bites, and inhalation; however, in 80% of the reported cases, no specific event was identifiably associated with infection.[1] In addition to infections, laboratory risks can also be associated with injury, depending on the operations of the laboratory. These risks include electrical, mechanical, and ergonomic hazards as well as hazards associated with chemical, radioactive, compressed gas, and cryogenic materials.

While no one standard approach for hazard assessment exists, the CDC proposed the following five steps to reduce or mitigate sources of risk: (**FIGURE 4–5**).

1. Identify the hazard associated with an infectious agent or material
2. Identify the activities that might cause exposure to the agent or material
3. Consider the competencies and experience of laboratory personnel.
4. Evaluate and prioritize risks
5. Develop, implement, and evaluate controls to minimize the risk of exposure

Universal Precautions

Universal Precautions is a term used in healthcare infection control and prevention in which all human blood and body fluid specimens are treated as if they are infectious. Both OSHA and the CDC recommend the use of universal precautions (or standard precautions) for the prevention of viral diseases such as human immunodeficiency virus (HIV) and hepatitis B, as well as bacterial pathogens such as Streptococcus and Staphylococcus species. As defined in OSHA's Bloodborne Pathogen Standard (29 CFR 1910.1030(b)), universal precautions should include:

- Preventing contact with potentially infectious blood or other potentially infectious material (OPIM)
- Where differentiation of body fluids is difficult, all body fluids shall be considered potentially infectious materials

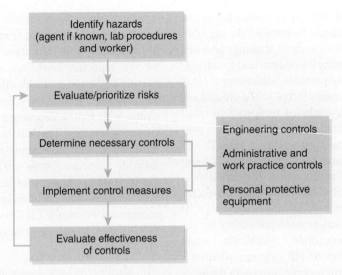

FIGURE 4–5 Risk assessment process for biological hazards.

Miller JM, Astles R, Baszler T, et al. Guidelines for safe work practices in human and animal medical diagnostic laboratories. Recommendations of a CDC-convened, Biosafety Blue Ribbon Panel. *MMWR Suppl.* 2012;61(1):1–102.

- Treat all blood and OPIMs with appropriate precautions:
  - Use gloves, masks, and gowns if blood or OPIM is anticipated
  - Use engineering and work practice controls to limit exposure

OPIMs are defined as human body fluids, including those predominately used in the immunodiagnostic laboratory, such as serum, cerebrospinal fluid (CSF), saliva, virally contaminated cell cultures, and any fluid visibly contaminated with blood. In addition, the CDC recommends the use of frequent handwashing as part of their standard precautions.

Handwashing

One of the most effective means of interrupting the transmission of infectious pathogens is through proper handwashing. While most clinical diagnostic laboratories require the use of gloves at all times, in the event of accidental chemical or biological exposure to the skin, the laboratorian should immediately wash his or her hands with soup and water. It is also typically recommended that lab personnel wash their hands at the beginning and end of every shift and when entering and leaving the laboratory. The creation of surfactants

that lift the bacteria from the skin and associate them with the soap are primarily responsible for the utility of handwashing. No additional benefits have been observed from washing with antibacterial soap.

Personal Protective Equipment

Personal protective equipment (PPE) is to be worn in all laboratory settings where pathogenic organisms are examined, and is recommended or required by a variety of biosafety oversight organizations such as OSHA, CDC, NAACLS, and WHO. These protections include disposable gloves; latex or nitrile, a lab coat, closed-toed shoes and other face, eye and extremity protection as needed for a given task including safety glasses, respiratory devices, and protective shields.

While protective gloves and lab coats/gowns are to be worn by all personnel who come into potential skin contact with biological specimens, other protective equipment is worn only under specific circumstances. These include activities in BSL-3 or BSL-4 facilities, or in situations in which specimen spills or splatter is more likely. An assessment of specific hazards and determination of equipment safeguards is part of the quality assurance process (described below).

For example, a respiratory protection standard may be written for work with airborne pathogens, e.g., aerosolized tuberculous specimens.

In almost all laboratory operations, medical examination gloves are used. Typically, gloves are either latex or nitrile. The use of latex-free gloves have has increased, due to the rising latex sensitivity among personnel. Gloves should be changed frequently, especially when contaminated with blood or body fluids.

Needle Precautions

Venipuncture is the most common source of blood in the laboratory. In many facilities, it is the job of the laboratory technologist to perform the blood draw to collect a specimen for analysis. In larger reference laboratories, blood draws for test controls are commonly performed by technologists as well. However, drawing blood is increasingly performed by a trained professional known as a phlebotomist, who replaces the labratorian and interacts directly with a patient population.

When phlebotomy is performed, it is important to properly label all collection tubes and to verify the patient whose blood is being drawn. In addition, universal precautions, including handwashing and the use of fresh gloves to prevent the transmission of disease should be employed. Selection of the appropriate collection equipment and patient positioning are both important before a blood draw. It is important to be cautious when using needles or other puncture devices. The vast majority of needles and puncture devices are now manufactured with safety features to prevent inadvertent/accidental punctures (**FIGURE 4–6**).

Needles should be inspected for imperfections and positioned, bevel up, before being inserted into a securely anchored vein. The needle should be removed after all blood is collected and after tourniquet pressure has been released. In most modern facilities, the needle, either a butterfly style or straight needle attached to a tube holder, will have a needle safety device attached. Depending on the model, these can be activated while in the vein (butterfly device) or immediately after the needle is removed to prevent inadvertent/accidental punctures. The needle is then

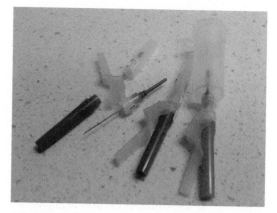

FIGURE 4–6 Contemporary safety needle (and needle in tube hub) used in phlebotomy.
Courtesy of Ian Clift.

immediately disposed of in a puncture-resistant **sharps** container.

In some situations, needles will come to the laboratory associated with a patient tube as part of a syringe set. Most contemporary syringe sets include a needle safety shield that should be activated to protect the user from inadvertent/accidental punctures. The needle should be removed and deposited in a sharps container. A blood-transfer device can then be attached to the syringe and the fluid transferred to an appropriate tube type. After the transfer, the syringe and blood-transfer device should be deposited in a sharps container.

Vaccinations

An important safety precaution for laboratory students, workers, and other healthcare employees is the development of a robust vaccination culture. Three to five cases per 1,000 laboratory workers are infected with hepatitis B, which is two to four times greater than the rate in the general population.[1] Prevention of LAIs such as hepatitis B is both a result of proper handwashing and universal precautions, as well as a regimented vaccination policy for laboratory workers. The WHO and CDC have made recommendations about them not all facilities mandate them. Others implement policies to increase voluntary vaccinations, via rolling vaccination carts to various hospital units facilitate vaccination of staff. An employee who declines to be vaccinated must sign an opt-out waiver.[9] There are some critical diseases for which there is no effective vaccine, e.g., AIDS, TB and malaria.

Generally, many vaccinations required of health care workers, including laboratory workers, are mandated by the state during their primary, secondary, and college educations as well. Proof of vaccination is usually requested by the clinical facility for its records. These include tetanus, diphtheria, pertussis, and the MMR (measles, mumps, and rubella) vaccines. Based on the high number of cases of hepatitis B in healthcare personnel, most facilities now require that laboratory personnel receive the three-dose hepatitis B vaccine as part of the condition of their employment requirements. In addition, it is recommended that a yearly influenza vaccine be administered. Other vaccines that may be required or recommended include varicella zoster (chickenpox), and meningococcal vaccines for microbiologists who may be exposed to N. meningitides.[10] Typically, the costs of vaccinations are covered by the employer or the state, but college students may have to pay for specific vaccines during schooling. Refer to your specific facility for more details.

Waste Management

Waste management and waste disposal in the clinical diagnostic laboratory are regulated by federal, state, international, and institutional standards and, therefore, cannot be delineated with authority for all situations. Several guidelines for managing waste are common and practical in most instances. Specifically, a division between hazardous and nonhazardous waste must be established. The most common hazardous waste in the diagnostic lab comes from patient specimens in the form of biohazardous materials. Decontamination of any contaminated waste must be a part of any facility design and operation.

Biohazardous Waste. Biohazardous waste is any waste that has the possibility of spreading disease. The Medical Waste Tracking Act, signed into law in 1988, set definitions for medical waste.

The Environmental Protection Agency (EPA) was assigned to track the disposal and treatment of waste. Rules concerning medical waste apply to a wide variety of healthcare facilities including clinical laboratories. Medical waste is defined as specific waste from a healthcare facility including solid waste that could transmit disease if improperly handled. Two approved methods for disposal of medical waste are through incineration and steam sterilization.

Every facility that handles medical/hazardous waste must follow these procedures:

- All facilities should develop an infectious waste disposal program (OSHA standard)
- All biomedical waste should be placed in a container marked with a biohazard symbol, with a secure lid to prevent leakage
- All needles, broken glass, and other piercing implements should be disposed in a puncture-resistant sharps container

Hazardous waste can be biohazardous or chemically hazardous. Chemical hazards include oxidizing and reducing agents, inorganic acids and bases, halogenated organic compounds, toxic heavy metals including chemicals, e.g., hydrocarbon solvents, amines, amides, esters, and others.[11] Disposal of these wastes must avoid contaminating water supplies or inadvertently causing injury or death.

Quality Assurance

Quality assurance (QA) is defined as an attempt to reduce errors in an effort to improve the quality of products and services (**FIGURE 4–7**). Approaches to error rates and quality assurance have shifted recently from a "laboratory-centered" focus on analytical errors toward a "patient-centered" focus on the process from preanalytical through postanalytical.[12] Often equated with "good laboratory practice," QA includes measures of reliability within an investigation: test selection, patient identification, proper procedures, and reporting of results. Because of the significant historical focus on the analytical phase, most errors in testing now occur outside of the analytical phase and have been greatly reduced due to the presence of

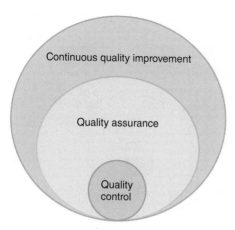

FIGURE 4–7 Relationship between continuous quality improvement, quality assurance, and quality control.

quality improvement processes and specialized laboratory professionals focused on monitoring quality controls. Approximately 68% of all errors are estimated to occur in the preanalytical phase.[5,6] In one hospital in the United Kingdom, almost 88% of all laboratory errors occurred in the preanalytical phase.[5]

A set of **quality indicators (QI)** has been adopted by quality assurance personnel in order to track and monitor performance in the diagnostic laboratory. QIs for the preanalytical phase include patient identification, sample identification, sample transportation conditions, and appropriateness of the test request.[12] In most clinical laboratories, it is the responsibility of the accessioning team to perform the first examination of these preanalytical indicators and divert mislabeled and inappropriate tests from the laboratory. A bad draw leading to a poor sample can still find its way into the laboratory. The medical technologist performing the tests is often responsible for performing a second examination of these identifiers before initiating the assay. In addition to reducing overall error rates that might lead to patient misdiagnosis, QA efforts also reduce costs from inappropriately performed tests. Technologists need to be able to detect poorly or incorrectly drawn specimens and document these conditions even if the test is going to be performed, so that corrective actions in other departments can be developed based on the logging of the evidence.

Steps involved in proper specimen collection are described in another section.

Quality can also be improved by implementing efficiency efforts, such as those provided in the Lean Principle (3P): *people, preparation, process.* For example, the Carolina HealthCare System laboratories were redesigned to place commonly utilized resources centrally, which decreased transit time for immunological specimens by 87%.[13]

Postanalytical errors can also be mitigated by careful observation, calculation, and report transcription onto established forms and/or online databases. In addition, most results are reported alongside a reference range for a given result, which allows both the technologist and physicians to establish whether a result is within a normal range and whether the result is reasonable.

Staff selection and training are an extremely important aspects of QA. Employees should be selected for aptitude and motivation and should be trained or retrained as needed. A biosafety officer or QA specialist may be assigned to oversee both QA and quality control (QC) activities; however, it is everyone's responsibility to be aware of laboratory quality policies in order to ensure accurate, timely, and safe results.

Quality Control

Quality controls are typically daily, weekly, or monthly measurements that indicate whether an assay or process is being performed within a designated standard. These daily maintenance tasks are documented and stored either manually or digitally, and periodically assessed by members of the quality assurance team for trends that may be indicative of a system heading in an inappropriate direction. QC is performed to validate whether an instrument is performing within specifications. At a specific intervals, e.g., at the beginning of a shift, or every 24 hours, QC is performed on the instrument by running one or several standard samples the results of which are then plotted in a graph. The selected type of QC depends on the type of instrument. For example, spectrophotometer function may be tested using a set of calibrated cuvettes at nominal values (**FIGURE 4–8**), which are capable

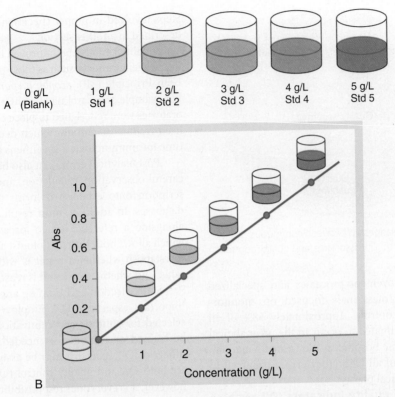

FIGURE 4–8 Spectrophotometer standards. Standards are used to insure instrument accuracy and can be used to determine the concentration of an unknown analyte. **(A)** Series of standards. **(B)** Standards plotted on an absorbance curve.

of testing wavelength and photometric accuracy, as well as stray light and photometric linearity over time. This kit comes with six standards for testing nominal absorbance that have been calibrated to five wavelengths from 440 nm to 635 nm,[14] and can therefore be used with a variety of spectrophotometer models. QC products should be run in the same manner as a patient specimen. Instruments that run anticoagulated blood, serum, urine, or other body fluids typically resemble the samples tested, and may contain preserved human biological material therefore they are handled within the same safety standards as other specimens.

Control charts have been in use since the early 1930s in manufacturing processes and were proposed for laboratory QC by Levey and Jennings in 1950.[15] These charts serve as the basis for assessing the control of an instrument or process. A series of six rules, called Multi-rules or Westgard Rules, for determining whether a clinical control is "out of control" are based on the position of the results on a Levey-Jennings chart. A control value in excess of three standard deviations (3s or 3SD) from the mean is considered out of control. These results can be defined both by chart position and by probability.[15] An in-depth examination of contemporary quality-control calculations is provided in other resources and will not be examined further here.[16]

Calibration. An assay or instrument calibration is performed to bring an "out of control" procedure back into control. Calibration is performed during the initial setup of an instrument and then periodically as part of general QA protocol. The testing of immunoreagents and development of immunoassays is augmented by the use of calibrants (or primary standards) and "working" standards (or secondary standards). Calibrants, also referred to as standards, often come from international reference materials prepared in accordance with regional, national, and international organizations such as the WHO, which allow for comparisons to be made between results achieved in different labs around the world. These materials may also be used in the development of laboratory proficiency tests, such as those provided by CAP.

Several basic rules apply to selecting standards:

- The standard material and the analyte should be identical or as similar as possible
- Any heterogeneity in analyte should be reflected in the standard preparation
- Standards should be chemically pure

The matrix (serum, urine, etc.) should be the same for sample and standards; the concentration of the standard should be confirmed by a reference assay; and the standard should be relatively stable. Often, a synthetic matrix is used to ensure that it mimics the true matrix but without the endogenous analyte. In many cases, such as in the testing of less-common body fluids, a synthetic matrix is not available and needs to be collected and purified inhouse. A collection of these fluids may be similar to that performed for method validation,[17] which is discussed elsewhere in this chapter. Additionally, normal clinically collected serum can be used where the tested analyte is found only in a pathological state. Matrix solutions can be created by removing endogenous analytes through various filtration methods, e.g., the use of a charcoal/cellulose column.

Standard Operating Procedures (SOPs). Every clinical laboratory requires lab professionals to follow a set of **standard operating procedures (SOPs)** to ensure quality and safety. A list of SOPs is usually found in a print or digital SOP manual. Each procedure provides detailed instructions for how a particular task should be performed. When commercial tests and reagents are used, the manufacturer's instructions are strictly followed during the development of the procedure. SOPs are revisited and revised each time new regulations and standards are implemented or when problems with the existing procedure are confronted. SOPs are the final step in the development before the implementation of a new procedure or protocol. Strict adherence to SOPs is fundamental to quality assurance within the laboratory; therefore, development or modifications to current SOPs must be conducted separately from any clinical, reportable results.

Documentation and Records. Quality assurance and regulatory compliance both mandate that appropriate documentation be kept on all quality indicators, including specimen collection, reagent lot and usage, dates, and lab personnel involved, in order to facilitate appropriate tracking and traceability in the case of an adverse event or required accreditation audit. Accurate record-keeping is critical to the investigation of past performance and to the initiation of performance and quality improvement initiatives.

Many labs have very specific rules for documenting results and errors. Results are to be documented at the time that they are performed including the lab personnel's initials and date. Erroneous results or documentation errors should be crossed out with a single line through the data and the correction written above the result, including the date and initials of the personnel involved, on print documents. Digital results also contain an audit trail indicating any changed outcomes and include the personnel involved in the change as part of the laboratory information-management system. Specific immunodiagnostic testing labs, such as the blood bank or transfusion medicine department, must also document information on patient and donor compatibility matching as well as the storage and chain of custody on FDA–controlled blood products.

Exposure Control Plan. Under OSHA guidance, employers must establish an exposure control plan (ECP) to document efforts to minimize and eliminate risks. This document should be reviewed annually to reflect new or modified SOPs in which an occupational risk of employee exposure may occur. The ECP must also document the consideration and implementation of safer medical devices that may eliminate or minimize occupational exposure.

Chemical Hygiene Plan. OSHA requires each laboratory to have a chemical hygiene plan (also known as the hazard communication plan **FIGURE 4–9**), which provides procedures and controls for reducing and preventing the risk of chemical exposure in the laboratory.

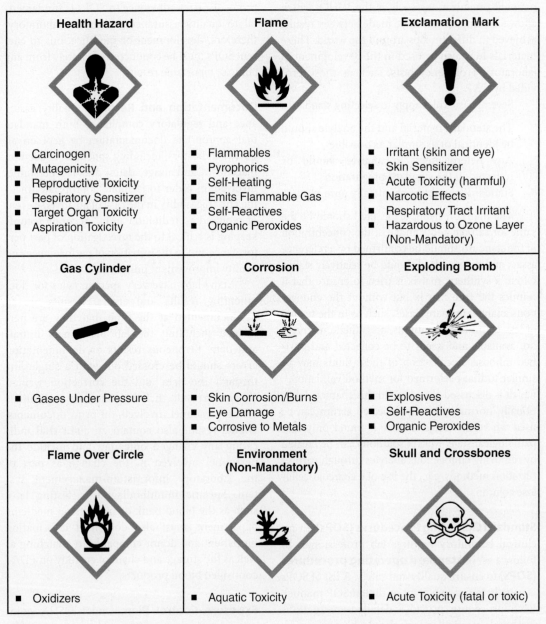

Health Hazard	Flame	Exclamation Mark
■ Carcinogen ■ Mutagenicity ■ Reproductive Toxicity ■ Respiratory Sensitizer ■ Target Organ Toxicity ■ Aspiration Toxicity	■ Flammables ■ Pyrophorics ■ Self-Heating ■ Emits Flammable Gas ■ Self-Reactives ■ Organic Peroxides	■ Irritant (skin and eye) ■ Skin Sensitizer ■ Acute Toxicity (harmful) ■ Narcotic Effects ■ Respiratory Tract Irritant ■ Hazardous to Ozone Layer 　(Non-Mandatory)
Gas Cylinder	Corrosion	Exploding Bomb
■ Gases Under Pressure	■ Skin Corrosion/Burns ■ Eye Damage ■ Corrosive to Metals	■ Explosives ■ Self-Reactives ■ Organic Peroxides
Flame Over Circle	Environment (Non-Mandatory)	Skull and Crossbones
■ Oxidizers	■ Aquatic Toxicity	■ Acute Toxicity (fatal or toxic)

FIGURE 4–9 OSHA's Hazard Communication Pictogram.

Hazard Communication Standard Pictogram, Occupational Safety and Health Administration, Retrieved from https://www.osha.gov/Publications/HazComm_QuickCard_Pictogram.html

SDS. The **Material Safety Data Sheet (MSDS)** must be available for examination by all personnel who come in contact with a hazardous material within a laboratory setting. An MSDS is provided by the chemical manufacturer. When specific chemicals are manufactured inhouse, the employer is required by law to have a document for each chemical in use. These documents are the major sources of information concerning potential hazards. Originally found as a printed document inside the laboratory, many MSDS databases are now online, and/or in a secure location accessible to all employees. CAP and other regulatory inspectors require all lab personnel to be able to find and access these files. The MSDS contains 16 sections: identification, hazard identification, ingredients, first aid procedures, fire-fighting procedures, accidental-release measures, handling and storage, exposure controls and protection, physical and chemical properties, stability and reactivity, toxicological information, ecological information, transport information, regulatory information, and other relevant information, including the dates of preparation and the last revision.

Emergency Plans. Most clinical laboratories and hospital institutions containing a clinical laboratory have an emergency management plan. Emergency situations can occur similarly in the laboratory as they occur elsewhere, and there is a high risk for specific emergencies including those resulting from fire, electricity, and chemical spills. The CDC has provided specific instructions for emergency preparedness and response regarding agents of bioterrorism in addition to chemical and radiation based emergencies. OSHA has established requirements for an emergency action plan (29 CFR 1910.38), which establishes contingencies for preventing fatalities, injuries and property damage, as well as a fire prevention plan and others. Plans should:

- Describe emergency reporting procedures
- Describe evacuation routes and procedures
- Designate critical operators during an emergency
- Contain a procedure for employee accounting after an evacuation
- Describe the role of employees performing rescue and medical duties
- Provide a resource for more information about the plan

To facilitate training for emergency situations, many organizations have developed mnemonic symbols and acronyms to help employees remember the significance. The elements of an emergency management plan can be neatly summarized in the acronym NEAR (See **TABLE 4–4**). The acronym PASS has been adopted in many major medical establishments to describe the proper usage of a fire extinguisher. P = PULL the pin, A = AIM the extinguisher at the base of the fire, S = SQUEEZE the handle, and S = SWEEP from side to side. Other acronyms used for emergency preparedness and PASS are included in the following table.

Method Validation. Method validation, also known as assay validation, is used to determine the precision profile, workable range, specificity, detection limit, and linearity of an assay, among other factors. A precision profile is developed

TABLE 4–4 Common Emergency Response Acronyms		
NEAR	Notify Evacuate Assemble Report	The key elements in an emergency management plan
PASS	Pull Aim Squeeze Sweep	Instructions for using a fire extinguisher in the case of an emergency
RACE	Rescue Alarm Contain Evacuate	Used in cases of hazardous spills and leaks

from repeat testing of a single sample or, more commonly a range of samples, to determine the variability between runs. The working range, also known as the specificity of an assay, is the range of values in which the assay is usable in workable practice. This is typically an extension of the standard curve. A workable range can be determined by completing a precision profile. For example, a workable range is sometimes established as values 20 to 30% less than those tested for in assay linearity. The detection limits, also known as sensitivity, determine the extreme values of detection for the assay and are also an important validation value.

For clinical assays, the most important component is the clinical sensitivity, or positivity in disease, but assay developers also look at the function sensitivity, i.e., true limits of detection. In immunodiagnostics, these terms should not be confused as an analyte's presence in a solution because they may not be equivalent to the quantity necessary for disease correlation. Finally, the linearity of an assay should be assessed by making dilutions of high-concentration specimens or by using spiked specimens.

If serum is the base solution, an analyte-free serum should be used for all diluted specimens, as changes to background may affect results. In addition to the above factors, assays must be validated for interfering substances and in conditions of antigenic excess. Clinical sample types should dictate if body fluids, in addition to blood, serum, and plasma should be validated for specific tests. Assays are valid only for conditions in which they are validated; therefore, even commercially available tests with external validation in serum or blood may require internal validation with commonly tested body fluids, e.g., drainage, CSF, peritoneal, pericardial, and pleural fluids.[17] Since these fluids are not typically available commercially, the specimens must be collected, sometimes over several months, for validation to occur. Standard method validation practices should be employed on any newly developed or adopted assay in order to ensure quality clinically-relevant results, and results should be reported only on validated specimen types, except under atypical circumstances.

Although not a part of method validation, another QA-related task may be participation in investigator- and manufacture-sponsored clinical validation. A clinical validation for an assay is used to determine the reference interval for a specific test, including differences in age, sex, and other factors. It may be used to establish "cut-off" values between normal and abnormal results, as well as clinical sensitivity (disease positivity) and clinical specificity (healthy negativity). This helps to establish the predictive value of an assay.

Proficiency Testing. An important aspect of external quality assessment is the performance of **proficiency testing** on commonly run assays. Proficiency testing is performed to ensure that laboratory personnel are accurately and appropriately performing tests. Proficiency testing is a required provision of the CLIA '88 regulations. Typically, each clinical diagnostic laboratory participates in at least one external control program. The most prominent of these tests are offered through CAP but can also be obtained through the CDC and others in the United States. Periodically, these organizations will send specimens to labs to be tested as a normal sample using routine procedures. The results are then returned to the program administrators, evaluated, and compared with other laboratories using the same or similar methods.

Training and Continuing Education. Like proficiency testing, training, and **continuing education** are a necessary part of laboratory QA. The ASCP and other clinical laboratory certifying organizations require continuing education to maintain certification. For example, the ASCP Medical Laboratory Scientist Generalist certification requires 36 continuing education credits in specific topic areas to be completed every 3 years as part of their certificate maintenance program. Due to the rapid advances occurring in laboratory and medical technologies, it is imperative that employees keep abreast of changes in technology and scope of practice.

Laboratory training is typically highly regulated through the use of competency checklists (BOX 4-1), to ensure quality and precision.

BOX 4-1 Example Competency Checklist

Task	Date	Student	Instructor
Specimens			
Evaluate and apply acceptance/rejection criteria			
Proper storage			
Measure volume			
Timed			
Calculate concentration vs time			
Keep work area neat and clean			
Replenish reagent/supply stocks before they are depleted			
Use phone in proper manner			
Practice safety at all times			
Correlate analytical results with patient condition			
Participate in workload documentation and analysis			
Recognize abnormal processes and take corrective action			
Make serial dilutions			
Keep records up to date			
Participate in inventory control			

(continues)

BOX 4–1	Example Competency Checklist			(Continued)

Task	Date	Student	Instructor
Maintain temperature records			
Check calibration of volumetric devices (e.g., pipettes)			
Manuals (location and contents)			
SOPs			
Safety			
MSDS			
Communicate critical results to appropriate person			
Correctly record assay results			

Beyond the essential competencies, such as understanding safe laboratory practices, all employees should be thoroughly trained in each assay that they conduct, and a record of that process documented. In each case, a competency checklist (Box 4–1), similar to the ones employed during training in a NAACLS-accredited clinical laboratory science program, will be completed by a previously trained laboratorian after a period of observation and assisted performance. Completion of this documentation is typically required for an individual to be deemed competent to perform an assay for use in diagnosis. Furthermore, periodic competency reviews are required in most instances.

Specimen Collection and Processing

The primary collected specimens for use in immunodiagnostics are determined by the diagnostic test to be performed. Peripheral blood and to some extent, urine, saliva, CSF and other body fluids are collected and processed for testing. This section covers the general procedures and safety precautions performed as part of several major types of immunodiagnostic laboratories. While many immunodiagnostic tests can be performed on cell and bacterial cultures, the predominant source of biological specimens used in clinical diagnostics still derives from a patient blood draw or body fluid collection. In the later chapters, many of the blood components commonly used in serology and immunodiagnostics will be described from the perspective of their biological activity and diagnostic utility.

Depending on their usage, the handling of blood products can be heavily regulated by a variety of agencies. For example, when blood is used in the practice of transfusion (discussed in detail in a later chapter), it is dispensed as a prescription drug within the United States and is regulated by the US Food and Drug Administration (FDA). Details regarding the regulating bodies and their impact on the clinical lab is found earlier in this chapter and in Chapter 15: Management, Regulation, and Clinical Translation in Immunodiagnostic Testing. However, safe handling of blood and body fluids requires the use of universal precautions and proper storage and transport of the product. Tubes should be opened only when proper safety precautions are in place, e.g., either with face and hand protection (gloves and glasses), and/or in a biological safety cabinet.

Aliquot

Aliquoting is the process of dividing a whole specimen or bulk reagent into smaller volumes (**aliquots**). When a single specimen enters the laboratory, several tests may be performed on the same tube. While it is sometimes possible to run several tests on a single tube sequentially, at other times, due to the nature of the assay or because of time constraints and/or logistics, a single patient tube must be divided. Specimen aliquoting is also performed when a specimen needs to be tested several times for validation purposes. Reagent aliquoting is also commonly performed to preserve agents that may lose efficacy through repeated freeze-thaw cycles or due to potential contamination. Aliquoting is the process of dividing a substance into equal smaller parts. The term is commonly misused, however, to describe all subdividing of specimens.

Specimen Labeling

Specimen tubes that enter the immunodiagnostic laboratory should be labeled by phlebotomy/or other specimen collection personnel at the time of collection, and should be double checked for accuracy upon arrival. If samples are to be aliquoted or transferred to another tube, the technologist should provide enough information on any secondary tube for a fellow technologist to continue his or her work. In many cases, these tests are critical for patient care. Incorrectly labeled tubes may lead to misdiagnosis or delayed diagnosis, sometimes with life-threatening consequences.

Specimen Storage and Transport

Methods of storage and transport should consider not only the stability of the specimen but also the risks that the specimen poses. Safe methods of management for infectious materials between and within the laboratory should attempt to contain agents to protect personnel from exposure. Containment is assured through good techniques, the proper handling of equipment, and through appropriate facility design and construction.

The four main storage temperatures are: liquid nitrogen, ultra-low, cold, and room temperature, and are applied for biological specimens depending on the specimen type and expected usage. Liquid nitrogen (LN^2) is often considered the "gold standard" for storage of biological specimens. It is ideal for long-term storage, as the specimen temperature is at –190°C, which is below the level at which any biological activity occurs, effectively preventing degradation of the specimen. Specimens in LN^2 are considered cryogenically frozen. Ultra-low storage freezers, common in any biological specimen processing and storage facility, keep specimens at between –70° and –80° C. A wide variety of biomarkers and serological immunomarkers have been maintained at these temperatures successfully for several years. Cold storage, at –20° to 5° C, is used for short-term storage for days to weeks. Many reagents cannot handle repeated freeze-thaw cycles, and are therefore, aliquoted in smaller volumes and stored at refrigerated or frozen temperatures. Finally, specimens are sometimes kept at room temperature, usually for short periods of time. Platelets, however, are typically stored at room temperature before therapeutic use in the blood bank. Although not considered a usual storage condition, when conducting ongoing cell culture experiments important for viral infection and some cellular function tests, laboratories sometimes must maintain a living culture at physiological body temperatures in an incubator.

CASE STUDY

Plague Infection From Unsafe Handling

This case has been adapted from a 2011 CDC report.[18]

A 60-year-old man with insulin-dependent diabetes mellitus arrived by ambulance through the emergency department (ED) with fever, a cough, and shortness of breath. Three days earlier, he had been observed with similar conditions at an outpatient center in which the physician noted similar symptoms. The patient was told to seek attention because of suspected influenza with respiratory infection. He did not seek further attention at the time. Within the ED, his body temperature was measured at 100.9°F, his pulse was elevated to 106 beats per minute, and his blood pressure was normal.

Initial Laboratory Analysis

A blood chemistry panel was performed and showed signs of renal failure (creatinine: 6.5 mg/dL; blood urea nitrogen: 73 mg/dL), incipient acidosis (bicarbonate: 17 mEq/L; PaCO2: 31mmHg; pH: 7.36), and elevated liver function enzymes (aspartate aminotransaminase [AST]: 794 IU/L; alanine aminotransaminase [ALT]: 160 IU/L). Complete blood count showed severe leukocytosis (white blood cells: 79.2 103/mL) with a left shift (22% band forms) and hemoglobin level and platelet count within normal limits. Extracellular bacteria were noted on a peripheral blood smear. He was treated for suspected heart failure with diuretics and antibiotics; however, his respiratory distress worsened and he was intubated. One hour later, he died of cardiac arrest.

24 hours after they were drawn, blood cultures revealed gram-negative bacilli (four of four bottles), gram-positive cocci (three of four bottles), and yeast (one of four bottles was presumed to be a contaminant). A day later, the gram-positive cocci was determined to be a nutritionally variant streptococcus (NVS). However, an autopsy revealed no signs of NVS infection. DNA sequencing performed on the gram-negative bacilli revealed it to be either *Yersinia pseudotuberculosis* or *Yersinia pestis* (the causative agent of the plague).

Patient History

The patient's work history was not noted on reports from either the outpatient clinic or the ED records. Days later it was determined that he had worked in a university research laboratory that conducted studies on select biological agents including an attenuated version of *Y. pestis*. An assessment of the laboratory environment identified no major deficiencies in engineering controls. A review of attendance records for university biosafety training showed deficiencies in staff attendance, including the patient. Discussions with coworkers revealed that the patient inconsistently followed the laboratory glove policy.

Final Diagnosis

The patient was not strictly following company policies for safety in the laboratory and was not attending all required safety training. The patient worked with an attenuated strain of *Y. pestis* (KIM D27) not known to cause infection, due to a deficiency in iron metabolism that stopped its ability to grow outside of specialized cultures. Preliminary PCR indicated that the patient was indeed infected with the KIM D27 strain and not the virulent CO92 strain of *Y. pestis*. Despite research-mediated modifications to the attenuated strain, the CDC found that they did not lead to an increased virulence. Yet the patient had lung nodules consistent with plague, and immunohistochemical tests using an anti-*Y. pestis* mouse monoclonal antibody found abundant staining of *Y. pestis* in blood vessels suggestive of systemic plague. Postmortem testing of blood revealed a total iron level of 541 mcg/dL which was well above reference range (40–160 mcg/dL), high iron saturation of 83.5% (reference range: 14–50%) and total iron binding capacity (TIBC) of 648 mcg/dL (reference range: 230–430 mcg/dL). A genetic test found that the patient had a mutation consistent with a diagnosis of hemochromatosis: an iron overload disease. The patient was not known to be aware of this condition, but investigators suspect that the high level of iron in the patient allowed the attenuated strain of *Y. pestis* to overcome its iron uptake deficiencies leading to its virulence in the individual.

▶ References

1. Miller JM, Astles R, Baszler T, et al. Guidelines for safe work practices in human and animal medical diagnostic laboratories. Recommendations of a CDC-convened, Biosafety Blue Ribbon Panel. *MMWR Suppl.* 2012;61(1): 1–102.

2. Krajewski M, Sztajnkrycer M, Báez A. Hospital disaster preparedness in the United States: new issues, new challenges. *The Internet Journal of Rescue and Disaster Medicine.* 2004;4(2):6.

3. Bundy KL, Foss ML, Stubbs JR. Transfusion service disaster planning. *Immunohematology.* 2008;24(3):93–101.

4. Delany JR, Pentella MA, Rodriguez JA, et al. Guidelines for biosafety laboratory competency: CDC and the Association of Public Health Laboratories. *MMWR Suppl.* 2011;60(2):1–23.

5. O'Kane M. The reporting, classification and grading of quality failures in the medical laboratory. *Clin Chim Acta.* 2009;404(1):28–31.

6. Hilborne LH, Lubin IM, Scheuner MT. The beginning of the second decade of the era of patient safety: implications and roles for the clinical laboratory and laboratory professionals. *Clin Chim Acta.* 2009;404(1):24–27.

7. DiBerardinis LJ. Impact of lab design onsafety, health, and productivity. *Medical Lab Management.* 2016;5(2):6.

8. World Health Organization. Laboratory biosafety manual. 3rd ed. Geneva: World Health Organization; 2004: http://www.who.int/csr/resources/publications/biosafety/WHO_CDS_CSR_LYO_2004_11/en/

9. Field RI. Mandatory vaccination of health care workers: whose rights should come first? *Pharmacy and Therapeutics.* 2009;34(11):615–618.

10. Healthcare Personnel Vaccination Recommendations. http://www.immunize.org/catg.d/p2017.pdf. immunize.org: Immunization Action Coalition; 2018.

11. Zubrick JW. *The organic chem lab survival manual: A student's guide to techniques.* 5th ed. New York: John Wiley; 2001.

12. Plebani M, Sciacovelli L, Aita A, Padoan A, et al. Quality indicators to detect pre-analytical errors in laboratory testing. *Clin Chim Acta.* 2014;432:44–48.

13. McElhiney B, Todd H, Longshore JW. Using Lean Principles to Design a Centralized laboratory. *MedicalLab Management.* 2016;5(10).

14. Product Specification: Thermo Scientic SPECTRONIC Certified Standards. www.thermoscientific.com: Thermo Scientific; 2015:4.

15. Carroll TA, Pinnick HA, Carroll WE. Probability and the Westgard Rules. *Ann Clin Lab Sci.* 2003;33(1):113–114.

16. Bishop ML, Fody EP, Schoeff LE. *Clinical chemistry: Principles, techniques, and correlations.* Eighth edition. ed. Philadelphia: Wolters Kluwer; 2018.

17. Cotten SW. Validating the Performance of Body Fluid Specimens. *MedicalLab Management.* 2016;5(5):6.

18. Centers for Disease Control and Prevention (CDC). Fatal laboratory-acquired infection with an attenuated Yersinia pestis strain–Chicago, Illinois, 2009. *MMWR Morb Mortal Wkly Rep.* 2011;60(7):201–205.

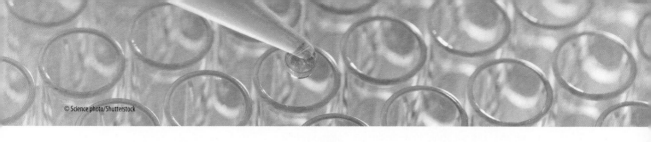

CHAPTER 5

Classic Principles in Immunodiagnostics

Ian Clift, PhD, MLS(ASCP)^{CM}

KEY TERMS

Affinity	Fab	Postzone
Agglutination	Fc	Precipitation
Agglutination inhibition	Hemagglutination	Precipitation curve
Avidity	Immunoelectrophoresis	Prozone
Coagglutination	Immunofixation electrophoresis	Radial immunodiffusion (RID)
Direct antiglobulin test	Immunoglobulins (Ig)	Rocket Immunoelectrophoresis
Double diffusion	Immunoreagents	Single diffusion
Electrophoresis	Indirect antiglobulin test	Turbidimetry
Epitope	Law of mass action	
Equilibrium constant	Nephelometry	

LEARNING OBJECTIVES

Upon completion of this chapter, the reader should be able to:

1. Define antibody identification and the principles involved.
2. Explain current technology used to identify antibodies.
3. Rank the probability of antibody formation resulting from epitope characteristics.
4. Break down the antibody structure based on binding locations and function.
5. Defend the use of antibodies as diagnostic tools; compare immunodiagnostics to alternative diagnostic approaches.
6. Differentiate between affinity and avidity.

(continues)

(Continued)

7. Restate the law of mass action as antibody and antigens.
8. Define the prozone and postzone responses in precipitation and agglutination.
9. Compare and contrast agglutination and precipitation curves.
10. Describe various immunodiffusion and precipitation techniques.
11. Diagram the steps involved with agglutination.

▶ Fundamental Principles

The broader field of clinical immunodiagnostics can be alternatively applied to a diverse range of diagnostic applications within the medical field. Some of the classical principles described within this chapter have an impact and are important for units/departments in the clinical lab with titles such as serology, immunology, blood banking/immunohematology, microbiology, and a number of other areas of study. However, in all cases, the procedures performed in these units are based on the detection of antigen and antibody interactions; classically, through agglutination and precipitation responses.

Antigens and Antibodies

Antigens are any surface product that stimulate the production of antibodies. Antibodies are specialized protein structures constructed by the body for an immunogenic purpose. A foundational understanding of the nature of antigenic and immunogenic substances, i.e., antigens and antibodies, is at the root of serology and immunodiagnostics. They will be discussed at some level in every chapter of this book. The basics of their structures are described here, as is their primary function in laboratory immunoassays. The development of antibodies in the immune system is a critical part of development that involves adaptive immune elements and lymphocytes. Antigenic targeting and expansion of antibody production occur after the stimulation of B-cell conversion to plasma cells. More specific details regarding antibody production in vivo can be found elsewhere in this text.

Basic Antigenic Structure

Immunodiagnosticians utilize antigens as detectors of specific antibodies within a body fluid and use various techniques to detect antigens in biological specimens as well. Pneumococcal antigens, for instance, can be used to indicate exposure to a specific serovar (subtype) of pneumococcus based on the titer of antibodies pulled out by the antigens in an assay of pneumococcal immunity.

A substance is termed antigenic, or an antigen, if its surface properties are recognized as foreign by the host immune system and elicit antibody production. Several properties aid in antigenic effectivity: stability, complexity, and as mentioned, most importantly, foreignness.

An **epitope**, or binding site, is the primary antigenic determinant of an antigen. Epitopes can consist of any molecular structure: primarily proteins but also sugar, fat moieties, and nucleic acids. Epitopes can elicit specific binding from antibodies or B-cell and T-cell receptors initiating an adaptive immune response. The structure of an antigen is, therefore, determined by its specificity for an antibody.

Stability

Effective antigens are both structurally stable and resistant to degradation. Molecules that are rapidly destroyed do not last long enough to form a robust immune response.

Complexity

Antigens can be composed of a variety of biochemical classes including glycoproteins and glycolipids, but are most commonly composed of protein due to their structural complexity and high molecular weight (MW). Lipids and carbohydrates alone are considered poor antigens due to reduced complexity and size, but when combined with other moieties such as proteins or carrier molecules, they can become antigenic. The more complex the structure, the greater the chance that it will produce a selective and specific antibody response.

Foreign

Antigens are detectable within a host organism if and only if they are determined to be foreign (or nonself) by the host immune system. Normally the host immune systems do not respond to self-antigens due to a negative selection of T cells in the thymus during development.

In addition to infectious disease antigens, antigens are useful for determining histocompatibility and blood groups, the presence of mutant proteins, increased protein production, and the determination of autoimmune disorders. A major arm of immunodiagnostics is focused on transfusion and transplantation compatibility. The surface proteins from an allogenic (genetically different) individual can elicit an immune response leading to tissue destruction and/or rejection of the tissue or organ. It is, therefore, vital that laboratorians test for these antigens prior to transfusion or transplantation. The most important of these antigens are known as major histocompatibility complex (MHC) antigens; glycoproteins, also referred to as human leukocyte antigens (HLA); and common blood group antigens (A, B, and H antigens). In addition to common allogenic antigens, another arm of immunodiagnostics is focused on detecting rare but often chronic conditions that occur as a result of autologous antibody formation resulting from autoantigens, called autoimmunity.

Basic Antibody Structure

The term antibody is used to define a specific group of glycoproteins known as **immunoglobulins (Ig)**. While five classes of immunoglobulins have been identified, only two immunoglobulins are commonly found in normal serum: IgG and, to a lesser extent, IgM (**FIGURE 5–1** and **FIGURE 5–2**). IgG comprises 70% to 75% of the normal Ig pool, and IgM accounts for roughly 10%. These two immunoglobulins are most commonly used in

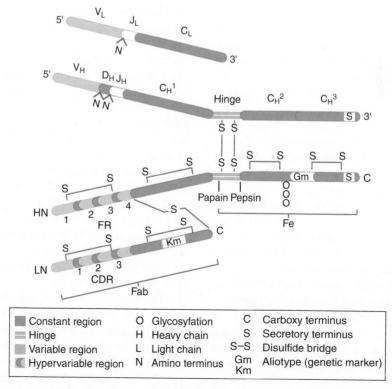

FIGURE 5–1 Basic immunoglobin (Ig) structures and domains. The Fab regions are named for their "antigen-binding" property and the Fc region is named for its "constant" property.

Modified from William E Paul. Fundamental Immunology, Lippincott Williams & Wilkins, 2012.

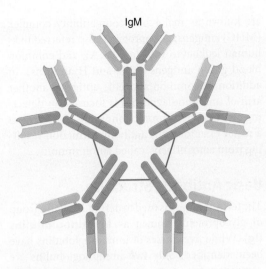

IgM

FIGURE 5-2 Structure of IgM.

Modified from DeLong, L., and Burkhart, N. General and oral pathology for the dental hygienist. Lippincott Williams & Wilkins, 2013.

immunodiagnostics. Although the most commonly utilized, all immunoglobulin classes, which also include IgA, IgD, and IgE, have their place in specific immunodiagnostic assays, particularly body fluid-specific immunoassays. For example, IgA, which constitutes roughly 15% of the total Ig pool, is found most commonly in tears, saliva, and colostrum/ breast milk; IgE increases against potential environmental allergens and, therefore, can be seen with more frequency during specific times of exposure. All Ig classes have several structural components in common that are important for their in vivo function as well as their utility as **immunoreagents** (Figure 5–1).

Antibodies are considered bifunctional. One end of the antibody is associated with the binding of antigen (typically 2), and the other is associated with the binding of host tissues of the immune system. The basic structure consists of four large chains linked through cysteine residues by disulphide bonds. These are referred to as the heavy (H) chains and light (L) chains. In addition, both heavy and light chains contain a conserved (C) region and variable (V) region. It is the V region that allows for the specificity of select antigens. An elaborate and unique system of recombination has evolved to allow for the nearly infinite combinations of antigenic targets used by the immune system in

the detection and defense against nonself. This process is the natural basis for almost all specific antibodies used in clinical diagnostics, with a small but growing subset established through advanced techniques in biological engineering.

The classic model of the Ig molecule is based on electron microscopy images of the IgG, which look like a Y and contain two antigenic binding sites. The light chains, common to all immunoglobulins, are composed of two subtypes called *kappa* and *lambda*, which, when separated by chemical disruption of the disulphide bonds, have been shown to be antigenically unique. The heavy chains can also be antigenically targeted. Many immunoassays have been expertly designed to take advantage of this process of targeting antibodies or regions of antibodies for use as secondary antibodies.

Fc and Fab Regions

The fundamental basic structure of the antibody is also practically divided into three globular regions: two **Fab** regions and one **Fc** region. These regions are linked by a flexible hinge. Pepsin is a natural enzyme used to cleave individual Fabs, while papain cleaves both Fabs together as a $F(ab)_2$ (**FIGURE 5–3**). These enzymes are used to cleave IgGs into pieces that can be useful in removing interfering agents from responding in a nonspecific manner within a particular immunoassay. For example, the Fc portion of the antibody, which is highly reactive, can be removed to increase selectivity. Microscopy studies have shown that the two Fab regions can swing freely, allowing for the antibody to bind two antigenic epitopes variously within one molecule, or to bind between two molecules. The existence of two Fab-binding regions is important for several techniques, including precipitation and agglutination described in this chapter and commonly performed in the diagnostic laboratory.

Two proteins, Protein A, from *Staphylococcus Aureus*; and Protein G, a type III Fc receptor, have a high affinity for the Fc portion of the antibody and are also commonly used to separate IgGs[1] (See **TABLE 5–1**). Some IgGs bind better to one of these proteins than the other and others do not bind at all. Many animal versions of IgG have been tested with both; lists are available to

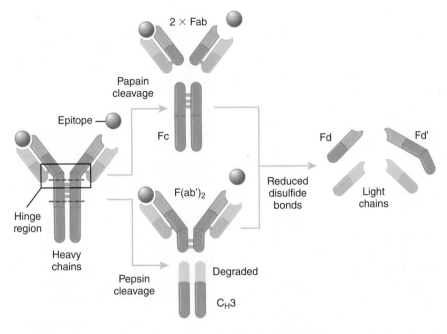

2 × Fab

Papain
cleavage

Epitope

Fc

Fd

Fd'

Reduced
disulfide
bonds

Light
chains

Hinge
region

F(ab')$_2$

Heavy
chains

Pepsin
cleavage

Degraded

C_H3

Heavy chains:		Light chains:	
Variable domain	V_H	Variable domain	V_L
Constant domain(s)	C_H1, C_H2,etc.	Constant domain(s)	C_L
Disulfide bond(s)			

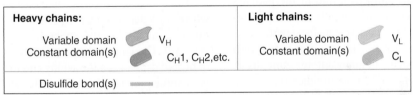

FIGURE 5–3 Papain and Pepsin Cleavage Sites.

TABLE 5–1 Protein A and Protein G Binding Affinity to IgG

Species	Protein A	Protein G
Human	High	High
Mouse	Medium	Medium
Sheep	Very low	High
Horse	Very low	High
Rabbit	High	High

aid in assay development and kits are sold commercially for many common assays.

Antigens and Antibodies as Reagents

Antibodies and antigens were not human inventions, but were discovered through biological and biochemical investigations. The studies of immune cells and subcellular structures are some of the best-studied in the biology, due to their fundamental importance in the treatment of disease and understanding of normal physiology. When antibodies or antigens are used in assays, including those utilized in clinical diagnosis as well as other fields such as forensics and environmental analysis, they are known as immunoreagents.

Immunoreagents can be purchased commercially, individually, in kits, manufactured in-house, or found in clinical patient and donor specimens in their natural form. Most immunodiagnostic assays use some combination of pre-established immunoreagents (antigens, antibodies, and other particles) as detectors, and natural immunoreagents (antigens, antibodies, or cellular components) for detection.

High titers of host antibodies or host antigens are often indicative of disease, but also may be used as indications of disease recovery and therapeutic efficacy. For example, in untreated syphilis patients, the presence of specific antitreponemal IgM antibodies can be detected using an enzyme-linked immunosorbent assay (ELISA). However, a more commonly performed test for syphilis infection is the reagin slide test. Reagin is an immunoreagent with the properties of an antibody that allow it to react with syphilis (treponemal) antigens found in the patient's heat-inactivated serum, providing for a qualitative detection of the disease-causing agent.

Antibodies are not always associated with invading pathogens; in many autoimmune disorders, antibodies called autoantibodies are formed against the host's own tissue.[2] Where possible, serological tests for these autoantibodies have been designed. For example, the autoimmune disorder myasthenia gravis can be detected through a reduction in acetylcholine (AcH) receptors, via an AcH-binding antibody through tissue examinations of the neuromuscular junction. However, in many cases, the antigens and antibodies for these disorders remain undefined.[3] Despite this caveat, nonspecific antibodies such as antinuclear antibodies (ANAs) can be used to detect an autoimmune disease. Specifically, ANAs are present in 99% of patients with untreated systemic lupus erythematosus (SLE).

Affinity and Avidity

The strength of antibody to antigen binding is determined by the **affinity**, the strength of a single antibody binding to a monovalent (single) antigen site, and **avidity**, the total binding strength of a molecule with more than one binding site. Higher affinity between antibody and antigen is important because less antibody is required. Higher-affinity antibodies will bind to lower quantities of antigen, which is important during the in vivo immune response to antigenic elimination and to the development of highly selective immunoassays.

The Law of Mass Action

As applied to antigen-antibody reactions, the **law of mass action** mathematically describes the equilibrium relationship between the soluble and insoluble reactants, i.e., the equilibrium between free and bound immunoreagents. The law states that all antibody-antigen responses are reversible, where the equilibrium constant (K) is defined by the rate of the forward rate (K_1, toward complex, AgAb) over the reverse rate (K_2, toward separation, Ag + Ab).

The **equilibrium constant** is thus defined as:

$$K = K_1/K_2 = [AgAb]/[Ab][Ag]$$

where bracketed quantities represent the concentration of complex (AgAb), antibody (Ab), and antigen (Ag). The content K is a measure of goodness of fit, and depends on the avidity and total strength of molecular interactions between the antibody and antigen. High affinity and high avidity both push toward an increase in complex or the rate of K_1.

▶ Precipitation

When antibodies and antigens are present in relatively equal proportions, the formation of precipitates is favored. The phenomenon of **precipitation** is observed when soluble antigens are combined with soluble antibodies to form a visible insoluble complex.[1] In general, the joining of an antibody to an antigen through specific antigenic-binding sites known as epitopes is required for precipitation. The final assay uses an excess of antigen where precipitation decreases as a result of more antigen, and can be used in a class of immunoassays known as competitive assays.

Precipitation is based on the number of epitopes that are present on the antigen, and the number of binding regions known as Fab regions, which are found on the antibody. Precipitation is also dependent on the proportion of antigens and antibodies present. At optimum, precipitation results from random and reversible reactions in which the numbers of antigens are bound by more than one antibody to form a lattice or organized network when the multivalent sites of the antigen are roughly equal. This is called the zone of equivalence and is determined by the affinity and avidity of the molecules. Outside of the zone of equivalence, the precipitation response declines, allowing for the establishment of the **precipitation curve**, traditionally described by the precipitin curve (**FIGURE 5–4**). At low levels of soluble antigen, where antibody levels are constant, a **prozone** phenomenon is seen. At high levels of soluble antigen, where antibody levels are constant, a **postzone** phenomenon is seen.

Precipitation is detected through the use of light scatter techniques and through passive and active diffusion techniques, such as Ouchterlony. It is one of the simplest methods for detecting antigen-antibody complexes. While some facilities still perform these assays manually, contemporary automated instruments and analyzers commonly incorporate these approaches into their system design.

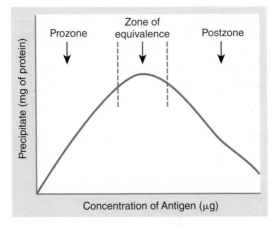

FIGURE 5–4 Precipitin curve. This traditional curve describes the complex formation (precipitate) as a relationship between a constant amount of antibody and increasing amount of analyte (antigen). The relative concentrations also describe the three precipitate zones: Prozone—relative paucity of antigen, zone of equivalence, and postzone—relative excess of antigen. *IC Clift.*

Light Scatter

Light scatter, in the form of **turbidimetry** and **nephelometry**, detects the formation of antigen-antibody complexes through changes in the direction, intensity, and angle of light passed through a sample cuvette.

Turbidimetry is a measure of the cloudiness (or turbidity) of a solution. A light source is passed through the sample cuvette and the light collected after it has passed through is measured and compared with a standard and calibrant; typically, both a baseline aqueous solution, often water, and an empty sample medium, such as a saline solution. Reductions in light detection are indicative of an increased percentage of antigen-antibody precipitate. Absorbance, a ratio of incident (starting) light to transmitted light, is recorded. Both spectrophotometers and advanced clinical analyzers utilize this principle. Spectrophotometers and turbidimeters come in two general varieties: those that measure light scattered in the forward direction, and those that measure light as a right angle to the incident beam.[4]

Nephelometry measures the amount of light that has scattered from the incident light source at a specific angle. Light scatter is measured in arbitrary units called "relative light scatter." Nephelometry must be performed after an initial linearity curve is created using set amounts of antibodies and increasing amounts of antigens. Experimentally, a set amount of one immunoreagent (either antigen or antibody) is used to detect the concentration of a variable (or unknown) amount of the other immunoreagent using this method. Nephelometry measures the concentration of the antibodies in suspension by passing a suspension of antibodies in water droplets through a laser. Relative light units can then be extrapolated to concentration of the unknown analyte based on the concentrations of the previously established standard curve. The antibodies will scatter that light and the amount of scatter is used to calculate the concentration of antibodies. The more the light is scattered, the higher the concentration of antibodies present. Typical nephelometry approaches can be used to measure the degree of light scatter between 10 and 90 degrees but can be increased using laser light to detect as little as a few degrees of change.

Nephlometry, performed using a nephelometer, is considered more sensitive than turbidimetry. Using advanced analyzer design, both endpoint nephelometry, detecting the antigen-antibody reaction at completion, and kinetic nephelometry, and detecting complex as analyte is added, have been successfully employed for the detection of serum proteins. Almost all quantifications of immunoglobulins are done by nephelometry because other methods are more labor intensive.

Passive Immunodiffusion

Diffusion is used to examine precipitates, which are seen as a visible line in a diffusion gel. Most gels are composed of agar, a high-molecular-weight polysaccharide derived from seaweed or agarose, a purified form of agar. Reagents are added to the gel and allowed to migrate by a passive process to form a line in which the antigen and antibody form a complex. Methods are distinguished based on the location of the immunoreagents, the number of reactants, and the direction of diffusion.

In **single diffusion**, pioneered by James Oudin in about 1951,[5] an antibody is incorporated into an agarose gel and solidified in a test tube. The antigen is layered on top and diffuses through the gel in proportion to the amount of antigen present. In a modified version of this process, a well is cut into a plated gel and the antigen is deposited in the well. The antigen diffuses in a radial fashion away from the well and, therefore, is called **radial immunodiffusion (RID)**.

In **double diffusion**, both the antigen and antibody are free to diffuse. Similar to some forms of single diffusion, wells are cut into a semisolid medium and filled with immunoreagents. In the classic, and still used Ouchterlony method, an incubation period up to 48 hours is employed in a moist chamber such as an incubator, and a detection of precipitin lines where the antigens and antibodies meet is assessed. In most cases, a multispecific antibody is placed in a central well, and six wells, placed at an equal distance, are filled with specific antigens to be tested. The precipitin bands from each antigen are then compared with one another. Patterns of lines indicate the presence of a common epitope between the antigens, forming a precipitin arc. Crossing the lines indicates separate epitopes for the antibody that are not identical. Finally, the fusion of lines with additional spurs from the line suggest a partial identity. Ouchterlony has found reduced utility in current practice primarily due to the labor intensity of the procedure and the difficulty in learning the interpretations, but it is still used in some facilities to identify fungal antigens such as *Aspergillus*, *Coccidioides*, and *Candida*. In addition, some reference laboratories perform laboratory-developed tests using modified double-diffusion assays.

STEP-BY-STEP PROCEDURE 5–1 Ouchterlony Double Diffusion Assay

The classic Ochterlony double-diffusion test was one of the first developed to determine the association of antibodies to specific antigens. A variety of setups can be used; for example, the antigen placed in the center with three to four surrounding unknown, whole serums to identify any that contain antibodies to the known antigen. Depicted below is a common five-well setup, allowing for the examination of one control and three unknowns, or other combinations. Ouchterlony provides us with a unique way to view the antigen-antibody complex.

Procedure:

1. Prepare sufficient volume of 1.2% agarose in appropriate assay buffer by boiling until agarose dissolves completely. (5 mLs of agarose solution for each Ouchterlony plate plus 10%)
2. Carefully pipet 5 mLs of cooled agarose (55°C) into each plate. Rotate plate to cover the bottom evenly

3. Allow plates to cool for 10 to 15 minutes
4. Use a well cutter (or gel punch) to place identical wells by using an Ouchterlony template
5. Remove agarose plugs with wooden stick or pipette tip
6. Repeat last two steps with all plates
7. Load approximately 30 µL of sample into the appropriate well using transfer pipette (two drops) or micropipette
8. Cover plates in humidified chamber for 24 to 48 hours at room temperature or 37°C incubator
9. Read results at 24 to 48 hours using overhead or alternate light source

Results:

Examine the plates for the presence of lines, called precipitin lines, between the wells of antigen and antisera. Three primary patterns are recognizable in the double diffusion assay.

- A pattern of identity, indicating that the two adjacent antigens are immunologically identical; the same
- A pattern of partial identity, indicating that adjacent antigens are partially cross-reactive; immunologically similar
- A patter of nonidentity, indicating that the adjacent antigens are immunologically different; they do not cross-react

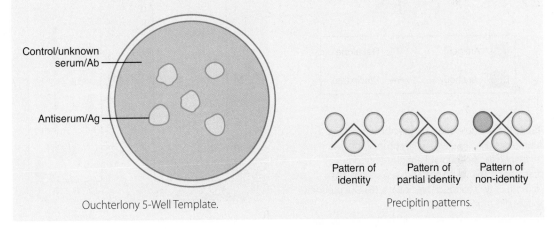

Control/unknown serum/Ab

Antiserum/Ag

Ouchterlony 5-Well Template.

Pattern of identity

Pattern of partial identity

Pattern of non-identity

Precipitin patterns.

Active Immunodiffusion

Electrophoresis, the application of an electric current, is used to assist diffusion (**FIGURE 5–5**). When performed in the presence of an electrical current, these techniques are typically referred to as *active immunodiffusion*, but may be classified by the method employed: electrophoresis. Electrophoresis separates molecules based on differences in their electrical charges because of the differences in protein size. Size may also play a role in the rate of diffusion through a semisolid medium. This can be used to augment both single- and double-diffusion assays. These are typically semiquantitative but can be used for qualitative

detection of antigens in a complex mixture as well through changes in size and charge.

Immunoelectrophoresis is a double diffusion technique in which the precipitin line develops as a right angle to the protein electrophoresis to perform a semiquantitation of a wide variety of antigens directly from serum (**FIGURE 5–6**). Antiserum is placed in a trough of a gel after the initial electrophoretic separation of proteins and allowed to incubate for 18 to 24 hours. Changes in the arcs and lines, including bowing and thickening of bands are indicative of abnormalities. Interpretation requires significant experience and can be used for a variety of qualitative and semiquantitative indications. Most commonly, it is used to

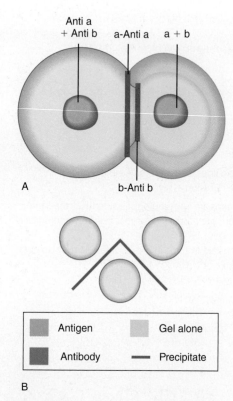

FIGURE 5–5 Double diffusion precipitation in the double-gel diffusion tests were some of the first developed for detection of antigen-antibody interactions. Two-plate methods are shown. **(A)** Diagram of two bands of precipitate. **(B)** Ouchterlony double diffusion in plates.

Adapted from Methods of Immunology and Immunochemistry, Volume III, Williams and Chase, 1971.

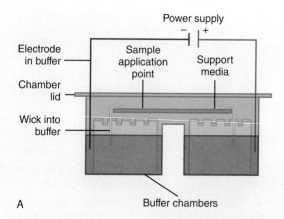

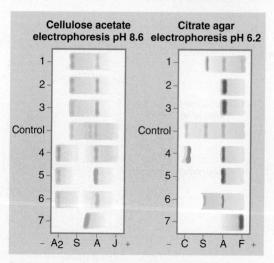

FIGURE 5–6 Electrophoresis chamber setup and blot. **(A)** Basic electrophoresis chamber (Bishop). **(B)** Example of common hemoglobin variants run by cellulose acetate and citrate agar electrophoresis.

(a) Modified from Bishop, Michael L., Edward P. Fody, and Larry E. Schoeff, eds. Clinical chemistry: principles, techniques, and correlations. Lippincott Williams & Wilkins, 2013; (b) Adapted from McClatchey, K.D., ed. Clinical laboratory medicine. Lippincott Williams & Wilkins, 2002.

detect differences in screening serum proteins including the major classes of immunoglobulins, as well as in the detection of immunodeficiencies, where bands may not appear when compared with normal serum.

Rocket Immunoelectrophoresis is an adaptation of the radial immunodiffusion (RID) technique developed in the 1960s by the Swedish chemist CB Laurell.[6] Like RID, antibody is diffused within a gel and antigen is placed in cut wells. However, electrophoresis is then used to facilitate and increase the speed of migration of the antigen into the agar (**FIGURE 5–7**). Its name is derived from the rocket-shaped expanding precipitin line that develops as a result of the changes in antigen concentration as the process of dissolution and reformation of the precipitate occurs. The concentration of antigen is directly proportional to the apex of the arc. Using a standard curve, a calculation of the antigen present can be determined in an unknown specimen. While faster than RID, typically taking only a few hours, the pH of the solution must be calibrated to prevent the movement of the antibodies and to maintain a negative charge for the antigens. When used to quantitate immunoglobulins, the pH is adjusted to 8.6.

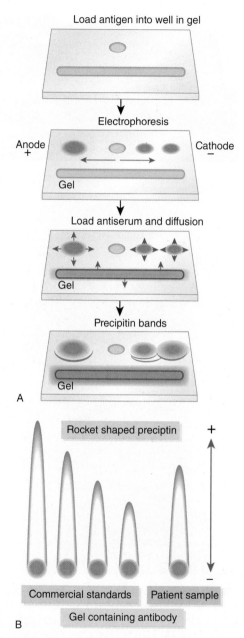

Load antigen into well in gel

Electrophoresis

Anode
+

Cathode
−

Gel

Load antiserum and diffusion

Gel

Precipitin bands

Gel

A

Rocket shaped preciptin

+

−

Commercial standards   Patient sample

Gel containing antibody

B

FIGURE 5–7 Immunoelectrophoresis and Rocket Immunoelectrophoresis. **(A)** Steps in immunoelectrophoresis. After running electrophoresis, antiserum is loaded into a well built into the gel and diffusion is allowed to occur, which leads to precipitin bands for select antigens now correlated with charge separation. **(B)** Laurell's Rocket immunoelectrophoresis, which is a single-stage quantifiable immunoassay through the use of a standard curve.

A third method, **immunofixation electrophoresis**, is similar to immunoelectrophoresis except that instead of the antigen being added to a trough, the antiserum is directly applied to the surface of the gel. Performed on both agarose and cellulose gels, the process is considerably shorter than immunoelectrophoresis, taking less than 1 hour to perform because diffusion is only across the thickness of the gel, typically 1mm. The technique is used most often to examine the presence or absence of an unknown patient antigen compared with a known set of specific antibodies. Thus, immunofixation can provide for the definitive presence of a disease-causing antigen if antibodies are selected correctly. Multiple lanes allow for investigation of several disease antigens at one time. Precipitates form only where specific antibody-antigen complexes have been formed. Subsequently, the gel is washed to remove excess and nonspecific proteins, and stained, often with secondary antibodies toward specific antibody heavy and light chains, to increase visibility of precipitates. Reference standards are also typically incorporated into the assay, for example, a reference lane in which an antibody directed at all serum proteins is added to confirm loading. Immunofixation is particularly useful in detecting hypogammaglobulinemias and low-volume antigens. Serum, cerebral spinal fluid, and urine are all commonly used as sources of patient antiserum. Dilutions of antiserum are often necessary for high-density antigens to remove zones of antigen excess. One of the most utilized modification of the immunofixation assay is the Western blot, which is used widely in clinical, academic, and research laboratories.

In comparison to Western blotting, immunoelectrophoresis does not require the use of labeled immunoreagents to aid in detection. Western Blotting will be described in more detail in relation to specific diseases in later chapters of this book and in relation to labeled immunoassays in Chapter 6: Immunoassay Design and with immunophenotyping in Chapter 8: Immunophenotyping.

Like all technology, the precipitation reactions predated the use of more complex methods of detection that are in use and being developed today. Passive approaches to precipitation such as detection by light scatter and immunodiffusion, predated the use of electrophoretic or active immunodiffusion. In all cases, however, the general principles of precipitation have been adopted and incorporated into more advanced techniques, such as labeled immunoassays, which will be described in more detail in Chapter 6: Immunoassy Design and with specific examples throughout this book. Additionally, the use of spectrophotometers and nephelometers, as well as the application of electric current for diffusion, would be used in developing advanced laboratory instrumentation and subsequently in the automation of the clinical laboratory.

▶ Agglutination

Agglutination differs from precipitation in that, instead of using soluble antigens, agglutination uses the visible aggregation of antigens bound to particles in the presence of specific antibody. Specifically, the use of a solid-phase support such as a latex bead or microwell, is required. Two commonly performed agglutination assays still performed as part of kit-based testing are the latex agglutination assays, including rheumatoid factor and *Staphylococcus aureus* detections (**FIGURE 5–8**).

Agglutination reactions are classified into categories such as direct, passive, reverse passive, agglutination inhibition, and coagglutination, and occur as a result of two steps: sensitization and lattice formation/enhancement. Because agglutination requires the use of carrier particles, a more detailed analysis of passive and covalent coupling to solid-phase supports is required for assay design and understanding. However, natural associations of antigens with specific cell types mean that agglutination can also be performed using only patient specimens. The discovery of the antibody's ability to clump cells was one of the earliest discoveries in immunodiagnostic history and led to the discovery of the A, B, and O blood types; agglutination is still one of the most common approaches used in A, B, and O blood typing. Agglutination occurs in several steps or phases including sensitization, lattice formation, and enhancement (**FIGURE 5–9**).

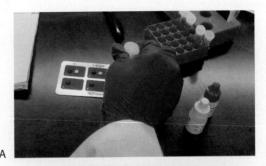

A

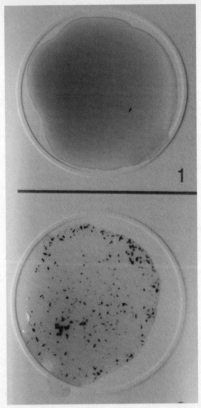

B

FIGURE 5–8 Latex Agglutination Testing. Latex particles can either be bound with antigens or antibodies leading to agglutination in the presence of specific particles in the specimen. **(A)** A lab technologist performs a rheumatoid factor latex agglutination test: latex beads are white and patient specimen is clear. **(B)** Results of a *Staphylococcus aureus* latex agglutination assay in which a colony of bacteria is mixed with *S. aureus* antibody-bound latex particle solution. The negative result (above) from a species other than *S. aureus* shows no agglutination, while the positive result (below) indicates the presence of bound coagulase found in *S. aureus* colonies.

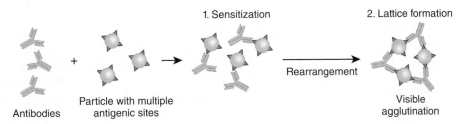

FIGURE 5–9 Stages of Agglutination. Antibodies are placed in association with a particle (i.e., latex bead, RBC). 1. Sensitization: Antibodies physically associate with antigens, the Ab-Ag complexes are rearranged (through mixing). 2. Lattice Formation: A rearranged visible agglutination response is observable.

Sensitization

Following the law of mass action, sensitization is the process of initial antigen-antibody complex through single antigenic determinants of the particle surface. Sensitization also involves a second step, whereby cross-linking forms the visible aggregates. Sensitization is affected by the nature of the immunoglobulin type. In addition, the antigenic binding sites are key to the process; the number and spacing of epitopes on the antigen surface play a significant role.

Lattice Formation and Enhancement

Lattice formation is dependent on the relative concentration of antigens and antibodies as well as the media and environmental conditions. In the case in which cells are the particles, the antibody must be able to span the gap between two cells in order for a lattice to be formed between the two cells. However, mammalian erythrocytes and bacterial cells have a slight negative charge and therefore tend to repel one another, complicating the process of lattice formation. Furthermore, in ionic solutions, erythrocytes tend to surround themselves with cations to form an ionic cloud. Therefore the ability to link cells in a lattice depends on the type of immunoglobulin and antibody type. For example, because of the larger general structure of IgM, which has a dimension of approximately 35 nm, larger than the distance between cells in an ionic cloud (25 nm), they form stronger agglutinins. IgG class antibodies are smaller and less flexible and may not span the distance between particles.

Some factors affecting agglutination include the pH of the solution, location and concentration of particle epitopes, and electrostatic forces from the particles and solution. Most importantly, agglutination is affected by the relative concentration of the antibodies and antigens. To overcome some of these barriers to lattice formation in agglutination, several enhancements to assay design have been employed, specifically, the use of low ionic strength saline and the addition of albumin to the medium help to reduce the effect of surface charges on cells. Additional method variations, such as changing the temperature or pH, have been used. Enzymes, such as papain, trypsin, and ficin have been used to reduce the surface charge on erythrocytes by cleaving specific chemical side chains. In addition, agitation and centrifugation can overcome surface charge barriers. Most commonly, blood cell-based agglutination and enhancement are seen and used in blood banking such as in **hemagglutination**.

Methods of Agglutination

Direct agglutination: Both bacteria and human cells have natural antigens on them. Direct agglutination occurs when serum antibodies are used to detect specific cells. Often, this is used to detect bacteria that are otherwise hard to culture. As an example, the Widal test is a rapid screen for the testing of typhoid fever, which includes salmonella O and H antigens that increase the antibody titer by up to fourfold. While this test has been replaced with more specific tests in developed countries, it is still used in developing countries due to reduced cost. When direct agglutination utilizes erythrocytes it is often referred to as hemagglutination. ABO blood typing is an example of this method, as the blood group antigens are arrayed on the surface of the cells. While titers can be performed by the performance of serial dilutions for a semiquantitative analysis, most commonly the response is graded from 4 to negative when performed in a tube (**FIGURE 5–10**). After centrifugation, one solid clump of cells is considered a 4+ and subsequently smaller clumps are rated down to 1+. A negative result is equivalent to no agglutination and is indicated by a smooth suspension. A slide method can also be used in which antigen and antibody are mixed on a slide and graded for clumping. For example, early

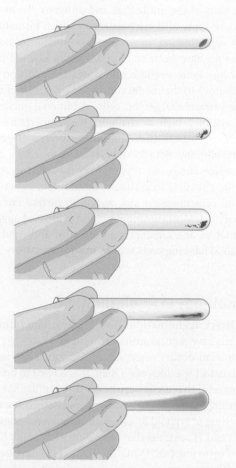

FIGURE 5–10 Tube agglutination can be graded using a manual inspection.

assessment of thrombosis can be done using a latex slide agglutination assay, where latex microparticles coated with monoclonal antibodies specific for D-dimer epitopes agglutinate in the presence of D-dimers, a breakdown product of coagulation. Numerous other kits have been developed for hemagglutination assays involving the detection of viral antigens such as HIV I and II, and several of the major hepatitis viruses.

Passive and Reverse Passive Agglutination: Passive agglutination is also called indirect agglutination (**FIGURE 5–11A**), and is related to the use of antigens that are not naturally found on the surface of a particle. In reverse passive agglutination, the antibody is attached to the carrier particle instead of the antigen. Organic, magnetic, and other polymer particles have been designed and utilized, the most common of which are latex, gelatin, and silicates. Erythrocytes have also been employed, but synthetic beads provide for consistency and stability. In many cases, passive adsorption to the particle is all that is needed and remains one of the most frequently used methods for immobilizing protein immunoreagents. For example, it was found that IgG naturally adsorbs to the surface of polystyrene (latex) beads. In other cases, chemical methods are utilized to add chemical bonding sites.

Large numbers of antibodies can bind to a single inexpensive latex bead, so the number of antigenic binding sites is large. Passive agglutination tests have been used to detect autoimmune factors such as rheumatoid factor, to bacterial products such as group A and B streptococcus, and to viruses such as cytomegalovirus and varicella-zoster. Commercial kits are available that employ the passive and reverse passive agglutination detection technique. They allow for the rapid detection of infectious organisms in as little as a few minutes with high specificity and sensitivity. For microbiological species, these rapid kits are useful for initiating earlier treatment, especially for slow or hard-to-culture organisms. The value of particle-coupled antibodies has also been extended to detecting fluctuations in a variety of normal serum proteins, and for detecting changes in hormones and other plasma proteins in response to therapy.

Coagglutination is the specific name of a series of reverse passive agglutination tests

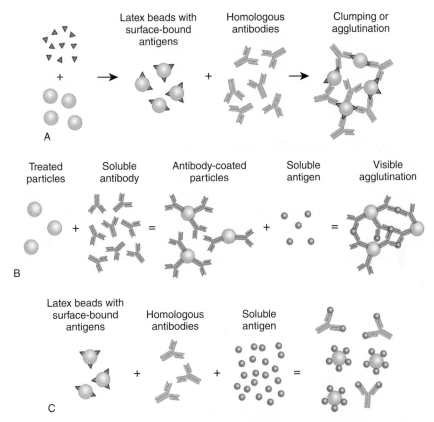

FIGURE 5–11 Passive, reverse passive, and agglutination inhibition. **(A)** Passive agglutination: particles with surface-bound antigen are used to detect antibodies from patient serum. **(B)** Reverse passive agglutination: antibody rather than antigen is attached to the particle. **(C)** Agglutination inhibition: agglutination is inhibited through the competition with soluble patient antigens.

(**FIGURE 5–11B**) in which bacteria, most commonly *Staphylococcus aureus*, is used as the inert particle. *S. aureus* is utilized because it has a unique protein called Protein A, which naturally adsorbs the Fc region of antibodies so that the antigen-binding Fab regions protrude from the surface. These particles tend to have greater stability to latex beads.

Inhibition of agglutination can also be used as a diagnostic tool when assessing the serum specimen. Typically, this type of **agglutination inhibition** is based on competition between a soluble (sample) antigen and a particulate (kit) antigen (**FIGURE 5–11C**). These common, kit-based assays lead to agglutination only in a negative response. The lack of agglutination is seen as positive. The patient sample is incubated for a period

of time with a kit antibody. If specific patient antigen is present, the antibody will bind all open-binding sites; if little or no antigen is present, the antibody-binding sites remain open. In step two, antigen-coated particles are added to the test reagents. Only open antibody binding sites will bind the kit particles and lead to agglutination (a negative test).

As agglutination methods become more complex, they approach the level of configurations used in the advanced, labeled immunoassays introduced in Chapter 6: Immunoassay Design. Antiglobulin tests, also known as the *Coombs' tests*, named for Robin Coombs, who first developed the test in 1945, look at a patient's normally nonagglutinating antibodies by using a secondary antibody targeting human globulin proteins. The

Coombs' test is most commonly associated with the testing for hemolytic disease of the newborn (erythroblastosis fetalis) in which the mother makes IgG antibodies against the Rh blood group antigen that target the newborns erythrocytes and mark them for destruction by the liver through an immune response. They are the most complex agglutination tests described in this chapter.

In general, the **direct antiglobulin test** (or direct Coombs test, as seen in blood bank serology) looks at erythrocytes directly from the patient's blood (**FIGURE 5–12A**). Cells are first washed to remove nonspecifically bound antibodies and then the cells are combined with anti-IgG antibodies (also known as the Coombs reagent). Visible agglutination is observed if IgG antibodies

are attached to the erythrocytes. A modification to this test can be performed with anti-complement antibodies to look for members of the complement cascade.

The **indirect antiglobulin test** (or indirect Coombs test) has been successfully employed to type human blood and to look for specific antibodies in patient serum (**FIGURE 5–12B**). It is a two-step process in which washed reagent (or patient 1) cells and patient antibody (typically patient 2) are allowed to incubate at 37 degrees C. When the Coombs reagent (antihuman globulin) is added, a visible reaction occurs during a positive test. This is commonly used in blood bank allotyping for compatibility testing before a blood transfusion. Reagent red blood cells can be used to

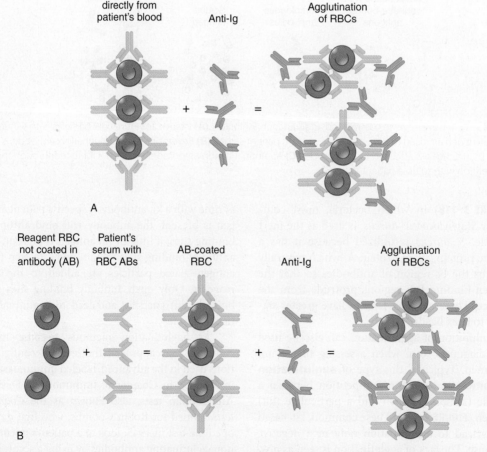

FIGURE 5–12 Direct and Indirect Coombs Test Mechanisms. **(A)** Direct Coombs Test. **(B)** Indirect Coombs Test.

test units for specific alloantibodies. Alternatively, a recipient's red blood cells can be tested against potential donor serum.

Automation

Although agglutination can be performed completely manually, many automated instruments have incorporated the principles of agglutination into their assay designs. Turbidimetry and nephelometry have been utilized to detect the endpoints of agglutination via light scatter. By adding *particle-enhancement*, used to define nephelometry-assisted agglutination, to detection methods, the sensitivity of antigen-antibody complexes detected can be increased from the microgram to nanogram level. Furthermore, many automated methods are orders of magnitude more sensitive to manual agglutination readings. The automation of most classic methods is nearly universal for detection of common diagnostic factors in large-scale facilities. For example, a commonly run assessment of diabetes I and diabetes II is the glycated hemoglobin (HbA1c), for which many methods of detection are employed, including agglutination on the Hemo One auto-analyzer (I.S.E. Srl Company), by first absorbing sample HbA1c to latex particles, which react with anti-HbA1c to yield agglutination.[7] While not as sensitive as the reference method of high-performance liquid chromatography (HPLC), the agglutination method is much less expensive to perform and similarly valid clinically. In smaller physician office facilities and in low-volume and resource-restricted communities, less-automated kit agglutination assays continue to be widely performed.

▶ References

1. Edwards R, Blincko S, Howes I. Principles of immunodiagnostic tests and their development: with specific use of radioisotopes as tracers. In: Edwards R, ed. *Immunodiagnostics: A Practical Approach*. Oxford University Press; 1999.
2. Glick B. The bursa of Fabricius: the evolution of a discovery. *Poult Sci*. 1994;73(7):979–983.
3. Robinson WH. Sequencing the functional antibody repertoire—diagnostic and therapeutic discovery. *Nat Rev Rheumatol*. 2015;11(3):171–182.
4. Optical analysis. In: Williams CA, Chase MW, eds. *Methods in Immunology and Immunochemistry; Volume II Physical and Chemical Methods. Vol 2*: Academic Press; 1968.
5. Augustin R, Hayward BJ, Spiers JA. Antigen-antibody reactions in agar. I. Experimental tests of current theories of Oudin's single diffusion method. *Immunology*. 1958;1(1):67–80.
6. Laurell CB. Quantitative estimation of proteins by electrophoresis in agarose gel containing antibodies. *Anal Biochem*. 1966;15(1):45–52.
7. Pocino K, Molinario R, Manieri R, Bianucci L, Capoluongo E. The hemo one autoanalyzer for glycated hemoglobin assay. *Lab Med*. 2016;47(2):119–123.

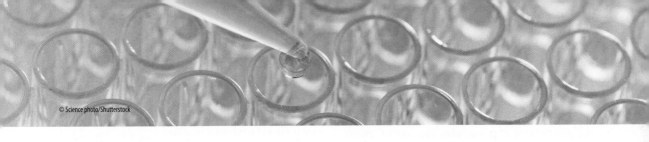

CHAPTER 6

Immunoassay Design

Ian Clift, PhD, MLS(ASCP)^{CM}

KEY TERMS

Adjuvant
Adsorption
Analyte
Antiserum
Calibrators
Chemiluminescence
Competitive
Confocal microscopy
Enzyme-linked immunosorbent
    assays (ELISA)
Enzyme immunoassay
    (EIA)

Enzyme Multiplied Immunoassay
    Technique (EMIT)
Flow cytometry
Fluorescein
Fluorescence immunoassays (FIA)
Fluorescence polarization
    immunoassays (FPIA)
Fluorochromes
Hapten
Heterogeneous assays
Homogeneous assays
Immunohistochemistry (IHC)

Lateral flow immunoassay (LFIA)
Liquid-phase
Noncompetitive
Precipitation
qRT-PCR
Radioallergosorbent test (RAST)
Radioimmunoassay (RIA)
Sandwich assay
Solid-phase
Solid-phase support
Western blotting

LEARNING OBJECTIVES

Upon completion of this chapter, the reader should be able to:

1. Categorize contemporary immunoassays based on label, specificity, reagent volume, and separation steps.
2. Compare and contrast noncompetitive and competitive assays.
3. Define the major labeled tracers used in immunodiagnostics.
4. Compare and contrast homogenous and heterogeneous assays.
5. Explain the recommendation to reduce the use of radioisotopes in immunoassay design.
6. Given a specific antigenic source, recommend the use of a specific immunoassay and labelled tracer.
7. Select the appropriate assay based on its characteristics.

▶ Fundamentals

Immunodiagnostics are typically defined as any diagnostic tool that employs the use of immunological agents, specifically, the use of antibodies to detect the presence of antigens. However, it can also be defined as any diagnostic that is used to interrogate a part of the immune system. An immunoassay is any laboratory method that employs one or several immune components (or immunoreagents) in its mechanism of action. Although there are many specific immunoassay preparations: the ELISA, Western Blot, FETIA, RIA, and others described within this chapter, three key reagents are used commonly in all labeled immunoassays.

1. Antibody or antiserum
2. Standards or calibrators
3. Labeled tracers

The sheer number of immunoassays is extremely broad. Furthermore, all areas of laboratory medicine utilize immunoassays for help in diagnostics in some capacity. In general, assays are named for the type of tracer that is employed and the type of assay performed, which is separated in two ways: either **competitive** or **noncompetitive**, or homophilic or heterophilic immunoassays, respectively (**FIGURE 6-1**). Additionally, general reagents and additives are used to optimize test solutions including nonspecific carriers such as serum albumin, salts such as sodium chloride, and specific proteins to eliminate "heterophilic" antibody effects such as gamma globulins. Other chemicals such as sodium azide as a preservative and ethylenediamine tetraacetic acid (EDTA) to reduce calcium ion interference are also common. Finally, a separation technique is often employed prior to detection.

We as diagnosticians are in a very real way adapting an extremely well-evolved natural foreign body detection technology for use in our own clinical diagnostics. As prior chapters, specifically Chapter 3: Lymphocytes in Adaptive Immunity, have pointed out, this technology has evolved within biological organisms to detect and thwart disease and degradation; it is only fitting that we discuss some of the ways in which this "alien" technology has been further engineered in our own efforts to thwart disease.

Antibody/Antiserum

The structure of the antibody and the in-vivo development of antibodies are discussed at length in other sections of this book. Here, we will focus on the role of antibodies and antiserum (solutions containing antibodies) as they are utilized in diagnostic immunoassays or immunodiagnostics.

When a specific antibody is contained within a serum, it is referred to as an **antiserum**. To produce specific antisera, an animal, commonly a rabbit, sheep, goat, or rodent, is injected with a protein with immunogenic properties. Immunogenicity is a product of the size and structure of the injected protein. Below 3,000 Daltons in size, the protein will most likely fail to produce antibodies against it unless attached to a

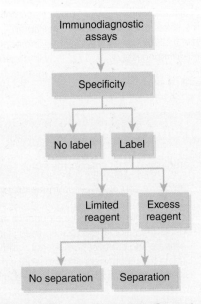

FIGURE 6-1 Immunodiagnostic Assay Categorization Schema.

larger molecule. Therefore, many man-made antisera require both the protein of interest and an **adjuvant**. Commercially available adjuvants include common carriers such as bovine serum albumin (BSA) or human serum albumin (HSA). Others such as rabbit thyrogobulin and keyhole limped hemocyanin (KLH) are considered better carriers for small molecules, but BSA has been found effective for the majority of peptides. Once conjugated to a carrier, the analyte/peptide is referred to as a **hapten**. Specific ratios of hapten to carrier have been shown to be the most successful, for example, a 10:1 ratio of hapten to BSA is recommended.[1] Either alone, or in combination with an adjuvant, the inoculation of an organism, such as mouse, rat, rabbit, or goat, remains the most common antisera production method. Specifically, the production of antisera is commonly a result of either polyclonal development in an animal or, alternatively, via hybridoma (cell) culturing for the production of monoclonal antibodies. In theory, genetic engineering and molecular in-printing have been proposed for antisera production but are currently not employed in most diagnostic production laboratories. Purified, specific antisera are then used for the manufacturing of immunodiagnostic assays. (See this book's Advanced Concepts Appendix for an article on antibody production methods).

Unlabeled Assays

The first immunoassays, many still used in clinical practice, were based on the scientific observation agglutination and precipitation. Agglutination and the related precipitation, i.e., falling out of solution as a result of complex formation, were the first visible signs used to determine antibody-to-antigen interactions. Furthermore, the complexing of antibodies to larger particles such as latex beads, required the development of the same principle techniques utilized in a wide area of labeling techniques described in detail below. Additionally,

unlabeled diffusion assay, including electrophoretic diffusion techniques such as serum electrophoresis and immunoelectrophoresis, were designed to provide further diagnostic specificity. However, there were limitations to these methods, primarily the need for large volumes of antibody-antigen (Ab-Ag) complex for visualization or detection. It was due, in part, to this limitation: the addition of labeled antibodies and/or antigens became important for advancing both scientific discovery and clinical diagnostics.

The First Labeled Immunoassays

The theory of immunoassay has been expounded in detail in many reports, but in general, the performance of an immunodiagnostic test is determined by three factors: affinity, concentration of binding sites, and specificity (**FIGURE 6–2**).

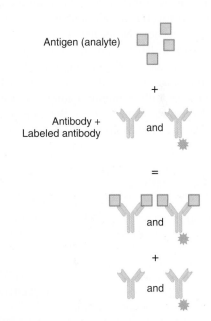

Antigen (analyte)

+

Antibody + Labeled antibody   and

=

and

+

and

FIGURE 6–2 All immunoassays rely on some combination of these factors. Both noncompetitive assays and competitive assays are constructed by adjusting the concentrations of these components. One unlisted variable is the addition of labeled antigens, which can be used in a variety of assays as well.

In all cases, antibodies form the analytical reagent to detect and sometimes quantify a specific **analyte**. Immunoassays utilize antibody specificity to detect levels of an antigen under study. The Ab-Ag compound is then visualized normally by conjugating the antibody to a reporter molecule or adding an antibody-conjugate (secondary antibody) that is specific to the antigen-binding antibody (primary antibody). Furthermore, immunoassays are also defined and limited by their structural specificity, i.e., antibody- and antigen-binding specificity. Unlabeled assays provide the basis for labeled immunoassays.

Some of the first labeled immunoassays were performed in the 1950s; specifically, Yalow and Berson developed the radioimmunoassay in 1959 to detect low concentrations of immune agents. Due to increased regulations on biohazardous waste, during the 1960s, radiological methods began to be substituted for less-labile and less-toxic substances. Chemiluminescent and enzymatic tracers allowed for safer nontoxic approaches. Nevertheless, much of the initial work in labeled immunoassays occurred first with radioisotopic labeling, broadly called radioimmunoassays (RIA), but also including the competitive immunoradiometric assays (IRMA) which came out in the late 1960s. Through these initial studies, it has been shown that the limitation in sensitivity for labeled analyte binding assays, such as immunoassays, is based not on the detectability of the label/tracer, but on the reactivity of the analytical reagent, i.e., reactivity of the antibody, as well as from experimental errors.[2] Ekins and others have mathematically defined the optimal sensitivity of immunoassays as a combination of the equilibrium constant of the reaction and the precision in which the assay is conducted (signal measurement error and manipulation error).[2]

Both core facilities and reference labs have some responsibility in assay design, development, and adoption. The central concerns, although sometimes empirical, are usually based on practical considerations such as the expertise of the personnel, reagent, supply costs, pre-existing systems, and overall costs (**BOX 6-1**). The steps that are important in assay development and design overlap with quality assurance considerations, such as comparisons of separation method and general reagent components, sample preparation, protocol optimization, and validation of assay performance, are discussed in Chapter 4: Safety and Standards. New laboratories in particular must consider the establishment or modification of standard protocols for the adoption of immunoassays, which, in part, go over the same terrain as the initial design considerations.

A DEEPER LOOK BOX 6-1   Mass Spectrometry vs the Immunoassay

Mass Spectrometry (MS) utilizes a measurement of the mass-to-charge ratio on ionized molecules to differentiate and quantitate a potential analyte, whereas immunoassays utilize specific antibodies with tracer elements for detection. Both methods have clinical laboratory applications and come with their own set of advantages and disadvantages.

Generally, mass spectrometry is capable of providing very precise analytical specificity and employs low-cost consumables. However, MS methods require specialized personnel and require batch processing, which increases turnaround time.

Immunoassays are much more easily automated, require less training to perform, and have been developed for a wide variety of uses. However, reagent costs are considerably higher and typically require considerably more analyte for detection than MS. These differences have led to both techniques being employed when attempting to detect a wide range of analyte concentrations; for example, testosterone, normally high in men, is commonly tested by immunoassay in males but is tested by MS in women and children, where it is very low.[3]

The majority of current assays use **solid-phase** reagents: antibodies and antigens attached to a particle structure such as a polymer bead or a vessel wall, with a vessel wall being the most used as it aids in separation. Various chemical methods can be used to remove the bound fraction, when necessary, after a wash step. Typically, either the bound or free fraction is of specific interest. A liquid phase has also been employed with success, specifically through the use of a secondary antibody. For example, an anti-rabbit antibody bound to a labeled tracer is administered if rabbit antibodies are used to bind the specific analyte. These secondary antibodies are often labeled commercially, allowing for a more streamlined approach to assay development.

Standards and Calibrators

Like all controlled assays and techniques, the use of standards and calibrators insures quality and accuracy. Analysis of label activity can be quantified only through the creation of a standard curve of specified, known concentrations of unlabeled analytes. The points of this curve, also known as a calibration curve, are determined through the use of **calibrators**, which are often commercially available.

Standards are also commercially available and can act as point references for determining the quality control of the assay. These standards may not be true analyte measurements, but are instead point references for the detector (i.e., fluorescent, spectrophotometric, or radiometric).

▶ Labeled Tracers

Light scatter, particle enhancement, radioisotopes, enzymes, fluorophores, and chemiluminescent particles are all potential labeling and detection methods for immunoassays. Labeling molecules, also known as tracer molecules, are used as detectors in most advanced immunoassays. The reaction itself, such as the agglutination response, is used as the detector in all unlabeled immunoassays, but is considerably less sensitive, often requiring the "eyeball" method or detection using light scatter instruments. In contrast, labeled tracers increase the analytic sensitivity of the immunoassay and therefore, are commonly employed in most manual and automated approaches to analyte detection. Detection of these assays occurs either as an observation of the extent of reaction of the analyte (antigen or antibody) or extent of reaction of the reagent (antigen or antibody).[2] Assays are named for the type of tracer that is employed and the type of assay performed, which is separated into competitive and noncompetitive immunoassays, i.e., as having limited antibody reagent (competitive) or excess antibody reagent (noncompetitive), which are further divided by the utility of separating free and bound fractions.[1]

Noncompetitive

Noncompetitive assays of this class have also been termed immunometric assays or excess reagent methods. Some of the earliest assays of this type were the radioisotopically labeled immunoradiometric assay and two-site immunoradiometric assay.[4] These assays can be performed with or without a solid support. A solid support includes a plate, tube, or polymer bead in which an antibody or antigen is bound. In a noncompetitive assay, the antigen is directly proportional to the labeled antibody. This relationship is linear up until high concentrations, at which time a hook effect is observed. They are often performed using various dilutions allowing for a dose response to be charted.

In noncompetitive excess reagent methods, the antibody is added in relative excess, pushing the reaction forward and shortening the incubation period (**FIGURE 6–3**). In one commonly performed assay, known as a sandwich assay (**FIGURE 6–4A** and **FIGURE 6–4B**), a bound antibody or antigen is used to capture the complementary analyte from a patient sample. After a round of washing to remove unreactive material, a labeled detector antibody is added.

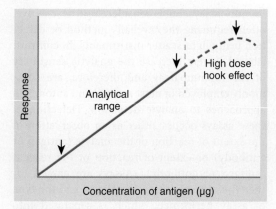

FIGURE 6-3 Non-competitive Immunoassay Dose-Response Curve.

Excess labeled antibody is washed away and the remaining tracer, when compared with a set of calibrators or standards, allows for a quantification of the target.

Competitive

While the term *immunoassay* has been used as a general descriptor of the entire class of antibody binding assays, *immunoassay* has also been used to specifically define competitive assays as a subclass. These were the earliest immunoassays, the first of which used radiolabeled antigens. In this assay design, a constant amount of labeled reagent antigen is added to an unknown quantity of combined unlabeled patient antigen and followed with a reagent antibody. As the concentration of unlabeled antigen increases, the amount of bound, labeled antigen decreases (**FIGURE 6-5**). This can be accomplished in one step in which labeled antigen (Ag*), unlabeled antigen (Ag), and reagent antibody (Ab) are simultaneously incubated together. Measurement can take place when the unbound and bound, labeled antigen are removed.

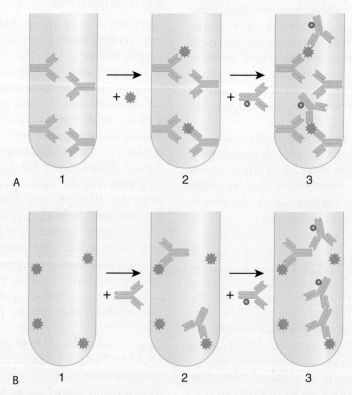

FIGURE 6-4 Noncompetitive Sandwich Assays. **(A)** Sandwich Assay for the Detection of Antigen. **(B)** Sandwich Assay for the Detection of Antibody.

Modified from Bishop, Michael L., Edward P. Fody, and Larry E. Schoeff, eds. Clinical chemistry: principles, techniques, and correlations. Lippincott Williams & Wilkins, 2013.

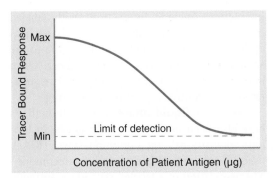

FIGURE 6–5 Competitive Immunoassay Dose Response Curve.

In a second competitive assay, sequential steps are used. First, reagent antibody and unlabeled antigen from a patient source are incubated together. Second, the labeled tracer antigen is added. After a separation step, the bound, labeled antigen is measured. Alternatively, the quantity of the unbound tracer can be measured. Indeed, the unbound tracer is the only variable, and is dependent on the unknown quantity of antigen from the patient and the finite number of antibody binding sites.

Additional factors, such as the order in which reactants are added and the specific fraction that is observed, are also considered in assay design and can affect the outcome. Finally, similar to nonlabeled assays, the avidity of antibody to antigen binding is an important factor regulating the performance of any assay.

Label Conjugation

The binding chemistry for label attachment is similar for most labels (chemiluminescent, fluorescent, or enzymatic) with some distinctions. For example, radiolabeling of immunoreagents (i.e., antigens or antibodies) may require only the substitution of tyrosine or histidine residues with radioiodine. This is typically performed through the oxidation of the radioiodine in the presence of the protein via several established methods including lactoperoxidase, chloramine T, and iodogen.[1,5] In most cases, oxidation is used to conjugate labeled tracers. Antibody conjugation

presents with its own unique challenges, as the conjugate-binding site may diminish the antibodies' ability to bind antigen. Specific early attempts to label antibodies through conjugation included coupling enzymes to amino groups within the immunoglobulin (Ig) chains using sodium periodate and glutaraldehyde; however, reports described the loss of antigen-binding activity as a result of these amino-directed labels.[6] Small molecules such as active esters, epoxides, isothiocyanates, isocyanates, and aldehyde can be activated so that they can form covalent bonds with amine groups on the enzyme.[7] In other cases, such as the use of beta-galactosidase and HRP, coupling can also occur with thiol groups. Further analysis showed that two factors influenced antigen binding to labeled tracers, the conjugation procedure itself, which could destroy the antigenic-binding sites, and steric hindrance, through the formation of large and irregular tracer-antibody complexes.[6]

Today, conjugations are most often performed through oxidation of the amino acid lysine, through its terminating primary amine ($-NH_2$). For example, succinimidyl ester methods are commonly used for fluorescent dye and enzymatic conjugation, and sodium periodate is still used because of its ability to activate horseradish peroxidase (HRP), one of the most popular enzymatic tracers. An older conjugation technique for HRP is described in SSP 6-1; however, these methods have been refined and commercialized in order to reduce time and complication. The Lightning-Link kit from Innova Biosciences provides a one-step conjugation strategy for attached various labels to antibodies (**FIGURE 6–6**). The use of bifunctional linker molecules is also employed in some commercial kits, for example, glutaraldehyde is a typical bifunctional agent with two active aldehyde groups, one to bind the enzyme and the other to bind the antibody.

Separation Techniques

Not all immunoassays require a separation technique. Some assays such as the fluorescence polarization immunoassays (FPIA), fluorescence

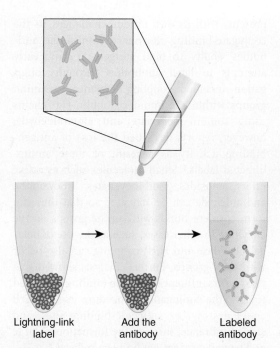

Lightning-link
label

Add the
antibody

Labeled
antibody

FIGURE 6–6 The Lightning-Link Antibody Conjugation System.

Courtesy of Expedeon Ltd.

excitation transfer immunoassay (FETIA), and enzyme inhibition technique (EMIT) require no separation and depend on a change in signal between bound and free fractions for detection.[4] These assays, sometimes called **homogeneous assays**, require no separation, while those requiring separation are called **heterogeneous assays**.[8]

However, even when a separation step is not required, the formation of an Ab-Ag complex and detection of a chemical or physical separation is measured. Separation of bound and free fractions is typically performed using some sort of **solid-phase support**. Solid-phase supports include many insoluble materials such as tubes, microtiter plates, beads, and columns made of polystyrene and other organic polymers to separate bound from free fractions of antigens and antibodies.[9] Solid-phase supports are used in immunodiagnostics to increase efficiency and to reduce non-specific binding (NSB). Non-specific

interactions include interactions with labeled immunoreagents, background signals such as optical and electrical noise, and binding to the sample matrix or assay vessel surfaces. Once bound, immunized immunoreagents are separated by decanting, aspirating, or washing.

However, **liquid-phase** separation methods have also been used. Many early assays, including conventional radioimmunoassays (RIAs), used a secondary antibody separation technique.[4] The association of a labeled secondary antibody is then used to facilitate the precipitation of the bound fraction and subsequent separation from the free fraction. Measurement can then be performed on either fraction, depending on the assay design. Immunoreagent-based, liquid-phase separation methods using specific monoclonal antibodies have also replaced traditional solid-phase methods such as protein A supports, in more recent enzymatic assays as well.[10]

Two of the earliest and simplest techniques for separation of free and bound fractions are **adsorption** and **precipitation**. Adsorption is the adhesion of the molecule, the adsorbate, to a solid surface, the adsorbent. Precipitation is the condensing of molecules from a solution. In both cases, the analyte of interest is then effectively isolated from other soluble components.

Immune precipitation described in some detail in Chapter 5: Classical Principles of Immunodiagnostics, has been used to examine the formation of larger immune complexes both with and without the addition of chemically and physically associated moieties such as latex beads. Non-immune precipitation occurs when the environment of the reaction is altered, leading proteins to lose solubility and fall out of the solution. Common compounds used to change solubility include polyethylene glycol, ammonium sulfate, sodium sulfate, and alcohols such as ethanol. In the ideal situation, both unbound antibodies and Ab-Ag complexes precipitate out after centrifugation and unbound antigens stay in the supernatant.

Adsorption uses a particle gradient to trap molecule size dependently. Porous particles such as charcoal combined with crosslinked dextran, silica, and Sephadex have all been used to create separation columns. The size of the pores determines the size of the molecule to be trapped. Unbound antigens, smallest in size, will filter through these columns first, followed by unbound antibody, and then Ab-Ag complexes. Columns have been designed to trap specific proteins as well. These so-called immunoaffinity separations depend on Ab-Ag reactions to remove selected analytes from patient samples. Similar to the sandwich assay described below, an immobilized specific antibody is used to capture the antigen of interest.[11] This can be used to accumulate a large amount of a low-volume antigen for quantification. Advances in technology have allowed these chromatographic columns to be placed in capillary-based microfluidic chambers embedded in a slide or chip.[11] Magnetic, particle-based separation methods have become very popular for both manual and automated immunoassays. Generally, with a tube-based system, an immune agent bound to a paramagnetic bead can be used to sequester analytes of interest while nonspecific particles can be removed through aspiration.

▶ Common Assays

Labeled assays have evolved away from the use of radiotracers toward enzymatic and fluorescent tracers, while many of the other aspects of their design have remained the same. Due to their historical importance, some detail has been given to the use of radiotracers in laboratory immunoassay development, as well as to illustrate the similarities among assay designs of more contemporary assays. It is also important to note that some facilities still use radiotracers in their diagnostic efforts, especially when it comes to reference methods and assays with the need for low levels of detection. However, contemporary assays are more often designed using enzymatic, fluorescent, and chemiluminescent tracers. Of additional importance, many of the assays have been adapted from their manual roots for incorporation in fully automated analyzers. For example, many drug-monitoring chemistry analyzers such as those produced by

COBAS, Siemens, and Abbott rely heavily on various immunoassays for detection including FPIA and EMIT tests.[12]

Radiological Assays

Radioisotopic labels are some of the oldest and still some of the most cost-effective and sensitive detection mechanisms for immunodiagnostics; however, they have lost some of their favor due to the health effects associated with radiation and complications associated with reagent disposal. The most common radiotracer is radioiodine (^{125}I). It is supplied as a high specific-activity sodium iodide from several commercial sources. This radioisotope was selected for most assays based on a compromise between obtaining high activity and extended shelf life; the shorter the radioactive shelf life, the more intense the radioactive emission (reduced detection limits).[2] Another commonly used diagnostic radioisotope is tritium (^{3}H), which has a particular use due to its ready incorporation into organic compounds through isotopic exchange with ^{2}H; however, the expensive process of liquid scintillation counting has reduced its number of practical applications.[13]

Radiolabeling occurs through one of several oxidation methods: the transfer of electrons from one molecule to another. The most common oxidation methods are lactoperoxidase.[1] Lactoperoxidase is thought to be the mildest oxidation method and reduces the possibility of damaging the tracer molecule. Conjugation methods are described further in a previous section.

Radioimmunoassay (RIA)

The **radioimmunoassay (RIA)** has seen significant usage in the pharmaceutical and toxicology industries due to its extreme sensitivity and precision, which is rivaled only by GC-MS and HPLC. Specifically, RIA is used for drugs of abuse testing and therapeutic monitoring. For example, drugs such as cocaine, morphine, and methadone can be determined through urine RIA, and everything from insulin to digitoxin can be tested in serum.[8] Generally, despite the radioactivity of this assay, it remains in common usage due to its extreme sensitivity; however, competition from nonradioactive assays such as FPIA and EMIT now account for a larger percentage of assays in many labs. Although of increased sensitivity, HPLC assays are still avoided due to time and resource constraints.[14]

RIA assays can be performed on multiple body fluids including serum, plasma, urine, and lysed whole blood. The sample is incubated with radiolabeled (^{125}I) antigen of interest, e.g., cyclosporine A; and an antibody against the antigen, e.g., ant-cyclosporine A[14]. Therefore, the radioactive antigen and patient antigen compete for antibody binding. The supernatant is decanted and the precipitate is measured for radioactivity using a gamma counter and compared with calibrators and controls. Alternatively, an indirect measurement of the free radioactive antigen can be measured from the supernatant to determine the patient's drug concentration.

Radioallergosorbent Test (RAST)

The **radioallergosorbent test (RAST)**, a variant of the RIA, has been commonly used in the detection of allergens, such as bee stings, penicillins, airborne allergens,[15,16] and parasitic infections[17] with a specific emphasis on Immunoglobulin E (IgE). IgE is associated with allergic responses and can be used to diagnose clinically relevant hypersensitivity. In the early

1980s, the RAST test was originally correlated to parasitic infections through a high concentration of IgE and is still considered the standard method; however, its utility has been challenged by IgE-specific ELISA testing.[17]

The RAST is performed by binding the antigen of interest, i.e., an allergen or parasite, to a gel filtration media such as Sepharose or other solid-phase support. This support is then incubated with patient plasma overnight, washed, and a radiolabeled (^{125}I) anti-human IgE antibody is applied and incubated.[17] After washing, the samples are counted using a gamma counter. The result is a quantification of analyte-specific IgE in the patient's plasma.

Immunoradiometric Assays (IRMA)

Immunoradiometric assays (IRMA) were the first immunometric assays to be developed (**FIGURE 6–7**). They are faster than their RIA counterparts because of the excess of reagent forces and the reaction toward equilibrium, which reduces incubation times.[4]

The earliest versions of immunoradiometric assays used an excess of polyclonal antibody and a solid support antigen (adsorbent) to bind and remove unreacted radiolabeled antibody.[4] Refinement of this method led to what is known as the **sandwich assay**, in which two identical antibodies were used, one labeled with the radioactive tracer and the other bound to the solid support. In this method, two incubations occurred, the first

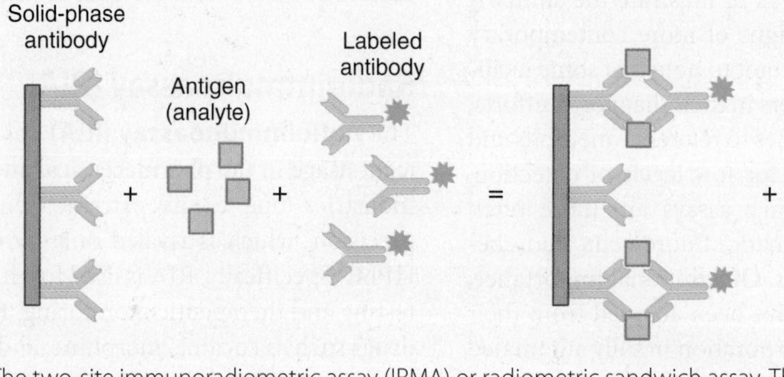

FIGURE 6–7 The two-site immunoradiometric assay (IRMA) or radiometric sandwich assay. This diagrammatic representation uses two antibodies, one attached to a solid phase and the other labeled with a radioisotopic tracer. Although the first of its kind, the design has been modified successfully with all tracer types.

with the solid support antibody and the patient sample, serum or plasma; and the second incubation, after several washes, with the radiolabeled antibody. This was further refined to include the use of the more-specific monoclonal antibody instead of the less-specific polyclonal variety.

Enzyme Assays

Enzyme coupling was initially developed because fluorescence was traditionally difficult to quantitatively assess, and radioisotopes had limited shelf stability and used radioactive materials, which are potentially harmful for lab workers.[18,19] Several natural enzymatic reactions have been co-opted by diagnosticians and scientists to aid in the identification and quantification of substances in body fluids. Some of the most common are β-gal (β-galactosidase), HRP, and ALP. β-gal, for example, also called lactase for its enzymatic activity on lactose, is a glycoside hydrolase that can catalyze hydrolysis of β-galactosides through the breaking of glycosidic bonds that have been used in both immunoassays and molecular studies as a reporter. An example procedure for coupling antibody to enzyme can be found in **SSP 6–1**.

Enzyme-labeled tests concurrently using colorimetric, fluorimetric, and chemiluminescent systems are some of the most widely used

---

STEP-BY-STEP PROCEDURE 6–1 HRP Antibody: Enzyme Conjugation with Succinimidyl Ester

Theory: Most enzyme-linked antibodies used in the clinical laboratory are available commercially. However, many reference-level laboratories may create their own conjugated antibodies. This procedure requires the availability of a free thiol group on the antibody used.

Materials: phosphate buffer (PB), phosphate buffered saline (PBS), specific IgG molecules at 10 mg/mL in PB, SATA: N-succinimidyl-S-acetylthioacetate (Pierce), hydroxylamine hydrochloride (Sigma Aldrich), 0.1 M sodium bicarbonate, purified HRP, dimethylformamide (DMF) (Sigma Aldrich), SMCC: succinimidyl-4-(N-maleimidomethyl) cyclohexane-1-carboxylate (Pierce), disposable Sephadex column (G-25 gel filtration on PD-10 columns), double distilled glassware.

Thiolation Reaction

1. Add 10 μL of SATA in DMF per mL IgG with mixing
2. Incubate for 30 minutes at room temperature
3. Separate IgG from smaller molecules using Sephadex PD-10 column using PB collection. This will dilute IgG 1.4 times approximately
4. Product can be stored long term frozen

Exposure of thiol

1. Add 100 μL hydroxylamine per mL of derivatrized IgG
2. Incubate for 1 hr at room temperature
3. Separate thiol-IgG by PD-10 column chromatography running in 0.1 M sodium biocarbonate

Enzyme Conjugation

1. Dissolve 9 mg of HRP in cold PBS to a concentration of 20 mg/mL
2. Add 3 mg SMCC in a minimum volume of DMF (0.025 mL approximately) with stirring
3. Incubate for 1 hr in refrigerator
4. Purify immediately through Sephadex column using cold PBS as elution buffer to remove unreacted SMCC
5. Pool enzyme fraction, which has a brown color
6. Adjust HRP concentration to 10 mg/mL
7. Add 8 mg of SATA-modified IgG (see above) in 1 mL PBS (the 4:1 molar ratio of enzyme:antibody will give high specific activity)

Additional purification steps may lead to increased activity.

immunoassay procedures. Specifically, an enzymatic response elicits a change in a secondary tracer, such as a change in color or fluorescence. Enzyme use allows sensitive detection of a small concentration of antigen, as well as reducing signal to noise ratio, as enzymes are signal amplifiers; each enzyme-Ab-Ag complex can catalyze multiple product-forming reactions, as opposed to the single signal molecule or direct fluoro- or radio-label conjugated to an enzyme. Currently, there are multiple, sensitive colorimetric substrates for each enzyme, including yellow PNPP absorbing at 405 nm for ALP, green ABTS absorbing at 410 and 650 nm, yellow-orange OPD absorbing at 492 nm, and TMB blue absorbing at 370 and 652 nm or at 450 nm with the addition of hydrogen peroxide for HRP. Changes in absorption are measured by a colorimeter. Additionally, there are multiple chemifluorescent and chemiluminescent substrates developed for enzymes that offer alternative reporting systems for enzyme-linked antibodies including luminals, polyphenol and acradidine esters and luciferin for HRP, AMPPD for ALP, and AMPGD for galactoside.[20–22] Enzymatic procedures, which found their start in immunostaining and gel-precipitin techniques, have been used in solid-phase separation systems, reagent-linked particle assays, a number of non-separation assays, and have been adapted for an increasing number of analyzers.[7]

Enzyme Immunoassay (EIA)

Analogous to the RIA, the **enzyme immunoassay (EIA)** uses a chemically associated enzyme as the label instead of a radioisotope. As with all enzymatic reactions, measurement is determined by examining the turnover of substrate into product. Often, this results from the conversion of a colorless chromogenic substrate into a colored product, through photometry, for instance, indicating the formation of an Ab-Ag complex. EIA has been successfully employed for the detection of antibiotics in circulation including commercially available kits for gentamicin, tobramycin, and neomycin.[8] EIA is also used for detection of bacterial infections such as *Clostridium difficile*,

the most common form of diarrhea in an adult population, through the detection of bacterial antigens in fecal samples.[23]

Enzyme-linked Immunosorbent Assays (ELISA)

Enzyme-linked immunosorbent assays (ELISA) have found many uses in research labs, diagnostic labs, and commercial settings to assess varied sample types, including serum, plasma, cells, whole blood, lysates, environmental samples, dried blood, and water. Many commercial ELISA kits have been developed (**FIGURE 6-8**). In a biological setting, they are often used to assess immune response, including cytokine secretion and quantified antibody levels to assess immune response to an allergen immunization. They have been used to assess levels of low-frequency T cells specific to cancer or other antigens, B-cell response, and humoral response as well.[21] Other diagnostic uses include assessing hormone levels (i.e., HCG, LH, estrogen), antibodies specific to infectious agents (i.e., syphilis, Tuberculosis), viral infection (i.e., rubella), or parasites.[24] Additionally, they can be used commercially to detect plant pathogens or food allergens in products. Due to the small volume of patient specimen needed, ELISA

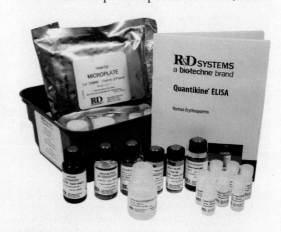

FIGURE 6-8 Commercial ELISA kits. ELISA Kits come with all the components necessary to perform the assay except for common lab consumables and supplies, such as pitetters and pipette tips. The microwell plate includes 96 reaction chambers.
Courtesy of R&D Systems, Inc.

was also one of the first immunoassays employed for multi-analyte analysis.[25] As a popular assay design, ELISA assays continue to be refined to increase sensitivity, reduce time, and automate processing, including new solid-phase systems such as multiplex bead assays, high temperature, and pressure-mediated approaches.[26,27]

ELISA offers a method to measure the amount of any molecule that can be recognized by an antibody. It is commonly considered a backbone method for diagnostic testing in infectious disease. This method of sensitive detection has broad commercial and clinical impact, as detection of an absolute level or change of a certain molecule can provide information about the sample or a sample's response to treatment. In ELISA, the labeled tracer is an enzyme conjugated to the antibodies. The enzymes most frequently used are conjugated via glutaraldehyde to an antibody, without loss of antibody-antigen binding or enzyme functionality, and catalyze a reaction in which the product is visually detectable.[28] The most widely used enzymes are horseradish peroxidase (HRP), alkaline phosphatase (ALP), and galactopyranoside. ALP activity, for example, is measured by the hydrolysis of 1 micromole of p-nitrophenyl phosphate per minute at pH 9.6 at 25°C.[7]

Levels of the patient antigen are quantified by enzymatic activity. Initially, the sample is exposed to the antibody-enzyme complex, allowing Ab-Ag-specific binding to occur (**FIGURE 6–9**). Following binding, bound molecules are immobilized, and unbound antibody and sample are washed from the formed complex. Bound sample is then exposed to the enzyme substrate, and an enzymatic reaction is allowed to proceed either for a set amount of time or to a set color density, at which point the reaction is quenched through washing. Relative levels of absorption or speed at which set absorption is reached can then be used to determine the number of enzymes present, which indicates the amount of Ab-Ag complex.[18,24]

ELISPOT

Generically, in ELISPOT, a capture antibody is coated overnight on a plate and then blocked with PBS with Tween. In one example procedure, after several washes, the ELISPOT assay is performed, whereby the antigens or cells of interest are added to the plate for a specified period of time. Biotin-labeled antibody against the antigen is then added, incubated, and washed before a three-reagent, HRP-conjugated streptavidin is added. The solution is then developed to reveal positive coloration when antigen/cells are present. In one use of this assay, HIV-particle-mediated CD8 T-cell granzyme B release was quantified in HIV patient cells.[29]

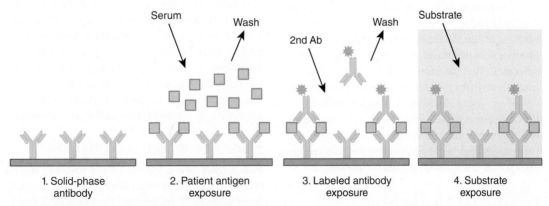

1. Solid-phase antibody
2. Patient antigen exposure
3. Labeled antibody exposure
4. Substrate exposure

FIGURE 6–9 Solid phase ELISA for antigen detection in four steps: In the solid-phase antibody, ELISA patient antigens in serum are added to solid-phase antibodies; excess serum is washed; and a secondary enzyme-linked antibody is added followed by substrate, which leads to a color change when patient antigen is present. An antibody-detection method is also employed to find patient antibodies (not shown) in which an antigen is bound to the solid phase; then the patient serum is added, followed by an antihuman IgG with label.

Enzyme Multiplied Immunoassay Technique (EMIT)

The **Enzyme Multiplied Immunoassay Technique (EMIT)**, also known as EMIA, is a variation on the EIA that has gained success in therapeutic and recreational drug monitoring.[8] In this assay, an excess of antibody is added and followed by an antigen-enzyme complex. Only unbound antigen-enzyme complex act upon the substrate.

Fluorescence Assays

Fluorescence immunoassays (FIA), also known as fluoroimmunoassays, again follow a similar design as the RIA assays with the exception of their fluorophore label instead of a radiolabel. Fluorophores, or **fluorochromes**, were first bound to antibodies in the mid-1940s, and were useful due to their ability to absorb energy from an incident light source and convert it to lower energy but longer wavelength light, thus allowing for light-aided detection of bound molecules. The two most common fluorophores used are **fluorescein**, which absorbs light at ~490 nm and emits at 517 nm (green), and rhodamine, which absorbs at 550 nm and emits at 580 to 585 nm (red) for tetramethyl-rhodamine (TMR). Fluorescence spectrometers, containing a source of radiant light, a sample holder, and a detection device, are used to produce incident light and detect emitted light.[30] More complex versions of this device have been manufactured to produce selective wavelengths of light and selective detectors. Multiple lasers and detectors allow for multiple analytes to be detected in a single sample.

FIAs come in several similar formats to the above-mentioned RIAs and EIAs including heterogeneous assays that include a separation step (two stage) and homogeneous assays that require no separation and one incubation (one stage).

Fluorescence Polarization Immunoassays (FPIA)

Fluorescence polarization immunoassays (FPIA) [FIGURE 6–10] are homogenous assays that do not require the separation of the free and complexed tracers. The advantage of this assay design is the reduced number of washing steps and additional manipulations when compared with assays such as the ELISA.[31] FPIA has been used for everything from detection of foodborne toxins[31] to serum pathogens.[30]

The principle of fluorescence polarization requires that, in addition to the excitation of the fluorophore by a plane-polarized light beam, the molecules must tumble during their fluorescent lifetime to emit light at a different angle.[30] In practice, this is achieved by taking measurements of fluorescent intensity at both vertical and horizontal positions using a fluorescence spectrometer.

Fluorescence Excitation Transfer Immunoassay (FETIA)

Heavily touted and refined in the late 1970s by Ullman and others,[32] FETIA has been used to detect IgG and C-reactive protein among other hormones, drugs, and proteins.[33] In general, this method uses two fluorochromes with overlapping spectra, such as fluorescein and rhodamine; one is used as the donor and the other as the quencher.[32] Typically, the antigen is labeled with the donor fluorochrome, also known as the fluorescer, and antibody is labeled with the quencher.[33] This negative response assay works by reducing the fluorescent signal as the two molecules antigen, and antibody, come within close proximity. This completive homophilic assay requires competing labeled antigen and nonlabeled patient antigen. Under high patient-antigen concentration, the quenching of fluorescence is decreased. Of note, the confocal technique known as FRET (Förster resonance energy transfer, or fluorescent resonance energy transfer) relies of the same principle.

Fluorescent Confocal Imaging

Pathologists use a variety of microscopic methods to make diagnostic determinations ranging from wide-field microscopy for examining fixed-tissue sections to traditional confocal microscopy, which is utilized to increase the optical resolution and contrast of a specimen by the elimination of out-of-focus light. These techniques have been enhanced considerably through advances in

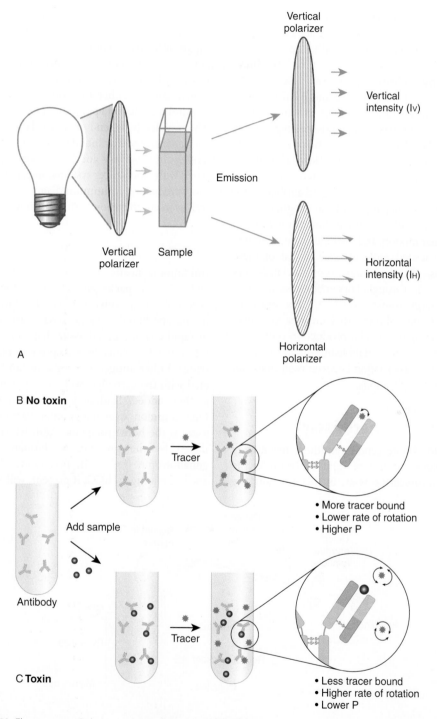

FIGURE 6–10 Fluorescence Polarization. A. In fluorescence polarization immunodiagnostic assays the reaction leads to a shift from vertical-light intensity to horizontal- (polarized) light intensity. When B; more tracer is bound there is a higher polarization (P) then when C; less tracer is bound.

Reproduced from Maragos, C. (2009). Fluorescence polarization immunoassay of mycotoxins: a review. Toxins, 1(2), 196–207.

fluorescence technology. Fluorescence-based sensing of cellular dynamics is a more advanced utility of labeled tracers in immunodiagnostic design, for instance. However, traditional **confocal microscopy** utilizes fluorescent, labeled antibodies to detect the presence and localization of specific surface and intracellular structures (antigens) in live and fixed-cell and tissue preparations (**FIGURE 6–11**). The precise specificity of antibodies toward their antigen and the development of a multitude of fluorophores has created a large number of commercially available tagged antibodies for use in confocal imaging. Confocal imaging is used to locate molecules in three-dimensional space, track cellular motion, and distinguish between two closely associated molecules.[34] The last of these utilizations—distinguishing close associates—was made possible through Förster/fluorescence resonance energy transfer (FRET).[35] For example, investigators have shown FRET imaging to be useful in detecting the cellular production centers for biomarkers of bone metabolism.[36] In all cases, the localization or association between molecules can have clinical implications.

Chemiluminescence Assays

Similar to fluorescence, another technology that employs the use of light emission is the **chemiluminescence** assay. In this reaction, the light is formed by a chemical reaction rather than by light stimulation. Assays of this form resemble the prior forms except that they can be performed similar to enzymatic assays and do not require a powered light source. However, the emitted light, which can last either for hours or milliseconds, requires a detection apparatus. These procedures, which typically depend on an oxidation response, such as are caused by the addition of hydrogen peroxide, can have very good sensitivity when compared with other tracer systems, and are being used more frequently in immunodiagnostic designs as well as in combination with other tracers.

Rapid Immunoassays

Immunodiagnostic assays have been commercialized and packaged to make them more accessible in a wider variety of locations. The membrane-based cassette assays are one type of rapid enzyme-based assay that can give quick reproducible results in a disposable plastic cartridge. Either antigen or antibody can be associated with the cartridge, wherein a patient sample is then added, leading to a colored response. One common over-the-counter version of this assay is the home pregnancy test, which is stimulated by the presence of human chorionic gonadotropin (hCG). In this sandwich, ELISA assay, the antigen, hCG, if present, will bind with

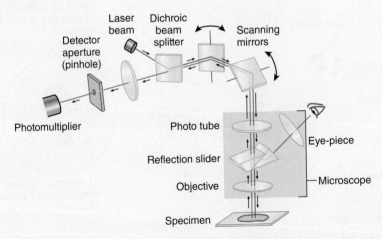

FIGURE 6–11 Structure and Beam Path of a Confocal Microscope.

Modified from Michael H Ross, Wojciech Pawlina. Histology: A Text and Atlas: With Correlated Cell and Molecular Biology, Lippincott Williams & Wilkins, 2015.

the anti-hCG-antibody on the surface of the cassette, leading to an enzymatic color-forming reaction. This test can be modified through a process called immunochromatography, in which the specimen migrates down an absorbent pad toward a detection zone. This is also known as a **lateral flow immunoassay (LFIA)**.[37] Antibodies or antigens immobilized in the detection zone lead to a color-forming response and a second, nonspecific immunoreagent is also used as a control.

Multimodal Assays

In addition to the multitude of single-label immunoassays in existence, multi-label and cross-labeled assays have emerged as well, many of which are proprietary in nature and built for use on specific devices. One example technique is the enzyme-linked fluorescent assay (ELFA), developed for the MiniVIDAS system for use in cortisol (and others) detection.[38] Some are very specialized and utilize overlapping methodologies, such as the Cloned Enzyme-Donor Immunoassay (CEDIA), which uses enzyme fragments that are combined to form a colored product,[8] and the utilization of nanoparticles and electrochemical methods, such as the amperometic immunosensor technology, which combines the enzyme action of HRP with gold nanoparticles for signal detection by electrodes,[39] or the combination of fluorescence with chemiluminescence technology in quantum dot FRET immunoassays.[40] Other complex assays have had a more long-lasting and a more broad reaching impact. The Western blot, for protein separation and detection, which has been used in research and diagnostics for more than 50 years, provides a good example of a technology that often overlaps as an immunoassay with complex diagnostic utilities. Immunohistochemistry also utilizes labeled immunoreagents for detection of changes in tissue surface profiles and has a strong place in immunopathological methods of disease diagnosis and detection. Finally, flow cytometry, a solely automated technique that utilizes fluorescence-labeled antibodies for cell-surface marker detection, is introduced here and discussed in more detail in Chapter 7: Instrumentation and Automation and Chapter 8: Immunophenotyping.

Western Blotting (Immunoblotting)

Western blotting is an electrophoretic technique focused on the motility of proteins, which is augmented by labeling with various reagents including antibodies. It is named for the similar technique for examining the migration of DNA developed by Edwin Southern, called the Southern blot. Similar to the technique of immunoprecipitation (discussed in Chapter 5: Classical Principles of Immunodiagnostics), Western blotting requires the use of an electrophoresis gel, typically through sodium dodecyl sulfate polyacrylamide gel electrophoresis (SDS-PAGE). Cell lysates or serum fractions are loaded into wells unlabeled and run on an SDS-PAGE to separate the proteins by size; various techniques are employed depending on protein type and structure being interrogated. The gel is removed from the electrophoresis device and transferred to a solid support, such as a nitrocellulose membrane strip (**FIGURE 6–12**). Antibodies against the solubilized and denatured proteins are applied (primary antibodies) and are followed by secondary antibodies against the immunoglobulin polymers of the primary antibody, which have been labeled with an enzyme (chemiluminescent, radioisotopic, or fluorescent) and visualized with the appropriate technique. The use of primary and secondary antibodies as well as the addition of a labeled tracer allows for the amplification of the signal. Western blots are commonly used in scientific-discovery efforts as well as the diagnostic laboratory.

The western blot has been used with success for the detection of human immunodeficiency virus (HIV) antibodies, for example. In this modification, a collection of HIV antigens is incorporated into the gel and allowed to run. The fixed antigens are then transferred to nitrocellulose paper, through the process of blotting, to preserve the antigenic signal. The patient serum is then overlaid and detection of antibodies against HIV can be detected, typically indicative of the disease.

Immunohistochemistry (IHC)

Immunohistochemistry (IHC) has a long history of usage in scientific and medical discovery and is used as a technique for the detection and

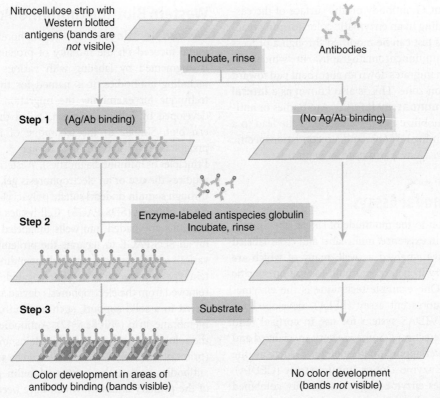

Nitrocellulose strip with Western blotted antigens (bands are *not* visible)

Antibodies

Incubate, rinse

Step 1 (Ag/Ab binding)

(No Ag/Ab binding)

Step 2 Enzyme-labeled antispecies globulin Incubate, rinse

Step 3 Substrate

Color development in areas of antibody binding (bands visible)

No color development (bands *not* visible)

FIGURE 6–12 Antibody bound to nitrocellulose strip after Western Blot. Antigens that have been electrophoretically separated via Western Blot are blotted on mitrocellulose paper.

Courtesy of Diane Leland, PhD, Professor Emeritus, Indiana University School of Medicine.

clinical diagnosis in many autoimmune diseases and a variety of cancers. Specifically, immuno-histochemical detection of CD138; IgG and IgM have been used successfully in differentiating various autoimmune liver disease such as autoimmune hepatitis from primary biliary cirrhosis.[41] It has become an essential tool in the field of surgical pathology.[42] Other immunofluorescent (IFL) technologies, similar to (IHC), have also been used quite successfully in the detection of autoimmune disorders.[43] Likewise, IHC is useful for the detection of tumor tissue through the development of directed antibodies focused on mutated proteins[44,45] or misexpressed surface receptors.[42] IHC is performed by applying a targeted antibody to a paraffin embedded, fixed, or nonfixed tissue specimen. A combination of multimodal labeled tracers can be used for detection. The use of positive and negative controls allows for determination of the patient-specimen status.

Flow Cytometry

Flow cytometric analysis, or **flow cytometry**, is most often performed with at least one, but usually more, fluorescently labeled markers. Fluorescent antibodies for a wide variety of surface and intracellular markers called cluster of differentiation (CD) markers are commercially available, and help in defining cellular subsets found in peripheral blood and bone marrow. Unlike IHC, which looks at specific tissue sections, flow cytometry is utilized to determine entire populations of cells in a specific body fluid, most commonly peripheral blood. It is also useful for disaggregated tissue samples. Laboratories routinely run assays to detect the absolute and relative numbers of immunological cells, such as T and B cells, in order to determine the patient's underlying immune status. The CD4/CD8 ratio, which flips during late-stage HIV infection, is one example of the clinical utility of flow cytometry.[46] A later chapter on immunophenotyping is dedicated to describing the CD markers useful for immune status determination, how these assays can aid medical practitioners in diagnosing both chronic and acute diseases, and a discussion of the method of performance.

Assay Validation

For every analyte to be examined in the clinical setting, a series of considerations is necessary before implementation. A key step in this consideration is what level of analytical sensitivity is necessary to provide the best clinical utility. Assay validation, also known as method validation, must be performed to ensure not just analytical significance but also clinical significance. Diagnostic laboratories rely on the thorough research performed by assay developers in determining the efficacy and working range of a particular immunoreagent. Prior to marketing a product, any analyte (biomarker) used in an immunoassay is first validated to have a clinical correlation to a given disease before undergoing a series of clinical trials.[25] Once marketed, it is the duty of the diagnostic lab to determine between viable commercial products or to build its own in-house product based on its own clinical needs, cost, time, and resource constraints.

CASE STUDY

Comparison of an EIA Immunoassay With qRT-PCR

This case report is adapted from Tate et al., *Emerg Infect Dis*, 2013.[47]

In a method comparison, two assays are examined for specific areas of analytical or clinical efficacy. Enzyme immunoassays (EIAs), such as the Premier Rotaclone product produced by Meridian Bioscience, are traditionally used for detection rotavirus in infants and children. Specifically, the EIA sandwich assay uses a monoclonal antibody against a rotavirus group, specific antigen produced by the sixth viral gene. For this assay, a fecal specimen is taken from children with acute gastroenteritis or diarrhea and dispensed into a microwell of the microtiter plate provided. This is followed by the addition of the enzyme conjugate included in the kit, incubation, washing, and addition of enzyme substrates that combine with the bound antigen to form a blue-colored response.[48] In the following report, this standard method was compared with quantitative reverse transcription polymerase chain reaction (**qRT-PCR**) (See **BOX 6–2**). See box for more details on this method.

Beginning in October of 2008, fecal specimens were collected from over 500 children less than 5 years old with diarrhea at three vaccine surveillance sites in the United States and tested via EIA for the rotavirus antigen. These values were compared with qRT-PCR, which measures the amount of viral RNA in the specimen.[47] Twenty-four percent of these children were found to be positive for rotavirus by EIA, but rotavirus was detected 10% more often by qRT-PCR.

Is qRT-PCR a Better Clinical Indicator of Rotavirus-Mediated Acute Gastroenteritis?

Although the qRT-PCR method was able to detect more rotavirus infections, i.e., providing greater analytical sensitivity, the subjects who were positive by qRT-PCR alone had lower viral loads and were less likely to have the whole genome detected than those who were positive by both EIA and qRT-PCR. Finally, a three-dose vaccination was effective only against those patients who were positive by EIA and qRT-PCR and not by qRT-PCR alone. This suggests that while more analytically sensitive, the qRT-PCR result was not as clinically relevant. In this case, the presence of viral RNA is not equivalent to the presence of viral protein in determining disease causality.

(continues)

CASE STUDY (Continued)

A DEEPER LOOK BOX 6–2 Quantitative RT-PCR (qRT-PCR) Method of Detection

In real-time reverse transcription polymerase chain reaction (RT-PCR), fluorescent molecules are used as reports of the production of amplified gene products. Thus, genetic amplification and detection are combined in a single step. Quantification of this process is based on the number of amplification cycles needed for the gene of interest to be detected reliably.[49] Therefore, the fewer cycles to fluorescent detection is an indication of more gene product in the original sample.

When compared with a traditional, protein-based immunoassay, two things are significant in interpreting our results. First, qRT-PCR detects gene products, most often mRNA, and immunoassays typically detect protein-based antigens. Second, the limit of detection using a PCR-based approach is substantially lower than an antibody-based detection method. However, in most cases, such as the case of viral disease, it is the protein product that is needed to facilitate the spread of disease, not the gene product alone. Gene products may be sequestered in a cell to prevent protein production, or be mutated in such a way as to produce a nonviable protein. Neither of these possibilities can be concluded from qRT-PCR alone.

Critical Thinking Questions

1. Why is there a difference in sensitivity between these two methods?
2. Why isn't sensitivity connected to disease correlation?

▶ References

1. Edwards R, Blincko S, Howes I. *Principles of immunodiagnostic tests and their development: with specific use of radioisotopes as tracers.* In: Edwards R, ed. *Immunodiagnostics: A Practical Approach*: Oxford University Press; 1999.

2. Jackson TM, Ekins RP. Theoretical limitations on immunoassay sensitivity. Current practice and potential advantages of fluorescent Eu3+ chelates as non-radioisotopic tracers. *J Immunol Methods.* 1986;87(1):13–20.

3. Mullins GR, Bazydlo LAL. *Technical Comparison of Immunoassay and Mass Spectrometry.* MedicalLab Management. Vol 5: Ridgewood Medical Media LLC; 2016.

4. Chapman RS. Immunoassays in Clinical Chemistry (Principle of Immunometric Assays). *In vitro radionuclide techniques in medical diagnosis*: International Atomic Energy Agency; 1998.

5. Bolton AE, Lee-Own V, McLean RK, et al. Three different radioiodination methods for human spleen ferritin compared. *Clin Chem.* 1979;25(10):1826–1830.

6. Jeanson A, Cloes JM, Bouchet M, et al. Comparison of conjugation procedures for the preparation of monoclonal antibody-enzyme conjugates. *J Immunol Methods.* 1988;111(2):261–270.

7. Howes I, Blincko S, Little J, et al. *Enzyme-labelled tests with colorimetric, fluorimwtric and chemiluminescent detection systems.* In: Edwards R, ed. Immunodiagnostics: A Practical Approach: Oxford University Press; 1999.

8. Darwish IA. Immunoassay methods and their applications in pharmaceutical analysis: basic methodology and recent advances. *Int J Biomed Sci.* 2006;2(3):217–235.

9. Blincko S, Rongsen S, Decun S, et al. *Solid-phase supports.* In: Edwards R, ed. Immunodiagnostics: A Practical Approach: Oxford University Press; 1999.

10. Hosoda H, Tsukamoto R, Tamura S, et al. Bound/free separation methods in steroid enzyme immunoassay with monoclonal antibody. *Chem Pharm Bull.* 1988; 36(9):3525–3531.

11. Peoples MC, Phillips TM, Karnes HT. Demonstration of a direct capture immunoaffinity separation for C-reactive protein using a capillary-based microfluidic device. *J Pharm Biomed Anal.* 2008;48(2):376–382.

12. Shipkova M, Petrova DT, Rosler AE, et al. Comparability and imprecision of 8 frequently used commercially available immunoassays for therapeutic drug monitoring. *Ther Drug Monit.* 2014;36(4):433–441.

13. Chapman RS. *Radiolabelling for Immunoassays*. In vitro radionuclide techniques in medical diagnosis: International Atomic Energy Agency; 1998.

14. Safarcik K, Brozmanová H, Bartos V, et al. Evaluation and comparison of therapeutic monitoring of whole-blood levels of cyclosporin A and its metabolites in renal transplantation by HPLC and RIA methods. *Clin Chim Acta*. 2001;310(2):165–171.

15. Green-Graif Y, Ewan PW. Diagnostic value of the skin-prick test and RAST assay in insect sting allergy. *Clin Allergy*. 1987;17(5):431–438.

16. Blanca M, Moreno F, Mayorga C, et al. The Nature of the carrier in the RAST assay influences the capacity for detecting IgE antibodies to penicillins. *J Clin Immunoassay*. 1994;17(3):166–170.

17. Wahyuni S, Van Ree R, Mangali A, et al. Comparison of an enzyme linked immunosorbent assay (ELISA) and a radioallergosorbent test (RAST) for detection of IgE antibodies to Brugia malayi. *Parasite Immunol*. 2003;25(11–12):609–614.

18. Lequin RM. Enzyme immunoassay (EIA)/enzyme-linked immunosorbent assay (ELISA). *Clin Chem*. 2005;51 (12):2415–2418.

19. Voller A, Bidwell DE. Enzyme-immunoassays for antibodies in measles, cytomegalovirus infections and after rubella vaccination. *Br J Exp Pathol*. 1976;57(2): 243–247.

20. Seydack M. *Immunoassays: Basic Concepts, Physical Chemistry and Validation*. In: Resch-Genger U, ed. Standardization and Quality Assurance in Fluorescence Measurments II. Vol 6: Springer; 2008.

21. Biological S. ELISA Encyclopedia. 2016.

22. Ricchiuti V. *Immunoassay-Based Technologies for the Measurement of Biological Materials Used for Biomarkers Discovery and Translational Research*. Biomarkers: In Medicine, Drug Discovery, and Environmental Health: Wiley; 2010.

23. Toltzis P, Nerandzic MM, Saade E, et al. High proportion of false-positive Clostridium difficile enzyme immunoassays for toxin A and B in pediatric patients. *Infect Control Hosp Epidemiol*. 2012;33(2):175–179.

24. Voller A, Bidwell DE, Bartlett A. Enzyme immunoassays in diagnostic medicine. Theory and practice. *Bull World Health Organ*. 1976;53(1):55–65.

25. Köhler K, Seitz H. Validation processes of protein biomarkers in serum—a cross platform comparison. *Sensors (Basel)*. 2012;12(9):12710–12728.

26. Comley DJ. Enzyme-linked immunosorbent assays (ELISA): recent innovations take analyte detection to new levels. 2012. http://www.ddw-online.com/screening /p191009-elisa-assays:-recent-innovations-take-analyte -detection-to-new-levels-fall-12.html.

27. Kannoujia DK, Nahar P. Pressure: a novel tool for enzyme-linked immunosorbent assay procedure. *Biotechniques*. 2009;46(6):468–472.

28. van Weemen BK, Schuurs AH. Immunoassay using antibody—enzyme conjugates. *FEBS Lett*. 1974;43(2): 215–218.

29. Rininsland FH, Helms T, Asaad RJ, et al. Granzyme B ELISPOT assay for ex vivo measurements of T-cell immunity. *J Immunol Methods*. 2000;240(1–2):143–155.

30. Nielsen K, Lin M, Gall D, et al. Fluorescence polarization immunoassay: detection of antibody to Brucella abortus. *Methods*. 2000;22(1):71–76.

31. Maragos C. Fluorescence polarization immunoassay of mycotoxins: a review. *Toxins (Basel)*. 2009;1(2):196–207.

32. Ullman EF, Schwarzberg M, Rubenstein KE. Fluorescent excitation transfer immunoassay. A general method for determination of antigens. *J Biol Chem*. 1976;251(14): 4172–4178.

33. Calvin J, Burling K, Blow C, et al. Evaluation of fluorescence excitation transfer immunoassay for measurement of specific proteins. *J Immunol Methods*. 1986;86(2):249–256.

34. Fritzky L, Lagunoff D. Advanced methods in fluorescence microscopy. *Anal Cell Pathol (Amst)*. 2013;36(1–2): 5–17.

35. Bunt G, Wouters FS. FRET from single to multiplexed signaling events. *Biophys Rev*. 2017;9(2):119–129.

36. Chung CI, Makino R, Ohmuro-Matsuyama Y, et al. Development of a fluorescent protein-antibody Förster resonance energy transfer probe for the detection and imaging of osteocalcin. *J Biosci Bioeng*. 2017;123(2): 272–276.

37. Connolly R, O'Kennedy R. Magnetic lateral flow immunoassay test strip development—considerations for proof of concept evaluation. *Methods*. 2017;116:132–140.

38. Proverbio D, Perego R, Spada E, et al. Comparison of VIDAS and radioimmunoassay methods for measurement of cortisol concentration in bovine serum. *ScientificWorldJournal*. 2013;2013:216569.

39. Hu W, Li CM. Nanomaterial-based advanced immuno-assays. *Wiley Interdisc Rev Nanomed Nanobiotechnol*. 2011;3(2):119–133.

40. Goryacheva OA, Beloglazova NV, Vostrikova AM, et al. Lanthanide-to-quantum dot Förster resonance energy transfer (FRET): application for immunoassay. *Talanta*. 2017;164:377–385.

41. Abe K, Takahashi A, Nozawa Y, et al. The utility of IgG, IgM, and CD138 immunohistochemistry in the evaluation of autoimmune liver diseases. *Med Mol Morphol*. 2014; 47(3):162–168.

42. Blind C, Koepenik A, Pacyna-Gengelbach M, et al. Antigenicity testing by immunohistochemistry after tissue oxidation. *J Clin Pathol*. 2008;61(1):79–83.

43. Bogdanos DP, Invernizzi P, Mackay IR, et al. Autoimmune liver serology: current diagnostic and clinical challenges. *World J Gastroenterol*. 2008;14(21):3374–3387.

44. Zagzag J, Pollack A, Dultz L, et al. Clinical utility of immunohistochemistry for the detection of the BRAF

v600e mutation in papillary thyroid carcinoma. *Surgery.* 2013;154(6):1199-1204; discussion 1204–1205.

45. Bruegl AS, Djordjevic B, Urbauer DL, et al. Utility of MLH1 methylation analysis in the clinical evaluation of Lynch Syndrome in women with endometrial cancer. *Curr Pharm Des.* 2014;20(11):1655–1663.

46. Clift IC. Diagnostic flow cytometry and the AIDS pandemic. *Lab Med.* 2015;46(3):e59–e64.

47. Tate JE, Mijatovic-Rustempasic S, Tam KI, et al. Comparison of 2 assays for diagnosing rotavirus and evaluating vaccine effectiveness in children with gastroenteritis. *Emerg Infect Dis.* 2013;19(8):1245–1252.

48. Premier Rotaclone: EIA for the detection of Rotavirus Antigen in Human Fecal Samples [package insert]. Cincinnati, OH, USA: Meridian Bioscience; 2015.

49. Bustin SA, Benes V, Nolan T, et al. Quantitative real-time RT-PCR—a perspective. *J Mol Endocrinol.* 2005;34(3): 597–601.

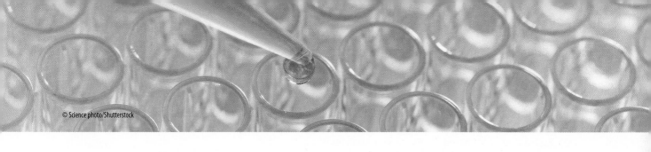

© Science photo/Shutterstock

CHAPTER 7

Serological and Immunodiagnostic Instrumentation and Automation

Ian Clift, PhD, MLS(ASCP)^{CM}

LEARNING OBJECTIVES

Upon completion of this chapter, the reader should be able to:

1. Examine the use of automation on test costs dependent on test volume.
2. Discuss equipment specifications important for the automation of immunoassays.
3. Explore the concept of total laboratory automation and assess its affect on laboratory operations and personnel.

(continues)

(Continued)

4. Compare several major analyzers that utilize immunoassays, based on their function, scope and system design.
5. Estimate test cost based on equipment/analyzer costs.
6. Discuss Flow cytometric use of antibodies.
7. Identify appropriate fluorescent antibodies based on laser availability.

▶ Instrumentation in Serology and Immunodiagnostics

Following the trends in technological innovation, the number of semiautomated and automated instruments in the clinical diagnostic laboratory has expanded exponentially since the middle of the 20th century.[1] In 2013, the estimated total market value for clinical automation was 3 billion U.S. dollars with the top shares of that market going to robotics-handling companies like Tecan (14%) and Perkin-Elmer (10%).[2] Signal detectors, include radioactive counters that measure gamma or beta radiation found in specimens; spectrophotometers, which measure absorbance or optical density of chromophores; fluorimeters, which measure intensity and polarization of emitted fluorescence; and **luminometers**, which measure luminescent light emission. They have historically been the instruments of choice in immunodiagnostic examinations.[3] It is also not surprising that the principles of serology and immunodiagnostics were adapted for utility in more advanced devices found in other parts of the clinical laboratory. Early attempts at automation for serological diagnostics handled simple, but time-consuming tasks, such as volume dispensing and titration (**FIGURE 7–1**). Indeed, some of the earliest serological techniques including **turbidimetry** and **nephelometry** are commonly used in a wide

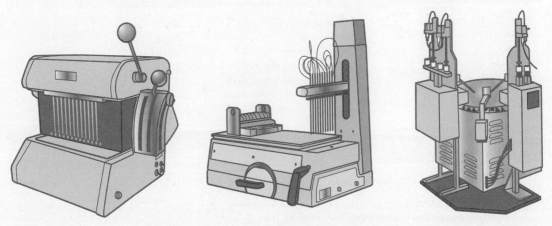

FIGURE 7–1 Early sera dispensers. The Weitz automatic titration apparatus, the Sequeira measured volume dispenser, and the Trotman diluent and reagent dispenser.

Reproduced from Taylor CE. Serological techniques. Journal of Clinical Pathology, 1969;s2–3:14–19.

range of clinical instruments; furthermore, ligand-based assays such as FPIA, EIA, RIA, and others have long been incorporated into clinical chemistry analyzers,[1] some of the first fully automated laboratory machines on the market. In addition, basic techniques, described in more detail elsewhere, have been modified and advanced upon using our more robust understanding of technologies such as electronics, optics, computing, and robotics.

In the 21st century, the field of immunodiagnostics is set to be disrupted by a series of low-cost and high-throughput approaches that will take testing out of the traditional laboratory and into the field, as well as see a consolidation of testing into regional and national laboratory and hospital organizations (**BOX 7-1**). Point-of-care testing (POCT), routinely seen in blood glucose monitoring and urinalysis, is now becoming more common for traditionally centralized serological and immunodiagnostic methods such as immunoassay-based hemoglobin A1c testing.[4] Fast, reliable communications to regional

centers have created an economic advantage for the development of centralized high throughput specialty centers as well. Both POCT and high throughput approaches rely on automation. Below are a few advanced techniques, traditionally incorporated into instruments and used in the clinical immunodiagnostic lab, which are now being incorporated into point-of-care and mobile devices as well as fully automated machines.

Biosensors

As in previous discussions of immunoassay design, the fundamentals of diagnostics require a method of detection, which, in immunodiagnostics, is traditionally via an antibody-antigen interaction. However, in automated systems, a conversion from human detection to computer detection is achieved via the use of what is known as a **biosensor**. Generally, biosensors, not to be confused with biomarkers, are analytical tools that convert a molecular target

---

A DEEPER LOOK BOX 7-1 POCT, Automation, and the Lab Profession

The rise of POCT, shortage of laboratory professionals, and increased assay automation has led to some concern over the future status of the lab profession. Indeed, a major decision by the Centers for Medicare and Medicaid Services (CMS) in April of 2016 expanded the definition of biological science degrees to include nursing degrees for the purpose of performing laboratory testing. Although this ruling was fought vigorously by laboratory professional organizations such as the ASCP and ASCLS,[5] including a petition signed by 35,000 individuals, it serves as an example of the changes that could disrupt the clinical laboratory profession. CLIA guidelines suggest that waived testing can be performed only by medical personnel without a biological science-based degree, yet increased automation means that more and more tests will be given CLIA-waived status in the near future.

POCT and automation have another potential disruptive effect on the laboratory profession as well, as they shift the focus away from hospital-based laboratory operations toward centralized laboratories, with fewer employees, and highly automated testing in decentralized clinics run by alternatively trained healthcare professionals, such as nurses and medical doctors. Unfortunately, these individuals are less well trained in the principles behind the testing performed or the variables that can invalidate a test result. In western European countries, such as Germany and Belgium, nearly 25% of all tests are POCT, and in Japan, known for its lower medical costs, most laboratory testing is performed in high-throughput, centralized facilities.[4] Cost plays a significant role in policy change in healthcare and will, therefore, undoubtedly favor the least costly strategies as long as patient safety does not become a factor.

into a measureable signal via a transducer. These have been successfully used in the detection of glucose levels, pregnancy, and various infectious diseases.[6] Similar to antibody-antigen detection, biosensors can be either labeled or label-free in design. The selectivity and sensitivity of immunoassays has made them the first choice in the development of biosensors such as the NRL (Naval Research Laboratory) Array Biosensor, devised for rapid, onsite detection and screening for biohazards through both kinetic and affinity-based binding interactions.[7] Three widely used label-free biosensors are optical, electrical, and mechanical **transducers**.[6] Optical transducers come in two main varieties: surface plasmon resonance (SRP), in which the signal is based on the total internal reflection of light leading to changes in returned light detection; and backscattering interferometry (BI), which consists of a laser light source focused onto a microfluidic channel leading to very specific interference patterns, which can be used to measure molecular binding/interfacing events.[6] All unlabeled transducers such as electrical transducers, which can be used to incorporate a signal into miniaturized hardware and mechanical transducers, such as quartz crystal microbalances that can measure changes in force and motion, have all been incorporated into advanced assay and instrument design.[6] However, the most commonly used biosensors are labeled. These sensors are traditionally designed with a solid support whereby a detector agent recognizes an analyte. In addition to the luminescent, fluorescent, radioactive, and chemiluminescent detectors described in association with manual immunoassay design, several other labelled detection systems have been incorporated into instrument design. These include biobarcoding, which uses barcode DNA (i.e., oligonucleotides) as a surrogate for signal amplification; metal nanoparticles, such as gold and silver used to enhance SRP of a specific molecule; and magnetic nanoparticles, used in a variety of methods for amplifying detection.[6]

Microfluidics

Microfluidics systems present a technology that could eventually reduce the size and cost associated with immunoassays, including in resource-strapped countries.[8] Microfluidics is one of the major technical components of the "lab of a chip" POCTs, along with miniaturization, wireless communications, and micromachining.[4] Microfluidic chips have commonly been designed from polymers, silicon, and glass. Despite most microfluidic devices continuing to be found in association with larger instruments, cartridge-based microfluidic systems have seen a dramatic growth in the past 5 years and, as of 2016, 23 cancer screening companion diagnostic (CDx) tests were available for the point-of-care market.[9] Though most of the systems are for non-protein biomarker detection, at least three protein based models are focused on detection via an immunohistochemical approach[9]. Several microfluidic-based systems including fluid nanoarrays, fluidic-integrated microarrays, and bead-based fluidic technologies, have emerged. Fluorescent barcodes have been designed for use in microfluidic systems that facilitate easier identification of specific antigens in immunoassays.[10] However, the costs associated with the lithography process remains labor intensive and costly to mass produce. Microfluidic systems can reduce the volume of liquid specimen from 100s of µl to the 2 to 5 µl range.[9] The use of relatively cheap electrochemical biosensors in combination with microfluidics in the performance of amperometric immunoassays has been used with some success.

Multiplexed Immunoassays

There is significant evidence that the analysis of multiple markers has a greater potential for diagnostics than single markers, specifically for cancer serology.[9,11] Although not always easily available, especially in resource-strapped countries,[8] multiplexed immunoassays have increased sensitivity and diagnostic productivity by reducing the turnaround time for antigenic detection. Due to the high heterogeneity among cancer cell populations, only 24 biomarkers have been approved by the U.S. Food and Drug Administration (FDA) and, therefore, it has been suggested that the testing of a group of biomarkers may be important for the successful detection of cancer.[9] The large majority of commercial tests that examine complex disease are either genetics-based or multiplexed, microtiter, plate-based immunoassays. However, a considerable number of experimental systems that include chemically etched arrays, printed electrodes, microfluidic systems, and 3D printing approaches have all been examined for creating low-cost automation that may breach into the POCT market.[9]

Principles of Automation

Automation is the process of increasing the utilization of equipment rather than manual labor for the performance of a production process. In the clinical diagnostic laboratory, automation is the process of reducing the number of manually performed tests through an increasing reliance on instrumentation and computer-controlled analyzers. However, in the current era, automation may also be indicated by a reduction of manual steps through using kit-based assays that require only limited intervention to obtain a result, e.g., requiring only the addition of a specimen and recording of a result. Even these assays can be further automated by computerizing the detection and analysis of the result. Furthermore, automation can be broken down into instrument automation and laboratory automation. Equipment automation is typically performed by incorporating manual assay elements within a machine that performs many of the steps required for processing the specimen to assay completion.

Most clinical analyzers typically incorporate elements common to the manual methods including computerized sample identification and worklist generation, transfer of samples to reaction vessels, incubations, signal generation, as well as calibration and quality control, in addition to report generation and export to laboratory information systems (LIS)[3] [**FIGURE 7–2**]. Adoption of instruments and analyzers in clinical immunodiagnostics are chosen based on the needs of the individual laboratory, including features such as the cost of operation, assay test menu, throughput, and space considerations. Additionally, contemporary analyzers are considered more valuable based on the flexibility of the hardware and software systems; specifically, functional, structural, and throughput flexibility of hardware should be considered when adopting a new piece of equipment.[12]

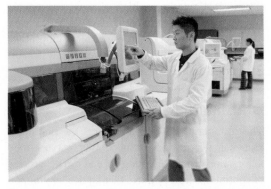
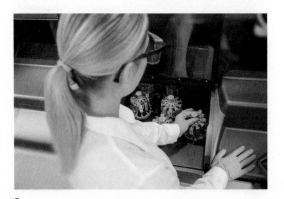

A   B

FIGURE 7–2 Automated instrument operations. Technologists enter data **(A)** and load specimens **(B)** on a VITROS analyzer.

Courtesy of Ortho Clinical Diagnostics and Allan Shoemake.

The first automated analyzers appeared in the mid-1950s with the demonstration of the Technicon, which could, in 2.5 minutes, produce results for sugar, calcium, and urea from a small quantity of blood[13] (**FIGURE 7–3**). As technologies mature, they are eventually incorporated into more complex instruments that utilize components of prior systems. As such, barcode readers, electronic pipetters, shakers, incubators, and reagent dispensing systems for example, still commercially available as stand-alone equipment, are now commonly incorporated into the front end and specimen processing units of complex analyzers. Furthermore, software tools, often called middleware, have facilitated the connection of previously separate operations.[13] **Middleware** has increased the utility of commercial analyzers by providing software that performs autoverification, automatic dilutions, and reflex testing, for example. These assembly-line-like analyzers increase workflow efficiency and reduce human error, and are often called semiautomated or fully automated analyzers.

Semiautomated analyzers often do not incorporate all of the steps required for specimen processing, most often excluding pre- and postanalytical steps, and sometimes excluding some analytical steps that require manual-specimen intervention prior to dispensing them within the analyzer. Fully automated analyzers often begin as early as removing the specimen from the specimen collection tube and dispensing it within a reaction vessel, and go as far as reporting the result within the LIS.

Laboratory automation, or total laboratory automation (TLA), emerged in the late 1980s when Dr. Masahide Sasaki at the Kochi Medical School in Kochi, Japan, began to use robots to load and unload analyzers, and transported samples by conveyor belts to analyzers in his laboratory.[14] Full laboratory automation has now been spearheaded by several commercial companies and is expected to continue to grow as an aging laboratory workforce and additional automation options pressure the market.

▶ Instrument Automation

As devices were seen to have reached maturity, the next step was the incorporation of more than one analyzer in a series, as was seen in the modular analyzers appearing at the end of the 20th century when, for instance, chemistry and immunoassay analyzers were combined into a single analyzer.[15] Instrument automation has been strongly advocated for in all areas of the laboratory, primarily due to the reduction in human errors, transcription errors, improved traceability, reductions in manual inputs, and reductions in turnaround times, particularly in high throughput operations.[16] Three instrumental designs have been employed with success in the clinical laboratory including continuous flow, discrete analysis, and centrifugal analysis systems.

Continuous Flow

The continuous flow system marks the first automated analyzers and provided the first test-tube automation from beginning to end.[17] The process of continuous flow requires that liquids be pumped through a system of tubing, air bubbles, and cleaning solutions, typically stored adjacent to the analyzer, separate samples as they are passed through the same network sequentially.[15] Multiple tests requiring the same parameters can, therefore, be run at an

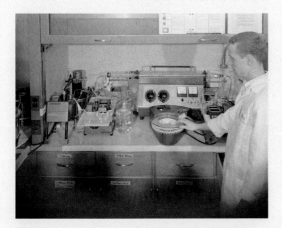

FIGURE 7–3 An early analyzer called the AutoAnalyzer produced by Technicon circa 1966. It used a continuous-flow analysis technique to determine protein-bound iodine.
Courtesy of C. Duncan/CDC.

extremely rapid rate; furthermore, advanced continuous flow analyzers can run multiple assays on a single sample. They have lost favor in the clinical diagnostic world due to issues with sample carryover and liquid reagent waste. However, technical improvements in design and materials have considerably reduced some of the issues with waste and carryover.

Discrete Analysis

With discrete analyzers, samples are separated into separate containers, i.e., tube or cuvettes, and are, therefore, capable of running multiple assays at the same time. They have become one of the most popular designs.

Centrifugal Analysis

Another useful instrumentation design feature utilizes centrifugation and is called centrifugal analysis. In centrifugal analysis, liquid samples are spun at a high rate of speed, and the sample reaction is read at the perimeter of the spinning rotor. The major advantage to centrifugal analysis is that samples can be run in a batch and read almost simultaneously. Laboratories that have a significant workload for a single assay may find these analyzers especially useful.

Liquid Handling Systems and Robotics

Most, if not all, laboratory analyzers must have the capacity to perform some liquid handling functions, from simple dispensing to aliquoting, mixing, and washing. Contemporary devices can typically aliquot a range of liquid volumes from either a sample or a reagent reservoir. Liquid handling systems can be seen in an array of clinical instruments from generalized chemistry analyzers to flow cytometers (**FIGURE 7–4**).

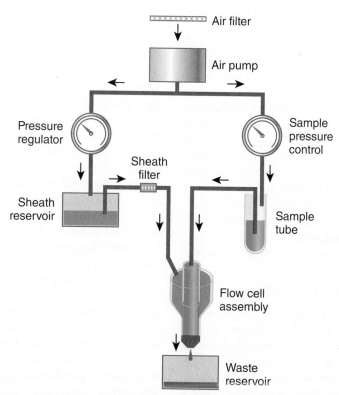

FIGURE 7–4 Simplified fluidics design for flow cytometers. From National Center for Infectious Diseases (NCID).

Robotic liquid handling systems have made significant advances due to their utility in clinical diagnostic analysis. For example, the use of microbeads functionalized for detection requires numerous time-consuming repetitive steps, such as repetitive pipetting, liquid exchange, washing, and mixing, that have been automated successfully using automated workstations from TECAN, Sartorius Stedim Biotech, and Perkin Elmer.[18] In the reference laboratory setting, the development of batches of functionalized microbeads for utility in laboratory-developed tests (LDT) using robots, such as the TECAN Freedom EVO, have played a role in increasing the utility of machines such as the fluorescence-based Luminex flow cytometric system.[19]

Liquid dispensing was one of the first processes to find a niche in the automation market. With all liquid handling technologies, overcoming surface adhesion resulting from dispensing viscous samples at nano- and microliter volumes has been dominant in performance.[20] Two significant methods have been developed to overcome surface adhesion: the first, called contact dispensing, in which surface tension is overcome by contact between the reservoir sample and dispensed sample using a drag back action; and noncontact dispensing, in which liquid is ejected under various forms of force.[20] **Noncontact dispensing** mitigates issues of cross-contamination between samples, and is performed using technologies derived from the ink-jet printing industry including solenoid; relying on the speed of a solenoid valve; piezoelectric, in which an electric signal leads to change in pressure within a capillary tube, allowing the release of nanoliter quantities; and **acoustic dispensing**, which uses focused acoustic energy to control the volume of ejected liquid.[20]

Liquid Handling Robot Design

Liquid handling robots are often built with one or two articulating arms that withdraw preprogrammed quantities of liquid using a modified multichannel pipettor, and which can move back and forth from sample reservoirs to microplates, dispensing and mixing the reagents. Other systems, such as the KingFisher from Thermo Electron,

use magnetics and disposable tips to move liquid-containing magnetic beads from one cuvette to the next.[18] Both well-designed dispensing parts such as actuators, dispensing heads, and substrates, as well as robotically controlled washing modules, sensors, and dispensing parts, are needed for accurate automation of liquid handling.

Total Laboratory Automation

Full laboratory automation has been underway in many high-throughput facilities around the world. Total laboratory automation (TLA) using robots to load and transport samples from analyzers and around the lab,[14] was first implemented in Japan by Dr. Masahide Sasaki. Full laboratory automation has now been spearheaded by several commercial companies, and is expected to continue to grow as an aging laboratory workforce and additional automation options pressure the market. Importantly, fully automated laboratories require personnel to be more adept at mechanical system maintenance than less automated environments.

Although currently found only in high-throughput laboratories, the aging laboratory workforce and increasing number of automation choices continue to increase the utility of total laboratory automation (TLA). Organizations such as the Clinical laboratory standards institute (CLSI) have produced guidelines for laboratory automation such as the AUTO03-A2, or Functional Control Model, which describes the relationship between devices, LIS, software, and hardware components.[14] Others, such as the American Society for Testing and Materials, have developed standardization guidelines for the integration of equipment within the laboratory space called the Laboratory Equipment Control Interface Specification (LECIS), which define a uniform computer control message passing communication protocols among devices, servers, and LIS systems.[21] These automated systems, often referred to as laboratory automation systems of LAS, are defined within the standards to include calculations of the aliquots for each sample based on tests ordered, the routing of samples to preanalytical processing equipment and analyzers, recapping of samples after testing, and the retention of samples for recall.

Total automation first found its way into centralized core facilities, where efficiency determined by turnaround time (TAT) has been shown to significantly increase in individual labs as a result. In one study, for example, the implementation of an automated tube registration and sorting system reduced the TAT for routine chemistry immunoassays, CBCs, and coagulation samples by a significant amount.[22] Automation has been spreading to other units of the clinical laboratory where immunodiagnostics and serological assays are more commonly performed, such as the blood bank and microbiology laboratory. In the case of blood banks, the serological systems must be integrated with components of the laboratory information systems that handle blood management and unit tracking and likewise; in microbiology, total automation reduces human intervention in the many specimen-processing steps prior to and after analysis of microbial cultures. Two companies, BD and Copan, have partial automation solutions available for the microbiology laboratory, while BD also provides a TLA package which provides for all steps in microbial specimen processing, incubation, and imaging, resulting in one automated setup.[23] However, total automation is focused more on workflow, computational, and mechanical operations of specimen processing, rather than on the serological and immunodiagnostic testing performed and is, therefore, only briefly referenced in this volume.

Laboratory Information Systems

One key automation technology found in most contemporary diagnostic laboratories is the LIS. The typical laboratory workflow now requires the uploading of clinical test results into a LIS system, whether they come from manual or automated systems. However, with many automated analyzers, these data can be set to upload to the system with or without the intervention of laboratory personnel or pathologists, depending of the type of test to be released. LIS systems require appropriate dedicated infrastructure including servers to store the data, and end-user devices, such as personal computers, monitors, scanners, and network access.[24]

At its core, an LIS is a database system that stores and allows access to data from the laboratory tests performed. These LIS directories provide definitions, terminology, test release criteria, and other formatting information that streamlines the workflow in the laboratory. Diagnostic tests, ordered by a physician, often move from a hospital information system to the LIS where specimens are registered, or accessioned, into the system in association with the patient. All specimens can be associated with a single patient reducing the inadvertent performance of duplicate tests, but individual specimens from a single patient are also designated with an individual identifier, allowing for the test results to be associated with the specimen.[24] Results stored in the LIS can be useful for tracking a number of metrics including test volume, average and shifting test values, specific assay turnaround times, and correlations of daily results with control and calibration schedules. Furthermore, LIS systems incorporated into laboratory automation systems can perform calculations that lead to reflex testing, notifications regarding abnormal values, and possible duplicate test orders.

▶ Serology Analyzers

As early as the 1960s, the automation of clinical serology was underway, and the term "automation" was in use, specifically with the advent of the so-called "automatic" pipette as well as automated serological dispensers, such as the Weitz automatic titration apparatus developed in 1967, and other automated dispensers developed for dilutions and reagent delivery[25] (**FIGURE 7–1**).

Many serological assays performed manually during the 20th century have found their way to automated analyzers. These assays, typically categorized as either microbial serology or transfusion serology, have been automated in a variety of ways. Starting at the turn of the century, very few semiautomated and automated analyzers for transfusion services, which reduced errors through saved results and less human error, made their way to market.[26] By the first decade of the 21st century, automated serological testing in the lab often led to lower costs when compared with manual methods. Factors that reduced the adoption of automated serology technologies included the abundance of well-trained technologists, and difficulties in designing automated serological methods used primarily in the blood bank.[27] However, with workplace shortages in laboratory science and the technical limitations overcome, the 21st century is likely to see widespread adoption of these analyzer systems.

Principles

In transfusion services, instruments are capable of performing ABO and Rh typing, antibody identification, antigen typing, direct antiglobulin testing (DAT), and donor confirmations.[26] The earliest instruments in this field set the standard for the currently available models by performing several common serological assays including hemagglutination, gel cards, and solid support screening.[26] The Ortho Vision® Analyzer, which received FDA premarket approval in 2015, is the descendent of the ProVue® system developed by Ortho Clinical Diagnostics and still utilizes the proprietary gel card system used in the ProVue® called the ID-mirotyping system (ID-MTS). This gel system first made its appearance as a popular modification to manual methods, in which cards could

be spun on specially made centrifugal systems and checked manually, before finding their place in semiautomated and, finally, fully automated instruments such as the Ortho Vision and Vision Max Analyzers (**FIGURE 7–5**). Other technologies, such as column agglutination, erythrocyte-magnetized, and the solid-phase, red-cell adherence assay, developed to overcome limitations in traditional blood bank tube assays, have also been incorporated into advanced analyzer designs.[16,28]

In microbiology, instrumentation became more readily available for identifying microorganisms. Many of these devices used DNA approaches to identification, but others continued to use immunodiagnostic approaches. Furthermore, serological assays for autoimmune diseases such as systemic lupus erythematosus and others have recently been examined using automated technologies compared with traditional methods.[29]

Device Design

Fully automated serology analyzers, like the ones implemented in blood bank (immunohematology) operations, have seen increased utility in order to deal with variability in workloads in high-throughput laboratories. Semi-automated and fully automated serology analysis systems have been FDA approved for use in blood bank

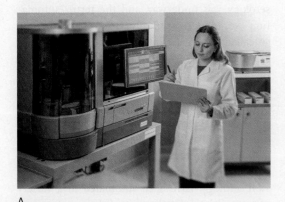
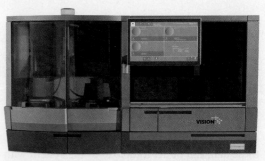

A   B

FIGURE 7–5 Ortho vision and vision max analyzers. **(A)** Ortho vision analyzer. **(B)** Ortho vision max analyzer. These examples of automated serology analyzers are found in association with high-volume blood bank laboratories and can be used on both patient and donor samples to perform assays including ABO/Rh testing, antibody screening/identifications.

(immunohematology) operations through several commercial manufacturers including Bio-Rad, Immucor, Grifols, Ortho-Clinical Diagnostics, and Diagast.[16] The Bio-Rad, Grifols, and Ortho-Clinical Diagnostic systems all use a column agglutination method consisting of a plastic card with between six and eight microtubes with subtle, but proprietary, differences in design. The steps required for specimen testing are similar among devices and, depending on the level of automation, many or all of the steps are performed by the analyzer including the creation of a weak RBC suspension (0.8%) that is mixed with plasma and incubated, if required, before centrifugation.[16] Two other device designs, solid-phase red cell adherence assays and erythromagnetic technology, have been employed in other commercial systems.

Analysis of autoimmune disorders, typically performed through physician-conducted microscopy and IIF (indirect immunofluorescence), have now been incorporated into more automated platforms as well, including the AKLIDES from Medipan, which works through a motorized inverse fluorescence microscope to record digital images that are interpreted via visual recognition algorithms.[29] Depending on the level of automation in these devices, considerations such as waste and slide management should be considered.[30]

Operations

The serological test specimen used by transfusion services differs from those used in hematology by the color of the tube, stopper. Both are EDTA tubes, but hematology specimens commonly arrive in purple-topped tubes, while nonclotted specimens used in transfusion services arrive in a pink-topped EDTA, specifically for differentiation and providing a slightly larger volume[26]. Historically, clotted specimens were used for some blood bank serology testing; this practice is mostly discontinued with automated and semiautomated equipment. Fully automated systems, such as the Erytra automated blood grouping system (Diagnostic Grifols S.A.), utilize whole blood specimens as well as RBCs, plasma, and serum derived from a variety of sources including from posttransfusion,

transplantation, and cord blood samples.[28] The Erytra DG gel card system, for example, may include reagent sera or RBCs, depending on the test to be performed. Automated platforms perform all of the detection steps, such as artificial vision detection in the case of gel card systems.

Several ideas should be considered during the adoption of these automated systems including reagent supply-chain issues, service support, and installation-related issues. Furthermore, adoption of new technologies within the laboratory will require some downtime related to staff training if it is to be implemented successfully. Due to the differences with device design, user interfaces, and testing performed, no general-purpose, operational guidelines can be comprehensive.

Analysis

In most blood banking operations, serological testing is performed using antihuman globulin (AHG) or other antisera. Using the card system, sensitized RBCs agglutinate in the presence of AHG and are trapped within the gel or bead matrix, whereas unsensitized cells fall to the bottom of the microtube. A positive or negative response can then be acquired via an artificial vision-detection system. Positive results can be further quantified using a 1+ to 4+ scale if appropriate coding and controls are incorporated. Results are stored electronically and can be repeated for individual specimen cards for up to 24 hours.

▶ Immunoassay Analyzers

Immunoassay analysis began with radioactive assays such as the RIA and progressed to other detection systems in the 1960s and later. Early players in the immunoassay analyzer market were DPC, now Siemens, and Abbott Diagnostics, which introduced the first commercial enzyme immunoassay and fluorescence polarization systems.[17] The next generation of these analyzers began to have features such as random access, allowing more than one assay at a time, and many other features such as liquid-level sensing, clot detection, barcoding, and on-board QC.[17] However, their major deficiency was that they were closed systems that did not allow for use of reagent sets from other manufacturers or for the optimization of assays. Today, analyzers that function as immunoassay only are rare, but can be found in laboratories and companies that perform exclusively or predominantly immunoassays, such as an immunology laboratory. In most cases, immunoassays are performed on other broad-spectrum analysis systems such as the chemistry analyzer. Some of the common immunoassay-based automated tests found on chemistry instruments are lipid tests such as Apo A, B C and E, inflammation markers such as complement components and CRP, nutritional tests such as ferritin and transferrin, as well as tests for serum proteins, allergy, coagulation, and others.

Principles

Lack of flexibility in commercial analyzer design continues to be one of the major concerns of end users[12]. The first step away from closed systems occurred with the development of the 96-well microplate and very simplified "xyz" coordinate robots in the 1980s.[17] In the current era, automated cartridge-based immunoassays have begun to make a larger impact on the market, as they allow users to pick and choose assays of interest and reduce the reliance on centralized equipment.

Immunoassay analyzers are a large subset of analyzer systems that incorporate the methods of ligand binding (i.e., antigen-antibody binding) into an automated framework. As with manual immunoassays, the steps to automation for immunoassays includes a series of preanalytical, analytical, and postanalytical steps starting with sample identification and ending with the export of results through a LIS. The principles of analyzer assay design vary in the same ways that immunoassays vary in manual methods of analytic detection. For example, analytical measurements of the quantities of disease-specific IgA and IgG for celiac disease can be quantified using a chemiluminescent or fluoroenzyme immunoassay with either a fully automated chemiluminescent immunoanalyzer or a fully automated microplate system, respectively.[31]

Despite differences in assay structure and analyte tested, immunoassay analyzers generally require four specific parts: liquid handling, assay-specific manipulations, data management, and additional logistics. Furthermore, devices can be built for broad or specific functionality depending on the end-user's needs. Automated immunoassays have the added advantage of precision fluidic systems, accurately controlled incubation times, and temperature control.[17]

Device Design

From the 1960s through the 1990s, the consolidation of technologies necessary for the automation of complex assays led to the instrument era of laboratory medicine. However, the consolidation and refinement of these technologies began to be supplanted by the technological miniaturization that also led the computer and telecommunications industries toward smaller footprints and mobilization.

Currently, the market is composed of a combination of high-throughput fully automated immunoassay analyzers, such as the DiaSorin LIAISON®. As well as integrated chemistry and immunoassay devices such as the Ortho Clinical Diagnostics VITROS and VITROS XT analyzers (**FIGURE 7–6**), as well as the Siemens ADVIA Centaur® assays used for high volume Vitamin D testing,[32] and semiautomated POC devices, such

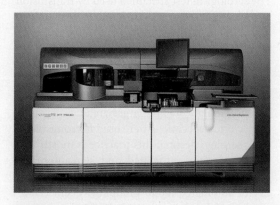

FIGURE 7–6 Ortho clinical diagnostics® VITROS XT 7600.

Courtesy of Ortho Clinical Diagnostics.

as an ELISA lab-on-a-chip device for detecting staphylococcal enterotoxin B.[33] For example, the DiaSorin LIAISON system performs chemiluminescent immunoassays using paramagnetic microparticles as a solid phase. Depending on the assays to be performed, a variety of reagent kits are purchased and loaded onto the instrument. Other instruments such as coagulation analyzers also use immunologic principles in their operation, along with chromogenic and clotting analysis; for example, D-dimers and protein fractions (C and S) are detected immunologically with thrombin and prothrombin assessments performed via ELISA.[34] In such cases, the immunological assays detect the presence of the antigens and should be correlated with functional assays.

More general-purpose systems such as Bio-Rads Bio-Plex array system, utilize xMAP technology (licensed from Luminex) to look at up to 100 analytes simultaneously[35] (**FIGURE 7-7**). Luminex xMAP immunoassays are performed through the combination of antibodies, antigens, or other specific detection reagents with beads coated with different combinations of two fluorescent dyes. The variation in bead color allows for the simultaneous detection of serum antibodies or antigens, whereby the bead acts as the substrate (solid-phase) for the assay.

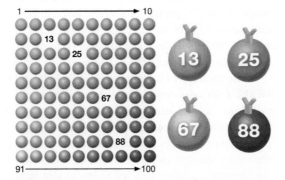

FIGURE 7-7 xMAP technology bead design. The BioRad xMAP technology is an example of a multiplex immunoassay technology whereby beads are labeled with two colors in various concentrations, allowing for up to 100 different targets in a single assay.

Brett Houser (2012) Bio-Rad's Bio-Plex® suspension array system, xMAP technology overview, Archives of Physiology and Biochemistry, 118:4, 192–196, DOI: 10.3109/13813455.2012.705301

Data acquisition occurs through a flow cell in which beads are separated similarly to cells within a traditional flow cytometer. Multiplexed bead detection assays can successfully replace traditional ELISA and Western blotting assays.

The first immunoassay-automated analyzers tended to use one or only a few methodologies with a limited selection of assay choices; this was a reflection of the high-throughput needs of clinical diagnostic operations, but did not allow for flexibility and innovation in the test menu.[36] In contrast, research labs are more likely to consider the automation of specific steps in the process, or open systems, that allow for more flexibility in assay design. The contrast between research methods and diagnostic methods has meant that many innovations developed in the research environment have not been incorporated into commercially available immunoassay analyzers. Furthermore, developers of novel immunoassays (researchers) still consider automation a late-stage goal of their research, with 39% suggesting that no automation was involved in their immunoassay setups, according to a 2014 survey.[36] Multiplexed bead technologies such as those described above can be used in both research and clinical evaluations. Other multiplexing technologies such as mass cytometry, digital ELISA, and automated microarray technologies, are also being produced commercially, which may create significant advantages in the automation of immunoassays.[37] In current practice, immunoassay analyzers use two approaches that have distinct advantages to the end user; the first is to fully integrate automation that allows for less hands-on technologist time and the second is the modular system, which requires more technologist intervention but provides for more versatility in assay selection.[38]

Operations

Immunoassay analyzers are not all created in a similar fashion and, therefore, operations vary depending on the device adopted. The DiaSorin LIASON XL system is capable of performing a variety of chemiluminescent immunoassays (CLIAs), such as the vitamin D test, described previously, and herpes simplex virus (HSV) 1 and 2 assays.[39] It uses reagent kits called "reagent integrals," which include all diluents required for the specific assay. Up to 25 "reagent integrals" can be loaded into the LIASON XL, and multiples of the same integral can be loaded as needed. A barcoded system on the side of the "reagent integral" cartridge allows the system to monitor the lot expiration, volume, and test numbers performed for each reagent component. Operators are responsible for loading up to 10 sample racks, which can hold 12 samples each. A barcode reader is used to identify all samples and track progress through the machine. Additional operator functions are to exchange reagents, dispose of single-use pipette tips used by the instrument, and remove and replace wash and waste solutions.

The Bio-Rad Bio-Plex is a semiautomated system that still requires some upfront preparation. For example, each capture bead must be incubated with an antigen standard or sample for a specific time, performed in a 96-well plate. Beads are then incubated with a reporter streptavidin-phycoerythrin conjugate. Each step is followed by removal of excess conjugate before the samples are run through the instrument. Like other commercial platforms, kits are available for purchase that contain the appropriate capture beads, but researchers can also develop their own; however, this requires significant validation and testing before becoming diagnostically useful.

Analysis

As with other semiautomated and automated analyzers, results are recorded electronically and can be triggered for release to a LIS system. As such, technologies are involved more often at the larger-level analytical operations of the laboratory including system comparisons, test validations, and population-level interpretations of results.

▶ Hematology Analyzers

Although not directly related to the study of serology or the use of immunodiagnostics, the original hematology analyzers were some of the first analyzers in common operation, and their design considerations were pivotal in the development of flow cytometers and the fluidic systems used in immunodiagnostic instruments. They are primarily utilized to perform the complete blood count and to detect variance within WBC and RBC populations in peripheral blood. Modern hematology analyzers, such as the Mindray® BC-6800, Beckman Coulter® LH750, and Sysmex® XN-2000, allow for the measurement of more than 30 hematological parameters.[40] In all cases, current analyzers examine at least three parameters: the hemogram; an examination of cellular characteristics such as mass and concentrations differential blood count; percentages of the most common leukocytes; and reticulocyte count utilizing whole blood anticoagulated with EDTA.[41]

Principles

Generally, determination of hematological parameters are detected using light scatter or electrical-impedance methods for separation. These methods are augmented by the use of staining with fluorescence or nonfluorescent dyes.[40] For example, the Sysmex® XN-2000 (Sysmex, Kobe, Japan) and others in their X-class series, utilize laser light scatter (forward scatter; FSC) and side fluorescent light (side scatter, SSC) to detect the size and shape of cells,[40,41] principles also employed in flow cytometry. Others such as the Coulter® LH750 and LH780 utilize electrical impedance to detect cell size and complexity.[40,41]

The measure of impedance (**FIGURE 7–8A** and **FIGURE 7–8B**) developed by Walter Coulter and called the Coulter principle was the first principle of automated measurement. It is based on changes in resistance as larger particles, such as cells, pass through a small opening between two electrodes (an aperture), leading to a reduction in electrical conduction compared with the diluent (liquid fraction).[41] The change in conductance is proportional to the cellular volume and therefore, the sum of the impulses can be plotted on a histogram. Smaller particles, such as platelets, lead to smaller reductions in electrical conductance (impedance); and

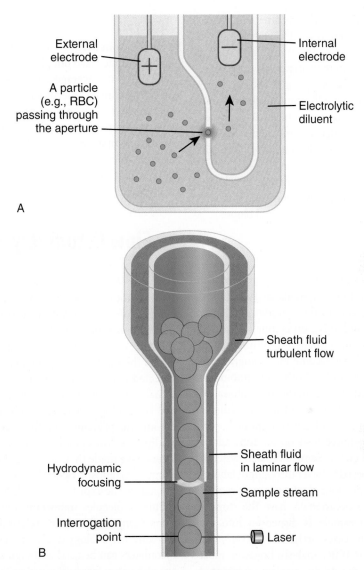

FIGURE 7–8 Impedance principle and hydrodynamic focusing. **(A)** Electrical impedance as used with small particles, such as cells, was first developed by Wallace Coulter for use in hematology analyzers. It has subsequently been applied to more advanced cellular analysis systems. **(B)** Hydrodynamic focusing allows for a single cell to pass through an aperture allowing for a clearer demarcation of cellular description.

larger particles, such as cells, lead to larger impedance, which can be quantified based on the total
volume of blood passed through the aperture.[41]
Important engineering discoveries, such as
hydrodynamic focusing further reduced error in
the system by reducing the duplicate counting of
cells by coincidence. Specifically, hydrodynamic
focusing, later employed in most flow cytometers,

incorporated a sheath fluid that reduced the size
of the opening to the size of a single cell.[41] Later,
system designs incorporated the principle of high-
frequency measurement, in which cells are exposed
to a high-frequency field, and impedance of all
cells is determined at the same time. This high-
frequency impedance depends on the size of
the internal structure of the cells and is typically

performed on WBC populations after the lysis of RBCs.[41] Special software is used to interrogate the signal and separate cells into mature and immature fractions based on their structural properties.

Hydrodynamic focusing is also used in other methods of cellular quantification, including scattered laser-light measurement, which has been used to measure RBCs, reticulocytes, and others. Systems such as the Cell Dyn® Sapphire utilize fluorescent laser light differentiation. The evolution of flow cytometric principles, discussed in more detail later, has led to more precise measurements and differentiation parameters for cells of peripheral blood.

Operations

Hematology analyzers have become one of the most ubiquitously found systems in the clinical laboratory setting, due to the extreme popularity of the basic CBC and WBC differential tests used for early investigations of patient health. As such, these instruments have become increasingly automated and can be found as both semi-automated and fully automated models. In the fully automated models, operations may consist of simply loading a tube onto a rack system with a preprogramed operation to run the required tests on the tube added to a computerized queue. Semiautomated systems, typically still employed in lower throughput laboratories due to a significant reduction in cost, require collection tubes to occasionally have the stopper removed before a sample is dispensed into the instrument. In some cases, prelysis of red cells may still be required for WBC analysis; however, most instruments have the lysing agents incorporated into the system design and perform this function when the appropriate test is indicated.

Minimally, a technician should be acquainted with the user interface, cleaning, and maintenance functions, and be capable of performing necessary quality-control testing on the machine. More and more often, troubleshooting, calibration, and long-term maintenance are performed by industry technicians specifically trained in maintaining the instrument. Furthermore, instruments are designed with online capacities, which allow some functions to be performed remotely by industry personnel.

Analysis

Analysis from these systems is typically conveyed using computerized dot plots and enumerations of cell counts and average cellular size. Despite their utility in clinical interpretations, caution should be exercised when comparing the results obtained among difference analyzers and analyzer designs. Studies comparing the results of many hematology parameters, such as reticulocyte count and WBC counts, have shown poor agreement among analyzers.[40]

▶ Flow Cytometry

Principles

Flow cytometry, known also as flow-through cytophotometry, consists of three different components including a fluidics system in which the cells are transported, optical components in which the fluorescent components of the cells are detected, and a data processing system allowing for visual processing and evaluation.[41] Advanced clinical hematology analyzers often incorporate flow cytometric principles in their design, and both traditional flow cytometers and hematology analyzers have made their way into the contemporary immunodiagnostic operations due to their ability to analyze the expression of cell surface and intracellular molecules important for disease correlations. Compared with the relatively closed design of many hematology analyzers, commercial flow cytometers can be used to design assays for a variety of heterogeneously expressed cell populations that allow multi-parameter analysis of single cells for the purposes of characterization, assessment of purity, and anomalous markers of cell populations.

Device Design

Patient-derived samples are first incubated in tubes or microtiter plates with unlabeled and fluorochrome-labeled antibodies (staining), and followed by analysis on the flow cytometer. Stained cells in a suspension buffer are extracted from sample reservoirs (tubes or microtiter plates) using an onboard

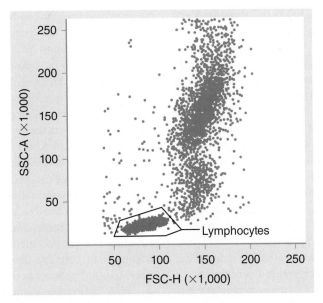

FIGURE 7–9 Example of forward and side-scatter differentiation of common hematological cells. These parameters are often the first used to separate cell populations prior to an examination of immunophenotypic markers. FSC is an indicator of particle (cellular) size and SSC is an indicator of complexity of the cell. In this plot, the proposed lymphocyte population has been gated for further analysis.

Modified from C. Hayden, https://commons.wikimedia.org/wiki/File:Flow_Cytometry_Chart.jpg

liquid handling system; they are hydrodynamically focused using a **sheath fluid**, which allows the cells to pass by a laser light source in a single file in a vessel called a **flow cell**. A number of detectors are used to count the cells, detect light scatter, one in the front and several to the side, and detect fluorescent emission of positively stained cells. Like hematology analyzers, forward scattered light detects cellular size, and side scattered light is used to detect the granularity of the cells. These size and complexity detectors are still a valuable tool in the differentiation of cell populations such as subtypes of immune cells in peripheral blood (**FIGURE 7–9**). The use of directly labeled or indirectly labeled antibodies toward specific cellular molecules are then used to further define and differentiate the cells, sometimes in combination with other markers or in combination with size and complexity parameters. Depending on the needs of the facility, instruments can be purchased with the capability to detect several to more than 20 parameters in a single tube, allowing for very complex immunophenotyping assays to be performed; however, most machines typically measure between 6 to 12 parameters at a time.[42]

A laser excites the fluorochrome to emit light at a specific wavelength. A series of mirrors and filters are used to direct the fluorescence and scatter light toward specific **photomultiplier tubes (PMTs)**. The PMT converts the photon energy into an electronic signal, which is then recorded in association with a single cell as part of a data packet. The commonly used fluorochrome FITC, when excited, releases light at approximately 519 nm, which is detected by a FITC channel PMT, for example; however, any emitted light at this wavelength will also be detected by this PMT. Filters can be set up in a series to allow for the passage of specific wavelengths of light, specifically, bandpass filters pass light only in a narrow range, short-pass filters pass light below a specified wavelength, and long-pass filters pass light above a specified wavelength. This can be compared to the principle of polarization in sunglasses. Mirrors have been designed to pass certain light and reflect other light. These so-called dichroic mirrors are situated at 45° angles to the light beam and allow for specified wavelengths to pass straight through, potentially to another mirror in a series, and for the rest of the light to be deflected toward a PMT for detection. Thus, a single beam of light can be used to detect multiple parameters almost instantaneously by creating a voltage pulse in the PMT known as an **event**. Hundreds of thousands to millions of cells from a single sample can then be analyzed in this way and then pass through the flow cell.

The popularity of flow cytometry and an increasing number of directed antibodies and fluorochrome choices have substantially increased the number and type of cytometers on the market. Newer fluorochromes, for instance, allow for the narrowing of emission spectra that has reduced the spillover effect seen with earlier fluorochromes.[42] In addition, more than a dozen commercial manufacturers have developed flow cytometric instruments utilizing various designs and focused on various functional needs and considerations such as lab footprint, throughput, upgradeability, software and technical support, and price point.[43] Systems have been optimized for the utilization of alternative fluorophores such as quantum dots, and have been created specifically for the detection of serological components that bind to fluorescent beads, and for the detection of a range of particle sizes such as smaller bacterial cells.

Operations

Before entry into the flow cytometer, cells must first be prepped through antibody staining. Four types of staining and detection are described: direct staining, indirect staining, intracellular staining, and detection of secreted proteins. Assays for each of these stains are available from commercial vendors such as Abcam, BD Biosciences, and others. The target, epitope, and fluorochrome are all important in the selection of these reagents.

Direct staining requires only the incubation of the antibody with the specimen for the manufacturer's suggested time; however, variations in incubation times can be used to increase the efficiency of staining in many cases. With indirect labeling, a non-tagged primary antibody to the specimen

target is used, and a secondary fluorescently tagged antibody against the primary antibody is then applied. This requires an incubation time for the primary, followed by a wash, and then an incubation for the secondary. Often, this method is used in the research setting or for esoteric diagnostic tests in which a directly coupled target antibody is not commercially available in the appropriate fluorochrome. The linking of antibodies can lead to reduced efficiency of binding and reduction in molecular quantification. Intracellular staining requires various fixation and permeabilization methods prior to the addition of the antibody. Cells prepped in this way are increasingly fragile, and variation in permeabilizaton, fixation, and incubation times should be attempted to optimize detection. Furthermore, a panel that incorporates both intracellular and surface molecules requires sequential labeling starting with surface markers, following with fix/perm steps, and finishing with intracellular labeling.[42] Finally, secreted proteins can be detected through additional steps that block the release of the secreted protein depending on its localization.

When detecting multiple analytes, a general practice is the coupling the dimmest fluorochromes, such as Pacific Blue or FITC to the most abundant molecules on the cell surface, and the brightest fluorochromes, such as PE or APC, to the least abundant or harder to detect analytes. Different instruments can detect different fluorochromes due to different lasers and filters, which can determine the intensity or ability of detection. **TABLE 7–1** provides a list of some of the most common fluorochromes and the laser source required for detection.

Before assays are run, the machine is evaluated through quality control with fluorescent beads of known fluorescent intensities in all wavelengths measured by the PMTs. When performing a multiparameter assay, compensation tubes should also be run on any fluorochrome used. Compensation tubes consist of a single-color tube used to optimize the fluorescent response and reduce any spillover effect. These tubes can be filled with a control specimen or with commercial antibody capture beads (CompBeads); ideally, anti-mIgGκ coated CompBeads are used for anti-human antibody conjugates.[42] Additionally, control tubes are

TABLE 7–1 Fluorochrome Excitation and Emission Chart

Fluorochrome	Excitation Range (nm)	Emission Range (nm)	Source LASER
FITC (fluoroscein isothiocyanate)	468–509	504–541	Argon ion LASER (488 nm)
PE (Phycoerythrin)	486–580	568–590	Argon ion LASER (488 nm)
APC (Allophycocyanin)	600–640	660 max	Helium-neon LASER (635 nm)
PE-Texas Red	486–75	610–635	Argon ion LASER (488 nm)
PerCP	490 max	677 max	Argon ion LASER (488 nm)
APC-Cy7	600–640	750–810	Helium-neon LASER (635 nm)
PE-Cy7	486–575	750–810	Argon ion LASER (488 nm)
Alexa Fluor 488	495	519	Argon ion LASER (488 nm)
Alexa Fluor 647	650	668	Helium-neon LASER (635nm)

necessary to determine accuracy of an assay and to compare results performed on a single day. These can be commercially available controls or provided via a donor sample. These controls can be used both to determine baseline for a "normal" sample and to establish appropriate gating parameters. Once established, gating parameters can be saved in most systems and loaded when future assays are performed. While specific gating is required for all new assays performed, gating strategies vary greatly between institutions and are based on the software suite used, which differs based on the specific instrument purchased and are therefore beyond the scope of this discussion.

Analysis

Flow cytometric analysis allows for the analysis of an overwhelming number of fluorochrome combinations and, therefore, needs to be carefully defined during assay development and implementation. Assay designers should determine ahead of time which parameters will be considered in their diagnostic and/or research applications. Dot plots presented on a biexponential scale are traditionally used in the initial analysis of flow data; however, this gating strategy approach may not be ideal for a fully refined representation of data, especially when a comparison of more than one gating parameter is diagnostically indicated. Typically, clinical flow assays have an incorporated template for analysis that is used for the extraction of analytical data. These data may be uploaded to the LIS system manually or through a computerized relay. However, in most cases, the complexity of flow cytometric data requires that an initial technologist analysis is performed, followed by a second technologist check, and finally, a critical review by a medical director, trained specialist, or pathologist is required before results are reported.

CASE STUDY

Case Report

The adoption of new technologies in the laboratory depends primarily on the per-unit test cost, as well as other factors such as upfront costs from equipment, personnel retraining, and validation. A study was conducted within the department of laboratory medicine at a national university hospital in Korea comparing the costs of performing manual ABO/Rh and unexpected antibody testing with the use of an automated serological system.[27] A manual tube test for both red cell typing of A and B antigens and serum screening for anti-A, anti-B, and anti-D isoagglutinins was performed. Unexpected antibodies were manually tested using a microcolumn agglutination technique found in a commercial LISS/Coombs gel card. The Ortho Clinical AutoVue Innova system was used to test ABO/Rh and unexpected antibodies in an automated system.

More than 2,000 samples were compared to determine the economic costs through workflow analysis. The average time to complete all steps in the manual ABO/Rh red cell typing and ABO serum processing was 5.65 minutes vs 8.4 minutes using the automated method. However, to perform a manual analysis of unexpected antibodies took 27.6 minutes vs 23 minutes using the automated method. The real advantage of the automated method was in performing both ABO/Rh testing with unexpected antibodies, which took only 24.7 minutes using an automated method vs 33.25 minutes via manual approaches.

The authors further analyzed the cost per test when 1, 5, and 12 tests were run simultaneously by manual method and compared to the unit cost for running a single test through an automated method. Labor costs were based on a set rate of pay multiplied by the tech time needed to run the assay. The cost of materials for the manual method was very low; however, the labor costs were much higher. Direct costs associated with materials were higher for automated analysis, while direct cost was lower for manual methods. Labor costs alone led to the increased cost of running a manual test, even when a large number of tests (up to 12) were run simultaneously.

Despite the study's findings, several major factors were not included in the cost estimates for the current comparison. Specifically, the costs associates with the initial analyzer purchase price should have been distributed across all tests performed using the assay over the amortization (debt payoff) period. Furthermore, the cost of new technology setup, including staff training and validation, should be brought into account.

Critical Thinking Questions

1. Which factors contribute to the unit cost of a diagnostic test?
2. How would cost per test be affected by increased test volume using an automated method compared with a manual method?
3. What effect does automation pose for the field of laboratory medicine?

▶ References

1. Armbruster DA, Overcash DR, Reyes J. Clinical chemistry laboratory automation in the 21st Century - amat Victoria curam (Victory loves careful preparation). *Clin Biochem Rev.* 2014;35(3):143–153.

2. Top Laboratory Automation Equipment Worldwide, 2013. *Market Share Reporter*. 26 ed. Gale Directory Library: Gale, Cengage Learning; 2016:844.

3. Howes I, Edwards R. *Equipment and Automation*. In: Edwards R, ed. Immunodiagnostics: A Practical Approach: Oxford University Press; 1999:215–242.

4. Abel G. Current status and future prospects of point-of-care testing around the globe. *Expert Rev Mol Diagn.* 2015;15(7):853–855.

5. BOC, ASCLS, and ASCP Meet with CMS on Nursing Degree Equivalency Rule 2016. http://www.ascls.org/communication/blog-society-news-now/339-boc-ascls-and-ascp-meet-with-cms-on-nursing-degree-equivalency-rule.

6. Sin ML, Mach KE, Wong PK, et al. Advances and challenges in biosensor-based diagnosis of infectious diseases. *Expert Rev Mol Diagn.* 2014;14(2):225–244.

7. Ligler FS, Sapsford KE, Golden JP, et al. The array biosensor: portable, automated systems. *Anal Sci.* 2007;23(1):5–10.

8. Gordon J, Michel G. Discerning trends in multiplex immunoassay technology with potential for resource-limited settings. *Clin Chem.* 2012;58(4):690–698.

9. Dixit CK, Kadimisetty K, Otieno BA, et al. Electrochemistry-based approaches to low cost, high sensitivity, automated, multiplexed protein immunoassays for cancer diagnostics. *Analyst*. 2016;141(2):536–547.

10. Han KN, Li CA, Seong GH. Microfluidic chips for immunoassays. *Annu Rev Anal Chem (Palo Alto Calif)*. 2013;6:119–141.

11. Madrid FF, Maroun MC. Serologic laboratory findings in malignancy. *Rheum Dis Clin North Am*. 2011;37(4):507–525.

12. Najmabadi P, Goldenberg AA, Emili A. Hardware flexibility of laboratory automation systems: analysis and new flexible automation architectures. *Clin Lab Med*. 2007;27(1):1–28.

13. Riben M. Laboratory automation and middleware. *Surg Pathol Clin*. 2015;8(2):175–186.

14. Hawker CD. Nonanalytic laboratory automation: a quarter century of progress. *Clin Chem*. 2017;63(6):1074–1082.

15. Greer RW, Straseski JA. *Principles of Clinical Chemistry Automation*. In: Bishop ML, Fody EP, Schoeff LE, eds. Clinical Chemistry : Principles, Techniques, and Correlations. Eighth edition. ed. Philadelphia: Wolters Kluwer; 2018:p. 139–158.

16. Bajpai M, Kaur R, Gupta E. Automation in immunohematology. *Asian J Transfus Sci*. 2012;6(2):140–144.

17. Allinson JL. Automated immunoassay equipment platforms for analytical support of pharmaceutical and biopharmaceutical development. *Bioanalysis*. 2011;3(24):2803–2816.

18. Enten A, Yang Y, Ye Z, et al. A liquid-handling robot for automated attachment of biomolecules to microbeads. *J Lab Autom*. 2016;21(4):526–532.

19. Rumilla KM, Winters JL, Peterman JM, et al. Development and validation of a fluorescent microsphere immunoassay for anti-IgA. *Immunohematology*. 2009;25(1):24–28.

20. Kong F, Yuan L, Zheng YF, et al. Automatic liquid handling for life science: a critical review of the current state of the art. *J Lab Autom*. 2012;17(3):169–185.

21. Staab TA, Kramer GW. *New Standards and Approaches for Integrating Instruments into Laboratory Automation Systems*. In: Layne SP, Beugelsdijk TJ, Patel CKN, eds. Firepower in the Lab: Automation in the Fight Against Infectious Diseases and Bioterrorism. Washington D.C.: Joseph Henry Press; 2001:243–260.

22. Ucar F, Erden G, Taslipinar MY, et al. Greater efficiency observed 12 months post-implementation of an automatic tube sorting and registration system in a core laboratory. *J Med Biochem*. 2016;35(1):1–6.

23. Croxatto A, Prod'hom G, Faverjon F, et al. Laboratory automation in clinical bacteriology: what system to choose? *Clin Microbiol Infect*. 2016;22(3):217–235.

24. Henricks WH. Laboratory information systems. *Clin Lab Med*. 2016;36(1):1–11.

25. Taylor CE. Serological techniques. *J Clin Pathol Suppl Coll Pathol*. 1969;3:14–19.

26. Butch SH. Automation in the transfusion service. *Immunohematology*. 2008;24(3):86–92.

27. Shin KH, Kim HH, Chang CL, et al. Economic and workflow analysis of a blood bank automated system. *Ann Lab Med*. 2013;33(4):268–273.

28. Roback JD, Barclay S, Moulds JM, et al. A multicenter study on the performance of a fully automated, walk-away high-throughput analyzer for pretransfusion testing in the US population. *Transfusion*. 2015;55(6 pt 2): 1522–1528.

29. Willitzki A, Hiemann R, Peters V, et al. New platform technology for comprehensive serological diagnostics of autoimmune diseases. *Clin Dev Immunol*. 2012;2012:284740.

30. Prichard JW. Overview of automated immunohistochemistry. *Arch Pathol Lab Med*. 2014;138(12):1578–1582.

31. Lakos G, Norman GL, Mahler M, et al. Analytical and clinical comparison of two fully automated immunoassay systems for the diagnosis of celiac disease. *J Immunol Res*. 2014;2014:371263.

32. Hsu SA, Soldo J, Gupta M. Evaluation of two automated immunoassays for 25-OH vitamin D: comparison against LC-MS/MS. *J Steroid Biochem Mol Biol*. 2013;136:139–145.

33. Yang M, Sun S, Kostov Y, et al. An automated point-of-care system for immunodetection of staphylococcal enterotoxin B. *Anal Biochem*. 2011;416(1):74–81.

34. Qari MH. High throughput coagulation analyzers review. *Comb Chem High Throughput Screen*. 2005;8(4):353–360.

35. Houser B. Bio-Rad's Bio-Plex(R) suspension array system, xMAP technology overview. *Arch Physiol Biochem*. 2012; 118(4):192–196.

36. Comley J. IMMUNOASSAY AUTOMATION: hands-free platforms set to change the workflow in research labs. *Drug Discovery World*. Winter 2014.

37. Mora J, Given Chunyk A, Dysinger M, et al. Next generation ligand binding assays-review of emerging technologies' capabilities to enhance throughput and multiplexing. *AAPS J*. 2014;16(6):1175–1184.

38. Ahene AB, Morrow C, Rusnak D, et al. Ligand binding assays in the 21st Century laboratory: automation. *AAPS J*. 2012;14(1):142–153.

39. Li Z, Yan R, Yan C, et al. Evaluation of an automated chemiluminescent immunoassay in typing detection of IgG antibodies against herpes simplex virus. *J Clin Lab Anal*. 2016;30(5):577–580.

40. Ciepiela O, Kotula I, Kierat S, et al. A comparison of Mindray BC-6800, Sysmex XN-2000, and Beckman Coulter LH750 automated hematology analyzers: a pediatric study. *J Clin Lab Anal*. 2016;30(6):1128–1134.

41. Lehner J, Greve B, Cassens U. Automation in hematology. *Transfus Med Hemother*. 2007;34:328–339.

42. Mahnke YD, Roederer M. Optimizing a multicolor immunophenotyping assay. *Clin Lab Med*. 2007;27(3):469–485.

43. Fung PA. 2016 Flow cytometry buyer's guide: a researcher's guide to selecting a flow cytometer. 2016. http://www.biocompare.com/186616-2016-Flow-Cytometry-Buyer-s-Guide/

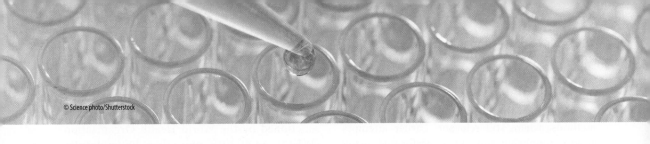

CHAPTER 8

Immunophenotyping

Ian Clift, PhD, MLS(ASCP)^{CM}

KEY TERMS

CD Markers
Erythrocyte

Immunofluorescence (IF)
Immunophenotyping

Lymphocyte

LEARNING OBJECTIVES

Upon completion of this chapter, the reader should be able to:

1. Define immunophenotyping.
2. Compare classical phenotyping analysis to contemporary methods.
3. Explain the origin and utility of the cluster of differentiation (cluster designation) markers.
4. Examine the role of immunohistochemistry and immunocytochemistry in phenotyping cancer.
5. Describe the use of fluorescence microscopy for imaging fixed and living cells.
6. Rank antigen selection based on utility in phenotypical analysis.
7. Review the preparation of blood sample for flow cytometric analysis.
8. Provide a rationale for the use of karyotyping in immunophenotyping.
9. Define the role of western blotting of intracellular proteins in phenotypic analysis.
10. List the major markers for erythrocytes, lymphocytes, and granulocytes.
11. Know the most common markers for differentiating T cells, B cells, and NK cells.
12. Use marker analysis to identify blast cells versus mature cells.

▶ Fundamentals of Immunophenotyping

Immunophenotyping is the process of specifying immune cell lineage and sub-lineages on the basis of cellular markers. Predominately, this is performed by an antibody-based assessment of surface proteins, but can also employ the use of antibodies targeting intracellular proteins, DNA, and other cell-specific molecules. Additionally, classical phenotyping occurs via the use of dyes that mark specific cellular organelles, based on content, or that bind to specific protein, lipid, and sugar moieties. Although typically less specific, these classical approaches are still employed in combination with antibody-based identification methods, where still relevant. Earlier attempts at immunophenotyping were performed using slide-based methods and fluorescent microscopy[1] and cellular morphology studies; however, today these assays are performed by flow cytometry more frequently.

In the last couple of decades, important technical advances in hardware, automation, and analytics have increased the utility of this process. Of note, phenotype can be determined through the assessment of a multitude of cellular factors including adhesion molecules, enzymes, chemokines and cytokines, signaling molecules, transcription factors, oncology products, and mutation-specific products.[1] Additionally, assays can be performed on a variety of specimen types from blood to tissue biopsies, depending on the method employed. This chapter provides some of the most commonly employed marker profiles used in immunophenotyping of normal immune cells and describes some introductory examples of phenotypic profile changes in disease. Prior to interpreting CD marker profiles, an understanding of the CD marker system and several of the major methods utilized in immunophenotyping, flow cytometry; blood, and bone marrow morphologies; immunohistochemistry; fluorescence microscopy; karyotyping; and western blotting should be examined. Where applicable, later chapters will discuss the use of immunophenotyping in specific subdisciplines of immunodiagnostics.

Clusters of Differentiation (CD) Markers: An Overview

With the relative success of flow cytometry has come a classification system used in the commercial development of monoclonal antibodies of common antigens, i.e., mAbs that target the same surface molecule, known as the cluster of differentiation (also cluster designations), or CD system.[2] The CD classification system has been adopted by other technologies utilizing monoclonal antibodies, including immunohistochemistry and confocal microscopy, and is sanctioned by the World Health Organization (WHO). As of 2015, more than 400 molecules have been designated by the CD system through 10 conferences of the Human Leukocyte Differentiation Antigen Workshops (HLDA).[3] Currently, markers range from CD1 through CD371 with some CDs covering multiple, closely related antigens designated by a lowercase letter, such as the case of CD1b. The CD1s are a class of glycoproteins related to MHC, which present lipid antigens to specialized T cells. Others are designated with an uppercase letter, such as CD45RA and CD45RO, representing splice variants of the protein CD45.[3] **CD markers** are most commonly utilized to determine cell lineage and sublineages of immune cells in circulation.[4,5] A complete list of CD designations can be found in Engel et al.[3] However, many phenotypic markers, such as mutation-specific and oncology-related factors, are not yet defined by the CD classification system. Nevertheless, attempts to map all cells of immune lineages, sometimes called the immunome, through comprehensive leukocyte immunophenotyping (CLIP), are underway utilizing CD markers.[6]

Blood and Bone Marrow Smears

Immunophenotyping is often used in the interpretation of precursor and mature cell populations found in the bone marrow and blood. One of the primary purposes for acquiring peripheral blood and bone marrow aspirates is for the identification of cellular morphologies indicative of disease. Therefore, they are still considered a first source of immunophenotypic diagnostic information. Peripheral blood spear examination is typically performed as part of the general operation of the hematology laboratory. Bone marrow aspirates are considered a surgical procedure, and are traditionally performed by a physician or nurse practitioner, but are sometimes done with the assistance of a member of the laboratory team, whose primary

Subset of CD Markers Used in Immunophenotyping

Antigen	Myelo-blasts	Pro-myelo-cytes	Matur-ing Grans	Mono-cytes	Eryth-roids	Mega-karyo-cytes	B Lym-phoid	T Lym-phoid	Comments
CD2	–	–	–	–	–	–	–	+	LFA-2; pan T-cell marker
CD3	–	–	–	–	–	–	–	+	OKT3; pan T-cell marker
CD4	–	–	–	–	–	–	–	Sub[b]	MHC-II associated; helper T cells
CD5	–	–	–	–	–	–	–	+	Leu-1; pan T-cell marker
CD7	–	–	–	–	–	–	–	+	Leu-9; pan T-cell marker
CD8	–	–	–	–	–	–	–	Sub	MHC-I associated; cytotoxic T cells
CD19	–	–	–	–	–	–	+	–	Leu-12; pan B-cell marker
CD20	–	–	–	–	–	–	+	–	L26; B-cell marker
CD22	–	–	–	–	–	–	+	–	BL-CAM; pan B-cell marker
CD79a[a]	–	–	–	–	–	–	+	–	MB-1; pan B-cell marker
CD13	+	+	+	+	–	–	–	–	Aminopeptidase N; pan myeloid marker
CD14	–	–	+	++	–	–	–	–	LPS receptor; bright on monocytes
CD15	–	+	+	–	–	–	–	–	LeuM1; maturing granulocytes
CD33	+	+	+	++	+	–	–	–	Sialic acid adhesion molecule; pan myeloid marker

(continues)

Subset of CD Markers Used in Immunophenotyping   *(Continued)*

Antigen	Myelo-blasts	Pro-myelo-cytes	Matur-ing Grans	Mono-cytes	Eryth-roids	Mega-karyo-cytes	B Lym-phoid	T Lym-phoid	Comments
CD36	−	−	−	+	+	+	−	−	GP IIIb/IV
CD117	+	+	−	−	+	+	−	−	c-kit; bright on mast cells
CD64	−	−	+	+	−	−	−	−	FC-γ receptor
MPO	Sub	+	+	−/+	−	−	−	−	Myeloperoxidase; definitive myeloid marker
CD71	−	−	−	−	++	−	−	−	Transferrin receptor; dim expression on activated cells
GlyA	−	−	−	−	++	−	−	−	CD235a; carries MN antigens on red cells
CD41	−	−	−	−	−	+	−	−	GP IIb; megakaryocytic
CD61	−	−	+	−	−	+	−	−	GP IIIa; megakaryocytic
CD10	−	−	+	−	−	−	Sub	+	CALLA, also expressed by hematogones
CD38	+	Var	Var	+	−	−	Var	Var	Broadly expressed
CD45	+	+	+	+	−	+	+	+	Leukocyte common antigen
HLA—DR	+	−	−	+	−	−	+	−	Class II MHC component
CD34	+	+	−	−	−	−	Sub	−	Adhesion molecule; marker of immature cells
TdT	−	−	−	−	−	−	Sub	Sub	Nucleotide transferase; marker of immature cells

Abbreviations: CALLA, common acute lymphoblastic leukemia antigen; GlyA, glycophorin A; GP, glycoprotein; LPS, lipopolysaccharide; MHC, major histocompatibility complex; —, absence of expression on normal bone marrow populations; +, presence of expression on normal bone marrow populations; ++, bright expression.

Reprinted from Peters JM, Ansari MQ. Multiparameter flow cytometry in the diagnosis and management of acute leukemia. *Arch Pathol Lab Med.* 2011;135(1):44–54. Copyright 2011 College of American Pathologists.

responsibility is to deposit the blood on a glass slide in a smear for microscopic examination. These specimens may be transported in tubes or on slides to the laboratory for further analysis. The smear is then examined for a complete blood count (CBC) and manual five-part differential of the WBC components. Bone marrow samples are traditionally collected in a non-anticoagulated tube, but can also be performed using EDTA tubes. Today, hematology analyzers are used for most peripheral blood CBCs and differentials, but smears are performed in the case of abnormal results using the same collection tube. A common stain for both blood and bone marrow smears is the Wright-Giemsa stain, which allows for differentiations of subcellular components such as organelles and granules.

Bone-marrow aspirate smears are still performed primarily in a manual fashion, as most hematology analyzers are not equipped to differentiate blast populations found in the bone marrow. All abnormal results are reported to the pathologist, who performs a second examination and provides any diagnostic information, including the ordering of more extensive testing such as immunohistochemistry, karyotyping, and flow cytometry.

In peripheral blood examinations, both the RBCs and WBCs are examined (**FIGURE 8–1**). RBCs are examined for abnormalities such as changes in shape or inclusion bodies. WBCs are counted based on morphology and size to be one of five common immune cell types: specifically lymphocytes, neutrophils, eosinophils, basophils, and monocytes. Typically, 100 cells are counted and the number is used to establish the percentage of the population for each cell type. Abnormal cells are also indicated during this analysis.

Bone-marrow aspirate smears are indicated only during suspected malignancy and are used for differentiating cells based on morphological features that are indicative of cellular maturation, myeloid-to-erythroid ratios, and malignancy.[7]

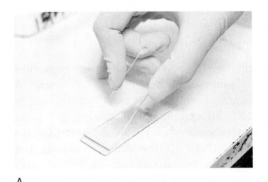

A

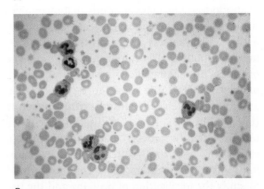

B

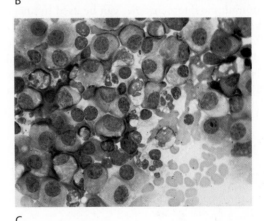

C

FIGURE 8–1 Examples of a Peripheral Blood and Bone-Marrow Aspirate Smear. **(A)** Technician performing a blood smear. **(B)** Peripheral blood smear using Wright stain, showing mostly erythrocytes, with six leukocytes (purple stain) and platelets (small spots). **(C)** Bone marrow aspirate smear at 100 × magnification using Wright Giemsa Stain, indicating multiple myeloma in a patient; cells are almost all immature plasma B cells.

Immunohistochemistry and Immunocytochemistry

Another technique which uses monoclonal antibodies designated by the CD system for immunophenotyping, is immunohistochemistry (IHC) for examination of tissues, and immunocytochemistry (ICC) for the examination of cells. IHC and ICC use antibodies to stain tissue samples for various cell types or the presence of specific proteins. IHC commonly uses two sets of antibodies: a primary antibody that recognizes the marker or protein of interest, and a secondary antibody that detects the Fc portion of the primary antibody and is conjugated to an enzyme or fluorochrome that allows imaging by confocal microscopy. IHC that uses fluorescently tagged antibodies is often called **immunofluorescence (IF)** (**FIGURE 8–2**). IF can be used as a clinical tool to identify cancers, pathological protein expression, and virally infected cells by staining for various markers. IF is commonly used to study the localization of proteins and the use of multiple fluorochromes can be used to image co-localization. Due to the relative ease in performing IF testing, many commercially available direct and indirect IF tests are used in the clinical lab for both phenotyping and disease detection. IF tests, for example, are commonly employed for the detection of viral infections through monoclonal antibodies directed at specific viral proteins, including respiratory syncytial virus (RSV), adenovirus, herpes simplex viruses, parainfluenza, and influenza.[8]

Unlike flow cytometry, variation in protein expression is not as easily quantified by IF; however, the association of proteins is spatially assessed, especially when combined with various forms of microscopy. The use of IF in IHC is commonly used for detection of tissue-based malignancies in the clinical pathology laboratory. However, it is a labor-intensive process that often includes specimen fixation, recovery from paraffin embedding, and other specimen-preparation steps, which have been somewhat overcome by the use of automated immunostainer machines.[1] This method is useful when both markers and morphology are needed for diagnostic interpretation.

Fluorescence Microscopy

Fluorescence microscopy, among other microscopy choices, has allowed for great advances in the imaging and diagnostics of fixed and living cells. It can be used to assess molecules in 3-dimensions, to identify close associations, and to examine cellular and molecular motion.[9]

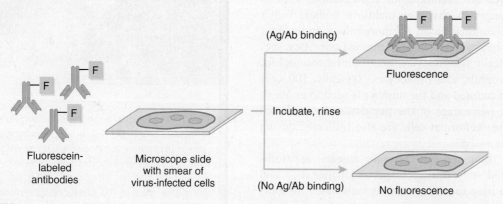

FIGURE 8–2 Immunophenotyping through direct immunofluorescence. Microscopic identification of cell phenotype can be accomplished by direct immunofluorescence (IF) by targeting cells with antibodies to specific surface markers on immune cells.

Image adapted from Diane Leland.

In addition, microscopy is used to detect the localization of surface and intracellular CD markers used in immunophenotyping. It can be used in isolation or in combination with IHC or flow cytometry. Fluorescent microscopy has seen a decline in clinical utility with the advent of flow cytometry, which is typically easier to perform and more characteristic of average cellular populations. In the case of flow cytometry, imaging cytometers allow for the combination of high-resolution digital microscopy images to contemporary flow cytometry, allowing for antigenic localization[1]

Flow Cytometry

The CD marker system was developed for use with flow cytometry technology. Flow cytometry is a common immunodiagnostic technology that uses lasers to excite fluorescently labeled antibodies to detect and quantify surface markers, intracellular proteins, size and shape, and other characteristics of the cells. Detection of monoclonal antibodies via flow cytometry is performed via antibody tagging with fluorochromes such as FITC, APC, and PE. Flow cytometry-based markers are developed via a process of antibody coupling to fluorochromes. The flow analyzer subsystems include modules for cellular isolation, utilizing a sheath fluid and hydrodynamic focusing for individual detection of fluorescent spectra recordings on single cells, which are then clustered to calculate averaged fluorescent intensities of gated regions within a defined range. In general, cells are read via a combination of histograms, a plot of a single parameter (color, size, or complexity) as a function of cell count, or as a dot plot (**FIGURE 8-3**), which separates a population by two parameters. Often, marker expression is also qualified by its localization on the dot plot. Specifically, cell types may be differentiated by the relative concentration of a marker. For example, they may be defined as dim, moderate, or bright (i.e., as CD16^{dim} or CD16^{bright}); alternatively, they could be defined as low or high (i.e., CD16^{low} or CD16^{high}) with a similar interpretation. Ultimately, all the data collected are interpreted to

define cellular populations in a tested population of cells. If immune cell differentiation is a primary function of the laboratory, flow cytometry should be considered an indispensable tool in the identification of these cells as well as malignancies of the hematopoietic system.

Flow cytometers can detect multiple, different antibodies conjugated to different colored fluorochromes, through the wavelength conversion of incident laser light, in order to establish a cell-surface profile that aids in identification of single cells in a population. The use of multiparameter flow cytometry has found significant utility in detection of hematopoietic malignancies as well as normal immune phenotypes.[10] For example, using a simple two-color or three-color system, T-lymphocyte populations can be distinguished both from other lymphocytes through presence of CD3 and as either CD4 (helper T cells) or CD8 (Cytotoxic T cells) positive; i.e., as CD3+CD4+CD8- or CD3+CD4-CD8+.

Using contemporary flow cytometers, such as the FACS Canto II from BD biosciences that has three lasers and detection of up to eight colors, much more elaborate cellular characterization can be performed with a single tube of cells.[11] Often, multiple tubes with different antibody cocktails are used to perform a more extensive cellular profile of a single patient. Flow cytometry is commonly used to profile peripheral blood cells,[12] such as RBCs and the subclasses of WBCs, but can also be used for detection of cells in bone marrow, cerebrospinal fluid and pleural fluid as well as for the detection of DNA, microbes, and even solid tissues that have been dissociated.[2] Furthermore, the increasing number of single fluorescent dyes such as APC (allophycocyanine) and PE (phycoerythrin) and tandem dyes such as Pe-Cy5 have increased the number of analytes that can be tested in a single tube. Generally, optimized analysis of immune cells can be classified by the frequency of the markers and assigning them to three categories: primary, secondary, and tertiary antigens.[13] Comparing the patient's cellular population profile to that of a normal population

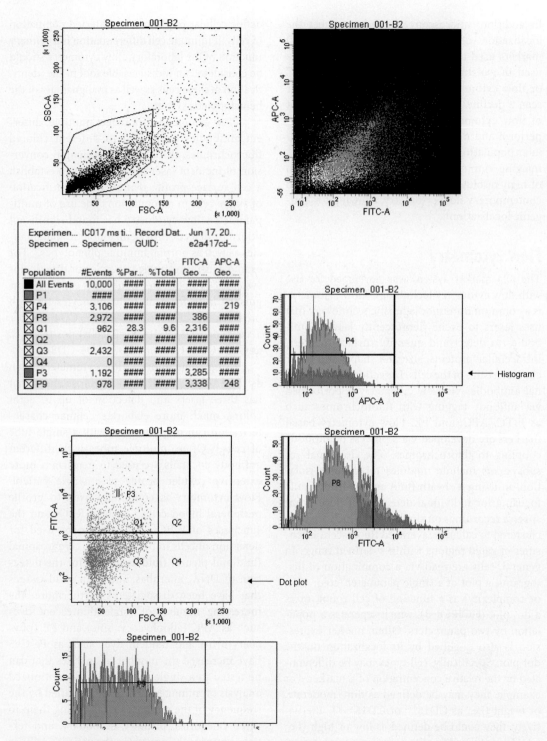

FIGURE 8–3 Example flow cytometry user interface. An example histogram, single parameter, and FACS dot plot; two parameters are indicated. *I. Clift.*

Immunophenotyping Optimization

Optimization of Immunophenotyping Panel Selections	
Primary antigens	Well characterized, broadly distributed, used to gate on a specific cellular subset. Either present or absent
Secondary antigens	High density per cell, also well characterized but found in a continuum from "low to high" or "dim to bright"
Tertiary antigens	Expressed at low levels only, used only if further differentiation is necessary

allows for a variety of applications, including assessment of pathological markers, therapeutic markers, and disease progression and diagnosis.

One caveat is that standardization in this field is still a work in progress,[14,15] specifically because new markers are being characterized, the large array of reagents commercially available, and the varying levels of expertise in clinical laboratories. In general, however, samples for flow cytometric analysis are obtained in heparinized or EDTA tubes, washed with PBS and BSA, and, in the case of WBC analysis, RBCs are first lysed using ammonium chloride or other lysis buffer before adding monoclonal antibodies.[16] Optimal sample preparation, in most cases, includes labeling antibodies at 4°C or room temperature. However, in some cases, lymphocyte enrichment using a Ficoll gradient and labeling at 37°C is more effective.[13] In some instances, such as in the FlowCellect Human CD4/CD8 T-Cell Assay developed through Millipore for use on the Guava EasyCyte and other instruments, whole blood specimens can be processed directly to detect CD4 and CD8 profiles.[17]

Karyotyping

Karyotyping was the first cytogenetic method used in clinical diagnostics of immunological malignancies and is still considered the gold

STEP-BY-STEP PROCEDURE 8–1   Preparing a Blood Control for Flow Cytometry Assays

Immunophenotyping laboratories commonly use either a patient sample or donor sample as a daily or weekly control for flow cytometric operations. However, untreated cells are prone to degradation and phenotypic changes; therefore, the following protocol describes how to prepare a blood control for long-term stability.

1. Collect specimen in EDTA tube
2. Determine the volume of collected blood
3. Add the appropriate volume of blood stabilization reagent (such as TransFix) using the manufacturer-provided ratios, e.g., 0.2 mL reagent to 1 mL of blood, as soon after collection as possible
4. Mix by inversion at least 10 times
5. Once treated, the sample may be aliquoted into smaller volumes to reduce cooling and heating of the specimen
6. The specimen can be stored for up to 14 days at 2–8°C
7. To use, warm specimen to room temperature and roll between hands 10 times and through inversion
8. Perform flow cytometry using manufacturer's instructions

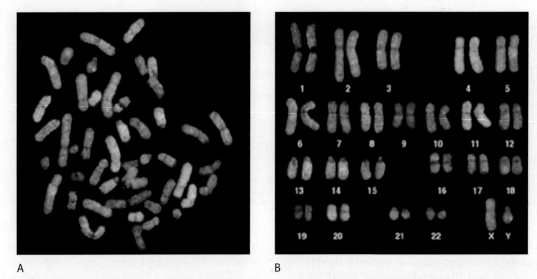

A   B

FIGURE 8-4 Normal male karyotype. Staining of each chromosome has been performed to further identify each chromosome pair. **(A)** Stained chromosome arrested in mitosis. **(B)** A karyotype where chromosome pairs are organized into groups.

From Reisner, H. (2017). Crowley's an introduction to human disease, 10e. Jones & Bartlett Learning.

standard (**FIGURE 8-4**). Although not technically an immunophenotypic method, this genetic technique has long been used along with immunophenotyping for the determination of inborne immunological malignancies, and any discussion of immunophenotyping techniques would be incomplete without its discussion. Genetic data have now become closely associated with the diagnostic and prognostic indications of neoplasms and are still particularly important in the work up surrounding hematological and immunological pathologies.[18] Following the culture of malignant cells from the bone marrow, metaphase-arrested chromosomes are harvested and prepared, including special staining and banding. The chromosomes are then examined by light microscopy to provide an overview of the chromosomal aberrations in a single tumor cell. Through karyotyping variants such as inversions, sectional duplications, translocations, and deletions of parts of specific chromosomes can be detected. A translocation, for example, is identified by the lower case letter "t" followed by the chromosomes involved, e.g., t(9;22). In addition, karyotyping can be used to detect trisomy and aneuploidy. The first abnormal chromosome detected was termed the Philadelphia Chromosome and is known as a hallmark of chronic myelogenous leukemia (CML).[18] Subsequently, many hematological and immunological tumors have been characterized using this method; thus, it remains an important immunophenotyping tool. Since the 1980s, newer genetic approaches to detection of genetic anomalies have begun to supplant karyotyping; namely, fluorescent *in situ* hybridization (FISH), in which labeled fluorescent probes are used to detect more specific regions of the genome. However, these advanced techniques are still less common for large-scale oncology screening due to reagent costs.[18]

Western Blotting

Antibodies are also used for Western blotting or immunoblotting. Western blots separate proteins by size from cellular lysates by running them through an agarose gel by electrophoresis. The proteins are transferred from the gel to a membrane where antibodies can be used to detect the protein of interest. Like IHC, typically, a primary antibody is used to detect the protein and a secondary antibody conjugated to an enzyme or fluorochrome that allows imaging of a band on the membrane. The band identified by the antibody provides a semiquantitative method of measuring the protein levels. One clinical use of Western blotting is during HIV testing. Common HIV proteins are separated on a gel and a patient's serum is used as the primary antibody. If the patient has HIV, he or she will have antibodies that recognize the proteins and bind to the membrane. Free antibody is washed away and a secondary antibody is used to detect if the patient has HIV-specific antibodies. Although traditionally less useful to immunophenotyping, due to the process of cell lysis that is required for antigenic isolation, isolated cell populations collected through cell sorting can be examined via Western blot analysis for intracellular markers of differentiation or pathogenesis, which have significant use in determining the etiology of malignancies.

Immunoprecipitations (IP) are a variant of the Western blot assay that uses antibodies. For an IP, antibodies for the protein of interest are conjugated to a bead. The beads are mixed with cell lysates and bind to the protein of interest. The beads can be spun down, pulling out the bound protein and anything else associated with the bound protein. The proteins precipitated out are separated by a Western blot. IPs are used to determine interactions among proteins.

▶ Erythroid Markers

Precursors to RBCs can occasionally be found in the periphery but are common in the bone marrow. Blasts can be characterized through flow cytometry via the expression of CD34, CXD38, CD45, CD117, and HLA-DR, and proerythroblasts are CD36+, CD38+, CD45+, CD71+, CD117+, CD235a+, and others.[19] They progressively lose expression of CD45 as they mature. In addition to traditional blood-group phenotyping, employed in the immunohematology or

blood-bank laboratory, there is a growing utility for the use of flow cytometry in the detection of **erythrocyte** markers.[20] Specifically, quantification of pretransplant group A and B antigens has been shown to have a prognostic value for long-term graft function.[20]

▶ Lymphoid Markers

Lymphocytes are critically important in the host defense against pathogens with B cells presenting antibodies to target disease-associated antigens and T cells acting in a regulatory role.[21] All lymphocytes are characterized by the presence of CD45. However, different, specific marker profiles are used by different commercial antibody suppliers for complete immunophenotyping of cell lineages such as B, T, and NK cells. A commonly ordered clinical panel assesses the populations of all three lymphoid populations, sometimes called the TBNK (T-cell, B-cell, and NK cell) assay. Cell lineage-specific antibodies such as CD20 for B cells and CD3 for T cells are traditionally recognized in these assays.[1] **Lymphocyte** populations are studied for their roles in chronic and acute genetic diseases, as well as in infectious disease correlations; in other words, for both primary and secondary immunological disorders.

Like other clinical assays, immunophenotyping of lymphoid populations is determined through defining a reference value range obtained through the assessment of a healthy control population.[12] Reference ranges are established within an institution based on the method employed, specimen type, and the age, sex, and other demographics pertaining to the patient population. Variation between facilities still remains in established reference ranges, and one important variable in reference-range determination is the removal of RBCs prior to analysis.[12] Another variable is based on CD panel design. However, despite differences between commercially available antibody panels, quantification of cell populations between panels has been shown to have good correlation.[16]

Reference Ranges for Common Leukocyte Antigens in Peripheral Blood (Adult Human)		
CD Marker	**Cell Lineage**	**Reference Range (%)***
CD3+	T Cells	49 to 85
CD3+CD4+CD8–	Helper T Cells	26 to 61
CD3+CD4–CD8+	Cytotoxic T Cells	10 to 31
CD16+CD56+ (or CD56–)	NK Cells	6 to 29
CD19+ CD20+ (or CD20–)	B Cells	7 to 23

*All data based on McCoy and Overton, *Cytometry*, 1994.

B-Cell Phenotyping

B cells represent between 7 and 23% of the peripheral lymphocyte population.[10] B cells have historically been identified through the expression of specific immunoglobulin heavy and light chains such as lambda (λ) and kappa (κ), which still serve some functional utility, as most B cells contain at least one of these chains in maturity.[21] Furthermore, heavy chain expression may represent a distinguishing feature in the argument that there are two B-cell lineages that can be distinguished by the presence of the N insertion in the rearranged V_H, DH, and J_H gene segments and the presence of CD5.[22] Currently, cells are most easily phenotyped by the presence of CD19, CD20, and CD22. CD20 is associated with the expression of the B-cell receptor. Both CD19 and CD20 generally represent B cells from the pro-B cell to pre-B cell phase until maturity.[21] Activated B cells can also be characterized by the upregulation of CD38.[23]

In addition to normal B-cell markers, plasma cells, also termed plasmablasts, are often identified by the presence of CD38 via flow cytometry; CD38 is also found in B-cell progenitors but is downregulated as the cells mature.[24] They are traditionally found in low levels in peripheral blood but can be found in the bone marrow and secondary lymphoid tissues such as lymph nodes.

Plasma cells in the bone marrow typically lack expression of traditional B-cell markers such as CD20. Plasma cells also upregulate CD138. The combined use of CD38 and CD138, in addition to other B-cell markers, is recommended for the identification of plasma cells found in multiple myeloma, a cancer of plasma cells.[24,25]

T-Cell Phenotyping

CD3 is the most commonly used T-cell marker as it is a major component of the T-cell receptor, which is thus far only found in T-cell populations. A cell that lacks CD3 cannot function as a T-cell.[4] In addition to CD3 there are several other pan–T-cell antigens, including CD2, CD5, and CD7, that can be used as a marker of T-cell lineage.[10] Despite this specificity, at least one CD3 chain, the zeta chain, has been found in other cells, specifically the NK cell.[4] This example illustrates the issue with utilizing a single marker for cell lineage specification. A CD3-only assay will not only pick up T cells, but also a population of NK cells, which could confound diagnostics. Thus, in T cells, as in any other cell lineage differentiation, diagnostic identification of cell populations is performed using multiple markers.

Several T-cell subpopulations are commonly examined for diagnostic purposes in a clinical setting. For example, it has been well established that a larger overall number of memory T cells and their subsets are a good prognostic indicator of vaccine efficacy.[26] All T cells are CD3+ cells, T helper cells (CD3+CD4+), cytotoxic T cells (CD3+,CD8+), and double negative T cells (CD3+, CD4-,CD8-).[23] The most classical separation of T cells is via the CD4 or CD8 antigens, which represent either class II (CD4) or class I (CD8) MHC identifying molecules. Among CD3 positive cells, approximately 75% are CD4+ while 25% are CD8+. A switch in the CD4/CD8 ratio was one of the earliest indicators of HIV's conversion to AIDS.[27] The double negative T-cell population is an indication of the quantity of immature T cells in circulation and is higher in childhood, peaking at around 2 to 6 years of age.[23]

More elaborate profiling techniques are used to examine the subpopulations and functional subtypes of T cells. Memory T cells, for instance, are characterized into two classes: central and effector cells, with central memory cells expressing CD45RO rather than CD45RA found in naïve populations.[26]

NK Cell Phenotyping

NK (natural killer) cells perform two very specific functions: cytolytic activity and cytokine production to eliminate malignant cells and viral infection. NK cells represent between 6 and 30% of circulating lymphocytes.[10] They typically lack expression of CD3, except occasionally when they present with CD3 zeta chain and are characterized by the expression of CD2 and CD16. However, they can be further subdivided by the fluctuation in expression of CD16 with CD56.[10,28] Fluctuations in the surface expression of CD marker CD56 is a strong indicator of NK cell activity. CD16[bright]/CD56[dim] cells are heavily involved in cytokine production while CD16[dim]/CD56[bright] cells, representing nearly 90% of the population, mediate cytotoxicity.[28] In traditional flow cytometry assays, NK cells are often characterized as CD3–, TcR–lymphocytes with either dim or bright CD56.[28] Whole blood samples have recently been used to detect the risk of colorectal cancer based on the

activity of NK cells in circulation via the expression level of CD56.[29] Another surface marker that is useful in identifying NK activity is CD69, which is considered an early activation marker.[28]

▶ Myeloid/Granulocyte Markers

Granulocytes found in bone marrow, peripheral blood, and other tissues are predominately part of the innate immune response to disease, and consist of the neutrophils, eosinophils, basophils, and monocytes. They are named for their morphological features including the presence of cytotoxic lysosomal granules, which were historically easy to stain using cellular dyes; one of the earliest methods employed for the phenotyping of immune cells, specifically, granulocyte populations. Lysosomal granules can contain lysozyme, myeloperoxidase, lactoferrin and others, and are either released during an immune response or are the target organelles used in eliminating potentially pathogenic molecules and bacterial cells. Accumulating evidence suggests an increased role for granulocytes, and in particular, neutrophils, in both bloodborne and solid-tumor pathophysiology.[30] Granulocytes and monocytes collected from bone marrow aspirates from individuals with suspected bone marrow malignancies, such as myelodysplastic syndrome (MDS), have begun to be analyzed clinically via flow cytometry using key CD markers such as CD45, CD10, and others as part of diagnostic workups.[31]

Neutrophils

Accounting for between 60 to 70% of peripheral leukocytes, neutrophils are traditionally known for their role in antimicrobial action; specifically in directed migration toward the pathogens, adherence and phagocytosis, and microbial killing.[21] They contain the most robust bactericidal lysosomal products of all the cell hematopoietic cells including lysozyme, myeloperoxidase, and lactoferrin.[32] The three classes of surface antigens suitable for detection and classification of neutrophils are the integrins, Fc gamma receptors (such as CD16), and the ectopeptidase CD10.[10] The beta 2 integrin (CD18) in combination with LFA1 (CD11a), Mac-1(CD11b), and/or p150 (CD11c), which are important for neutrophil recruitment to inflammatory sites, are common antibody targets.[10] Additionally, neutrophils have a very high and broad side scatter on dot plots and are often identified via the marker profile CD15+CD11b+ CD16+CD10+, which includes a combination of the above markers and the less-well-understood, granulocyte-specific carbohydrate CD15. In addition to their well-established role in microbial elimination, emerging evidence indicates a role of neutrophil expansion in poorer prognosis for patients with a variety of cancers, including ovarian, breast, and pancreatic cancer.[30]

Basophils

Basophils are the least-common granulocyte, representing less than 1% of circulating WBCs. However, they are found increased in circulation during inflammatory and allergic disease responses. Basophils are characterized as CD9+, CD13+, CD22+, CD25^{dim}, CD33+, CD36+, CD38^{bright}, CD123^{bright}, and are very low in SSC plot.[19]

Eosinophils

Eosinophils are typically easy to characterize via morphological studies due to their high density of acidophilic granules, which are stained red in the presence of the dye eosin. They consist of approximately 1 to 3% of total circulating WBCs in the normal population. In contrast to neutrophils, eosinophils can be characterized by a higher expression of CD45 and absence of CD16. In addition, they are recognized by having high SSC and low FSC. They are positive for CD11b, CD11c, CD13, CD15, and CD33.

Monocytes

Monocytes are known to be the circulating form of the tissue-invading macrophages, an important component of the innate immune response. Along with their distinctive size and shape on side and forward scatter plots (SSC and FSC) using traditional hematology analyzers, CD14, a co-receptor for the Toll-like receptors (TLRs),[33] is a prominent surface marker for monocytes. A useful panel for the immunophenotyping of monocytes is CD14+, CD13+, CD33+, CD36+, CD38+, CD163+, and HLA-DR. They are also positive for CD11b, CD11c, and CD64 with possible expression of CD2 and CD4.[19]. However, they share expression of some of these factors with other populations. For example, CD36 is also an expression on RBCs and platelets. Furthermore, two types of monocytes have been described: CD16– and CD16+.[10] CD16, an important Fc receptor subtype, is also expressed on other antigen-presenting cells such as the neutrophil. Monocyte markers are also useful for the identification of tissue-invading macrophages and other cells derived from this lineage including osteoclasts, Kupfer cells in the liver, dendritic cells, mast cells, and Langerhans cells.[19,34] Bone marrow mast cells can be differentiated from other cell types, for example, via the strong presence of CD117 and FcεRI when in the absence of CD138, CD34, and CD38.[35]

▶ Blast Markers and Markers of Development

Cells that will eventually become mature immune cells are characterized immunophenotypically by the presence of CD34, CD133, CD184, and HLA-DR.[19] As they mature, they lose expression of some of these early markers. Lymphoblasts and myeloblasts are typically isolated to the bone marrow in normal populations; however, during the course of malignancy, blast populations are commonly found in the peripheral blood and are often the first indicator of disease. In some clinical cases, pathologists are expected to determine a diagnostic and prognostic workup for a leukemia based on peripheral blood immunophenotyping alone, despite significant differences in the population of these cells in the bone marrow.[36] Many laboratories perform a single panel to detect both lymphoid and myeloid neoplasms, which are first gated on the total CD45 population. However, specific markers are indicative of different disease etiologies and most practitioners recommend using a standard, upfront panel followed by a more disease-specific panel.[1] Historical staging of differentiation was performed through morphological assessment of the cells of the bone marrow via microscopy. Flow cytometry has greatly aided in the quantification of these populations through the cytometric assessment of patient bone marrow specimens. Furthermore, the presence of lymphoid or myeloid precursor populations in peripheral blood is diagnostically indicative of specific disease processes.

Lymphoblast Markers

Like the general case for blast markers, initial indications are made through an examination of CD45. Both T and B lymphoblasts have similar morphological features on blood and bone marrow smears, including a variation in size from mature lymphocytes and the presence of low to moderated basophilic cytoplasm. Unlike mature cells, blast cells contain the potential presence of a number of CD markers. Indeed, the classification of lymphoblasts, based on marker profiles, is typically used to determine the age and maturity of these cells. Characterization of lymphoblasts by immunophenotyping often occurs only in the identification of malignancies. B lymphoblasts often contain CD10, CD19, and CD79a, which are used as correlative indicators of B-cell malignancies such as B-ALL (acute lymphoblastic leukemia). T-ALL, in contrast, can be marked by the presence of CD3, CD5, and CD7. Most lymphomas are B-cell lymphomas characterized by CD20. Peripheral T-cell lymphomas (PTCLs) are uncommon malignancies with both an aggressive clinical course and poor prognosis but consist of 15% of Non-Hodgkin lymphomas and a variety of clinically identifiable leukemic, cutaneous, extranodal, and nodal neoplasias.[37]

Myeloblast Markers

Myeloblasts, which also differentiate from a common hematopoietic progenitor cell type, continue to express CD34 and HLA-DR and upregulate the expression of CD38, CD117, CD4, CD13^{dim}, and CD33.[19] In normal development, myeloblasts are the progenitors to the class of predominately innate immune cell types known as granulocytes, which include neutrophils, eosinophils, basophils, and monocytes. They are normally present in large quantities in the bone marrow with a very rare presence in peripheral blood. Similar to lymphoblasts, the further staging of myeloid progenitors can be determined by the presence or lack of key markers. This is often clinically useful in determining the cause of specific disease conditions. For instance, myeloid-derived granulocytic suppressor cells have been found in cancer patients.[30]

▶ Major Clinical Utility and Disease Correlations

The major utility of immunophenotyping is in the detection and diagnosis of immune lineage malignancies such as chronic lymphocytic leukemia (CLL), acute myeloid leukemia (ALL), and acute lymphoblastic leukemia (AML). These malignancies have been profiled and classified by the World Health Organization (WHO) into either leukemias or lymphomas. Leukemias are defined as malignant bone marrow or blood-forming organs, which produce an increased number of immature leukocytes. Lymphomas are defined as a specific cancer of the lymph nodes; however, many diseases can be defined by both categories.

Recent advances in immunophenotyping and genetics have resulted in a significant reliance on these technologies in the detection of hematopoietic neoplasms.[36] Panels are used to determine the cell lineage, stage of differentiation, and clonality of a given cell population.[1] Panels for the detection of increased blasts in circulation have been used in the determination and therapeutic intervention of CLL,[38] for example. Other diseases, such as Burkitt lymphoma and mastocytosis, are defined by the presence of specific markers such as CD2 and CD25 in mastocytosis.[1] Organizations such as the

European Leukemia Net (ELN) and EuroFlow Consortium suggest comprehensive panels, not all of which have been deemed essential, in order to isolate these acute and chronic immune malignancies.[1] More recently, an emphasis has been given to the prognostic utility of immuno-phenotyping as well. A detailed examination of the phenotypic markers of hematopoietic malignancies of the myeloid lineage can be found in Gorczyca et al. 2011.[19]

Chronic Lymphocytic Leukemia

CLL is most often a B-cell leukemia (B-CLL) characterized by the overexpression of CD38. However, overexpression of CD38 is not a definitive marker of only CLL and, therefore, a panel of cellular surface markers have been variously proposed for determining the immunophenotype of CLL and prognostic indicators of the disease.[38] In particular, immunoglobulin variable heavy chain mutation has been shown to be prognostic for an aggressive course of the disease. Specifically, nonmutated variable heavy chain is considered to be the more aggressive form.[38] Other factors contributing to phenotyping include karyotype analysis and DNA microarray analysis.[39] CD5, CD23, CD43, Cd49d, and Zap-70 have all been seen in CLL, occasionally with prognostic value, and other markers have been assessed for diagnostic and prognostic value in the current literature. Besides other pan-B cell markers, CLL is typically characterized clinically via the CD19+, CD5+, Cd23+, CD22−, CD79b− phenotypes.[39] While no specific etiologic agent has been attributed to CLL, some evidence suggests that in the case of B-CLL, the retrovirus human T-lymphotropic virus type 1 (HTLV-1) has preceded the development of CLL in some patients, and may be the result of a B-cell transformation in response to that virus.[40] Marker panels are also used to differentiate CLL from other forms of lymphocytic disorders including mantle-cell lymphoma, hair-cell leukemia, and follicular-cell lymphoma.

Acute Myeloid Leukemia

AML is characterized by the presence of CD19 and PAX5 positivity but includes a diversity of malignancies with various characteristic markers. One variant of AML is acute promyelocytic leukemia (APL), which is associated with a high mortality rate without prompt intervention, and can be characterized by the presence of several key immunodiagnostic markers; for example, a new case of AML lacking CD34, and HLA-DR may be a case of promyelocytic leukemia.[5] In a recent study, more than 96% of patients with APL were found to be positive for CD9.[41] Of note, CD2+, CD56+, and CD34+ APL is associated with increased incidence of early death and lower overall survival.[41] In general, AMLs are low in SSC and express moderate CD45; they are also positive for myeloid markers in the majority of cases.[19]

Acute Lymphoblastic Leukemia

Most ALL are within the B-cell lineage. B lymphoblasts often contain CD10, CD19, and CD79a, which are used as correlative indicators of B-cell malignancies such as B-ALL. The existence or absence of certain CD markers may be indicative of a specific form of B-ALL. One variant of ALL, called early T-cell precursor ALL, which accounts for 15% of all T-lymphoblastic leukemia/lymphoma, is specifically characterized by expression of CD7, cytoplasmic CD3, weak or absent CD5—the stem cell associated CD34—and the absence of CD1a and CD8, as well as the aberrant expression of several myeloid-associate antigens.[1]

Nonmalignant Disorders

In addition to detection of hematopoietic malignancies, immunophenotyping can be used in the diagnosis of nonmalignant disorders such as septic infections, large granular lymphocyte increases as a result of neutropenia or anemia, disorders of glycosylphosphatidylinositol (GPI), and hypereosinophilia syndrome.[10] Other immune disorders, such as common variable immunodeficiency (CVID), which is associated with at least a third of primary immunodeficiency cases in the United States, are often coupled with a clonal lymphoproliferation of one or more T- or B-cell populations, which can be detected via immunophenotypic analysis.[42]

The ultimate goal of immunophenotyping in the clinical setting is to determine the causative cellular population affecting the patients' health and, when possible, to establish timely therapies that also monitor changes in the patients' cellular profiles.

CASE STUDY

Lymphoma to Leukemia

This case is based on Steussy et al., 2016, *Lab Medicine*.[43]

A 52-year-old Caucasian woman was being seen at an Iowa hospital for a stage IV grade 1 follicular lymphoma, the second most common B-cell lymphoma seen clinically. She was being treated with bendamustine, an anticancer chemotherapy drug, and rituximab, a monoclonal antibody therapy targeting CD20, with partial success, followed with rituximab for a period of 2 years. CT scans showed no evidence of disease; however, the patient did seek treatment for bruising, dyspnea, pancytopenia, and coagulopathy.

Laboratory Findings

Smears of the blood and bone marrow revealed extremely large cells with folded nuclei that had abundance of basophilic cytoplasm with scattered granules that stained strongly for myeloperoxidase. These findings raised suspicions of a potential promyelocytic leukemia. Immunophenotyping via flow cytometry revealed cells that were CD45+, CD64+, CD38+, CD15(partial)+, and CD71(partial)+ with negativity for other myeloid and lymphoid markers, including CD14, CD33, and CD34. A core biopsy revealed 100% cellular marrow entirely replaced with tumor cells, and IHC studies revealed cells positive for CD4, lysozyme, and CD31^{dim}, but lacking expression of CD79a, CD68, and CD163. A FISH study for translocation t(15;17) was negative. Karyotypic evaluation, however, revealed cytogenetic abnormalities leading to an additional FISH study that revealed a t(14;18) translocation involving the BCL2 gene and an extra immunoglobin (Ig)H with loss of BCL2. DNA extracts from the recent bone marrow specimens and the original follicular lymphoma from the patient showed similar heavy-chain rearrangement indicative of a clonal relationship. A repeat CT scan showed new widespread lymphadenopathy not present 2 months prior, which was suspicious for acute myeloid leukemia.

Discussion

The authors report that this was the first reported case of a leukemic transdifferentiation of follicular lymphoma into an acute histiocytic leukemia. The finding of a t(14;18) translocation and the same-size IgH rearrangements in the case suggested transdifferentiation instead of coincidental sporadic leukemia. Furthermore, they suggest that this provides evidence that there is plasticity among these tumors with a preference toward a specific differentiation from lymphomatous B cells into leukemic macrophages. They also point out that this case provides evidence that a more thorough examination of under-recognized subsets of transdifferentiated tumor may need more robust elucidation.

Critical Thinking Questions

1. What role did flow cytometric immunophenotyping play in the characterization of tumor transdifferentiation in this case?
2. What other methods were employed to phenotype changes in the patient's tumor?

▶ # References

1. Heel K, Tabone T, Röhrig KJ, et al. Developments in the immunophenotypic analysis of haematological malignancies. *Blood Rev.* 2013;27(4):193–207.

2. Virgo PF, Gibbs GJ. Flow cytometry in clinical pathology. *Ann Clin Biochem.* 2012;49(pt 1):17–28.

3. Engel P, Boumsell L, Balderas R, et al. CD Nomenclature 2015: human leukocyte differentiation antigen workshops as a driving force in immunology. *J Immunol.* 2015;195(10):4555–4563.

4. Zola H. Markers of cell lineage, differentiation and activation. *J Biol Regul Homeost Agents.* 2000;14(3):218–219.

5. Peters JM, Ansari MQ. Multiparameter flow cytometry in the diagnosis and management of acute leukemia. *Arch Pathol Lab Med.* 2011;135(1):44–54.

6. Biancotto A, McCoy JP. Studying the human immunome: the complexity of comprehensive leukocyte immunophenotyping. *Curr Top Microbiol Immunol.* 2014;377:23–60.

7. Chai CC. Bone Marrow Procedure, Examination, and Reporting. In: Farhi DC, ed. *Pathology of bone marrow and blood cells.* Philadelphia: Lippincott Williams & Wilkins; 2004:15–25.

8. Leland DS. Virus isolation in traditional cell cultures. *Clinical Virology.* Philadelphia: Saunders; 1996:xi, 236 p.

9. Fritzky L, Lagunoff D. Advanced methods in fluorescence microscopy. *Anal Cell Pathol (Amst).* 2013;36(1–2):5–17.

10. Béné MC, Le Bris Y, Robillard N, et al. Flow cytometry in hematological nonmalignant disorders. *Int J Lab Hematol.* 2016;38(1):5–16.

11. Boldt A, Borte S, Fricke S, et al. Eight-color immunophenotyping of T-, B-, and NK-cell subpopulations for characterization of chronic immunodeficiencies. *Cytometry B Clin Cytom.* 2014;86(3):191–206.

12. McCoy JP, Jr., Overton WR. Quality control in flow cytometry for diagnostic pathology: II. A conspectus of reference ranges for lymphocyte immunophenotyping. *Cytometry.* 1994;18(3):129–139.

13. Mahnke YD, Roederer M. Optimizing a multicolor immunophenotyping assay. *Clin Lab Med.* 2007;27(3):469–485.

14. Maecker HT, McCoy JP, Nussenblatt R. Standardizing immunophenotyping for the Human Immunology Project. *Nat Rev Immunol.* 2012;12(3):191–200.

15. Wood B, Jevremovic D, Béné MC, et al. Validation of cell-based fluorescence assays: practice guidelines from the ICSH and ICCS - part V - assay performance criteria. *Cytometry B Clin Cytom.* 2013;84(5):315–323.

16. Preijers FW, Huys E, Favre C, et al. Establishment of harmonization in immunophenotyping: a comparative study of a standardized one-tube lymphocyte-screening panel. *Cytometry B Clin Cytom.* 2014;86(6):418–425.

17. Flow Cellect Human CD4/CD8 T-Cell Kit. Revision 2 ed. Darmstadt, Germany EMD Millipore Corporation; 2015.

18. Wan TS. Cancer cytogenetics: methodology revisited. *Ann Lab Med.* 2014;34(6):413–425.

19. Gorczyca W, Sun Z-Y, Cronin W, et al. Immunophenotypic Pattern of Myeloid Populations by Flow Cytometry Analysis. In: Darzynkiewicz Z, Holden E, Orfao A, Telford W, Wlodkowic D, eds. *Recent Advances in Cytometry, Part B Advances in Applications.* Vol 103: Elsevier Inc.; 2011:221–266.

20. Sundbäck M, Grufman P, Teller J, et al. Quantification of blood group A and B antibodies by flow cytometry using beads carrying A or B trisaccharides. *Transplantation.* 2007;84(12 suppl):S24–S26.

21. Fleisher TA, Tomar RH. Introduction to diagnostic laboratory immunology. *JAMA.* 1997;278(22):1823–1834.

22. Wortis HH. Surface markers, heavy chain sequences and B-cell lineages. *Intern Rev Immunol.* 1992;8(2–3):235–246.

23. Tosato F, Bucciol G, Pantano G, et al. Lymphocytes subsets reference values in childhood. *Cytometry A.* 2015;87(1):81–85.

24. Flores-Montero J, de Tute R, Paiva B, et al. Immunophenotype of normal vs. myeloma plasma cells: toward antibody panel specifications for MRD detection in multiple myeloma. *Cytometry B Clin Cytom.* 2016;90(1):61–72.

25. Pojero F, Flores-Montero J, Sanoja L, et al. Utility of CD54, CD229, and CD319 for the identification of plasma cells in patients with clonal plasma cell diseases. *Cytometry B Clin Cytom.* 2016;90(1):91–100.

26. Saade F, Gorski SA, Petrovsky N. Pushing the frontiers of T-cell vaccines: accurate measurement of human T-cell responses. *Expert Rev Vaccines.* 2012;11(12):1459–1470.

27. Clift IC. Diagnostic flow cytometry and the AIDS pandemic. *Lab Med.* 2015;46(3):e59–e64.

28. Butterfield LH, Whiteside TL. Measurements of natural killer (NK) cells. *Crit Rev Oncog.* 2014;19(1–2):47–55.

29. Jobin G, Rodriguez-Suarez R, Betito K. Association between natural killer cell activity and colorectal cancer in high-risk subjects undergoing colonoscopy. *Gastroenterology.* 2017;153(4):980–987.

30. Dumitru CA, Moses K, Trellakis S, et al. Neutrophils and granulocytic myeloid-derived suppressor cells: immunophenotyping, cell biology and clinical relevance in human oncology. *Cancer Immunol Immunother.* 2012;61(8):1155–1167.

31. Moon HW, Huh JW, Lee M, et al. Immunophenotypic features of granulocytes, monocytes, and blasts in myelodysplastic syndromes. *Korean J Lab Med.* 2010;30(2):97–104.

32. Strobl H, Knapp W. Myeloid cell-associated lysosomal proteins as flow cytometry markers for leukocyte lineage classification. *J Biol Regul Homeost Agents.* 2004; 18(3–4):335–339.

33. Raby AC, Labéta MO. Therapeutic boosting of the immune response: turning to CD14 for help. *Curr Pharm Biotechnol.* 2016;17(5):414–418.

34. Teodosio C, Mayado A, Sánchez-Muñoz L, et al. The immunophenotype of mast cells and its utility in the

diagnostic work-up of systemic mastocytosis. *J Leukoc Biol.* 2015;97(1):49–59.

35. Escribano L, Orfao A, Villarrubia J, et al. Immunophenotypic characterization of human bone marrow mast cells. A flow cytometric study of normal and pathological bone marrow samples. *Anal Cell Pathol.* 1998;16(3):151–159.

36. Almarzooqi S, Crumbacher J, Firgau E, Kahwash SB. Immunophenotypic comparison of peripheral blood (Pb) versus bone marrow (Bm) blasts in pediatric acute leukemias. *Modern Pathol.* 2010;23(2):328–328.

37. Bisig B, Gaulard P, de Leval L. New biomarkers in T-cell lymphomas. *Best Pract Res Clin Haematol.* 2012;25(1):13–28.

38. Zucchetto A, Cattarossi I, Nanni P, et al. Cluster analysis of immunophenotypic data: the example of chronic lymphocytic leukemia. *Immunol Lett.* 2011;134(2):137–144.

39. Dillman RO. Immunophenotyping of chronic lymphoid leukemias. *J Clin Oncol.* 2008;26(8):1193–1194.

40. Holmer LD, Bueso-Ramos CE. Chronic Lymphocytic Leukemia and Related Lymphoproliferative Disorders. In: Harmening D, ed. *Clinical hematology and fundamentals of hemostasis.* 5th ed. Philadelphia: F.A. Davis Co.; 2009:440–465.

41. Xu F, Yin CX, Wang CL, et al. Immunophenotypes and immune markers associated with acute promyelocytic leukemia prognosis. *Dis Markers.* 2014;2014:421906.

42. Williams SA, Moench LE, Khan F, et al. Clonal lymphoproliferations in a patient with common variable immunodeficiency. *Lab Med.* 2016;47(4):318–325.

43. Steussy B, Lekostaj J, Qian Q, et al. Leukemic transdifferentiation of follicular lymphoma into an acute histiocytic leukemia in a 52-year-old Caucasian woman. *Lab Med.* 2016;47(2):155–157.

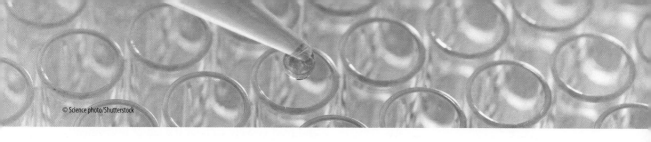

CHAPTER 9

Viral Serology

Diane Leland, PhD; **Ian Clift**, PhD, MLS(ASCP)CM

KEY TERMS

Acquired immunodeficiency
  syndrome (AIDS)
Adenovirus
Arbovirus
Burkitts lymphoma
California encephalitis group
Chikungunya virus
Coronaviruses
Cytomegalovirus (CMV)
Dengue virus
Eastern equine encephalitis
Enterovirus

Epstein-barr virus (EBV)
Flaviviruses
Guillain-barre
Hepatitis viruses
Herpes simplex virus
Human immunodeficiency virus
  type - 1 (HIV-1)
Human T-cell lymphotropic viruses
  (HTLV)
Influenza virus
Measles
Noroviruses

Petechiae
Respiratory syncytial virus (RSV)
Retroviruses
Rhinoviruses
Rotavirus
Rubella
Varicella zoster virus (VZV)
Western equine encephalitis virus
West nile virus
Zika virus

LEARNING OBJECTIVES

Upon completion of this chapter, the reader should be able to:

1. Classify viruses by family.
2. List diseases associated with commonly infectious viruses.
3. Indicate whether viral antigen detection methods are available and/or clinically utilized.
4. Describe major arboviruses detected clinically.
5. List the major herpes Family Viruses and indicate the most infective cell type.
6. Review the history and derivation of Human Immunodeficiency Viruses.
7. Describe antigen testing for respiratory viruses such as influenza and parainfluenza.

▶ Introduction to Viral Serology

Methods for direct detection and identification of viruses have improved dramatically in the last several decades. Molecular methods for detecting viral DNA and RNA are now available for many viruses and are easy to use. Viral antigen detection is also available for many viruses in immunofluorescent and immunochromatographic (lateral flow) formats suitable for use in point-of-care settings and for rapid viral antigen detection in the clinical laboratory. Virus isolation in culture has also improved with the advent of centrifugation-enhanced inoculation of cells grown on coverslips contained in shell vials, allowing for detection of many viruses after only 24 to 48 hours of culture incubation.

Despite these advances in direct virus detection methods, the serologic approach, which is based on detecting antibodies produced against the virus during infection, continues to be useful in many situations. This is especially true for viruses for which molecular methods or antigen-detection methods are not widely available, those that do not proliferate in standard cell cultures, and those that pose a hazard for laboratory personnel. Methods for antibody detection are often much easier to standardize and automate, require less technical expertise, take less time to perform, are more cost-effective, and do not require an invasive collection of samples for as only a peripheral blood sample collected by venipuncture is needed. Often, a serologic method is used as a screening test, which will then be followed by confirmatory or molecular testing if samples yield a positive screening test result.

Serologic testing is based on detecting/identifying antibodies by their capacity to react with the antigen that stimulated their production. Thus, serologic assays, regardless of assay format, involve exposing a known viral antigen to the patient's serum in order to allow the corresponding antibodies, if present, to bind to the antigen. Then, depending on the assay format, this binding is detected and measured to confirm the presence of the antibody. Serologic assays can be very simple direct methods, or require multiple steps performed by sophisticated instrumentation. Some of the simple assays can be performed manually on a disposable card and read visually without the aid of instrumentation. In these assays, many of which are based on the serologic principle of passive agglutination, a particle (usually a latex particle or an erythrocyte) is coated with the viral antigen. The coated particles are then mixed on a slide with the patient's serum. Visible agglutination of the particles signals the presence of the viral antibody of interest. These assays can be completed in 1 or 2 minutes.

More complex assays are often based on the principle of solid phase enzyme-linked immunosorbent assay (ELISA or EIA). Such assays feature a multistep process in which the known viral antigen is coated on a solid surface such as the wall of a test tube or microwell or the surface, of a microbead. The patient's serum is then exposed to the solid surface, allowing viral antibodies in the serum to bind to the viral antigen coated on the surface. After washing away any unbound components, a preparation of enzyme-labeled antibodies directed against human antibodies—usually human IgG—is added and will attach to antibodies that bind to the viral antigen in the first step of the assay. After washing away unbound components, a substrate solution—which will change color when acted upon by the enzyme attached to the bound antibodies—is added. After a suitable incubation period, the amount of color change is evaluated and interpreted as positive or negative for the presence of the viral antibody of interest. These ELISA assays typically take 1 to 2 hours or more to complete and may require sophisticated instrumentation.

Other serologic methods, usually blotting methods employing viral antigenic components separated based on their molecular weights, are designed to detect antibodies against specific viral epitopes; this sort of detection is needed to differentiate antibodies produced against the infecting virus from those produced against closely-related viral strains. Other viral serodiagnostic methods rely on qualitative detection of antibodies expressed at various stages of the infection in order to determine whether the antibodies are related to acute, chronic, or resolved infection or are vaccine-related.

These examples of serologic assays are just a sampling of the concepts employed in serologic determinations. The principles of additional serologic assays are explained and their formats are further described in Chapters 5 and 6 of this volume.

Exactly how the serologic approach is employed in diagnosis and management of viral infections varies from virus to virus. Assays that detect virus-specific IgG antibodies can be used quantitatively to measure changes in IgG level between acute and convalescent samples collected 2 to 3 weeks apart. A significant increase in IgG level signals a current or very recent infection. Other IgG assays are performed qualitatively for use in immune status determinations. Typically, if antibodies are absent, the individual is identified as "susceptible" to further infection. If antibodies are present, the individual is expected to be immune to further infection with that particular virus. When some viruses that establish latency after the primary infection, the presence of IgG indicates previous experience with the virus but does not indicate protection from further viral activity. These viruses have the capacity to react and produce disease symptoms when the host is stressed. In congenital infection, IgG testing can be helpful. Although maternal IgG crosses the placenta and can be detected in the serum of the infant, sequential testing for IgG antibodies will help differentiate antibodies of maternal origin from those produced by the infant. Sequential testing for infant IgG over a 6-month period will demonstrate a marked decrease in IgG level, probably to undetectable, if the antibodies are maternal in origin; these diminish simply due to the half-life of circulating antibodies. In contrast, if the infant is actually infected, sequential IgG testing will not show a decrease in IgG level. Instead, the IgG level will remain steady or will increase over a 6 month period. This shows that the infant is actually infected and is producing the IgG.

Some serologic assays are designed to detect only virus-specific IgM class antibodies. A positive result with these assays indicates current or very recent viral activity. A negative result may rule out current or recent infection. IgM-specific testing is also useful in determining congenital infection. Because maternal IgM does not cross the placenta, any IgM detected in an infant indicates that the infant is producing the IgM and is infected with the corresponding virus. Unfortunately, IgM-specific methods are not perfect and also are not available for many viruses.

Traditional serologic testing has been performed on serum samples diluted in serial two-fold dilutions, e.g., 1:2, 1:4, 1:8, 1:16, 1:32, etc. The antibody level, or "titer," was assigned to the highest dilution that produced reactivity; this result was called the "endpoint," and was expressed as the dilution factor of the highest dilution-producing reactivity, e.g., an endpoint, or titer, of 1:4. In assays that required comparing antibody levels of two samples, at least a four-fold difference was required in order to define a significant difference, e.g., 1:4 vs. 1:16. This strategy worked well until EIA testing became popular. EIA results are reported as continuous-scale numbers rather than serial dilution titers. The manufacturer of the particular EIA assays must define how much numerical difference must be shown between two samples in order to confirm that there is a significant difference.

Serologic testing can be complicated by cross-reacting antibodies as well as technical issues involved with assay performance. In addition, patients who are immunocompromised may not produce a typical antibody response in viral infections. Despite such issues, the serologic approach can often be very helpful in identifying infecting agents and providing information that is vital for effective patient management.

The purpose of this chapter is to provide information on the current uses of the serologic approach for diagnosis of viral infections, with emphasis on those viruses for which antibody detection remains the primary diagnostic approach. The role of serology for viruses typically diagnosed by other methods is reviewed, and the pros and cons of using the serologic approach for diagnosing/monitoring each infection is presented.

▶ Arboviruses

Arbovirus is a generalized name for any viruses that are passed or transmitted by arthropods; most commonly, the tick, the culex mosquito, which is a known vector for Japanese encephalitis and

West Nile, and the Aedes mosquito, which is the source or dengue virus and yellow fever virus. The arboviruses include any arthropodborne viruses primarily consisting of a member of the Flaviviridae, Togaviridae, Bunyaviridae, and Reoviridae families.[1] A preliminary diagnosis is based on clinical presentation and symptoms, while a definitive diagnosis is made in the laboratory through a combination of blood-based immunological and serological techniques, as well as genetic testing.

These viruses will not proliferate in standard cell cultures, and tests for detection of viral antigens are not widely available. The diagnosis relies on serologic testing of paired sera. Such serologic testing is usually available at public health laboratories and reference centers and is not offered at most clinical facilities.

Antibody-based detection of both dengue and zika virus, technically classified as **flaviviruses**, small enveloped RNA viruses, are available; however, there is a high degree of protein overlap from these two viruses leading to cross-reaction of many available antibodies, which is particularly important in dengue virus endemic areas where zika is also increasing.[2] The serological detection of flavivirus infection occurs via a measurement of IgM and IgG antibodies, commonly in an ELISA framework, which appear around a week after initial symptoms are observed with IgG detection being the method of choice. The high levels of cross-reactivity between dengue and zika leads to an increased rate of false positive results. Therefore, confirmatory diagnosis is required through viral neutralization assays in a BSL-3 facility. Very recent studies, which have shown that an almost identical sequence in the envelope, called the fusion loop in all flaviviruses, is the source of cross-reactivity. Attempts to overcome this barrier but are still in the experimental phase.[2]

Dengue Virus

Dengue virus is a flavivirus that occurs in four known serotypes: DENV-1, DENV-2, DENV-3, and DENV-4, which are antigenically similar but different enough not to confer immunity to the other serotypes.[3] It is the most significant viral disease transmitted by arthropods. Its single-strand

RNA genome consists of M and E structural proteins and seven nonstructural proteins including the NS1 protein, which interacts and elicits a host T-cell response often used as a diagnostic marker of infection. The WHO has reported over 1.5 million cases worldwide with a significant portion in the lower United States and Mexico.[3]

The early febrile stage of dengue fever may be clinically indistinguishable from other febrile illnesses, but the increase in **petechiae** during a tourniquet test may increase the likelihood of dengue diagnosis, as does a decrease in white blood cell count.[3] During the critical phase, which lasts 24 to 48 hours, the fever subsides and is often accompanied by an increase in bleeding and hematocrit. Blood tests indicate a decrease in platelet count, overall leukopenia, and neutropenia with accompanying lymphocytosis. Loss of plasma volume may lead to increased risk of shock and potential progressive organ deterioration that may lead to death. However, if the critical phase passes, the total WBC count increases, including an increase in neutrophils and decrease in lymphocytes, it indicates entry into the recovery phase.

Chikungunya Virus

Chikungunya virus is the causative agent of chikungunya fever, a sudden fever with skin rashes and joint pain; it is an RNA virus in the alphavirus genus with three dominant lineages with different antigenic features.[3] Roughly 25% of adults are asymptomatic as are approximately 35% of neonates. In others, chikungunya fever presents with a sudden onset and is accompanied by joint and body pain, which is more severe than in other febrile diseases. It is complicated by comorbidities including cardiovascular, neurological, and respiratory issues, as well as hypertension and the prior administration of nonsteroidal anti-inflammatory drugs (NSAIDs). Severe forms of the disease are more common in neonates and the elderly.

West Nile Virus

The **West Nile Virus**, like most arboviruses, does not require humans as a normal host in its life cycle. It is typically spread between *Culex pipiens* and other mosquitos to bird species such as the finch. However, if a human is bitten by a mosquito, the human dendritic and macrophage cells will take up the virus and result in its replication, but humans are a dead-end host for the virus.[1] Dissemination of the virus through the lymph organs is thought to be the source of CNS infection. Both the direct infection of neurons and the subsequent immune response play a role in neuronal cell death and CNS injury. The majority of West Nile infections (80%) are asymptomatic, while 20% have febrile responses, and fewer than 1% develop encephalitis and other neuroinvasive diseases, typically in older individuals.[1] Diagnosis of neuroinvasive West Nile is through specific IgM ELISA.

Zika Virus

Zika virus, the causative agent of the rapidly emerging zika fever most prevalent in South America, primarily Brazil, is an RNA virus most similar to dengue and is in the *Flaviviridae* family.[3] The symptoms are nonspecific and provide a challenge for differential diagnosis, as they can be similar to both dengue and chikungunya in many regards. Symptoms, including fever, maculopapular exanthema, conjunctivitis, body pain, headache, and others, occur within 3 to 12 days of infection, and only one in five patients develop them.[3] However, zika has been seen to be highly neurotropic, leading to complications seen predominantly in the nervous system, including many described cases of **Guillain-Barre** syndrome.

The diagnosis of these arboviral diseases is mainly clinical, through a combination of patient medical history, physical signs, blood work, and finally, serological testing. Specifically, dengue is serologically confirmed via ELISA detection of the NS1 antigen, which is present in high levels during the first 5 days of infection for any of the four serotypes of the disease. However, this glycoprotein is present in all flaviviruses and thus may lead to possible misdiagnosis with zika. The IgM ELISA is the test of choice. Chikungunya is also detectable via both IgG and IgM ELISA techniques from 4 days after disease onset. Zika is currently detected through a generalized IgM ELISA

for flavivirus. In many cases of epidemiological monitoring, these diseases may be further defined serotypically through reverse transcriptase PCR (RT-PCR). For zika, RT-PCR is still the test of choice. However, due to the long-known complication of cross-reactivity in these three viral diseases, attempts have been made experimentally to increase specificity of testing systems including through IgG and IgM identification of the NS1 protein and the E protein found in all flaviviruses.[2]

Encephalitis Viruses

Encephalitis, a syndrome of altered mental state with potential fever, seizures, and neurological deficits, can be caused by a number of viruses discussed in this chapter including members of the herpes virus family such as HSV-1, HSV-2, and VSV, as well as measles, mumps, and rubella, which are discussed later. In addition, the arboviruses: dengue, chikungunya, West Nile, and zika, described above, may result in encephalitis. This section covers some of the more common arboviral causes of encephalitis. In all cases, a serological evaluation of CSF IgM may help in the differential diagnosis.[4] While many of these viruses have been endemic in South and Central America, their increased emergence farther north has raised concerns in Mexico and in the United States.

California Encephalitis Group

The **California Encephalitis Group** is a group of viruses in the genus Bunyavirus, including California encephalitis virus, Jamestown Canyon virus, La Crosse virus, and Tahyna virus. The La Crosse virus, originally named for a child who died of encephalitis in La Crosse, Wisconsin in 1965, remains the most common cause of disease in the California encephalitis group. Both La Crosse and California cause encephalitis mainly in children.[1] Clinical analysis of this group reveals increased leukocytosis and hyponatremia in the peripheral blood. While the detection of IgM or a fourfold increase in paired sera, patient sera drawn 14 to 21 days apart for IgG is considered diagnostic for infection.

Eastern Equine Encephalitis Virus (EEEV)

Eastern Equine Encephalitis is endemic to the eastern United States and the Caribbean. Patients infected with this virus will present with nonspecific symptoms similar to other viral encephalitis causes including fever, malaise, and chills. These symptoms are followed by either a recovery phase or the onset of encephalitis with confusion, vomiting, and headaches as well as common brainstem involvement leading to gaze palsies and pupillary abnormalities. Mortality is 33% of all infections, which rises to 50% in patients older than 60.[1] Diagnosis is made via detection of IgM antibodies in the CSF via ELISA, as well as serum IgM detection, and fourfold increase in IgG in paired acute and convalescent sera. Antiviral therapies are not yet proven for EEEV.

Western Equine Encephalitis Virus (WEEV)

Western Equine Encephalitis Virus is an alphavirus in the Togaviridae family. Like EEEV, and the related Venezuelan equine encephalitis virus, it is transmitted from mosquitos to both humans and horses, causing a range of reactions from fever to encephalitis and death. It is derived from a recombination between the EEEV and the old world virus Sindbis but has a reduced incidence of mortality in humans compared with EEEV, estimated at 3 to 7%.[5] It is an enveloped RNA virus with two envelope proteins, E1 and E2, which form trimer of E1-E2 dimers on the viral surface leading to a spiked appearance.[5]

The most common treatment for EEEV, WEEV, and other arbovirus infections is still prevention of mosquito bites in endemic areas.

CASE STUDY

Case courtesy of Laurel J. Glaser, MD, PhD
University of Pennsylvania Perelman School of Medicine

Viral Mediated Rash and Fever

History

A 23-year-old female visits her doctor in the summer, complaining of a rash that started on her trunk 5 days previously and is now spreading toward her extremities. In addition of to the rash, she has fever, fatigue, and a dry cough. She returned from a Caribbean island 10 days ago, where she had been vacationing for the week. While she was there, she visited the beach, swam in the ocean, and spent time hiking and rafting. She did use an insect repellent and remembers numerous mosquito bites. There is a known measles outbreak on the island, but she has not had any sick contacts and no one else she traveled with had similar symptoms. High doses of anti-histamines (used to treat allergic reactions) have not helped. She is otherwise healthy and takes no medications. She does not know if all of her vaccines are current.

Physical Exam

Vital signs: Pulse 83 (nrl); Temp 100 F (high); Respiratory rate 16 (nrl); Blood Pressure 100/65 (nrl)
Mouth/Throat: Oropharynx is clear and moist. No Koplik spots.
Eyes: Conjunctivae are red.
Neck: Neck supple.
Cardiovascular: Normal rate, normal heart sounds, and intact distal pulses.
Pulmonary/Chest: Effort normal and breath sounds normal. No respiratory distress. She has no wheezes.
Lymphadenopathy: She has no cervical adenopathy.
Skin: Rash noted.

Diffuse morbilliform rash on torso and extremities.
Family History: Mother with hypertension.
Social History: Works in an office as a receptionist; no smoking or illicit drugs, occasional alcohol use. Patient
 has a male partner and they have sex without condoms.

Assessment and Plan

The travel with rash and conjunctivitis raises the suspicion for measles. The differential diagnosis also includes
mononucleosis (EBV), acute HIV infection, and arboviral infection (dengue, chikungunya, and Zika viruses). The
health department was notified due to the concern for measles, and the patient is asked to stay in her home
and away from other people until testing is completed. An in-office heterophile antibody test is negative, and
a panel of diagnostic tests is ordered.

2 days later, the following results are available:
Measles IgM 0.26 AU (negative <0.79)
Measles IgG 35 AU (negative <24.9)
EBV IgG capsid 5 (negative <0.8)
EBV Early antigen 0.2 (negative <0.8)
EBNA 2.4 (negative <0.8)
HIV antibody/antigen screen: reactive
HIV antibody assay: negative for HIV-1 and HIV-2 antibodies
Zika IgM MAC ELISA: pending
Dengue IgM/IgG: pending
Chikungunya IgM/IgG: pending

Critical Thinking Questions

1. Does the patient have serologic evidence of current or past infection with any viruses?
2. Should any additional tests be ordered?
3. Does the patient have evidence of Zika virus, dengue virus? Both? What additional tests could
 be considered?

▶ Hepatitis Viruses

The viruses called "**hepatitis viruses**" are
named hepatitis A, B, C, D, and E. These
viruses all cause disease, primarily in the liver,
but have little else in common. Acute infections
with any of these hepatitis viruses cannot be
differentiated on clinical characteristics alone.
Because none of these viruses efficiently proliferates in standard cell cultures, the serologic
approach, rather than direct detection, remains
the approach of choice. However, the ways in
which serology are used in diagnosis vary, with
different combinations of serologic assays used
and various testing algorithms in place in the
United States. Each of these viruses is discussed
individually.

Hepatitis A Virus (HAV)

Transmission of HAV ("infectious hepatitis")
is by the fecal-oral route, with most infections
due to fecal contamination of food. The incubation period ranges from 2 to 6 weeks after exposure. Up to two-thirds of HAV infections may be
asymptomatic, especially in children. Symptoms
may include jaundice, fever, anorexia, vomiting, and fatigue. Dark urine and pale stools are
associated with the beginning of jaundice. Acute
disease usually lasts about 1 week and is generally
mild. Recovery usually takes 2 to 4 weeks, and the
infection is rarely life-threatening; the mortality
rate is approximately 0.1%. Chronic carriers are
not found. Acute infection rates in the United
States have declined by more than 95% since the
implementation of HAV vaccine programs.[6]

At the onset of symptoms, IgM antibodies are detectable. These reach a maximum titer in 1 to 3 weeks and fall to undetectable levels in 3 to 6 months. IgG is detectable shortly after IgM and persists for years, usually at high titer. In the clinical laboratory, testing for HAV includes determinations specific for HAV IgM and those that detect total (IgG and IgM) HAV antibodies. The finding of HAV IgM is highly diagnostic of current or very recent HAV infection in symptomatic patients. A positive result in the total HAV antibody test may signal either current or past infection. Testing for total HAV antibody is primarily used to determine previous exposure to HAV.

Assays for HAV IgM and total HAV antibodies are typically based on EIAs and are often highly automated. Screening for HAV antibodies is routinely a component of a "hepatitis screen" in patients with jaundice.

Hepatitis B Virus (HBV)

HBV is the number one cause of hepatitis associated with exposure to blood and body fluids and is often called "serum" hepatitis. Infections occur following transfusions of infected blood or contact with infected body fluids such as semen and saliva. Symptoms appear within 6 weeks to 6 months following infection and include hepatosplenomegaly and jaundice. HBV infection may result in a variety of syndromes: subclinical infection; acute hepatitis with resolution of illness; fulminant hepatitis or subacute hepatic necrosis with possible death within 3 months; chronic active hepatitis frequently resulting in cirrhosis; chronic persistent hepatitis; or a silent carrier state with minimal (or absent) liver damage. Of those individuals who develop chronic HBV infections, all continue to shed the virus. However, some chronic cases simply persist with benign consequences, while chronic active infections may involve severe liver necrosis and may result in the development of primary hepatocellular carcinoma. Safe and effective HBV vaccines have dramatically reduced the incidence of HBV.

Although molecular testing is used for monitoring HBV DNA levels during treatment,

serologic tests for HBV antigens and HBV-specific antibodies are used for initial hepatitis screening of patients with jaundice to determine the stage of HBV disease and to confirm immunity after HBV vaccination. HBV has a complicated serologic profile (**FIGURE 9–1**). HBV surface antigen (HBsAg) is the first detectable marker in a new HBV infection, usually detectable 4 weeks after exposure to the virus (CDC, http://www.cdc.gov/hepatitis/hbv/hbvfaq.htm) and is the hallmark of current or recent infection. The viral core-related e antigen (HBeAg) is also detectable in the early stages of infection. The first antibody produced is the antibody against the HBV core (HBcAb), which appears during acute infection and persists for years. Both HBc IgM and total (IgG + IgM) HBc antibody are measured in the laboratory. The next marker to appear is the antibody against the HBV-core-related e antigen (HBeAb), which is followed months or years later by the development of the antibody against the HBV surface antigen (HBsAb). The presence of HBsAb signals the late stages of disease and the development of immunity. In chronic HBV, HBsAg remains detectable, and HBsAb fails to develop. The serologic profiles seen in the various stages of HBV disease are shown in **TABLE 9–1**.

Of interest serologically, is a period in the course of HBV infections when HBsAg is thought to form immune complexes with HBsAb produced as part of the recovery process. This immune complexing of antigen and antibody may render both the HBsAg and HBsAb undetectable. During this time, the only serologic markers that are reliably positive are the HBc IgM and total HBcAb. This time period is often called the "core window." Additional factors that may result in this pattern of HBcAb positive in the absence of HBsAg and HBsAb include past infection, immunosuppressive therapy, and antiviral therapy for hepatitis C virus. Fortunately, HBV DNA testing can be used to differentiate active from resolved HBV infection in these situations (CDC, https://www.cdc.gov/hepatitis/hbv/hbvfaq.htm).

Molecular testing for HBV DNA may be useful for monitoring the level of HBV DNA in confirmed cases of HBV infection or to confirm/rule

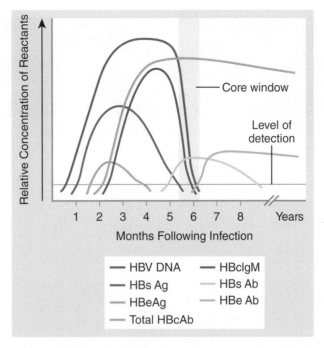

FIGURE 9–1 Hepatitis B Virus (HBV) serologic marker profile in uncomplicated infection. Antibody and antigen markers associated with HBV infection can be detected in this order: surface antigen (HBsAg); core-related e antigen (HBeAg; core antibodies (HBcIgM and total [IgG and IgM]) HBcAb; antibody to core-related e antigen (HBeAb); and surface antibody (HBs Ab). The core window may occur when HBsAg declines to undetectable and before HBsAb is detectable, leaving HBcIgM and total HBcAb as the only serological markers that are reliably positive. HBV DNA is detectable before any of the antigen/antibody markers; however, this is not usually tested for routine diagnostic purposes.

Modified from Leland DS. Clinical virology. Philadelphia: Saunders; 1996. Used with permission from Diane Leland.

out infection in cases where serologic results are confusing. In a new acute infection, HBV DNA can be detected before HBsAg (Figure 9–1). However, molecular testing is seldom performed unless the patient has a positive HBsAg or total HBcAb screening test result.

HBV reactivation may be encountered. This is an abrupt reactivation or rise in HBV DNA in a patient with previously inactive or resolved HBV. Reactivation can occur spontaneously or when the patient is undergoing cancer chemotherapy, taking immunosuppressive therapy, undergoing organ transplantation, or is coinfected with hepatitis C virus (CDC, https://www.cdc.gov/hepatitis/hbv/hbvfaq.htm).

HBV assays, both antigen and antibody, are typically EIAs, and many testing systems are marketed commercially. Most are completely automated and are reported to produce high-quality results. HBsAg and total HBc antibodies are tested on each unit of blood and organ donated in the United States, along with HBV DNA.

Hepatitis C Virus (HCV)

HCV infections occur worldwide. Parenteral transmission through transfusions of blood and blood products, organ transplantation, and intravenous drug abuse are the most well-defined routes, although other routes of transmission have not been ruled out. Approximately 1% of the U.S. population is thought to be HCV infected.[8] Most infected persons are asymptomatic during the early years of infection. In symptomatic individuals, mild gastrointestinal symptoms and jaundice may be seen, but a

TABLE 9–1   Hepatitis B Virus (HBV) Serologic Profiles[a,b]

Stage of Infection	Serological Markers					
	HBsAg[c]	HBeAg	HBc IgM	Total HBcAb	HBeAb[d]	HBsAb
Acute Infection						
Incubation period	+	+	0	0	0	0
Acute	+	+	+	+	0	0
Early Convalescent	+	0	+	+	+	0
Convalescent	0	0	+	+	+	0
Late Convalescent	0	0	0	+	+	+
Resolved infection	0	0	0	+	+/0	+
Chronic Infection (active, persistent, carrier)	+[c]	+/0[d]	+/0	+	+/0[d]	0
HBV Immunization	0	0	0	0	0	+
No Past or Present HBV Infection or Immunization	0	0	0	0	0	0

[a]Table modified from Niesters et al., 2016; CDC https://www.cdc.gov/hepatitis/hbv/; and Leland, 1996.

[b]Abbreviations: HBsAg=HBV surface antigen; HBeAg=HBV e antigen; HBc Ab=antibody to HBV core; HBsAb=antibody to HBV surface antigen, +=present, 0=absent, +/0=may be present or absent.

[c]HBsAg-negative chronic infection may occur.

[d]Liver disease in chronic infection is seen more frequently in the presence of HBeAg than of HBeAb.

small percentage can progress to severe disease. Approximately 80% of HCV patients develop chronic disease; these are at risk for cirrhosis and hepatocellular carcinoma. Various HCV genotypes have been identified, each with a different response to antiviral therapy. However, recent success with HCV antivirals have rendered all HCV infections potentially curable.[8]

Laboratory diagnosis of HCV involves serologic screening for HCV total antibodies, which become detectable 4 to 6 weeks after infection. Testing systems typically use recombinant HCV core antigens NS3, NS4, and NS5 in the antigen system. Reactivity of patients' sera with these cloned antigens usually indicates that the patient has past or present HCV infection. The algorithm currently recommended by the U.S. Centers for Disease Control and Prevention (CDC) requires additional testing by a molecular method that detects HCV RNA for all samples yielding positive results in the initial antibody screening test (**FIGURE 9–2**).[9]

A positive HCV RNA test result indicates current, active HCV infection. Patients with positive HCV RNA test results are referred for treatment. During treatment, HCV RNA testing in a quantitative format is repeated sequentially to monitor response to treatment. A negative HCV RNA test result on a sample that produced a positive result in initial HCV antibody screening may signal

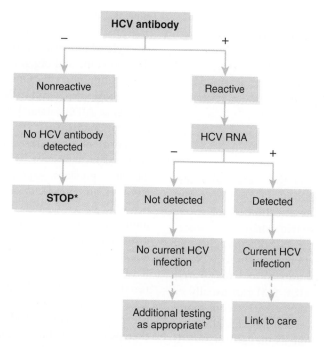

FIGURE 9–2 Recommended testing sequence for identifying current hepatitis c virus (HCV) infection. Initial HCV antibody tests detect HCV IgG and IgM. If this is nonreactive, no further testing is performed. If this is positive, HCV RNA testing is performed. A positive result confirms current HCV infection. *A negative result rules out current infection, but further testing may be needed for persons who might have been exposed to HCV within the past 6 months or for persons who are immunocompromised. †To differentiate past, resolved HCV infection from biologic false positivity of HCV antibody screening assays, testing with another HCV antibody assay can be considered. Repeat HCV RNA testing if the patient is suspected of having HCV exposure within the past 6 months or has clinical evidence of HCV disease, or if there is concern regarding the handling or storage of the test specimen.[9]

Centers for Disease Control and Prevention (CDC). Testing for HCV infection: an update of guidance for clinicians and laboratorians. *MMWR Morb Mortal Wkly Rep.* 2013; 62(18):362–365.

several different clinical circumstances: past HCV infection that cleared without treatment, successfully treated HCV infection, or a false-positive HCV antibody screening assay result. If this latter situation is suspected, the sample should be tested again for HCV antibodies using a testing method that is different from the one used in the initial screening. A positive result with a second assay rules out a false-positive initial screen result and is consistent with the patient having experience with HCV. A negative result with a second assay confirms a false-positive initial assay result and should eliminate concern for HCV infection in the patient. False-positive results in initial screening tests may be due to antibodies directed against the vector or fusion proteins associated with the HCV recombinant antigens used in the test system.

Numerous EIAs and chemiluminescent assays are available for HCV antibody screening. Most have shown good sensitivity and specificity. Testing for HCV antibodies and RNA is performed on all donated blood and organs in the United States.

Hepatitis D Virus (HDV)

HDV infection, called "delta hepatitis," occurs only in the presence of active HBV infection. HDV is an incomplete virus and requires the helper functions of HBV. The symptoms of HDV are similar to those of HBV. Chronic HDV-HBV infection often results in progressive liver disease and fulminant hepatitis. HDV may be diagnosed by detecting HDV antibodies or HDV RNA.

Typically, this testing is not performed except in patients who are infected with HBV and are from countries in which HDV is prevalent (e.g., the Mediterranean, the Middle East, Central Asia, West Africa, the South Pacific, and others). HDV testing is available only at public health, reference, or commercial laboratories.

Hepatitis E Virus (HEV)

HEV is transmitted via the fecal-oral route, often in waterborne outbreaks; person-to-person spread is minimal. The infection is not severe except in pregnant women where HEV infection may result in death of both the fetus and the mother. HEV infection is seen in Asia, North and West Africa, and Mexico and only rarely in the United States. HEV IgM can usually be detected within 3 to 4 days after onset of symptoms and persists for several months. HEV IgG appears at the same time as the IgM or shortly thereafter and persists for 14 or more years, although the titer declines. Although reagents for HEV antibody testing are available commercially in the United States, comparisons of results show discordance among the various products. Also, cross-reactivity with IgM antibodies of cytomegalovirus and Epstein-Barr Virus has been shown.[10]

▶ Herpes Family Viruses

Infections with viruses in the family *Herpesviridae* are widespread and frequently encountered. The most well-known of these viruses are cytomegalovirus, herpes simplex virus types 1 and 2, varicella zoster virus, and Epstein-Barr virus. Some of these viruses proliferate well in cell cultures, and viral antigen detection methods are available. Regardless, antibody detection may be useful under certain circumstances. All of these viruses establish latency within the host after initial infection and can be reactivated when the host is stressed. Although disease due to reactivation in seropositive individuals is usually not as severe as primary infections, such reactivation infections may be devastating in immunocompromised individuals. This is usually observed during disease-related processes or therapy including cancer chemotherapy and organ transplant-related therapies. Immunocompromised individuals, especially those with T-cell deficits (organ transplant recipients, AIDS patients), are especially prone to reactivation disease.

For all of these viruses, a positive IgG result—often called a positive "immune status" result—indicates previous experience with the virus. However, in contrast to a positive immune status result for most other viruses, which indicates immunity to further infection and disease, a positive immune status result for a herpes family virus does not guarantee that further disease is ruled out. Because these viruses establish latency, they can reactivate at any time. Immune status determinations for these viruses are often performed prior to organ transplantation or other immunosuppressive therapies so that the treatment plan can include antiviral therapy to keep the herpes viruses from reactivating due to the immunosuppression.

Cytomegalovirus (CMV)

Cytomegalovirus (CMV) infections are spread from human to human through contaminated blood and body fluids such as urine, saliva, semen, breast milk, and cervical secretions. Most CMV infections in immunocompetent, otherwise-healthy individuals are subclinical or insignificant, although a mononucleosis-like syndrome has been reported, which includes sore throat, fatigue, and lymphadenopathy. CMV-related mononucleosis can be differentiated from classic Epstein-Barr virus infectious mononucleosis through serologic evaluations (See the Epstein-Barr Virus section of this chapter). The most important CMV infection in otherwise healthy individuals involves pregnant CMV seronegative women who have a primary CMV infection during pregnancy. In approximately 30% of these cases, the fetus will be infected by CMV, with 10% of these having CMV-specific symptoms such as hepatosplenomegaly, chorioretinitis, deafness, microcephaly, or mental retardation.[11]

In immunocompromised individuals, CMV may cause serious infections in both CMV seronegative and seropositive individuals. Infections may be due to reactivation of the individual's own latent CMV or to infection by a heterologous strain of the virus. The infections are often severe, usually beginning with pneumonia and ending with a multi-system infection.

CMV proliferates in standard cell cultures, but it is slow growing. Molecular methods for detection of CMV DNA in peripheral blood and other tissues are becoming widely available and are usually the diagnostic method of choice. Molecular testing may also be performed quantitatively in order to monitor disease progression or effectiveness of antiviral therapy.

In the laboratory, testing is available for both CMV IgG and CMV IgM. Both of these are routinely reported in a quantitative format. CMV antibody levels may increase in primary as well as in reactivation disease, so quantitative testing of IgG levels in paired sera may be helpful in disease diagnosis. However, most CMV IgG testing is performed for immune status evaluations. CMV IgG persists lifelong after infection. The presence of CMV IgM is thought to confirm current CMV activity.

Many commercial products are available for CMV antibody determinations; most detect either CMV IgG or CMV IgM, rather than both together. EIA is the most common format for these determinations.

Epstein-Barr Virus (EBV)

Epstein-Barr Virus (EBV) is transmitted by oral secretions and also through blood transfusions. It may produce subclinical infections or mild cold or flu-like illness, but it is most well-known as the agent of classic infectious mononucleosis (IM). This syndrome occurs most frequently in teenagers and young adults and presents routinely with a low-grade fever, sore throat, lymphadenopathy, and fatigue. The virus has also been implicated as the agent of malignancies, including **Burkitts Lymphoma**, nasopharyngeal carcinoma, lymphoma, and leukemia. Once infected with EBV, humans harbor the virus lifelong, with reactivation disease possible upon stress.

Because EBV does not proliferate in standard cell cultures, and antigen-detection methods are not available, laboratory confirmation of EBV infection usually begins with testing for antibodies. In EBV IM, heterophile antibodies are produced in 80 to 90% of patients and are detectable within 2 weeks of onset of symptoms. Heterophile antibodies are antibodies that react with antigens, which are different from and phylogenetically unrelated to the antigens responsible for their production. The heterophile antibodies of IM are capable of reacting with sheep erythrocytes. Although IM heterophile antibodies are not the only heterophile antibodies that have been identified in humans, they are the most common type, and assays are widely available for detecting these antibodies and differentiating them from other non-IM heterophile antibodies. In heterophile assays based on agglutination of sheep or horse erythrocytes, absorbing the patient's serum with a guinea pig kidney extract eliminates reactivity of two known non-IM heterophile antibodies, Forssman and serum sickness. Antibodies that agglutinate erythrocytes after guinea pig kidney absorption are assumed to be the heterophile antibody of IM. Heterophile antibodies are not typically produced in CMV mononucleosis, so this testing can aid in differentiating EBV and CMV mononucleosis.

Erythrocyte-based IM heterophile antibody testing is routinely performed in a manual slide format and is widely available as "monospot" testing. The patient's serum is added to a slide, along with a drop of guinea pig kidney extract, and these are stirred together. Erythrocytes are then added, and the mixture is observed for agglutination of the erythrocytes, indicating the presence of the heterophile antibodies of IM. Some manual methods no longer include the guinea pig absorption step because both Forssman and serum sickness heterophile antibodies are now quite rare. These assays typically feature latex particles coated with an erythrocyte extract; heterophile antibodies of IM will agglutinate the coated particles. These methods are known to yield false positive results in the presence of serum sickness heterophile antibodies. Heterophile antibody testing is sometimes included in large, automated, multiplex, bead-testing panels, along with EBV-specific antibody assays.

Because heterophile antibodies are produced in only 80 to 90% of EBV IM cases, 10 to 20% of infected individuals will yield negative heterophile test results. The diagnosis of heterophile-negative IM relies on detection of antibodies directed against components of EBV itself. Testing for at least four types of EBV-related antibodies is widely available; these include antibodies, both IgG and IgM, against viral capsid antigens (VCA), antibodies against viral early antigens (EB EA), and antibodies against nuclear antigens (EBNA). There are several types of EBNAs, but antibodies against EBNA-1 are the most frequently tested. The sequence of appearance/disappearance of the four types of antibodies in classic IM is shown in **FIGURE 9–3**. VCA IgM is first to appear

and becomes undetectable within 4 weeks. VCA IgG also appears very early in the infection, and, although it may decline somewhat, it persists at detectable levels for life. EB EA antibodies also appear during the acute phase of the infection; these decline to undetectable within 3 to 6 months after onset of disease, although persistence of EB EA IgG has been demonstrated. Antibodies against EBNA-1 are the slowest to appear; they are rarely present during the acute phase of the illness but increase during convalescence and are maintained in most individuals for life. In acute EBV IM, VCA IgM should be detectable, and EBNA-1 antibodies should be absent. In other EBV-related conditions, the pattern of reactivity of the four types of EBV antibodies may be atypical and difficult to interpret. **TABLE 9–2** shows typical antibody-response patterns in the various EBV-related conditions. Testing paired, acute and convalescent sera is not useful to differentiate recent and past EBV infections because the antibody response occurs rapidly

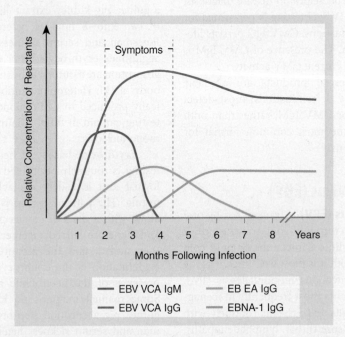

FIGURE 9–3 Epstein-Barr Virus (EBV) Antibody Response. At Least Four Types of Antibodies Can Be Monitored. They appear in this order: immunoglobulin M (IgM) against viral capsid antigen (EBV VCA IgM; G against viral capsid antigen (EBV VCA IgG); antibody against early antigen (EB EA IgG); and antibodies against nuclear antigen (EBNA-1 IgG). EBV VCA IgG and EBNA-1 IgG persist lifelong after infection.

Modified from Balfour et al., 2016,[13] Gartner and Preiksaitis, 2016,[14] and Leland, 1996.[7]

TABLE 9–2 Epstein-Barr Virus (EBV) Antibody Profiles in EBV-Related Syndromes[a,b]

EBV-Related Syndrome	EBV-Related Antibodies Present/Absent			
	EBV VCA IgM	EBV VCA IgG	EB EA IgG	EBN A-1 IgG
No past or present EBV	0	0	0	0
Acute Primary Infection	+	+	+	+/0[c]
Convalescent-phase Primary Infection	+/0	+	+/0	+
Past infection	0	+	0	+
Reactivation	+/0	+	+/0	+
Burkitt's lymphoma, Nasopharyngeal carcinoma, others?	0	+	+	+

[a]Table Modified from Balfour et al., 2016; Gartner and Prieksaitis, 2016; and Leland, 1996.
[b]Abbreviations: EA=EBV early antigen, EBNA=EBV nuclear antigen, VCA=EBV viral capsid antigen, +=present, 0=absent, +/0=may be present or absent.
[c]EBNA antibodies are the last to develop, so they may be undetectable in the early stages of infection.

during primary EBV infection. Thus, serologic testing may done too late in the infection to detect this antibody increase.[12]

Most EBV antibody assays are now in EIA formats and performed by automated systems as part of multiplex panels. Once past or present EBV infection has been confirmed through antibody testing, further EBV antibody testing is seldom helpful in clarifying diagnoses or guiding patient management in complicated non-IM EBV infections/diseases. Instead, molecular testing is used to follow the level of EBV DNA to monitor disease status and effects of therapy.

EBV immune status is determined by testing for EBV VCA IgG. This is performed prior to organ transplantation or other immunosuppressive therapies to ensure that the patient's treatment plan includes monitoring for EBV reactivation in seropositive individuals and protection from new EBV infections in seronegative patients.

Herpes Simplex Virus (HSV), Types 1 and 2

There are two major types of **Herpes Simplex Virus** (HSV): HSV type 1 (HSV-1) and HSV type 2 (HSV-2). Both oral and genital infections are common, with HSV-1 more common in oral infections (cold sores, fever blisters) and HSV-2 more common in genital infections; lesions will heal without treatment. Although these lesions are painful, unsightly, and inconvenient, they are usually not life-threatening. Occasionally, meningitis or encephalitis may develop due to severe HSV infection. Congenital HSV infection occurs both *in utero* and during delivery in women with genital HSV, and perinatal infections may also be serious. The virus establishes latency, and reactivation can occur lifelong when the host is stressed. In immunocompromised individuals, reactivation of HSV can be extremely serious.

HSV proliferates rapidly and vigorously in traditional cell cultures; HSV antigens are detectable in clinical materials by several techniques, and molecular methods are also available for detecting and differentiating HSV 1 and 2 DNA. Detection of HSV via culture, antigen detection, or molecular methods is most important for confirming acute disease when lesions are present. Serologic methods are seldom used in this setting.

In settings in which HSV lesions are absent, antibody detection can confirm current infection or determine immune status. A conversion from HSV IgG negative, to antibody positive, or a significant increase in HSV IgG titer in paired sera is consistent with current infection. There are also methods for detection of HSV IgM, but these are not widely available. Using methods based on glycoprotein G, many EIA methods are able to differentiate HSV-1 and HSV-2 antibodies, despite their extensive cross-reactivity.

Evaluations of HSV immune status are complicated by the fact that HSV establishes latency. Therefore, the presence of HSV antibodies indicates prior experience with the virus but does not confirm current acute infection or signal immunity to subsequent infections or reactivations. Recurrent infections are common due to reactivation of latent HSV. Screening for HSV IgG is performed prior to organ transplantation and other immunosuppressive therapies to ensure that appropriate prophylaxis is used for HSV seropositive individuals.

Many methods are available commercially for HSV IgG testing. EIAs are most common, and sensitivity and specificity of most are very good.

Varicella Zoster Virus (VZV)

Varicella Zoster Virus (VZV), also called varicella or herpes zoster, is the etiologic agent of the classic childhood disease chickenpox. The infection is characterized by vesicular lesions with indented centers. Once individuals have experienced chickenpox, antibodies are produced, which persist lifelong. However, the virus persists indefinitely within the body, being sequestered in nerve cells, and may reemerge to produce another clinical syndrome, shingles. In shingles, large, painful, vesicular lesions are produced on the skin that overlies the pathway of a nerve. Lesions are restricted to the specific area and may produce a burning sensation and intense pain. Shingles is a frequent complication in both pediatric and adult transplant recipients, cancer patients, and others who are immunocompromised.

VZV proliferates in standard cell cultures, and VZV antigens can be detected in materials from lesions. Molecular methods are also available for detecting VZV DNA. These methods are the preferred approach for confirming acute VZV disease.

VZV IgG antibodies are detectable by many methods, but most laboratories rely on automated EIA methods. VZV IgM methods are available at some reference and commercial laboratories. Presence of VZV IgG indicates prior experience with the virus and immunity to chickenpox. A seroconversion from antibody negative to positive or a significant increase in VZV IgG level in paired sera can be used to confirm current infection. The primary usefulness of serologic evaluation of VZV IgG testing is to determine immunity to chickenpox. This evaluation is required routinely for many healthcare personnel and others who may be exposed to the virus. Any seropositive individual is at risk for developing shingles upon stress or immunosuppression. Serologic testing is not helpful in confirming a diagnosis of shingles. Instead, scrapings from the lesions should be tested for VZV DNA or antigen. A safe and effective VZV vaccine is available for children, and a shingles vaccine is available for adults.

▸ Human Immunodeficiency Viruses and Other Retroviruses

The **retroviruses** that infect humans were not brought to prominence until the early 1980s when a link for some of these viruses with

acquired immunodeficiency syndrome (AIDS) patients was established. Initially, five of these viruses were described and were named **human T-cell lymphotropic viruses (HTLV)** 1-5. With progress in AIDS research, two of these, HTLV-3 and HTLV-4, were renamed human immunodeficiency virus (HIV) 1 and 2, respectively. The other three HTLVs retained their name and numbers and, at this writing, are as follows: HTLV-1, agent of adult T-cell leukemia/lymphoma (ATLL), tropical spastic paraparesis (TSP)/HTLV-1-associated myelopathy (HAM), and HTLV-1 associated uveitis (HAU); HTLV-2, no confirmed disease association; and HTLV-5, no confirmed disease association. Descriptions of some of individual retroviruses follow.

Because the retroviruses do not proliferate in standard cell cultures, their diagnosis relies largely on initial detection of virus-specific antibodies. Testing for antibodies of HIV-1 and -2 is available at most clinical laboratories and is also performed on all transfused blood and donated organs in the United States. Confirmatory testing is required in follow-up for any sample yielding a positive antibody screening test result. Once a diagnosis is confirmed, response to therapy and disease progression are monitored via molecular assays that provide a quantitative measurement of the level of circulating HIV RNA.

Testing for antibodies of HTLV-1 and 2 largely follows the same protocol as that used for HIV-1 and -2 antibody testing; these antibodies are also monitored in all transfused blood and donated organs in the United States. However, this testing is not routinely available for diagnostic purposes in most clinical laboratories.

Human Immunodeficiency Virus, Type 1 (HIV-1)

After the initial **Human Immunodeficiency Virus type - 1 (HIV-1)** infection, the patient may experience a mononucleosis-like syndrome, which includes fever, lymphadenopathy, headache, and sore throat. The symptoms last only a few weeks and are followed by a lengthy asymptomatic period. As the infection progresses to AIDS, the immune system is depressed, specifically through inactivation or destruction of T-lymphocytes of the CD4 subset. This immunodeficiency produces dramatic alterations in the individual's ability to respond to infection. Infecting agents that would be of little significance in otherwise healthy individuals often produce significant infection in HIV-1 infected patients, and these patients often suffer recurrent infections that are seldom experienced by immunocompetent individuals. Although HIV-1 infection can be confirmed through laboratory tests, the diagnosis of "AIDS" is not made until the evidence of an immunocompromised state manifests itself through susceptibility to infections. HIV-1 is by far the most important AIDS virus in the United States.

Retroviruses establish infections that persist for life. The period between infection and antibody production, which typically averages 3 weeks in HIV-1 infection, is often called the "window" period. During the window period, HIV-1 antigen can be detected in the serum of infected individuals. With newer testing methods, HIV-1 antigen may be detected as early as 16 days after infection in many individuals. HIV-1 antigen presence in serum is transient, and when antibodies become detectable, the antigen usually becomes undetectable. The antigen remains routinely undetectable in serum until the patient's disease becomes severe, and the presence of detectable antigen typically signals increased viral replication and poor prognosis. HIV-1 RNA is also detectable in the serum prior to antibody production, often within 10 to 11 days of infection. HIV-1 RNA may be detectable throughout the infection, and quantitative molecular assays are useful in monitoring effectiveness of treatment and disease progress.

Most diagnostic testing is conducted when patients begin to show signs of immunodeficiency, which is typically 10 years after initial infection. At this point, the antibody response is well developed, so the primary means of diagnosing HIV-1 infection is by detecting HIV-1 antibodies. At present, a fourth generation combination EIA that detects both HIV-1 and HIV-2 antibodies as well as HIV-1 p24 antigen is used widely in the United States. Most HIV methods marketed at present in the United States also detect antibodies to HIV-1 group O, a subtype of HIV-1 not detected by earlier versions of HIV-1 antibody assays. This subtype is rare in the United States and is typically restricted to persons originating from Cameroon, Gabon, and Equatorial Guinea.

Each manufacturer of HIV antibody/antigen detection systems has a carefully defined protocol for performing the specific assay; these protocols must be followed without modification or alteration if the assay is expected to yield accurate results. Although three analytes (HIV-1 antibody, HIV-2 antibody, and HIV-1 p24 antigen) are detected with the 4th generation assays, the result is simply reported as positive or negative—there is no indication which of the three analytes was detected. All initially positive samples are tested

in duplicate by the same assay in another run of testing. Although a repeatedly positive screening HIV EIA result may be presumptive evidence of HIV-1 infection, falsely positive EIA results are possible. These may be related to autoimmune or histocompatibility-related antibodies in some human sera or to antibodies directed against vector-related antigens (usually *Escherichia coli* or *Bacillus* species). Confirmatory testing is required following repeated reactivity in the HIV EIAs.

The protocol for HIV confirmatory testing used now in the United States is the CDC protocol that was established in 2015 and updated in 2018 (**FIGURE 9–4**). Confirmatory assays detect and differentiate HIV-1 and HIV-2 antibodies by their reactivity to certain viral epitopes. The BioRad Geenius Assay (Bio-Rad Laboratories, Redmond, WA) is one approved assay for confirmation of HIV-1 and HIV-2 antibodies. This is an

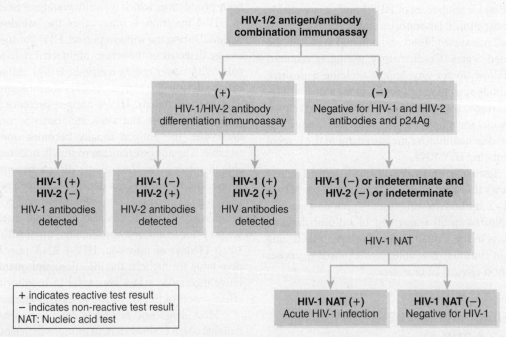

FIGURE 9–4 Recommended human immunodeficiency virus (HIV) testing algorithm. Initial screening tests detect HIV-1 and HIV-2 antibodies and HIV-1 p 24 antigen in a combination immunoassay. If this is negative, no further testing is routinely performed. If this is positive, an additional assay that detects/differentiates HIV-1 and HIV-2 antibodies is used. Various possible result patterns are shown. If results are negative or indeterminate, nucleic acid testing for HIV-1 RNA is used.[15]

Centers for Disease Control and Prevention (CDC). 2018 Quick reference guide: recommended laboratory HIV testing algorithm for serum or plasma specimens. Laboratory Testing for the Diagnosis of HIV Infection 2018; https://stacks.cdc.gov/view/cdc/50872. 2019.

immunochromatographic (lateral flow) method. It features a cassette holding a membrane strip that has HIV-1 and HIV-2 antigenic epitopes bound in distinct bands along the strip. The antigens used are HIV-1 p 31 polymerase peptide, HIV-1 gp 160 envelope recombinant protein, HIV-1 gp 41 group M and O envelope proteins, and HIV-1 p24 core recombinant protein and HIV-2 gp 36 envelope peptide and HIV-2 gp 140 envelope peptide. The patient's sample is applied to a port in the cassette. The serum migrates along the strip with Protein A (a protein that binds to antibodies) labeled with colloidal gold dye particles. As HIV antibodies bind to their homologous antigen epitopes on the strip, the protein A binds to the bound antibodies to produce a pink/purple line. An instrument evaluates the intensity and location of the bands of reactivity and provides an interpretation of the result as positive for HIV-1 antibodies, positive for HIV-2 antibodies, or negative for HIV-1 and HIV-2 antibodies. Indeterminate results are also seen. If either HIV-1 antibodies or HIV-2 antibodies are identified by the confirmatory assay, these results are then reported. If results are negative for both HIV-1 and HIV-2 antibodies or indeterminate, molecular testing for HIV-1 RNA is needed.

Indeterminate reactions in confirmatory HIV testing may signal mixed infections or other more-complicated situations. Both HIV-1 and HIV-2 antibody results may be negative in early HIV infection when antigen and RNA are circulating but antibodies have not yet been produced at detectable levels. This result pattern would also be seen if the HIV screening test result was false-positive. Molecular testing will confirm/rule out HIV-1 infection. HIV-2 molecular testing is not included in the CDC algorithm; any patient with risk factors consistent with possible HIV-2 infection can be tested for HIV-2 RNA at a public health or reference laboratory.

Human Immunodeficiency Virus Type 2 (HIV-2)

HIV-2, often called "the other AIDS virus," was discovered in 1986 in an AIDS patient. HIV-2 infections are largely confined to Western Africa,

but cases have been identified in Europe, India, and the United States—primarily in individuals with an epidemiological link to West Africa. HIV-2 is less pathogenic than HIV-1, and disease does not progress in most infected individuals. In cases that progress, pathology is very similar to HIV-1 infection.[16]

Although HIV-2 accounts for less than 0.01% of HIV infections in the United States, testing is in place to ensure its detection. Diagnostic testing for HIV-2 infection follows the same testing algorithm as HIV-1 testing (Figure 9–4), although current 4th generation screening combination tests, which include testing for HIV-1 p24 antigen, do not include testing for HIV-2 antigen. Molecular testing for HIV-2 RNA may be needed to confirm confusing or mixed HIV-1/HIV-2 infections.

Human T-Cell Lymphotropic Virus, Type 1 (HTLV-1)

HTLV-1, the cause of ATLL, TSP/HAM, HAU, and possibly others, is most common in Central Africa, South Japan, and the Caribbean. Many HTLV-1 infected individuals remain disease free throughout their lifetime, with only 2 to 6% developing disease. Typically, the incubation period for HTLV-1 infection/disease is very long, usually spanning a number of years.[16]

Although HTLV-1 infection is rare in the United States, a comprehensive testing algorithm is in place that is very similar to the one used for detecting HIV-1 and HIV-2. One major difference in testing is necessitated by the biology of HTLV infections. HTLVs never release virions into the plasma. Because of this, testing for HTLV antigen or HTLV RNA is not needed. However, the blood of infected individuals contains high levels of cells carrying HTLV provirus, which can be used as a target for molecular testing in difficult cases.

HTLV screening relies on detection of HTLV-1 and HTLV-2-specific antibodies, usually in a combination EIA. Samples with positive screening test results are subjected to confirmatory testing by methods that measure antibody reactivity with p24 *gag* and gp 46 and/or gp 68 *env* proteins. HTLV antibody detection methods are not widely available for diagnostic purposes in clinical laboratories. Public health and reference laboratories provide HTLV-1 and HTLV-2 antibody assays. However, HTLV-1 and HTLV-2 antibody testing is included in infectious-disease screening of all donated blood and organs in the United States.

Human T-Cell Lymphotropic Virus, Type 2 (HTLV-2)

Although HTLV-2 has been isolated sporadically in cases of hematologic anomalies (e.g., elevated platelet, lymphocyte counts, and hairy cell leukemia), no link has been confirmed. It is less pathogenic than HTLV-1. HTLV-2 has been found in intravenous drug users in North America, Europe, and Asia and in Native-American Indian tribes in North, Central, and South America.

Diagnostic testing for HTLV-2 is as described for HTLV-1. The two are routinely detected in combination assays that detect both HTLV-1 and HTLV-2 antibodies.

▶ Measles, Mumps, and Rubella Viruses

Measles virus, mumps virus, and rubella virus infections were included in the common diseases of childhood in the United States prior to the implementation of nationwide immunization programs starting in the 1960s. Infections due to these three viruses are now relatively rare in the United States, and most clinical laboratories have little to offer for diagnosis of acute infection. All three of these will proliferate in standard cell cultures, although they do so very slowly, and the types of cell cultures available in most clinical laboratories are not optimal for their recovery. Viral antigen detection tests are not available for detection of any of the three. Molecular testing and IgM-specific antibody testing, both of which are useful in confirming acute infection, are not typically available in most clinical laboratories.

In cases in which these infections are suspected, it is best for clinical laboratories to work with public health or reference laboratories to obtain high-quality direct testing.

Serologic testing for virus-specific IgG for each of these three viruses is available at most clinical laboratories. In acute infection, in addition to working with a public health or reference laboratory to obtain high-quality direct testing, it is recommended that sera be collected at onset of symptoms and 2 weeks later. A conversion from IgG antibody negative to antibody positive or a significant increase in antibody level is evidence of current infection.

Because antibodies are expected to persist lifelong following immunization or infection with any of these three viruses, immune status determinations are often performed. It is important for healthcare workers and others who will be exposed to these viruses to ensure they have antibodies present. Typically, if IgG antibodies are present, the individual is expected to be immune to further infection/disease. If IgG antibodies are absent, the individual is susceptible to infection and should be immunized. Most clinical laboratories offer testing for IgG of all three viruses. Assays are commonly based on EIA or multiplex-bead immunofluorescence principles and test for IgG only.

For each of these three viruses, partially immune individuals present a greater diagnostic challenge, in that signs and symptoms of infection may not be typical. Partial immunity may result from presence of transplacental antibody, from presence of antibodies due to administration of immune serum globulin, from immunizations with partially inactivated vaccines, or from atypical response to immunizations. In these situations, simple immune status determinations may not be useful.[17] More information about each of the three viruses follows.

Measles Virus

Measles (formerly called rubeola) virus is highly contagious and causes fever, cough, conjunctivitis, an oral rash of bluish-white lesions of the buccal mucosa (Koplik spots), and a maculopapular rash on the skin, lasting 6 or more days. Less than 0.2% of infections involve complications such as encephalitis and secondary bacterial otitis media. A rare, late-occurring fatal sequelae, subacute sclerosing panencephalitis (SSPE), which involves a progressive encephalitis that occurs 4 to 17 years after the initial infection, occurs roughly once in each 1 million cases. Measles cases are being seen in the United States now due to a cohort of unimmunized children.

Mumps Virus

Classic mumps, caused by the mumps virus, is spread from human to human through respiratory droplets and is highly contagious. Mumps infection may be subclinical in 20 to 40% of infections but when symptomatic, it is characterized by low fever, inflamed pharynx, and swollen parotid glands, with swelling lasting 7 to 10 days. Most mumps cases are uncomplicated, but 10 to 20% of the infections in postpubital males involve the testicles, and about half of all cases involve the central nervous system, with only 1 to 10% showing clinical symptoms. Mumps has been seen in sporadic outbreaks in the United States in the last decade. Most of these outbreaks are in highly vaccinated populations; the reason for this is poorly understood (Leland and Relich, 2013). Detection of reinfection in immunized individuals is difficult. IgM antibodies may be detected within 3 days of onset of symptoms, although only 15% of previously immunized individuals may test positive for IgM. The virus may be isolated from samples collected at that same time. Testing outside of this narrow timeframe is not likely to be successful.[17]

Rubella Virus

Rubella virus is the agent of "German measles" or "three-day measles." The virus is transmitted from person to person through aerosols and is highly infectious. Rubella typically produces mild symptoms for 3 days including low-grade fever, headache, mild conjunctivitis, lymphadenopathy, and rash. Complications of rubella infection in children are rare.

The most serious aspect of rubella infection involves pregnant women, particularly those in the first trimester of pregnancy, who become infected with the virus. The infection in the mother is not remarkable, but, during maternal viremia, the virus crosses the placenta and replicates within the fetus, leading to disseminated infection of fetal organs. Anomalies produced in the fetus by rubella virus infection include heart lesions, ocular complications, ear malfunctions, hepatosplenomegaly, meningoencephalitis, and lesions of the long bones. Cases of congenital rubella in the United States are exceedingly rare. Although direct methods such as molecular testing are typically used for confirmation of congenital rubella infections, sera collected from the newborn at birth and sequentially during the next 5 to 6 months can be used to confirm/rule out congenital infection. Using rubella IgG quantitative methods, levels in these samples are compared. Rubella antibodies detectable at 6 months at levels equal to or higher than levels at birth indicate that the infant is producing the antibodies, thus confirming congenital infection. When rubella antibodies drop to very low or undetectable levels at 6 months, the antibodies are confirmed as being of maternal origin, and the decline is simply indicative of the natural half-life of antibodies. This combination of results rules out congenital infection. Rubella IgM-specific antibody testing methods are available at public health and reference laboratories. Detecting rubella IgM in an infant is evidence that the infant is actually infected by the virus. Reminder: Maternal IgM does not cross the placenta.

▶ Respiratory and Enteric Viruses

Respiratory Viruses

In the past several decades, a variety of rapid, easy-to-use, accurate, and cost-effective assays that can be performed by clinical laboratories and point-of-care settings for direct detection of many respiratory viruses have become available commercially. These are a variety of techniques including viral antigen detection, molecular methods, and rapid viral cultures using centrifugation-enhanced culture inoculation and staining with monoclonal antibodies for detection. For many respiratory viruses, these developments provide for accurate respiratory virus detection within 15 to 60 minutes. The serologic approach is seldom used for confirmation of acute infection due to the slow turnaround time for comparing antibody levels in paired sera, the lack of availability of IgM-specific methods and the very nature of the immune response to infections produced by most respiratory viruses.

Although most respiratory viruses stimulate an immune response, the response may be slow to develop and not strong. Also, because many respiratory viruses are closely related antigenically, antibodies may cross-react, making serologic diagnosis a challenge. In addition, antibody may be transient and often does not confer long-lasting immunity. Conversion from antibody negative to antibody positive or a significant increase in antibody level can be evidence of current infection.

At this writing, most clinical laboratories do not offer antibody testing for respiratory viruses. This testing is typically conducted at public health, reference, or research laboratories and is focused more toward epidemiologic studies, vaccine development, and outbreak management. Additional information for some of the common respiratory viruses follows.

Adenovirus

Adenovirus (at least 51 serotypes) infections produce symptoms ranging from mild cough and pharyngitis to acute respiratory disease/pneumonia and ocular infections. Conversion from antibody negative to antibody positive, or a significant increase in antibody level is evidence of current adenovirus infection. Adenovirus antibodies are serotype-specific and long lasting. Antibody testing typically uses a group antigen that detects all serotypes, so additional testing by more sophisticated methods is needed for detecting antibody to the various serotypes.

Coronaviruses

Coronaviruses, along with **rhinoviruses**, are the major cause of the common cold, causing 5 to 10% of colds in adults and children. Their infections are typically self-limiting and confined to the upper respiratory tract. Although most infections are diagnosed on clinical grounds alone, newer molecular panels testing for more-recently-recognized pathogenic strains of coronaviruses, such as 229E, OC43, HKUI, and NL 63, provide rapid direct diagnosis. Serologic detection is not used. Remarkable among coronaviruses are two strains recently involved with pandemic disease: severe acute respiratory syndrome (SARS-CoV), and Middle East respiratory syndrome (MERS CoV). Both cause severe, life-threatening, lower respiratory tract infections. Diagnosis of SARS and MERS is by molecular methods. Serology is not used in acute disease diagnosis because antibodies develop too slowly.

Influenza A and B

Influenza virus type A (Flu A) and type B (Flu B) cause more life-threatening respiratory tract disease than any of the other respiratory viruses. Infections occur from December to March in the Northern Hemisphere. Many rapid, direct-detection methods are available, so serology is seldom useful. Also, the presence of low levels of antibody may not be sufficient to determine immunity, so immune status determinations are not used routinely. Public health and reference laboratories may use sophisticated and cumbersome antibody testing methods to differentiate/characterize Flu A and Flu B strains.

Parainfluenza 1, 2, 3, and 4 (Para)

Para 1, 2, and 3 usually cause upper respiratory symptoms including rhinitis and pharyngitis and may result in croup. Para 4 is encountered much less frequently and produces milder disease. Although para viruses infect individuals of all ages, they are second only to respiratory syncytial virus in frequency of severe illness in children. EIA and other types of serologic assays are not effective for para antibody detection, so alternate, more cumbersome, sophisticated methods are used and are available only at reference or research laboratories. There is extensive cross-reactivity among para types, so antibody titers may not effectively indicate which para type is involved in an infection.

Respiratory Syncytial Virus (RSV)

Respiratory Syncytial Virus (RSV) is found worldwide and is the single most important cause of severe respiratory infections in infants and young children. It has been reported that all children are infected with RSV before they reach 4 years of age. The serologic approach is seldom useful in diagnosis, and antibody testing is not offered by most laboratories. RSV antibodies do not protect against infection, and reinfection is common, although less severe than initial infection.

Rhinovirus

Rhinoviruses (more than 100 distinct serotypes) are believed to cause ¼ to ½ of all mild upper respiratory infections, better known as the "common cold." Serious, acute, lower-respiratory disease or involvement of other organ systems is rare in rhinovirus infections. In general, the diagnosis of rhinovirus infection in otherwise healthy individuals is made on a clinical basis, and laboratory testing is not usually undertaken. Molecular testing is available for diagnosis of severe, acute infection. Antibody detection methods are not used routinely for confirming infection. Such methods are not available commercially and are not offered at most clinical laboratories.

Enteric Viruses

Infections with enteric viruses are usually diagnosed by direct methods. The serologic approach is seldom used for confirmation of acute infection. Most clinical laboratories do not offer antibody testing for enteric viruses. As with respiratory virus serologies, enteric virus serologic testing is typically conducted at public health, reference, or research laboratories and is focused more toward epidemiologic studies, vaccine development, and outbreak management. Additional information for some of the common enteric viruses follows.

"Enteroviruses" (Coxsackievirus, Poliovirus, Echovirus, and Others) and Parechoviruses

The **enterovirus** group, previously divided into coxsackie A virus, coxsackie B virus, echovirus, and poliovirus, and now simply called "enteroviruses," have been characterized and numbered and include at least 68 strains. Poliovirus is the most well-known, producing classic paralytic polio. Coxsackie A viruses have been associated with vesicular pharyngitis (herpangina), hand-foot-and-mouth disease, infantile diarrhea, aseptic meningitis, and paralysis. Coxsackie B viruses have been implicated in pericarditis and myocarditis as well as in infections similar to those of coxsackie A virus. The echoviruses (E=enteric, C=cytopathogenic, H=human, O=orphan) have been isolated in various types of infections, but, as the "orphan" part of the acronym-based name suggests, the role in disease production is not well defined. Additional enteric viruses that produce clinical signs and symptoms similar to those of the enteroviruses have been grouped together and named "parechoviruses."

Identification of enterovirus and parechoviruses is challenging due to the extensive cross-reactivity and inter-relatedness of the numerous types and strains. Fortunately, differentiation among the enteroviruses has little impact on patient management. Enteroviral antibody detection methods are seldom offered, and their use is not encouraged. A method called neutralization is the most effective but is cumbersome and very slow. It is most effective when acute and convalescent sera are tested to evaluate changes in antibody level. Because some individuals have low levels of antibodies against some enteroviruses and because enterovirus antibodies tend to cross react, a single antibody assay is not usually helpful.

Norovirus

Noroviruses are the agent of sporadic gastroenteritis in older children and adults and are usually associated with contaminated food. Molecular testing is used for diagnosis and outbreak management. Antibody testing is not useful.

Rotavirus

Rotavirus, which is transmitted primarily by the fecal-oral route, is one of the many agents that produce diarrheal disease in humans. Onset of symptoms is usually sudden, beginning with low fever and vomiting, which are followed by watery diarrhea. The young (6 months to 3 years) and the elderly are the two groups who experience the most severe symptoms.

There may be an antibody response to rotavirus infection, but it is not always seen. Additionally, antibody production has been demonstrated in asymptomatic individuals. For these reasons, rotavirus antibody testing is not usually performed in the diagnostic laboratory.

▶ ## References

1. Beckham JD, Tyler KL. Arbovirus Infections. *Continuum (Minneap Minn)*. 2015;21(6 Neuroinfectious Disease):1599–1611.
2. Rockstroh A, Moges B, Barzon L, et al. Specific detection of dengue and Zika virus antibodies using envelope proteins with mutations in the conserved fusion loop. *Emerg Microbes Infect.* 2017;6(11):e99.
3. Beltrán-Silva SL, Chacón-Hernández SS, Moreno-Palacios E, et al. Clinical and differential diagnosis: dengue, chikungunya and Zika. *Revista Médica del Hospital General de México.* 2016;81(3):146–153.
4. Tyler KL. Acute viral encephalitis. *N Engl J Med.* 2018;379(6):557–566.
5. Liu JL, Shriver-Lake LC, Zabetakis D, et al. Selection of single-domain antibodies towards Western Equine Encephalitis Virus. *Antibodies.* 2018;7(44).
6. DA A, NA C. Hepatitis A and E viruses. In: Jorgensen JH, Pfaller MA, Carroll KC, American Society for Microbiology, eds. *Manual of clinical microbiology.* 11th ed. Washington, DC: ASM Press; 2015:1584–1598.
7. Leland DS. *Clinical virology.* Philadelphia: Saunders; 1996.
8. Mallory M, Hillyard D. Hepatitits C virus. In: Loeffelholz MJ, Hodinka RL, Pinsky B, Young SA, eds. *Clinical virology manual.* 5th ed. Washington, DC: ASM Press; 2016:351–361.
9. Centers for Disease Control and Prevention (CDC). Testing for HCV infection: an update of guidance for clinicians and laboratorians. *MMWR Morb Mortal Wkly Rep.* 2013;62(18):362–365.
10. Vaughn G, Purdy M. Hepatitis A and E viruses. In: Loeffelholz MJ, Hodinka RL, Pinsky B, Young SA, eds. *Clinical virology manual.* 5th ed. Washington, DC: ASM Press; 2016:329–339.
11. Pancholi P, Martin S. Cytomegalovirus. In: Loeffelholz MJ, Hodinka RL, Pinsky B, Young SA, eds. *Clinical virology manual.* 5th ed. Washington, DC: ASM Press; 2016:373–385.
12. Centers for Disease Control and Prevention (CDC). Epstein-Barr virus and infectious mononucleosis. 2018; https://www.cdc.gov/epstein-barr/laboratory-testing.html, 2019.
13. Balfour H, Hogquist K, Verghese P. Epstein-Barr virus and cytomegalovirus. In: Detrick B, Schmitz JL, Hamilton RG, eds. *Manual of molecular and clinical laboratory immunology.* 8th ed. Washington, DC: ASM Press; 2016:563–577.
14. Gartner BC, Prieksaitis J. Epstein-Barr virus. In: Jorgensen JH, Pfaller MA, Carroll KC, American Society for Microbiology, eds. *Manual of clinical microbiology.* 11th ed. Washington, DC: ASM Press; 2016:1738–1753.
15. Centers for Disease Control and Prevention (CDC). 2018 Quick reference guide: recommended laboratory HIV testing algorithm for serum or plasma specimens. *Laboratory Testing for the Diagnosis of HIV Infection* 2018; https://stacks.cdc.gov/view/cdc/50872. 2019.
16. Schüpback J. Human immunodeficiency viruses and human T-lymphotropic viruses. In: Loeffelholz MJ, Hodinka RL, Pinsky B, Young SA, eds. *Clinical virology manual.* 5th ed. Washington, DC: ASM Press; 2016:527–544.
17. Leland D, Relich R. Measles, mumps, and rubella. In: Detrick B, Schmitz JL, Hamilton RG, eds. *Manual of molecular and clinical laboratory immunology.* 8th ed. Washington, DC: ASM Press; 2016:610–619.

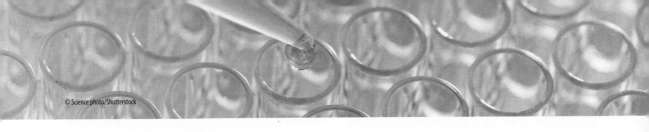

© Science photo/Shutterstock

CHAPTER 10

Bacterial Serology and Immunodiagnostics

Barbara Spinda, MS, MLS(ASCP)CM

KEY TERMS

Agglutination
Anamnestic response
Cilia
Clinical laboratory improvement amendments
Colonize
Conjugated
Direct agglutination assays
Direct fluorescent antibody (DFA)
Direct transmission
Enzyme-linked immunosorbent assay (ELISA)

Enzyme immunoassay
Flocculation
Fluorescein isothiocyanate (FITC)
Fomites
High complexity
Indirect agglutination assays
Indirect fluorescent antibody (IFA)
Indirect transmission
Lyme disease
Lysosome
Microbiome
Mode of transmission

Moderate complexity
Normal flora
Pathogens
Phagocytes
Phagolysosome
Phagosome
Reservoir
Resident colonizers
Transient colonizers
US food and drug administration (FDA)
Waived

LEARNING OBJECTIVES

Upon completion of this chapter, the reader should be able to:

1. Summarize the history of immunodiagnostics used for microbial identification.
2. Define Clinical Laboratory Improvement Amendments (CLIA) test complexity as it relates to immunodiagnostic methods.
3. Differentiate immunodiagnostic methods commonly used for the detection and diagnosis of bacteria.
4. Explain the host response to bacterial infections.
5. Describe the etiology, epidemiology, and pathogenesis of given medically important bacteria.
6. Compare and contrast conventional, immunodiagnostic, and molecular methods for the detection of given medically important bacteria.

The rapid detection and accurate identification of bacterial agents is paramount to ensuring effective treatment of infected individuals. In the clinical microbiology laboratory, the gold standard for the identification of bacterial agents has long been culture. With the advent of immunodiagnostic methods, bacterial identification has become almost routine under some circumstances. Many immunodiagnostic methods have been adapted to detect microorganisms, resulting in a plethora of commercially available immunoassays. While some immunoassays are designated for screening purposes, such as rapid testing for streptococcal pharyngitis, others are used as the primary means by which infections are diagnosed, including Lyme disease, cryptococcal meningitis, and syphilis. Due to their ease of use, rapid turnaround time, cost-effectiveness, and generally high specificity, immunoassays are also showing increased prevalence in point-of-care (POC) settings outside of the traditional laboratory.

▶ History of Immunodiagnostics for Microbial Identification

The first immunoassays were developed in the early 1940s, requiring a visual observation of antigen-antibody precipitation bands. These assays, referred to as immunodiffusion assays, are able to detect milligram to microgram quantities of analytes.[1] Immunodiffusion assays are described further in Chapter 11: Fungal and Parasitic Serology and Immunodiagnostics. The first significant improvements to immunoassays occurred in 1959 when Solomon Benson and Rosalyn Yalow created the radioimmunoassay (RIA). Their historical discovery of human antibodies to insulin and, subsequently, development of an immunoassay to detect these antibodies when linked to a radioisotope led to their receipt of the Nobel Prize in Medicine in 1977.[2] The RIA became the method after which all future immunoassays were modeled. The immunoassay continued to advance after the discovery of monoclonal antibodies by Kohler and Milstein in 1975 enabled the production of RIAs with an increased specificity. Improved RIAs using monoclonal antibodies expanded the range of immunoassays available for measurement. RIAs were considered one of the most sensitive immunoassay techniques available; however, they presented laboratorians with many significant challenges including the need for well-trained, attentive technologists.[1] The radioisotope used in RIAs is a hazardous substance and must be disposed of in accordance with federal guidelines. Due to these and many other challenges, the RIA has been replaced in clinical laboratories by avidin-biotin assays, chemiluminescent assays, fluorescent immunoassays, and other enzyme-linked detection systems.

Today, the world of immunoassay testing is very different from that less than a century ago. Advances in immunoassay design have led to the use of small, solid-phase matrices to which either an antibody or antigen is adhered. These methods have become so abundantly used in clinical laboratories that diagnostic companies have packaged microtiter plates and bead technology into "kit tests" that are commercially available to the clinical laboratory. They contain all components necessary to perform the test, including the solid-phase matrix, reagents, and controls. Automation has also entered the immunoassay arena, allowing more specimens to be tested with decreased turnaround times and requiring less technologist time, making them more cost-effective. The commercially available "kit tests" have also been modified to allow for analysis on large, automated instruments where multiplex testing can occur. The most recent innovation to the world of immunodiagnostic testing is the introduction of molecular technology. Molecular methods have significantly advanced both the level of sensitivity of assays and the range of their utilization. This has ultimately lead immunoassays to be some of the most popular and widely used testing platforms in the clinical laboratory.

▶ Immunodiagnostic Methods for Identification

Test Complexity

The **Clinical Laboratory Improvement Amendments** of 1988 (CLIA) mandate that all clinical laboratory test systems are assigned a complexity category. The **US Food and Drug Administration (FDA)** uses the criteria provided by CLIA during the pre-market approval process. The final score given by the FDA will determine if the system is categorized as **waived**, **moderate complexity**, or **high complexity**. Any test that is developed inhouse or is a modification of the approved manufacturer's instructions is automatically classified as high complexity.[3] When evaluating a new or updated test system, the FDA generates a score based on established criteria. Diagnostic test systems may be categorized as waived if they are simple to use and have little chance of providing incorrect information or causing harm if performed incorrectly. All other test systems are categorized as either moderate or high complexity. There are seven categories with specific criteria used to assign a score. **TABLE 10–1** includes a brief summary of the criteria used.

Each criterion is assigned a score ranging from one to three, based on the definitions, with one indicating the lowest level of complexity and three indicating the highest level of complexity. All seven scores are added together; scores of 12 or fewer are categorized as moderate complexity; scores higher than 12 are categorized as high complexity.[4]

Agglutination

Immunodiagnostic systems that employ agglutination reactions are widely used in the clinical laboratory. There is a plethora of **agglutination**-based diagnostic methods commercially available for the microbiology laboratory. Assays use a latex particle, such as a bead, bound with either antigens or antibodies, to identify antibodies or antigens found in clinical specimens. In the microbiology laboratory, agglutination methods are widely used to identify species of bacteria, either grown on agar plates or found in direct clinical specimens. **Direct agglutination assays** use latex beads coated with antibodies that bind directly to the antigen on the surface of the bacterium (**FIGURE 10–1A**). When the latex reagent is mixed with the bacterial suspension, antibodies on the latex bead and bacterial antigens will form an insoluble matrix, which can be seen visually (**FIGURE 10–2**). This method is used often in clinical microbiology laboratories to definitively identify *Staphylococcus aureus* and beta hemolytic streptococci isolates grown in culture. **Indirect agglutination assays** are available to identify antibodies found in serum that have been created in the presence of specific bacterial antigens (**FIGURE 10–1**). Indirect agglutination assays are able to detect both IgG and IgM antibodies, although IgM antibodies form a better agglutination matrix. These methods are often used to identify current or recent infections of bacterial, viral, and fungal agents that are not easily cultured in the clinical laboratory.

Flocculation

In contrast to the large aggregates seen in direct and indirect agglutination methods, **flocculation** tests form a fine precipitate as a product. The soluble antigen bound to antigen is visible only because the product is confined to a small space. Flocculation testing is used often in screening serum and cerebrospinal fluid for syphilis. A detailed description of flocculation assays for syphilis serology can be found later in this chapter when syphilis is discussed further.

Enzyme Immunoassays

The **enzyme immunoassay**, (EIA), also referred to as **enzyme-linked immunosorbent assay (ELISA)**, is the most utilitarian of all immunodiagnostic methods in the clinical microbiology

TABLE 10–1 Criteria Used to Categorize Test Complexity, as Defined by CLIA[4]	
Criterion	**Description**
Knowledge	Scientific and technical knowledge required to perform the preanalytic, analytic, and postanalytic phases of testing. Test systems requiring more scientific and technical knowledge are assigned a higher score.
Training and experience	Training and experience needed to perform preanalytic, analytic, and postanalytic phases of the testing process. Test systems requiring specialized training and substantial experience to perform are assigned a higher score.
Reagents and materials preparation	Stability and reliability of reagents and materials. Reagents and materials that require special handling, storage, or manual steps to prepare are assigned a higher score.
Characteristics of operational steps	Operational steps are characterized as automated or manual. Test processes requiring close monitoring or control, special specimen preparation, precise timing of steps, accurate pipetting, or extensive calculations are assigned a higher score.
Calibration, quality control, and proficiency testing materials	Availability and stability of calibration materials, quality-control material, and proficiency testing materials. Tests with calibration materials, quality-control materials, and proficiency test materials that are labile, if available, are assigned a higher score.
Test system troubleshooting and equipment maintenance	Complexity of test system troubleshooting and equipment maintenance. Test systems requiring decision-making and direct intervention to resolve most problems or maintenance that requires special knowledge or skills are assigned a higher score.
Interpretation and judgment	Amount of interpretation and judgment required to perform prenalytic, analytic, and postanalytic processes. Test systems that require extensive interpretation and judgment are assigned a higher score.

Modified from U.S. Food and Drug Administration. CLIA Categorizations. Medical Devices. https://www.fda.gov/MedicalDevices/DeviceRegulationandGuidance/IVDRegulatoryAssistance/ucm393229.htm. Updated: March 22, 2018. Accessed: October 1, 2018.

laboratory. The basic EIA method consists of enzyme-conjugated antibodies that are able to detect either another antibody or an antigen, and catalyze a discernible colorimetric result. The use of enzymes for immunodiagnostic methods has a number of advantages. The enzyme is not changed during the testing process, therefore, allowing it to catalyze the reaction of many substrate molecules and amplify the results. Enzyme-conjugated antibodies are stable and can be stored for a long time.[5] Commercially available test kits often either have a shelf life that is stable at ambient temperature (15–30°C) or refrigerated (2–8°C) for at least 6 months. The generation of a colored end product allows for direct observation of results or being read on a spectrophotometer.[5]

Since its humble beginnings, the EIA has expanded to multiple platforms including solid-phase immunoassays and membrane-bound, solid-phase immunosorbent assays, both of

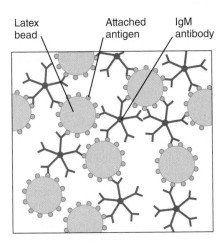
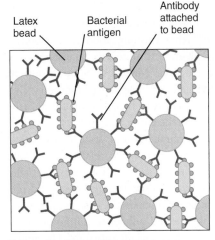

A Reaction in a positive passive agglutination test for antibodies

B Reaction in a positive passive agglutination test for antigens

FIGURE 10–1 Agglutination reactions. **(A)** Indirect agglutination reaction showing antigens bound to a latex bead that bind IgM antibodies in serum. **(B)** Direct agglutination reaction showing antibodies bound to a latex bead that bind to a bacterial antigen.

From Pommerville, J. C. (2017). Fundamentals of Microbiology, 11e. Jones & Bartlett Learning.

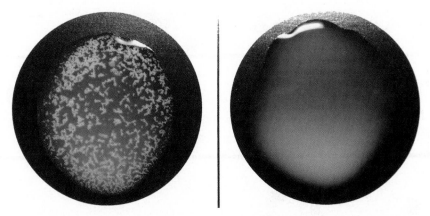

FIGURE 10–2 Latex agglutination test for *Staphylococcus aureus*. When *S. aureus* bacteria are mixed with the latex reagent, the antibodies on the surface of the latex beads will bind to the antigens on the surface of *S. aureus*. A positive result will show agglutination (left), while a negative result will not show agglutination (right).

Courtesy of Gunnar Flayten, Bionor Laboratories AS.

which are widely used in the clinical laboratory. Assays are available for a wide variety of bacterial, viral, parasitic, and fungal infectious agents. The designs of both methods permit small amounts of specimen to be tested. The EIA is intended to give rapid detection of an infectious agent in a clinical specimen. The solid-phase immunoassay is designed with antibodies firmly attached to a solid surface, whether it is the inside of a microtiter well or the surface of a plastic or metal bead. If antigen is present in the specimen, an antigen-antibody complex will be formed. After washing, a second antibody conjugated with an enzyme substrate is added and sandwiches the antigen between the two antibodies. Alkaline phosphatase and horseradish peroxidase are two enzymes used frequently. After washing unbound antibody, an enzyme substrate is added to catalyze the colorimetric reaction. Microtiter-based assays may be read visually or by spectrophotometry. Bead-based assays are read by instrumentation, which may automate the entire assay process.

The membrane-bound, solid-phase, enzyme immunosorbent assay, also referred to as lateral flow assays, use an absorbent material that allows the specimen to flow through the solid-phase assay. Antigens present in the specimen pass along the membrane and adhere to antibodies conjugated with a chromogenic substrate. The antigen-antibody complexes are then moved along the solid matrix where they bind to another antibody and develop a visual test result. Remaining antibody, not bound to antigen, flows past the test result and adheres to another antibody, where it becomes a control result, indicating the test was performed correctly. **FIGURE 10–3** demonstrates an example of one such method.

Immunofluorescent Assays

The immunofluorescent assay is frequently used in the clinical microbiology laboratory to detect microorganisms that are difficult or impossible to culture. Commercially available test methods use glass slides, to which the antigen in the patient's specimen is adhered with formalin, methanol, ethanol, or acetone, depending on the manufacturer's instructions. Monoclonal or polyclonal antibodies are used to detect the antigen in either a **direct fluorescent antibody (DFA)** technique or an

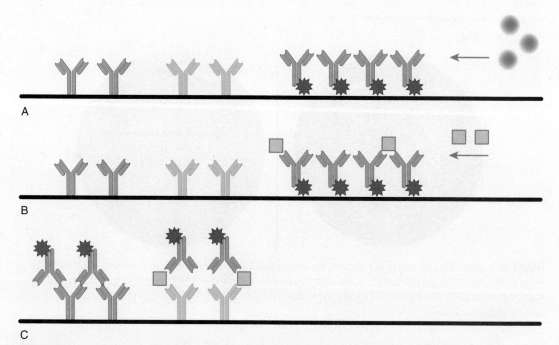

FIGURE 10–3 Membrane-bound, solid-phase sandwich EIA. **(A)** Specimen is added to a solid phase (black line) containing a mouse monoclonal antipathogen antibody bound to a chromogen (red) as the testing reagent, antipathogen antibodies bound to the solid phase (test line), and antimouse antibody (control line). **(B)** As the pathogen antigen flows along the solid phase, it binds to the antipathogen antibody. **(C)** The antipathogen antibody/pathogen antigen complex binds to the antipathogen antibody adhered to the solid-phase, resulting in a positive test result. Any additional antibodies, not complexed with antigen, bind to the antimouse antibody, resulting in an internal control line, indicating the test was performed according to manufacturer's instructions.

indirect fluorescent antibody (IFA) technique. In the DFA method, antibodies are **conjugated** to fluorescent dyes and applied to the test specimen. After appropriate incubation and washing, a counterstain is then applied to stain the background. In the IFA method, an antibody directed against the antigen is first applied, incubated, and washed. A second antibody is then conjugated with fluorescent dye is applied to bind to the first antibody, thus creating a two-step or sandwich technique. After appropriate incubation and washing, the counterstain is applied to stain the background. Regardless of method used, stained slides must be examined using a fluorescent microscope with filters specific to the dye used to excite the fluorescence. Many of the kits used in the clinical microbiology laboratory use **fluorescein isothiocyanate (FITC)** as the fluorescent dye, which appears bright apple green under excited light.

The IFA is also widely used in the clinical laboratory to detect antibodies in a patient's serum when the microorganism is difficult to cultivate. Antigens corresponding to the desired antibody are fixed to the test slide. When the serum is added, antibodies will attach to the antigens on the slide. After incubation and washing, a fluorescein-labeled, anti-human antibody is added to visually see the patients' antibodies under fluorescent light. Commercially available test kits can detect antibodies to a wide range of microorganisms including syphilis (*Treponema pallidum*), pertussis (*Bordetella pertussis*), Legionnaire's disease (*Legionella pneumophila*), as well as a plethora of viral, parasitic, and fungal agents. Test kits often include test slides with the antigen fixed, positive, and negative controls, fluorescent-labeled conjugate, diluent for patient serum, and wash buffer.

Immunofluorescent methods, both direct and indirect, come with a number of advantages and disadvantages for use. Tests can be performed in a timely manner and are cost-effective, although the cost of a fluorescent microscope is more substantial than a brightfield microscope. The assay also allows the adequacy of the specimen to be visually assessed. For example, using a chlamydial DFA test, the technologist can determine if the specimen was collected from the columnar epithelial cells at the opening of the cervix. Examining and interpreting immunofluorescent assays does require training and practice for laboratory personnel to become proficient. Fluorescent dyes also fade rapidly over time, thus requiring digital imaging for result archiving. It is for these reasons that manufacturers have conjugated antibodies to other markers, allowing for visual identification without the need for a fluorescent microscope. These colorimetric enzymes include horseradish peroxidase, alkaline phosphatase, and avadin-biotin, which create a colored end product that can be seen using a Brightfield microscope[5]. The pigment does not fade with storage and allows slides to be permanently mounted with a coverslip.

Membrane-bound, solid-phase assays are available that use immunofluorescence to identify antigens in clinical specimens. Unlike the visual results that can be interpreted from an enzyme immunoassay, the immunofluorescent assay requires an instrument to read the results of the test cassette.

▶ Bacterial Infections

Host Response to Bacterial Infections

Microorganisms are everywhere, and human encounters with them are inevitable. It seems that almost immediately after a microorganism is identified and its abilities and natural products understood, humans begin using the microorganism in various ways. Today, microorganisms are seen in a wide range of industries including food and fermentation, agricultural insecticides, waste biodegradation, and even antimicrobial production. The interactions that occur between humans and bacteria are exceptionally complex and, despite extensive research into the human **microbiome**[6], there is still much to learn. What is known is that humans and microorganisms have found ways to coexist in a symbiotic relationship, with both gaining benefit from the other. However, at the same time, microorganisms share the same goal of survival as humans; and through their search for food, shelter, and the ability to replicate, microorganisms outside of the human microbiome are often the cause of disease. Microorganisms that are able to cause infection and disease are known as **pathogens**.

Understanding the complex relationship of the microorganism and host emerges when the specific steps of the interaction are examined. General stages in the host-microorganism interaction include: (1) the physical encounter between the host and the microorganism; (2) the colonization of the host with the microorganism, internal or external, and the subsequent survival of the microorganism; (3) entry, invasion, and dissemination of the microorganism into deeper tissue and organs of the host; and (4) resolution or outcome of the host-microorganism interaction.[5] The knowledge gained from examining these interactions plays an important role in the development and use of immunoassays for the identification of medically important bacteria.

Humans encounter bacteria through exposure, often as the result of a person's activities or behaviors. The means by which the human acquires infection is known as the **mode of transmission**. **Direct transmission** of microorganisms occurs when one acquires the microorganism from another, serving as the **reservoir**. The reservoir may be a human, animal, or insect. A classic example is seen when a neonate leaves the sterility of the mother's womb and passes through the birth canal, which is heavily colonized with a variety of microorganisms. This occurrence is the first interaction of the newborn with microbial agents. In many cases, this interaction provides bacteria to the newborn that will survive synergistically to the benefit of both the host and microorganism. However, not all direct interactions are beneficial to the host. If the mother is a carrier of *Streptococcus agalactiae*, the newborn will likely become infected with the organism and may develop sepsis or meningitis. **Indirect transmission** occurs when microorganisms are acquired through contact with a contaminated vehicle, such as water, food, air, medical devices, or other inanimate objects known as **fomites**.

Once contact is made, the microorganism attempts to colonize the host; however, the human body has natural defenses to protect vital tissues and organs from infection. The first defenses of the human body are the external and internal surfaces that come in direct contact with the infecting agent. The surfaces include the skin and mucous membranes of the oral cavity, respiratory tract, gastrointestinal tract, and the genitourinary tract. The skin acts as a physical barrier, preventing the penetration of microorganisms into the body. Colonization of microorganisms is hampered by the dry, cool environment of the skin, constant shedding of skin cells, natural antibacterial substances such as sebum and sweat, and even by natural colonizers of the skin microbiome. The mucous membranes of the respiratory tract, gastrointestinal tract, and genitourinary tract are constantly exposed to outside microorganisms. The major protective component of all mucous membranes is the production of mucous, which traps bacteria before they can reach the inner surface of cells, lubricates cells to prevent bacteria from adhering, and distributes antibodies and antibacterial agents. Saliva found in the oral cavity not only physically flushes microorganisms away but it also contains antibacterial substances such as IgA and lysozyme to assist in the destruction of microorganisms. The upper respiratory tract has the advantage of cells lining the trachea containing fingerlike projections known as **cilia**. These cilia work in a sweeping motion that moves microorganisms trapped in mucous upward and outward away from the cells of the lungs. Within the gastrointestinal tract, the low pH and proteolytic enzymes of the stomach create an inhospitable environment for many microorganisms. The urethra of both males and females have a natural microbiome that is able to survive in the lower pH and fight any foreign invaders. The physical action of urination also acts to prevent microorganisms from migrating up the ureters into the kidneys.

Despite efforts of the body's first line of defense, microorganisms manage to **colonize** and even invade. As was previously described, the human microbiome, also referred to as **normal flora** or normal microbiota, encompasses microorganisms that are natural colonizers of the inside and outside surfaces of the body. These organisms may be **transient colonizers** that are able to survive but do not replicate and are frequently shed through the natural loss of host cells. **Resident colonizers** are the microorganisms that are able to survive and thrive in and on the surface of the host. While most of these microorganisms do not cause disease under normal circumstances, it is when normal microbiota or foreign microbiota penetrate the outer barriers that infection is seen. Once the surface barriers are disrupted, numerous other host defense mechanisms are activated.

The response of the host immune system to microbes within the underlying tissue may be specific or nonspecific. Nonspecific occurs no matter what the invading organism and is either biochemical or cellular. Biochemical responses act to remove nutrients essential to the survival of the microorganism. A cellular response includes the action of **phagocytes**, cells that are able to ingest and destroy bacteria and other foreign materials. Phagocytic cells include polymorphonuclear neutrophils, macrophages, and dendritic cells. These cells ingest microorganisms through a process known as endocytosis and ingest them in a **phagosome**. The phagosome then fuses with a **lysosome**, becoming a **phagolysosome**. Three outcomes may result from this action: (1) the microorganism is able to survive long-term in the cell, (2) toxic chemical and destructive enzymes in the phagolysosome destroy the bacteria and release fragments, or (3) the phagocytic cell is destroyed as a result of bacterial destruction.[5] The presence of phagocytic cells is an important observation in the diagnosis of infection by microorganism.

In addition to the nonspecific cellular and biochemical responses of the immune system, the human host is able to mount a specific protective response in the presence of invading microorganisms. Antibodies are specifically produced by activated B cells in response to a foreign antigen. Bacterial antigens are chemicals or toxins produced by the invading microorganism or components of the organism's structure. During the first encounter with an invading microorganism, B cells become activated and a series of events mediated by helper T cells and the release of cytokines occur. Antibodies are then created to correspond with the antigen seen. It is only after memory B cells are created and remain quiescent in the body that an **anamnestic response** occurs upon subsequent exposure to the same antigen, and antibodies are created rapidly to fight the infection. In bacterial immunodiagnostics, the presence of these antibodies (IgG or IgM) in a patient's serum are diagnostic of infection.

Streptococcus Pyogenes (Group A Streptococcus)

Etiology

Streptococcus pyogenes are facultative anaerobic gram-positive, nonmotile, nonspore-forming, catalase negative, cocci that grow in chains and are part of the genus, *Streptococcus*. Streptococci are divided by their ability to cause hemolysis on trypticase soy agar with 5% sheep red blood cells. *S. pyogenes* are one of many streptococci that cause beta-hemolysis. Beta-hemolytic streptococci are further differentiated by carbohydrates found in their cell walls. These carbohydrates are used to divide streptococci into 20 defined groups based on the work of Dr. Rebecca Lancefield. The Lancefield grouping is based on these group-specific carbohydrates that can be identified serologically. *S. pyogenes* belongs to the Lancefield group A and is commonly referred to as group A streptococcus.[5] While most beta-hemolytic streptococci are seen as part of the normal flora in humans, *S. pyogenes* is not considered normal microbiota. *S. pyogenes* inhabits the skin and upper respiratory tract in humans and is often carried in the nasal and pharyngeal mucosa. Isolation of *S. pyogenes* is always clinically significant.

Epidemiology and Pathogenesis

S. pyogenes is the most aggressive beta-hemolytic streptococcus isolated in the clinical laboratory, and a frequent cause of acute pharyngitis and many other cutaneous and system infections such as impetigo, scarlet fever, necrotic fasciitis, and streptococcal toxic shock syndrome. Infectious organisms are transmitted person-to-person either by direct or indirect contact through droplet nuclei.

S. pyogenes produces a number of factors that contribute to its virulence including streptolysin O and streptolysin S. Both of these factors are capable of lysing erythrocytes, leukocytes, and platelets, with streptolysin S possessing functionality in the presence of ambient air while streptolysin O is broken down by the presence of oxygen and will lyse only cells in the absence of oxygen. Streptolysin O is also inhibited by cholesterol found in skin lipids, resulting in an absence of protective antibodies during skin infections.[5] Both streptolysins are responsible for the organism's hemolytic actions.

S. pyogenes often initiates autoimmunity after acute infection if not treated properly with antibiotics. The resulting sequelae of acute rheumatic fever and poststreptococcal acute glomerulonephritis have been responsible for substantial morbidity and mortality in all parts of the world.[7] In rheumatic fever, antibodies produced in response to the M protein antigen found in the cell wall of *S. pyogenes* cross-react with heart muscle proteins such as myosin, tropomyosin, and vimentin. This molecular mimicry causes an autoimmune reaction, leading to rheumatic heart disease.[5,8] In contrast, acute glomerulonephritis is caused by the deposition of antibody-streptococcal antigen complexes in the kidney that result in damage to glomeruli.[5]

Immunodiagnostic Methods

When infected with group A streptococci, the host mounts an immune response with specific antibodies to both extracellular and intracellular antigenic components of the bacteria. Streptococcal serological tests have been developed to identify these biomarkers. Streptococcal serology tests play a useful role in diagnosing secondary disease seen as a result of streptococcal infection for a number of reasons. For example, the postinfective nature of rheumatic fever and glomerulonephritis means the acute infection has already passed. Serologic tests for streptococcal infection are not applicable for acute pharyngitis as it is not clinically practical to wait 2 to 4 weeks for a convalescent specimen.[9] The extracellular antigens streptolysin O and DNase B continue to be the most useful serological markers of previous streptococcal infection despite being a nonspecific marker of group A infection. The

anti-streptolysin O (ASO) serologic assay was first developed by Todd in the 1930s. The classic method for ASO is a dilution assay for measuring the ability of human serum to neutralize the hemolytic activity of the streptolysin O regent. Results were originally reported as Todd units until the World Health Organization (WHO) standardized ASO reporting in 1961. Most laboratories now report ASO results as international units per milliliter (IU/mL). Latex agglutination, nephelometry, and turbidity methods have been developed based on the classic neutralization method. The fist anti-DNase B immunoassay was developed a decade after the ASO assay and was also a neutralization method. The assay measured the ability of diluted serum to neutralize the effect of DNase B on a DNA substrate. The substrate is complexed to colored dye and results are inversely proportional to the highest dilution that blocks the loss of color expressed by the digested substrate. Latex agglutination and nephelometry methods have also been developed for anti-DNase detection. Anti-DNase immunoassays are often used along with ASO immunoassays for detection of antecedent group A streptococcal infections. Positive results are determined by demonstrating a rise in titer from acute to convalescent (2 to 4 weeks apart) specimens.[9] The cellular components of the bacteria elicit an immune response specific to streptococcal infection; however, they are not used for clinical assessment of infection, but are utilized in clinical research related to acute rheumatic heart disease.[7]

The gold standard for the identification of *S. pyogenes* pharyngitis and systemic infection continues to be the cultivation and isolation of the organism. The first rapid immunodiagnostic methods for definitive identification of *S. pyogenes* isolates were seen in the early 1980s with the Directigen Strep A Test Kit leading the way. Studies at that time demonstrated a 91 to 99% sensitivity and 98 to 99% specificity. The test took 60 to 75 minutes to complete and must have been performed from a well-isolated colony from nutrient growth agar.[10,11] Technology behind the Directigen Strep A Test Kit has been modified and updated over the last 30 years; today there are multiple commercially available test kits for the identification of groups A, B, C, F, and G beta-hemolytic streptococci. All available immunoassays employ the same method: (1) extraction reagents lyse the organisms releasing the group-specific antigens, and (2) latex beads with attached antibodies to each specific streptococcal group, that (3) display agglutination when the lysed organism is mixed with the corresponding group-specific latex beads. Testing must be performed from an isolated beta-hemolytic streptococcus colony and can be completed in under 5 minutes.[12–14] Although the streptococcal latex typing immunoassays are relatively rapid once the organism is isolated, it often takes 24 to 48 hours to isolate the organism.

Rapid enzyme immunoassays (EIA) for the detection of *S. pyogenes* organisms directly from patient specimens have become the standard screen for all patients with acute pharyngitis. Rapid EIAs allow for a quicker (usually 15–20 minutes) result than many physician offices can perform as most tests are considered CLIA-waived. A quick search of "Streptococcus, group A" in the CLIA registry of the FDA website shows 284 registered immunoassays for direct testing of *S. pyogenes* from throat swabs. In 2019, 37 immunoassays have been registered: 23 waived, 13 moderate complexity, and only one designated high complexity.[15] This increase in immunoassay production, with a substantial portion holding moderate complexity designation, is most likely due to advancements in rapid molecular technology.

Whether the solid-phase test platform is developed as a stand-alone test strip or encased in a cartridge that may be read by an analyzer, the lateral flow EIA design is similar from one assay to another. A two-swab pharyngeal specimen is collected from the patient. One swab is placed in a tube of lysing reagents to release the *S. pyogenes* surface antigens present in the specimen, similar to the reagent used in the latex agglutination identification methods. The second swab is reserved for culture, if required. Either the stand-alone test strip is placed in the tube of fluid or the fluid is placed in the cartridge, allowing it to flow along the solid matrix. Many different solid-phase platforms are commercially available and are either interpreted manually by the user or electronically by an instrument. Due to the lower sensitivity of most rapid immunoassays for direct *S. pyogenes* detection, strong recommendations by the Infectious Disease Society of America require that all specimens with negative rapid immunoassay results have a backup throat culture for *S. pyogenes*, as it is the gold standard method.[16] With this recommendation, clinical laboratory inspection agencies, Centers for Medicare and Medicaid Services (CMS), College of American Pathologists (CAP), and The Joint Commission (TJC), have all included backup culture as a requirement to achieve accreditation.

Molecular Diagnostic Methods

The advent of rapid molecular-based methods for direct *S. pyogenes* identification has created a new paradigm in laboratory testing. Molecular testing methods, by nature, are more sensitive to the analyte in question; therefore, eliminate the need for a backup culture of any negative specimens. As seen in the CLIA search, more molecular platforms are approved for clinical diagnostic use each year.[15] The two most significant limitations of molecular testing, thus preventing adaptation in all laboratories, are the cost and assay time. As in all clinical laboratory testing, molecular methods incur an increased cost to perform, including the reagents and instrumentation. In addition, the time required to perform a rapid molecular-based assay for *S. pyogenes* is anywhere from 1 hour to 4 or more hours; some methods are random access while others are batch-testing only. When diagnosing and treating a patient in an urgent care setting, speed and accuracy are of the essence. This creates a balance of necessity, seen in many areas of the laboratory, where the challenge becomes identifying an immunoassay that possesses both of these attributes.

Mycobacterium Tuberculosis
Etiology

Mycobacterium species are the only genus within the family *Mycobacteriaceae* in the actinomycetes class of microorganisms. Within the genus, organisms are further speciated based on genotypic properties; however, for many years, they were differentiated based on phenotypic characteristics. *Mycobacterium* species are traditionally grouped based on the speed of their cultivation, with rapid growers taking fewer than 7 days and slow growers requiring more than 7 days for colony production. The organisms are aerobic, nonspore forming, nonmotile, very thin, slightly curved bacilli. Mycobacteria are easily differentiated from many other microorganism genera by the acid fastness of their cell walls. The cell wall contains N-glycolylmuramic acid instead of N-acetylmuramic acid. This difference in cell-wall structure results in a high lipid content and creates a hydrophobic permeability barrier.[5] The traditional Gram Stain procedure produces a faintly staining Gram-positive bacillus, demonstrating a beaded pattern due to the inability of the crystal violet to efficiently penetrate the cell wall. However, they do resist decolorization with acidified alcohol (3% hydrochloric acid) after prolonged application of a basic fuchsin dye (**FIGURE 10–4**). Carbolfuchsin is selected as a primary stain to detect acid-fast organisms in direct specimens and confirm mycobacterial growth on plated media.

Epidemiology and Pathogenesis

Mycobacterium tuberculosis is the cause of most cases of human tuberculosis, and is one of 10 species collectively termed the *Mycobacterium tuberculosis* complex. Differentiation of species within this complex rarely occurs because distinction is complicated and is of little or no clinical importance. Specimens are reported as *M. tuberculosis* complex and speciated only when required for epidemiologic or public health reasons. Organisms within the complex are not able to replicate in the environment; therefore, humans and other warm-blooded animals are the only reservoir. An estimated one-quarter of the world's population is infected with tuberculosis.[17] According to the Centers for Disease Control and Prevention (CDC), a total of 9,093 new tuberculosis cases were reported in the United States in 2017. This was a 1.8% decrease compared with cases reported in 2016 and was the lowest on record. The decrease in tuberculosis has been attributed to an increase in public health measures to identify and treat active cases. Despite aggressive measures, the goal of tuberculosis eradication in the United States will not be attainable as 69.8% of cases seen were among foreign-born persons and represent reactivation of latent tuberculosis infections. In 2016, four of the top five foreign countries of origin reported to the CDC were considered high tuberculosis burden countries by the World Health Organization (WHO): China, India, Philippines, and Vietnam.[18] In the United States, tuberculosis is typically seen among the poor, the homeless, intravenous drug users, alcoholics, elderly, and the medically underserved communities. Transmission of tuberculosis is person-to-person via inhalation of droplet nuclei

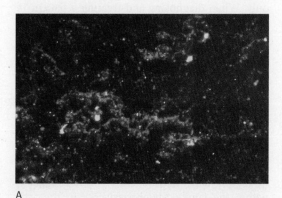

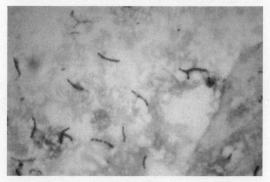

A

B

FIGURE 10–4 **(A)** Auramine-Rhodamine stain under florescent microscopy. **(B)** Light microscope image showing *M. tuberculosis* cells (red) stained with the acid-fast procedure. Cells often show growth in thick bead-like strings in sputum specimens.

(a) Courtesy of Ronald W. Smithwick/CDC; (b) Courtesy of Dr. George P. Kubica/CDC.

from persons with pulmonary tuberculosis, and in clinical laboratories during the manipulation of specimen and cultured organisms. The infectious dose of *M. tuberculosis* is only 10 tubercle bacilli.

Tuberculosis often manifests clinically as pulmonary disease that may mimic others, such as pneumonia, neoplasm, or fungal infections. Primary tuberculosis commonly presents symptoms including low-grade fever, night sweats, fatigue, anorexia, and weight loss. Patients often have a productive cough, chills, myalgia and sweating, symptoms similar to influenza, acute bronchitis, and pneumonia. Pulmonary infection elicits migration of T cells and macrophages to the lungs where mycobacteria are phagocytized by the macrophages. Organisms are capable of intracellular multiplication. The host is typically unable to eliminate the organisms, resulting in a systemic hypersensitivity to *Mycobacterium* antigens. Hard tubercles, termed granulomas, form in the lungs consisting of lymphocytes, macrophages, and cellular material (**FIGURE 10–5**). Elevated concentrations of *Mycobacterium* antigen may lead to tissue necrosis, caused by enzymes released from the macrophages. In a small percentage of pulmonary tuberculosis patients, disease may spread via the lymphatic system or hematogenously, leading to miliary tuberculosis.[5] Extrapulmonary tuberculosis may extend into the genitourinary tract, lymph nodes (cervical lymphadenitis), central nervous system (meningitis), bone (osteomyelitis), joint (arthritis), peritoneum, pericardium, larynx, and pleural lining (pleuritis). Patients with latent tuberculosis are noninfectious and asymptomatic as organisms are sequestered in granulomas. Reactivation to active disease can occur at any time, typically after an incident in which cellular immunity is suppressed or damaged. This may be a result of a change in lifestyle or other health conditions. Commonly used antibiotics for the treatment of tuberculosis include isoniazid and rifampicin. Spontaneous mutations are being seen to cause resistance to these and other available antibiotics, resulting in multi-drug resistant tuberculosis (MDR-TB) and, even extensively, drug-resistant tuberculosis (XDR-TB) strains.

Conventional Methods

In patients with active tuberculosis, specimens are collected from the source of infection, typically pulmonary, but may include body fluids or tissue. Specimens are processed with N-acetyl-L-cysteine (NALC) to digest mucous and decontaminate normal flora if present. Specimens are cultured for up to 6 weeks on media selective for *Mycobacterium* species, due to the relatively slow growing nature of *M. tuberculosis*. To expedite treatment, processed specimens are first stained with either auramine or auramine-rhodamine and examined under fluorescence. Suspect specimens are then stained with a basic fuchsin stain for confirmation. While the identification of a *Mycobacterium* species is crucial for the initiation of treatment, definitive identification of *M. tuberculosis* cannot occur until growth is obtained.

Immunodiagnostic Methods

The tuberculin skin test has been used as a screening tool for latent infection for more than a century since it is a proven method for identifying infection with *M. tuberculosis* in persons who do not have disease. The immunologic basis for the tuberculin skin test is based on the principle that infection with *M. tuberculosis* elicits a delayed-type hypersensitivity reaction to certain antigenic components.[19] The purified protein derivative (PPD) tuberculin, used in most skin tests, is extracted from culture filtrates by protein precipitation. A large, single lot of PPD, produced in 1939, has become the international standard with which all subsequent preparations are compared for biological reactivity. The effective testing concentration has been determined so that 0.1 mL will be biologically equivalent to 0.1 μL of the PPD standard, or 5 tuberculin units. An immunologic reaction occurs in response to intradermal injection of 0.1 mL PPD on the inside surface of the forearm using a 26- or 27-gauge needle with the bevel facing up. When injected properly, the skin becomes raised with a 6- to 10-mm wheal that subsides within a few minutes after the PPD has dispersed into the tissue. The skin reaction is read at 48 to 72 hours, looking for a characteristic raised immunologic reaction.

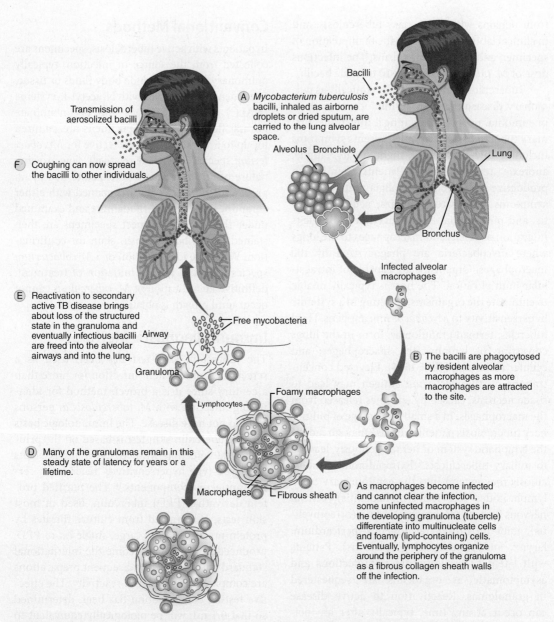

FIGURE 10–5 The stages of Mycobacterium tuberculosis infection. After the aerosolized bacilli are inhaled, the bacteria invade the alveoli of the lungs, where the cells are engulfed by macrophages. The immune system is unable to eliminate the infection, and lymphocytes attempt to "wall off" the bacilli. When disease is activated, the bacteria rupture to granuloma and enter the alveoli where they are coughed up and transmitted to another susceptible person.

The diameter of induration is measured, not the area of erythema (**FIGURE 10–6**). Three cutoff levels have been recommended for positive reactions of the PPD test, based on its sensitivity and specificity. The 5-mm cutoff is used for high-risk patients such as those exposed to tuberculosis and immunocompromised individuals. The 10-mm cutoff is used for other high-risk

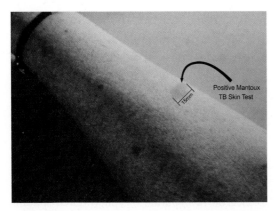

FIGURE 10–6 Tuberculin skin test. This is a positive reaction to the Manatoux skin test. The induration must be more than 15mm to be considered positive.

Courtesy of Donald Kopanoff/CDC.

patients such as recent immigrants and injection drug users. The 15-mm cutoff is used for patients with no risk factors.[20] Sensitivity ranges from 75 to 90% sensitivity with 10-mm indurations,[20] to 99% in patients with latent tuberculosis infection with normal immune reponse.[19] False-positive test results may be seen in patients who have been vaccinated with Bacilli-Calmette Guérin (BCG). The BCG vaccine is widely used in European and African countries, but not the United States; therefore, false-positive results are often seen in immigrants from these countries. False-negative results occur in at least 20% of patients with active tuberculosis infection due to the general illness and malnutrition that may reduce delayed hypersensitivity reactions.[19]

Interferon gamma release assays (IGRAs) were developed with the first assay gaining FDA approval in 2001. The Quantiferon-TB assay (Cellestis Limited) was developed as an enzyme-linked immunosorbent assay (ELISA) to measure the amount of interferon-gamma (INF-γ) released in response to PPD compared with controls. Despite using *M. avium* as a control for nontuberculosis mycobacteria and saline as a negative control, the specificity was less than that of the traditional tuberculin skin test. The Quantiferon-TB assay has not been on the market since 2005. To improve sensitivity, a new IGRA was developed, the Quantiferon-TB Gold. This assay assessed INF-γ response to synthetic peptides that represent specific *M. tuberculosis* proteins, early secretory antigenic target-6 (ESAT-6), and culture filtrate protein 10 (CFP-10). These proteins are present in all *M. tuberculosis* and are absent from the BCG vaccine, removing the possibility of a false positive from vaccination. As antigens, these proteins also offer improved specificity compared with PPD.[21] Qiagen purchased Cellestis Limited in 2001, gaining access to the patent-protected Quantiferon technology. In June of 2017, Qiagen received FDA approval for their updated Quantiferon-TB Gold Plus assay (QFT-Plus).

The QFT-Plus assay builds on its predecessor. Patient immune cells are stimulated with the proteins ESAT-6, CFP-10, and the new addition, TB7.7 (p. 4). Specimen collection occurs in four specially designed tubes, in which only 1 mL of blood is required in each. The Nil tube serves as a negative control while the Mitogen tube serves as the positive control, which may also indicate insufficient lymphocytes or reduced lymphocyte activity in the patient. The TB1 and TB2 tubes each contain ESAT-6 and CFP-10 peptides to elicit a response from CD4+ T-helper lymphocytes; the TB2 tube also contains p4 peptide targeted to elicit a response from CD8+ cytotoxic T lymphocytes. The assay is dependent on sample tubes being collected in the required order (Nil, TB1, TB2, and Mitogen) to prevent the crossover of antigens inside the tubes. Immediately after filling, tubes must be shaken 10 times, coating the entire inner surface of the tube and dissolving antigens on the wall. Tubes are incubated at 37°C in an upright orientation for 16 to 24 hours before testing. Tubes are then centrifuged to separate plasma from cells so it may be harvested. Plasma from each tube is incubated, with conjugate bound to anti-human INF-γ antibodies, in a microtiter well coated with anti-human INF-γ monoclonal antibody. INF-γ present in the sample will be captured between both to anti-human INF-γ antibodies. After adequate washing and further incubation with an enzyme substrate, followed by the addition of a stopping solution, the optical density of each well is read with a microplate reader. A patient is considered positive when the TB1 or TB2 tube has an INF-γ value ≥0.35 IU/mL and the value is ≥25% of the nil value, when values are subtracted from the Nil tube value. The reported sensitivity and specificity are 88.7% and 98.11%, respectively.[22]

The only other FDA-approved IGRA is the T-Spot.TB (Oxford Immunotec), which received FDA approval in 2013. The T-Spot.TB measures the amount of INF-γ released from CD4⁺ and CD8⁺ effector T cells in response to stimulus of a combination of peptides simulating markers of *M. tuberculosis*, ESAT-6 and CFP-10. The test is based on an enzyme-linked immunospot (ELISPOT) method. Whole blood is collected in standard lithium heparin vacutainer tubes, centrifuged within 8 hours of collection, and the buffy coat is removed for testing. After sufficient washes to endure only peripheral blood mononuclear cells (PBMCs) are remaining, a cell count is performed. Once the concentration of PBMCs is determined in the stock cell suspension, 500 μL of the final cell suspension at a concentration of 2.5×10^5 cells/100 μL is prepared. Once at the final concentration, cells are incubated in a well containing a membrane coated with anti-human INF-γ antibodies. Four wells are required for each patient with reagents nil, panel A, panel B, and positive control added separately. Samples are then incubated for 16 to 20 hours to elicit INF-γ release in response to stimuli. After incubation with conjugate and substrate added, with washes before and after each step, the membrane is allowed to dry completely. Results are determined by counting distinct dark blue spots on the membrane. A patient is considered positive if panel A or panel B has ≥8 spots. The reported sensitivity and specificity are 94.4% and 97.1%, respectively.[23]

With the adoption of IGRAs in many hospital and clinic settings the CDC issued updated guidelines for using IGRAs to detect *M. tuberculosis* infection. General recommendations include ensuring specimens are collected according to protocol, sent to the laboratory immediately, and tested in a timely manner. They also state that IGRAs should not be used for testing low-risk individuals. Even though specificity reaches almost 99% for both assays, the prevalence of *M. tuberculosis* infection is ≤1%; many positive results will be false positive results.[21]

Molecular Diagnostic Methods

The GeneXpert MTB/RIF molecular assay (Cepheid) is a completely self-contained test cartridge using real-time reverse transcriptase polymerase chain reaction (PCR) and real-time PCR assays for use with the GeneXpert platform. The assay simultaneously identifies *M. tuberculosis* complex and rifampin resistance by amplifying a specific portion of the *rpoB* gene and probing for five different known gene mutations that translate for rifampin resistance. Testing may be performed on raw sputum or concentrated sputum specimens using 2 mL of specimen or less. Patient testing is complete and reportable within 4 hours of specimen receipt in the laboratory, when specimen testing is not delayed. Two negative specimens, collected 1 day apart, are indicative of a patient no longer demonstrating active tuberculosis infection. The patient may be removed from airborne isolation.[24] The use of molecular-based direct methods for *M. tuberculosis* identification has great utility in a hospital setting. Direct smears for acid-fast bacilli have reported sensitivities ranging from 68 to 90%.[25,26]

Syphilis

Etiology

Syphilis is a venereal disease caused by the microorganism *Treponema pallidum* subsp. *pallidum*. *T. pallidum*, a spirochete of the family *Spirochaetaceae*, and is a long, slender, helically curved, gram-negative bacillus. The organism is microaerophilic and stains poorly with Gram stain and Giemsa methods. The organism is best observed using dark-field or phase-contrast microscopy. Culture for *T. pallidum* has not been developed for clinical use. The generation time for *T. pallidum* is 30 to 33 hours, unusually slow for bacteria. The organism does not survive outside of the mammalian host. Virulence is lost from the organism within a few hours to days of harvesting. For experimental purposes, *T. pallidum* must be cultured in a rabbit host. Researchers have not been able to propagate the organism in a tissue environment for an extended time, resulting in complete loss of viability within seven generations.[27]

Epidemiology and Pathogenesis

Following inoculation, infection is asymptomatic with an incubation phase ranging from 3 to 90 days, with an average of 21 days.[28] Syphilis is transmitted from person to person through sexual contact or congenitally from mother to fetus. Syphilis affects all ages, genders, and races. The disease is divided into different stages that may manifest clinically throughout the infected life of the patient. The clinical presentation of the stages are varied, complex, and often mimic other diseases. Primary syphilis presents with the characteristic hard chancre lesion that develops at the site of infection; the genitalia are most common. This stage is extremely infectious due to the lesion containing an abundant amount of viable organisms (**FIGURE 10–7**). During this stage, disease may not be visually detected in inconspicuous portions of the body since lesions are typically painless. Within 3 to 6 weeks of initial inoculation, the chancre will heal spontaneously without treatment. During this stage, dissemination of the organism occurs until it reaches a sufficient number to progress into secondary syphilis. Complete dissemination typically occurs within 2 to 24 weeks.[5]

It is during secondary syphilis that patients typically seek medical care. Common symptoms are flulike and include fever, sore throat, and lymphadenopathy; half of patients experience symptoms such as weight loss, malaise, and loss of appetite. Visual diagnosis of syphilis is easier during this stage because skin is the most common organ affected. Patients experience widespread rashes often seen on the face, scalp, palms, and soles of the feet; patchy hair loss may also be seen. Like primary syphilis, secondary syphilis is also a highly infectious stage due to the large amount of spirochetes present. For some patients, this stage may be very mild and go unnoticed and undiagnosed. Symptoms may disappear in some patients. After the disappearance of symptoms, the patient is identified as having latent-stage syphilis. During the latent stage, the patient is asymptomatic but the organisms are not necessarily dormant. Relapsing active syphilis often occurs during early (<1 year) latent-stage syphilis, while late (>1 year) latent syphilis is usually asymptomatic and noninfectious.[5] During this stage, patients are often diagnosed using serological methods.

Untreated cases of syphilis develop into tertiary syphilis, the tissue-destructive stage of disease. This stage appears 10 to 25 years after initial infection in approximately 35% of untreated patients. Complications of this stage are more severe than earlier stages of disease and often include central nervous system disease (neurosyphilis), cardiovascular abnormalities, eye disease, and granuloma-like lesions found in the skin, bones, or visceral organs. These lesions are soft, painless, and noninfectious.[5]

Congenital syphilis is transmitted from mother to fetus during any stage of infection, most often seen during early syphilis. The unborn fetus may develop symptomatic or asymptomatic infection. With symptomatic infection, deafness, blindness, and notched peg-shaped teeth may be seen, known as Hutchinson triad. Bone formation may be poor, resulting in bowing of the tibia (saber shin) and a deformed maxilla (bulldog appearance). In advanced infections, neurosyphilis or neonatal death can occur.[5]

Infections with syphilis can span decades when left untreated. Primary and secondary syphilis represent the earliest stages of infection, reflect symptomatic disease, and are considered indicators of incident infection. The reported rates of primary and secondary syphilis have steadily increased

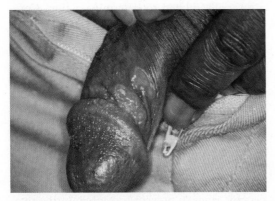

FIGURE 10–7 Syphilis. The chancre of primary syphilis occurs mainly on the genitalia. It has a raised margin and is usually painless.

Courtesy of M. Rein, VD/CDC.

annually from 2000 to 2016 after only 2.1 cases per 100,000 population in 2000 and 2001, the lowest rate reported since reporting began in 1941. In 2016, a total of 27,814 cases of primary and secondary syphilis were reported in the United States, representing a rate of 8.7 cases per 100,000 population. This rate is a 17.6% increase compared with 2015 data and a 74.0% increase compared with 2012 data. Rates of infection increased in all age groups, in every race and ethnic group, and in all regions of the United States. Highest incidents of reported primary and secondary syphilis were seen among men who have sex with men (MSM), men in the western region of the country, and among African-American men. An increase in primary and secondary syphilis infections reported in women is also of concern, as congenital syphilis cases tend to trend upward in parallel. Congenital cases have increased in recent years, after a decline during 2008 to 2012. In 2016, a total of 628 cases of congenital syphilis were reported including 41 syphilitic stillbirths. The national rate was 15.7 cases per 100,000 live births in 2016, representing a 27.6% increase relative to 2015 and an 86.9% increase relative to 2012.[29]

Infections with *T. pallidum* elicit a strong humoral and cell-mediated immune response, often resulting in inflammation and tissue loss. Two different categories of antibodies are produced in response to infection: treponemal and nontreponemal. Treponemal antibodies are produced in response to antigens on the organism itself. Nontreponemal antibodies are produced in infected patients but are targeted to components of mammalian cells rather than the treponeme. These nontreponemal antibodies, referred to as regain antibodies, are also produced in patients with other bacterial, viral, and parasitic infectious diseases, as well as noninfectious conditions such as drug addiction, autoimmune disorders, pregnancy, and recent immunization.[5] Both treponemal and nontreponemal antibody detection are the basis of serological diagnosis of syphilis.

Conventional Methods

Since its isolation in 1905 and confirmation as the causative agent of syphilis in 1912, *T. pallidum* has challenged laboratorians. The organism's near inability to be cultured has removed this classic gold standard method for diagnosis from the list of available options. Scientists have been required to utilize alternative methods for detection and identification. Initial direct detection was made using dark-field microscopy to identify spirochetes in tissue and lesion specimens.[30] Throughout the 1900s, both treponemal- and nontreponemal-based serological methods were developed and are currently in use today for routine syphilis testing.

Immunodiagnostic Methods

The two most widely used nontreponemal serological assays are the rapid plasma reagin (RPR) and Venereal Disease Reference Laboratory (VDRL) tests. The RPR assay is more often used than the VDRL assay for initial screening of patients for syphilis. The RPR assay is based on the presence of regain, a nonspecific anti-lipid antibody. When syphilis infection breaks down tissue, the fatty substances released are combined with *T. pallidum* proteins to form an antigen, thus resulting in specific and nonspecific antibody formation. The antigen used in the RPR assay is cardiolipin-lecithin-coated cholesterol bound to charcoal particles. Upon mixing of patient serum or plasma with the RPR reagent and rotation at 100 rpm for 8 minutes, flocculation will be visible in specimens positive for antibody production.[31] (**FIGURE 10–8**) Positive RPR patient specimens are serially diluted to determine a titer. Commercially available RPR test kits allow testing to occur without heating the specimen using a specially coated card that is disposable once used. The VDRL assay identifies the same antibody response as the RPR assay; however, the VDRL assay uses an antigen containing cardiolipin, lecithin, and cholesterol in suspension rather than bound to a solid particle. The patient serum or cerebrospinal fluid is mixed with the VDRL reagent and rotated for 4 minutes at 180 rpm on a slide. Test slides for serum contain paraffin or ceramic rings to prevent spreading during rotation, while test slides for CSF have concave test areas. The slide is observed under microscopy for flocculation. Positive patient specimens are serially diluted and tested, and a titer is reported.[32]

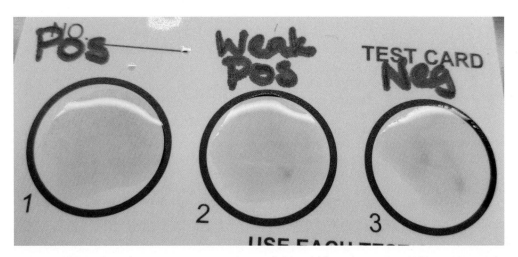

FIGURE 10–8 RPR Test. Flocculation is seen in a positive result (1), mild flocculation in a weakly positive result (2), and no flocculation in a negative result (3). The negative result demonstrates the characteristic "tail" that is seen when rotation of the test card occurs.

STEP-BY-STEP PROCEDURE 10–1 RPR Test for Syphilis

Purpose: The RPR test is a nontreponemal procedure for the serologic detection of syphilis.

Principle: Patients with syphilis produce an antibody-like substance, reagin. A cardiolipin antigen bound to carbon particles is used to detect this substance in serum. When bound to the reagin, the cardiolipin-carbon antigen will form floccules upon mixing.

Specimen: Serum or plasma (EDTA, heparin, potassium oxalate, or sodium fluoride)

Procedure:

1. Dispense 50 µL of serum or plasma onto a test card containing an 18 mm circle designed for the RPR test
2. Spread the specimen, filling the entire surface of the circle
3. Place one free-falling drop of antigen onto each test area
4. Rotate card for 8 minutes (±30 seconds) under humidifying cover, on a mechanical rotator at 100 ± 2 rpm
5. Following rotation, view test area using a high-intensity incandescent lamp to identify floccules. Brief rotation or tilting of the card (3 to 4 times) may be required.

Results:

- Reactive: characteristic clumping ranging from slight but definite, to marked and intense
- Nonreactive: showing no clumping

Positive patient results may be tested using a semiquantitative method to determine a titer

1. Using a clean test card, label circles 1 through 6
2. Place 50 µL of 0.9% saline onto circles 2 through 6, each. Do not spread the saline
3. Place 50 µL of serum or plasma onto circle 1
4. Place 50 µL of serum or plasma into the saline drop on circle 2. Prepare a twofold dilution by drawing the saline-specimen mixture up and down 5 to 6 times to mix. Avoid formation of bubbles
5. Transfer 50 µL of the 1:2 mixture into the saline drop on circle 3. Prepare a twofold dilution by repeating the previous step

(continues)

STEP-BY-STEP PROCEDURE 10–1 RPR Test for Syphilis *(Continued)*

6. Create serial twofold dilutions through circle 6 by performing the previously described steps
7. After preparation of the final dilution (circle 6), discard 50 μL
8. Spread each specimen, filling the entire surface of the circle and using a different spreader for each specimen
9. Place one free-falling drop of antigen onto each test area
10. Rotate card for 8 minutes (±30 seconds) under humidifying cover, on a mechanical rotator at 100 ± 2 rpm
11. Following rotation, view test area using a high-intensity incandescent lamp to identify floccules. Brief rotation or tilting of the card (3 to 4 times) may be required
12. The final titer is determined by the last circle showing visible flocculation
13. Additional dilutions may be tested for specimens that exceed a titer of 1:32

	Circle 1	Circle 2	Circle 3	Circle 4	Circle 5	Circle 6
Saline		50 μL	50 μL	50 μL	50 μL	50 μL
Specimen	50 μL	50 μL	50 μL of 1:2 dilution	50 μL of 1:4 dilution	50 μL of 1:8 dilution	50 μL of 1:16 dilution
Titer	1:1	1:2	1:4	1:8	1:16	1:32

Quality Control: With each batch of patient specimens tested, reactive, weakly reactive, and nonreactive controls must be included to verify test performance.

With each new lot number of RPR antigen and with each change of the dispenser needle, the needle must be tested to verify delivery of 30 ± 1 drops.

The RPR assay is often selected over the VDRL assay for routine patient screening due to ease of use and interpretation and overall cost of the testing equipment and supplies. The VDRL assay has one advantage over the RPR assay; it is available for the diagnosis of congenital syphilis.

Several assays are available for the detection of antibodies produced against the organism. The *Treponema pallidum*-particle agglutination (TP-PA) and Fluorescent Treponemal Antibody-Absorption (FTA-ABS) assays are the most often used treponemal assays for confirmation of a positive nontreptonemal assay. The TP-PA assay uses gel particles sensitized with a *T. pallidum* strain. The gel particles are placed in a microtiter well and mixed with the serially diluted samples of patient serum or plasma. After sufficient incubation, the microtiter plate is observed from the bottom for agglutination. When a sample contains anti-*T. pallidum* antibodies, the antibodies will form a lattice with the gel particles. When antibodies are not present in a sample, the gel particles will sink to the bottom of the well, forming a button. This method is intended to replace the microhemagglutination assay for antibodies to *T. pallidum* (MHA-TP). The FTA-ABS assay is an indirect fluorescent assay that uses a microscope slide to which *T. pallidum* organisms have been fixed. Prior to testing, the patient serum or CSF is mixed with a sorbent to remove antibodies to any other *Treponema* species that may be present as they would interfere with the test, producing a false-positive result. The patient's sample is then seeded on the slide and allowed to incubate. When antibodies are present, they attach to the *T. pallidum* organisms fixed to the slide. Subsequent incubation with FITC-labeled anti-human immunoglobulin and wash steps result in visible fluorescence of positive results when viewed using a fluorescent microscope[5] (**FIGURE 10–9**).

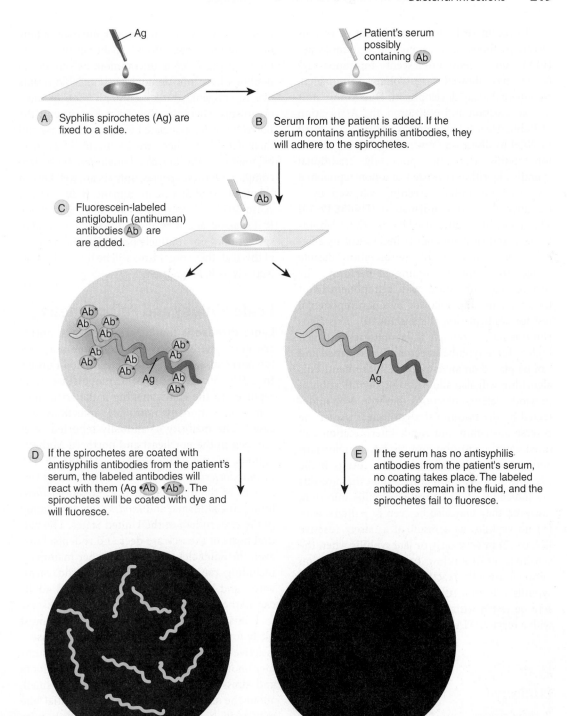

A Syphilis spirochetes (Ag) are fixed to a slide.

B Serum from the patient is added. If the serum contains antisyphilis antibodies, they will adhere to the spirochetes.

C Fluorescein-labeled antiglobulin (antihuman) antibodies Ab are are added.

D If the spirochetes are coated with antisyphilis antibodies from the patient's serum, the labeled antibodies will react with them (Ag •Ab •Ab*). The spirochetes will be coated with dye and will fluoresce.

E If the serum has no antisyphilis antibodies from the patient's serum, no coating takes place. The labeled antibodies remain in the fluid, and the spirochetes fail to fluoresce.

FIGURE 10–9 Indirect fluorescent antibody (IFA) for the diagnosis of syphilis. The syphilis bacteria are visible fluorescently.

From Pommerville, J. C. (2017). Fundamentals of Microbiology, 11e. Jones & Bartlett Learning.

In recent years, the development of various testing methods, such as enzyme immunoassays (EIA) and chemiluminescent immunoassays (CIA), has allowed large-volume, automated, treponemal assay development. Due to this shift in test selection and utilization, the Association of Public Health Laboratories (APHL) convened in 2009 to discuss a "reverse" testing algorithm for syphilis. Until this point, the traditional syphilis algorithm consisted of a nontreponemal test used for initial screening followed by a treponemal test for confirmation. (**FIGURE 10–10**) This algorithm is often used by clinicians, laboratorians, and epidemiologists because of its cost-effectiveness and ease of interpretation, despite being more time consuming to perform. The reverse algorithm starts with a treponemal test used for screening, followed by a nontreponemal test for confirmation (Figure 10–10). This algorithm is more attractive to laboratories in which high-volume syphilis screening is performed and can be placed on an automated instrument. This algorithm will also allow for the identification of previous (latent) infections that would be undetected by the traditional algorithm.[30] Use of the reverse algorithm and result interpretation can often cause confusion and anxiety in clinicians and patients, especially when the results if the EIA and RPR are conflicting. Often these results are indicative of past, treated syphilis infection; however, they may also be seen in patients with (1) no syphilis, as a result of a falsely reactive EIA or (2) in very early or late syphilis when the sensitivity of RPR is low. To aid in differentiation between a falsely reactive EIA and early or late syphilis infection, the CDC has recommended sera be tested with TP-PA assay for any patient with a reactive EIA and nonreactive RPR.[33]

Lyme Disease
Etiology

Borrelia species, spirochetes of the family *Spirochaetaceae*, are the causative agents of tickborne and louseborne relapsing fever and tickborne Lyme disease in humans. In contrast to *Treponema* species, *Borrelia* stain well with Giemsa stain and

have been grown in vitro under microaerophilic or anaerobic conditions.[5] Laboratory testing for relapsing fever is uncommon, as serological methods have not demonstrated reliable results due to antigenic shifts commonly seen in these organisms. Therefore, this text will cover only the *Borrelia* species associated with Lyme disease and their detection. There are 14 species of *Borrelia* belonging to the *Borrelia burgdorferi* sensu lato complex. Of these species, only six are well known agents of Lyme disease in humans: *B. burgdorferi* sensu stricto, *B. garinii, B. afzelii, B. spielmanii, B. lusitaniae,* and *B. valaisiana.*[5] Differentiation of species does not routinely occur. For the purpose of this text, these organisms will be referred to collectively as *B. burgdorferi.*

Epidemiology and Pathogenesis

Lyme disease is found throughout the northern hemisphere and is the most common vector-borne disease in North America and Europe. In 2015, 36,429 cases of Lyme disease were reported to the CDC, making it the sixth most common, nationally notifiable, infectious disease.[34] The majority of annually reported cases are seen in the northeast and northern Midwest regions of the United States (**FIGURE 10–11**). *B. burgdorferi* is transmitted to humans by two species of the blacklegged tick: *Ixodes pacificus* found in California, and *Ixodes scapularis* found in the eastern half of the United States. The natural hosts of the tick are deer and rodents; however, the adult tick will feed on other mammals, including raccoons, domestic and wild carnivores, and birds. The larva, nymph, and adults can harbor the spirochete and transmit disease to humans and pets. The nymph is the most likely form of tick to transmit disease because it is active and feeding during the spring and summer months when people are active outdoors and dress lightly. The nymph is quite small, about the size of a pinhead, and the initial bite may easily be overlooked. The tick does require at least 24 hours of attachment prior to transmitting disease.[5]

Direct inoculation of the organisms through skin by the vector is responsible for the clinical

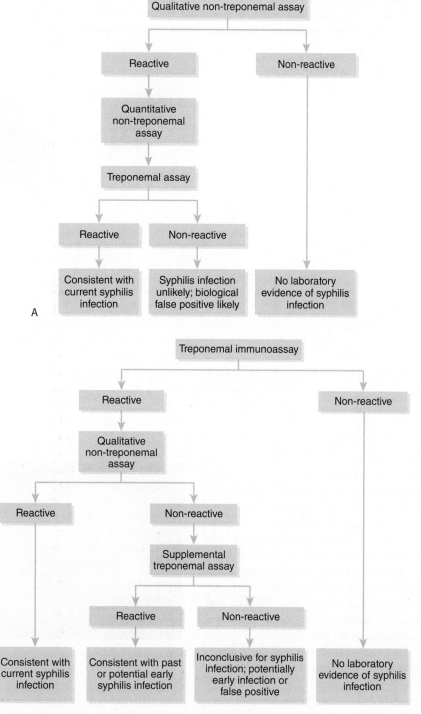

FIGURE 10–10 Traditional **(A)** and Reverse **(B)** Syphilis Serology Testing Algorithms.

APHL Sexually Transmitted Disease Subcommittee. Suggested reporting language for syphilis serology testing. Silver Spring, MD: Association of Public Health Laboratories; 2015. Used with permission from Association of Public Health Laboratories.

Each dot represents one case of Lyme disease and is placed randomly in the patient's county of residence. The presence of a dot in a state does not necessarily mean that Lyme disease was acquired in that state. People travel between states, and the place of residence is sometimes different from the place where the patient became infected.

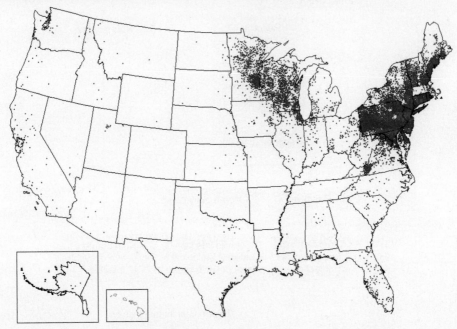

FIGURE 10–11 Reported cases of Lyme Disease—United States, 2016.

Courtesy of Centers for Disease Control and Prevention. About C. neoformans infections. Fungal Diseases. Accessed at https://www.cdc.gov/lyme/datasurveillance/maps-recent.html

manifestations of Lyme disease. The spirochete changes its antigens after initial infection, resulting in a continual production of IgM antibodies by the host. This abundance of IgM antibodies with changing variable regions may induce an auto-immune process, avoid complement attack, and avoid the host immune response.[5] All of these contribute to the pathology of the disease. Clinical manifestations of the disease vary and may affect dermatological, neurological, cardiac, and musculoskeletal systems. The initial symptom, and clinical hallmark of Lyme disease, is erythema migrans, a red, ring-shaped skin lesion with a central clearing that first appears at the site of the tick bite (**FIGURE 10–12**). It is seen in approximately 60 to 80% of patients with Lyme disease.[35] Patients may also experience fever, headache, malaise, and muscle and joint pains during this first stage.

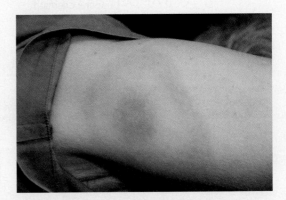

FIGURE 10–12 Erythema migrans. The rash that accompanies 80% of cases of Lyme disease. The rash consists of a large, central patch with an intense red border. The rash is usually hot to the touch and will expand in size with time.

Courtesy of James Gathany/CDC.

Dissemination of *B. burgdorferi* begins weeks to months after infection with the most important features being neurological disorders and carditis. During this stage of the disease, spirochetes spread hematogenously to organs and tissues. Patients often experience one or more of the following symptoms: arthritis, multiple erythema migrans lesions, carditis, meningitis, meningoencephalitis, and facial palsy.[35] In untreated patients, late Lyme disease may develop months to years after onset of disease. This stage is characterized by chronic arthritis or acrodermatitis chronica atrophicans (ACA), a rash of fibrosing skin.[5] The Infectious Disease Society of America (IDSA) has published treatment guidelines for patients with Lyme disease, including antibiotic therapy for initial infection, extended antibiotic therapy for late-stage disease, and anti-inflammatory treatment for those with major tissue damage and chronic conditions.[36] Patients exhibiting the classic erythema migrans, especially those who recall tick encounters, do not require laboratory testing for the diagnosis of Lyme disease. However, depending on which part of the body the tick bite occurred, visible symptoms may disappear before the patient seeks medical attention. In these patients, laboratory testing is necessary for diagnosis.

Conventional Methods

Although *B. burgdorferi* may be cultivated using nutritionally rich media in a microaerophilic environment, the procedure is cumbersome and unreliable. To recover the viable organism, the patient's plasma, CSF sediment, or ground tissue biopsy is inoculated into modified Kelly's broth media and incubated at 30 to 34°C for up to 12 weeks in a microaerophilic environment ($4\% \ O_2$, $5\% \ CO_2$, $5\% \ H_2$, and $86\% \ N_2$). Each week, blind subcultures are performed from the bottom portion of the broth to fresh media. A sample from each culture is also examined by dark-field microscopy or stained with acridine orange and examined by fluorescent microscopy for spirochetes. Due to the low sensitivity and long-incubation time, culture is rarely performed in a clinical laboratory. Specimens are often sent to a reference laboratory when culture is the diagnostic method of choice.

Direct identification of *B. burgdorferi* organisms may be performed in tissue sections stained with Warthin-Starry silver stain. The number of spirochetes in blood, synovial fluid, and CSF of patients with Lyme disease is below the detectable limits of microscopy[5].

Immunodiagnostic Methods

Serology continues to be the standard for diagnosis of Lyme disease. As seen in many immunologic responses, IgM antibodies are the first to be developed. These antibodies are created in response to the OspC membrane protein, the flagellar antigens (FlaA and FlaB), or the fibronectin-binding protein (BBK32). While IgM-antibody levels peak after a few weeks, they may be detectable for several months. The immune response with IgG antibodies develops more slowly over the first several weeks of disease and increases when antibodies respond to Osp17 (decorin-binding protein), p39 (BmpA), and p58 proteins.[5] As disease develops, antibodies are generated in response to additional surface antigens of *B. burgdorferi*. A variety of serological assays are commercially available; however, the performance characteristics of these assays vary because standardization of testing methods has not been established. The most common tests seen are indirect immunofluorescent assays (IFA), ELISA, and Western blot. ELISA are commonly used for screening because they are easy to use, quick, and relatively inexpensive.

IFA methods are still commercially available but are being replaced by ELISA and Western blot immunoassays. IFAs have a high false-positive rate, often due to cross-reactivity. Patients with syphilis, HIV, leptospirosis, mononucleosis, parvovirus infection, rheumatoid arthritis, and other autoimmune disorders commonly show false-positive results to Lyme disease when tested with IFA methods. Serum may be adsorbed with *Treponema phagedensis* sonicate (IFA-ABS) prior to testing to enhance specificity.[5] IFA tests use cultured organisms fixed to a glass slide. Patient serum is diluted and incubated on the slide. Antibodies present in the serum adhere to the fixed organisms. FITC-labeled, anti-human IgG and IgM antibodies are added, allowing for antibodies to be detected by fluorescent microscopy. In general, antibody titers ≥64 (with adsorption) and ≥256 (without adsorption) seen with IFA are considered positive.[35]

The most common immunoassay used for the detection of *B. burgdorferi* antibodies is the ELISA, and, more recently, rapid EIA methods. ELISA and EIA tests are available for IgG or IgM detections, with some detecting both antibodies in one test cartridge, and may be interpreted calorimetrically, whether manually or on an instrument, or fluorescently by an instrument. One of the newest commercially available rapid EIAs for Lyme disease is the Sofia Lyme FIA. This assay is a rapid, solid-phase, bidirectional, lateral flow assay that is not only able to detect both IgM and IgG antibodies to *B. burgdorferi* but also to differentiate them. This assay is tested and interpreted by the same Sofia analyzer utilized by influenza A/B, RSV, and *Streptococcus* A rapid assays, allowing for multiple tests performed on a single platform with rapid turnaround times. The assay also uses a small amount of serum or plasma (30 μL) and presents a result in under 15 minutes.[37]

Regardless of the advancements made in Lyme disease detection, the CDC recommends a two-tier testing process for serological diagnosis. The two-tier algorithm (**FIGURE 10–13**) begins with screening by either an EIA or IFA method. Patients negative by one of these methods are considered negative for Lyme disease; however, if the patient has been showing signs or symptoms for less than 30 days, a convalescent specimen is recommended. If a patient specimen is determined positive by a screening method, confirmation by Western immunoblot should follow. The use of IgG and/or IgM Western immunoblot for confirmation is determined by how long the patient has been displaying symptoms.[38]

Rickettsial Infections
Etiology

Rickettsia species and *Orientia tsutsugamushi* (formerly *R. tsutsugamushi*) are members of the family *Rickettsiaceae*. These organisms are tiny,

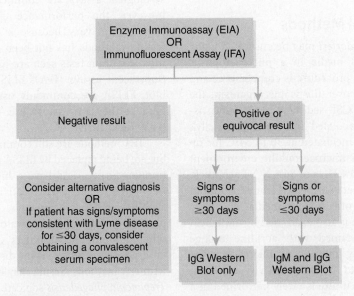

FIGURE 10–13 Two-Tiered Testing for Lyme Disease.

only 0.3 μm × 1–2 μm, pleomorphic, gram-negative bacilli. They are fastidious obligate, intracellular bacteria that multiply only intracellularly and survive outside of a host for a brief amount of time.

Epidemiology and Pathogenesis

The rickettsias and rickettsia-like organisms are generally categorized into three groups based on the type of diseases they cause. **TABLE 10–2** describes characteristics of important *Rickettsia* species and *Orientia*.[5] For the purpose of this text, only *R. rickettsii* will be discussed in further detail.

Humans are considered an accidental host in most cases, when an arthropod vector transmits the organism from a wild animal host. The organism is deposited directly into the bloodstream of the human host through the bite of the arthropod vector. The rickettsiae will then coerce the endothelial cells of the host's blood vessels to engulf it. The organism is then carried into the cell's cytoplasm by way of a vacuole. Organisms within the genus *Rickettsia* do not experience an intracellular developmental cycle. Without this requirement, organisms easily escape the vacuole and become free in the cytoplasm. *Rickettsia* spp. are then able to replicate and cause cell death by lysis during exit of the host cell. The following endothelial cell damage results in the symptomatic changes seen throughout the body.[5] Disease is considered when the triad of fever, headache, and rash are seen, especially when following known exposure to ticks, lice, fleas, or chiggers.

TABLE 10–2 Characteristics of *Rickettsia* and *Orientia* Species

Organism	Disease	Vector	Location(s)
Spotted Fever Group			
Rickettsia conorii	Mediterranean and Israeli spotted fevers; Indian tick typhus; Kenya tick typhus	Ticks	Southern Europe Middle East Africa
Rickettsia	Rocky Mountain Spotted Fever	Ticks	North and South America
Rickettsia parkeri	Mild illness with no reported fatalities	Ticks	North and South America
Typhus Group			
Rickettsia prowazekii	Epidemic typhus	Lice	Worldwide
	Bril-Zinsser disease	None	Worldwide
Rickettsia typhi	Murine typhus	Fleas	Worldwide
Scrub Typhus Group			
Orientia tsutsugamushi	Scrub typhus	Chiggers	South and Southeast Asia South Pacific

Rocky Mountain Spotted Fever (RMSF), caused by *Rickettsia rickettsii*, is the most commonly seen spotted-fever disease in the United States. The organism is most often transmitted via bite of the American dog tick, *Dermacentor vriablilis*, which is found primarily on the eastern, central, and Pacific coasts. Transmission is also seen in the western United States by the Rocky Mountain wood tick, *Dermacentor andersoni*, and more recently, in Arizona and the United States-Mexico border, by the brown dog tick, *Rhipicephalus sanguineus*.[39]

Symptoms of RMSF generally show 3 to 12 days after a bite from the tick or 4 to 8 days after discovering a tick still attached. The incubation period is generally 5 days or fewer, and initial symptoms present with sudden onset of fever, headache, chills, malaise, and myalgia. The infected individual may also experience nausea or vomiting, abdominal pain, anorexia, and photophobia. The classic rash associated with RMSF begins as a small (1–5 mm), pink macule on the ankle, wrist, or forearm that spreads up the arms and legs and to the soles and trunk. Infections with *R. rickettsii* lead to systemic infections that, if untreated, can result in end-organ damage with sever morbidity or even death.[39]

Beginning January 1, 2010, the reporting of rickettsial disease shifted from individual disease reporting to a new category of Spotted Fever Rickettsiosis (SFR). This new group includes Rocky Mountain Spotted Fever (RMSF), *Rickettsia parkeri* rickettsiosis, Pacific Coast tick fever, and rickettsialpox. The change to this grouped reporting of rickettsial disease reflects the inability of commonly available serologic tests to differentiate the agents of disease.[40] The change in reporting does little service to identifying the true number of RMSF and separating them from other, less-severe spotted fevers. In 2016, there were 4,269 cases of spotted fever rickettsias reported in the United States. Infections with RMSF and other rickettsias are seen seasonally, with the majority of cases reported from May through August, during periods when the adult dog tick is most active. Infections have been reported throughout much of the United States. Five states: North Carolina, Oklahoma, Arkansas, Tennessee, and Missouri, account for more than 60% of spotted fever rickettsia cases reported[40] (**FIGURE 10–14**).

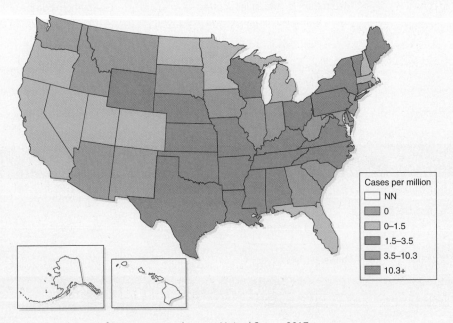

Cases per million
- NN
- 0
- 0–1.5
- 1.5–3.5
- 3.5–10.3
- 10.3+

FIGURE 10–14 Reported cases of *Neisseria gonorrhoeae*—United States, 2017.

Courtesy of CDC. Centers for Disease Control and Prevention. Epidemiology and Statistics. Rocky Mountain Spotted Fever (RMSF). Accessed at https://www.cdc.gov/rmsf/stats/index.html

Conventional Methods

Cultivation of the *R. rickettsii* bacteria is considered to reference standard for microbiologic detection and diagnosis of RMSF. However, the organisms are obligate intracellular pathogens and must be grown using cell culture methods, such as embryonated eggs and tissue culture. Specimens for culture include heparinized whole blood or punch biopsies of skin or eschars.[5] *R. rickettsii* is classified as a biosafety level 3 (BSL-3) organism. Attempts at culturing must occur in a laboratory equipped with BSL-3 equipment and adhere to acceptable practices.[39] The combination of safety requirements and specialized techniques limits the ability of most laboratories to perform culture. Therefore, the availability of culture is limited to a few specialty laboratories. Gram stain and Wright-Giemsa stains of blood are not useful for the diagnosis of RMSF.

Immunodiagnostic Methods

Commercially available immunodiagnostic methods are limited to detection of IgG and IgM antibodies to *R. rickettsii*. A review of FDA-approved methods shows a slew of antibody identification kits produced in 1993, with moderate or high complexity designation. A lull in available methods was seen until 2010, when Focus Diagnostics produced a Rickettsia IFA IgG and IgM test; this method is also obtaining high complexity designation. In 2017, DiaSorin Molecular gained high complexity designation for their IFA for IgG or IgM antibodies to *R. rickettsia*.[41] The IFA slides are designed to detect antibodies to both *R. rickettsii* and *R. typhi* in a sandwich method. The commercial market does not offer other immunodiagnostic methods that can be purchased by hospital or reference laboratories.

Molecular Diagnostic Methods

The only molecular diagnostic method to hold FDA approval is the Centers for Disease Control and Prevention Rickettsia Real-time PCR assay. This assay is available only for laboratories designated as Laboratory Response Network (LRN) facilities that hold high complexity designation.[41]

Helicobacter Pylori

Etiology

Helicobacter pylori are gram-negative bacilli that are microaerophilic and spiral in shape. They closely resemble *Campylobacter* species in such a manner that when first discovered in 1983, the organism was named *Campylobacter pylori*. Only after additional testing was the genus *Helicobacter* established and the organism renamed in 1989.[5] *H. pylori* is now considered a significant human pathogen and recognized as probably the most common bacterial infection seen in humans, infecting approximately 50% of the world's population.[42]

Pathogenesis

H. pylori is distributed worldwide, naturally inhabits the human gastric mucosa, and appears to be normal microbiota. It is recognized as the primary cause of chronic gastritis in humans. Untreated infections often develop into gastric and duodenal ulcers. Infections occur in all human populations with an observed incidence of infection ranging from 30% in developed countries to more than 90% in some developing countries. Infections are often seen in children in developing countries and, if treatment does not occur, chronic infections may be seen throughout the life of the individual. Chronic *H. pylori* infections are recognized as a significant risk factor for gastric carcinoma and mucosa-associated lymphoid tissue (MALT) lymphoma.[42] The exact mode of transmission is unknown; however, a number of possible routes have been suggested including oral-oral, fecal-oral, and a common environmental source. Evidence suggests transmission occurs between members of the same family and from mother to child.[5] The prevalence of *H. pylori* infections, gastritis, and gastric carcinoma increase in populations with lower socioeconomic status and the elderly.[42]

H. pylori is capable of colonizing the mucous layer of the antrum and fundus of the stomach but is unable to inhabit the epithelium. The organism produces urease, hydrolyzing urea-forming ammonia, resulting in a significant increase of pH around the infection site. This change in pH protects the organism from the acidic environment created by gastric secretions. The motile nature of the organism allows it to escape the acidity of the stomach, enabling colonization of the gastric mucosa in close association with the epithelium. Infection with *H. pylori* elicits an intense release of phagocytic cells that attempt to eliminate the organism by releasing large amounts of oxygen metabolites.[43] However, *H. pylori* survives this oxidative stress by producing catalase to neutralize this phagocytic mechanism. *H. pylori* also possesses a number of genes that enhance the virulence of the organism (**TABLE 10–3**).[5]

Conventional Methods

Conventional methods for *H. pylori* detection and identification include both invasive and noninvasive testing. The urea breath test and fecal antigen test are commonly used noninvasive, nonserological methods. Biopsy culture and histology examinations are invasive and reserved for patients with a positive initial result of a noninvasive method. Culture for *H. pylori* is not as routine a practice, as cultivation is time-consuming and often requires selective media. Gastric-tissue biopsies must be processed and incubated for up to a week in a microaerophilic environment (4% O_2, 5% CO_2, 5% H_2, and 86% N_2) at 35 to 37°C before growth is seen. Cultures must be reviewed daily for a minimum of 10 days before reporting as negative. Once growth is obtained, organisms are presumptively identified based on typical cellular morphology and positive test results for oxidase, catalase, and rapid urease. In lieu of culture, gastric biopsies are often embedded in a small piece of agar containing urea and a pH indicator such as phenol red, referred to as a CLO (Campylobacter-like organism) test. The specimen is then incubated at 35–37°C for up to 24 hours, with initial observation at 4 hours. If *H. pylori* is present, the organism will produce urease, which will hydrolyze the urea into ammonia, and subsequently increase the pH changing the indicator from yellow (negative) to pink-red (positive). The biopsy specimens sent to the histology laboratory are immunostained specifically for *H. pylori* in addition to routine hematoxylin and eosin stains. Results of histological tests will vary depending on the number and location of biopsy samples, the experience of the pathologist, and stains used.

TABLE 10–3 *H. pylori* Genes and Their Possible Role in Enhancing Virulence	
Gene	**Possible Role**
VacA	Exotoxin (VacA) Creates vacuoles in epithelial cells, decreases apoptosis, and loosens cell junctions. Only 50% of all strains express toxin.
CagA	Pathogenicity island Encodes a type IV secretion system for transferring CagA proteins into the host. Proteins affect host cell gene expression, induce cytokine release and alter cell structure, and interact with neighboring cells, enabling *H. pylori* invasion of gastric epithelium.
BabA	Encodes outer membrane proteins and mediates adherence to blood-group antigens on the surface of gastric epithelial cells.
IceA	Presence associated with peptic ulcer disease in some populations.

Immunodiagnostic Methods

There is a variety of immunodiagnostic methods commercially available for the detection of *H. pylori* infection without need of the invasive collection of a gastric biopsy. One commonly used method is the *H. pylori* stool antigen test. The colonization of *H. pylori* in the gastrointestinal tract tends to result in specific antigens that are found in the stool. Rapid diagnostic immunoassays utilizing monoclonal or polyclonal antibodies to these specific antigens demonstrate sensitivities and specificities comparable to the urea breath test. Monoclonal antibody tests show high sensitivity reaching 95%. The stool antigen test is recommended as a noninvasive test method of diagnosis before and after eradication therapy.[42] Rapid, CLIA-waived assays are available that utilize anti-*H. pylori* antibodies for detection of the organisms in a stool sample within 10 minutes.

Infections with *H. pylori* elicit an immune response that is characterized by circulation IgG, IgA, and acutely IgM antibodies. Spontaneous eradication of *H. pylori* and treatment of disease is rare. The presence of any *H. pylori*-specific antibody in the blood is indicative of active infection. However, since most individuals are asymptomatic at the time of infection, assays that identify IgM antibodies have shown little clinical utility. In addition, there are few reported cases of individuals with IgA antibodies that do not have IgG antibodies. Therefore, most assays for *H. pylori*-specific antibodies are designed to detect IgG only. ELISA are considered the method of choice because they are noninvasive, easy to perform, relatively rapid, and cost-effective when compared with invasive methods such as gastric biopsy. Generally, *H. pylori* ELISA use at least one of four *H. pylori*-specific antigens that are seen in almost all individuals infected with *H. pylori*. When combining more than one antigen into the assay, sensitivity and specificity usually exceed 95%.[42]

A number of rapid serological immunodiagnostic methods are commercially available for the detection of *H. pylori*-specific antibodies in serum, plasma, and whole blood. Rapid, solid-phase lateral flow immunoassays vary in their antibody detection. Many commercially available assays are selective for only IgG anti-*H. pylori* antibodies.[44,45] The Acceava *H. pylori* test is able to detect the presence of IgG, IgM, and IgA antibodies, but the test is unable to differentiate them.[46] There is a mix of commercially available CLIA-waived and CLIA-moderately complex rapid immunoassays. It appears that CLIA-waived status is designated for assays in which whole blood is tested. When testing is performed on serum or plasma, the assay is deemed moderately complex. Instrument-based, automated, immunoassay methods detect IgG antibodies in serum, and show greater sensitivity and specificity than rapid immunoassays when compared with biopsy culture and histology.[44-47]

Molecular Diagnostic Methods

DNA-based molecular methods have been developed over the last decade. While they are able to identify *H. pylori* with a higher sensitivity than other methods, these methods cannot differentiate living from dead organisms. Currently, there are not any molecular-based methods that have received FDA approval for diagnostic testing.

Neisseria Gonorrhoeae and *Chlamydia Trachomatis*
Etiology

Neisseria gonorrhoeae and *Chlamydia trachomatis* are sexually transmitted infections (STIs) that are often spoken of and tested for together. Therefore, for the purpose of this text, they will be discussed together as many current immunodiagnostic tests are designed to detect at least these two STIs together, if not more.

Neisseria gonorrhoeae, the causative agent of gonorrhea, is a small, gram-negative diplococcus that is a clinically significant pathogen found in the urogenital tract. *N. gonorrhoeae* can be found in the mucous membranes of the genitalia, anorectal area, or propharynx, and conjunctiva during times of infection. Humans are the only natural host, and the asymptomatic carrier often disseminates infections throughout the population through sexual contact, although infection may be spread from mother to child during birth.

Chlamydia trachomatis is an obligate, intracellular bacterium that requires the biochemical resources of eukaryotic cells to grow and replicate. It is this requirement for metabolism that formerly categorized them as viruses. The lipopolysaccharide cell wall makes them similar to gram-negative bacilli; however, they have little endotoxin activity. *C. trachomatis* has a life cycle reminiscent of parasites. In a normal life cycle, which takes approximately 48 to 72 hours, the bacterium undergoes two morphologic rearrangements and is seen in two forms. The elementary body, or infective form, is ingested by the host cell where it resides in the phagosome. The elementary body then reorganizes and transforms into the reticulate body, or replicative form. This change occurs within 6 to 8 hours of ingestion. The reticulate body then divides by binary fission within the host cell. This causes the phagosome to enlarge into a structure known as an intracytoplasmic inclusion. After approximately 48 to 72 hours, the reticulate body reverts to the elementary body form. The elementary body then lyses the host cell, causing cell death, and is then able to infect more cells. There is evidence that the reticulate body may cease to divide and not differentiate into the elementary body form. They form persistent bodies, leading to chronic infections and disease. It is suggested that this form ensues due to increased interferon-gamma (INF-γ) and reduced tryptophan in the host cell. Removal of INF-γ or increased tryptophan will stimulate the persistent body to the reticulate body form, thus allowing replication.[5] *C. trachomatis* infects humans almost exclusively, and the difference in major outer membrane proteins (MOMP) results in the variety of disease seen with these organisms.

Epidemiology and Pathogenesis

The CDC reports gonorrhea as the second most reported notifiable disease in the United States. In 2017, there were 555,608 cases of gonorrhea reported in the United States, resulting in a rate of 171.9 cases per 100,000 population. The number of reported cases increased 18.6% from 2016 to 2017, and 75.2% since the historic low in 2009. As seen with chlamydia, the highest prevalence of gonorrhea infections is seen in the southern portion of the United States (**FIGURE 10–15**).[48] Infections with *N. gonorrhoeae* are often localized to the mucosal surface where the host is initially exposed to the microorganism, whether it is the cervix, anorectal area, conjunctiva, oropharynx, or urethra for males. The purulent discharge seen with gonorrhea infections often initiates a visit to the physician's office for males; however, the discharge may not be noticed in females. Annual screening is recommended for all sexually active women under the age of 25 and for older women at increased risk for infection.[49] If left untreated, gonorrhea infections may cause pelvic inflammatory disease (PID), which can result in tubal scarring and lead to infertility and ectopic pregnancy. Disseminated infections are uncommon but may result in serious morbidity and mortality, including arthritis, bacteremia, endocarditis, and meningitis.

C. trachomatis is the most commonly reported notifiable disease in the United States. In 2017, there were 1,708,569 cases of chlamydial infections reported, corresponding to a rate of 528.8 cases per 100,000 people. *C. trachomatis* is the most commonly seen of all sexually transmitted infections in the United States. Prevalence of the organism is seen highest in the same geographic regions as *N. gonorrhoeae* (**FIGURE 10–16**).[50] Infections with *C. trachomatis* are seen in a variety of forms.

In both men and women, genital chlamydial infections often present with no symptoms. Asymptomatic carriage may occur for months without diagnosis. However, genitourinary tract infections from *C. trachomatis* may cause urethritis, cervicitis, infections of Bartholin glands, proctitis, salpingitis (infections of the fallopian tubes), and epididymitis.[5] Both *C. trachomatis* and *N. gonorrhoeae* are major causes of pelvic inflammatory disease, which have resulted in a rising rate of infertility and ectopic pregnancy in

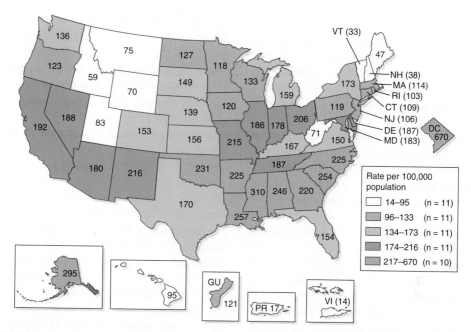

FIGURE 10–15 Reported cases of *Neisseria gonorrhoeae*—United States, 2017.

Courtesy of CDC. Centers for Disease Control and Prevention. Gonorrhea. Sexually Transmitted Disease Surveillance 2017. Accessed at https://www.cdc.gov/std/stats17/gonorrhea.htm

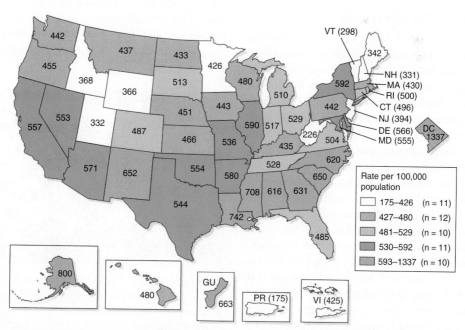

FIGURE 10–16 Reported cases of *Chlamydia trachomatis*—United States, 2017.

Courtesy of CDC. Centers for Disease Control and Prevention. Chlamydia. Sexually Transmitted Disease Surveillance 2017. Accessed at https://www.cdc.gov/std/stats17/chlamydia.htm

young women.[51] Perinatal infections are seen in one-fourth to one-half of infants born to women infected with *C. trachomatis*. Infants often develop inclusion conjunctivitis but may present with chlamydial pneumonia up to 6 weeks after birth.[5]

Infections also occur in the form of ocular trachoma, which affects more than 84 million individuals worldwide. Significant portions of these infections result in blindness. Hyperendemic regions are found in areas of rural Africa, Asia, Central and South America, Australia, and the Middle East, where prevalence rates range from 60 to 90% in preschool children. The organism causes inflammation of the conjunctiva, with increased irritation, pain, and discharge. Repeat infections may lead to blurred vision, photophobia, and even scarring of the inner eyelid, resulting in the eyelid turning toward the eye (entropion). This eventually allows the eyelashes to scratch the surface of the eyeball leading to scarring, ulceration, and loss of vision.[5] Lymphogranuloma venereum is a sexually transmitted form of disease that is rarely seen in North America.

Conventional Methods

The traditional method for identifying *Neisseria gonorrhoeae* is culture. Although *N. gonorrhoeae* is able to survive well in the mucosa of the human body, there are special requirements for collection and cultivation of the organism. A Dacron or rayon-tipped, plastic-shafted swab may be used if the specimen will be plated to media within 6 hours of collection, optimally within 30 minutes. If the specimen must be transported for analysis, a transport media containing charcoal should be used to inhibit toxic fatty acids found in the fibers of the swab. Ideally, specimens for *N. gonorrhoeae* should be inoculated on media designed to appease the fastidious nature of the organism. *N. gonorrhoeae* does not grow on the traditional trypticase soy agar with 5% sheep blood cell that is routinely used in the microbiology laboratory. It can be recovered from chocolate agar; however, an enriched media is best for optimal recovery. A selection of enriched media is commercially available, including modified Thayer-Martin (MTM) medium, Martin Lewis medium, and

New York City medium, to name a few. Medium should be incubated at 35–37°C in 5–7% CO_2 for up to 72 hours. Humidity will enhance growth. Organisms can be definitively identified as *N. gonorrhoeae* by growing on an enriched medium, showing gram-negative diplococci by Gram stain, demonstrating a very strong reaction with superoxol (30% H_2O_2), and having expected results with rapid fermentation sugars (glucose positive, maltose negative, lactose negative, sucrose negative, and fructose negative).[5] In addition, a Gram stain of a direct specimen collected from a male may be definitively identified as *N. gonorrhoeae* if polymorphonuclear neutrophils are seen with intracellular gram-negative diplococci (**FIGURE 10–17**). The sensitivity and specificity of the Gram stain from urethral discharge specimens reaches 95% for symptomatic males.[49]

Cultivation of *C. trachomatis* requires recovery in a cell culture line, such as McCoy, HeLa, or monkey kidney cells. Cycloheximide-treated McCoy cells are most often used in a shell vial assay. The specimen, collected in viral transport media, is shaken with 5 mm glass beads to lyse cells, centrifuged, and seeded onto the cell monolayer. This typically occurs on a coverslip in the bottom of a vial. After 48 to 72 hours, the monolayer is stained with fluorescent antibodies that

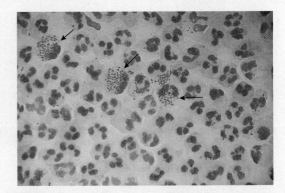

FIGURE 10–17 Gonococcal Urethral Smear. A Gram stain of a male urethral discharge showing many polymorphonuclear neutrophils and Gram-negative diplococci (gonococci). The intracellular bacteria (arrows) are diagnostic of *N. gonorrhoeae* in this specimen.

Courtesy of Joe Miller/CDC.

are either species-specific, targeting the MOMP, or genus-specific, targeting the lipopolysaccharide cell wall.[5] While it is the recommended diagnostic method in some situations, cell culture is not routinely performed in most clinical laboratories.

Immunodiagnostic Methods

In many clinical laboratories, the testing for infections with both *N. gonorrhoeae* and *C. trachomatis* is performed at the same time, often from the same sample. Serologic methods, while once performed to detect system immune responses, are no longer recommended due to the lack of precision in the detection of an active infection. Enzyme immunoassay tests are also no longer recommended for the detection of *N. gonorrhoeae* or *C. trachomatis* in urogenital specimens. The cost and performance characteristics of EIA tests for *N. gonorrhoeae* have not allowed them to be competitive with other tests available on the market. EIA tests for *C. trachomatis* detect chlamydial lipopolysaccharides. The cell wall of other microorganisms, specifically Gram-negative bacilli often seen in the urogenital tract, can give a false-positive result.[51] In fact, the last EIA to obtain FDA approval was in 2004.[15]

The only FDA-cleared, recommended, immunodiagnostic method for the detection of either *N. gonorrhoeae* or *C. trachomatis* is the use of direct fluorescent antibody (DFA) tests for the identification of *C. trachomatis* in ocular infections. Specimens are directly inoculated onto a slide, which is then stained with a fluorescent monoclonal antibody to either the MOMP or the lipopolysaccharide molecule. Stained organisms are identified by fluorescent microscopy. This technique requires an experienced technologist, is labor-intensive, and is time-consuming. There are no DFA tests available for the detection of *N. gonorrhoeae*.[51]

Molecular Diagnostic Methods

The recommended method for routine screening and diagnosis of infections with *N. gonorrhoeae* and *C. trachomatis* is the nucleic acid amplification test (NAAT). There are currently five major manufacturers of NAAT: Abbott, Beckton Dickinson, Cepheid, Hologic, and Roche.[51] Each company offers dual testing in a cost-effective, high-throughput platform. The available tests are able to detect small amounts of each organism from a single sample that ranges from endocervical or vaginal swabs in women, urethral swabs in men, and urine specimens from both women and men. FDA-cleared specimen types and specimen transport and stability vary from one manufacturer to another. For additional information, refer to the package insert for each individual assay as manufacturers update their testing capabilities often. It is also important to be familiar with the performance characteristics of the assay chosen. While NAATs are considered greatly superior to traditional culture and nonculture diagnostic methods, there is still a possibility for false positive and false negative results from molecular methods. These inaccuracies are often the result of incorrect specimen collection, test operation, and laboratory environment. Nevertheless, NAATs usually demonstrate sensitivities well above 90% and specificities ≥99%. Studies have shown NAATs often detect 20 to 50% more chlamydial infections that culture and preceding nonculture methods.[51]

CASE STUDY

Rapid Strep A

A 3-year-old child is brought to his pediatrician after the mother noticed the child crying when eating or drinking, causing a loss of appetite. Upon examination, the physician noted a fever of 101.3°F, red throat, and swollen lymph nodes in the neck. A throat swab was collected and a rapid strep A screen was performed

(continues)

CASE STUDY (Continued)

in the physician's office. The results were negative and a second swab was sent to the laboratory for culture confirmation. The child was given oral amoxicillin and sent home.

Critical Thinking Questions

1. Why might a rapid strep A screen give a negative result despite clinical symptoms leading to strep throat?
2. The results come back showing a pathogenic bacteria that is Gram positive, occurs in pairs or chains, and exhibits beta hemolysis on blood agar. What is the most likely identification of this organism?
3. If the patient is not treated, what sequelae may occur because of this infection?
4. What diagnostic method is more sensitive and will give a diagnosis quicker than the method used by the physician?

▶ References

1. Theel ES, Carpenter AB, Binnicker MJ. Immunoassays for Diagnosis of Infectious Diseases. In: Jorgensen JH, Pfaller MA, Carroll KC, et al., eds. *Manual of Clinical Mictrobiology, Eleventh Edition.* Washington, DC: ASM Press; 2015:91–105.

2. Annesley TM. It's about the journey, not the destination: the birth of radioimmunoassay. 1960. *Clin Chem.* 2010;56(4):671–672.

3. Centers for Disease Control and Prevention. Test Complexities. Clinical Laboratory Improvement Amendments (CLIA). https://wwwn.cdc.gov/CLIA/Resources /TestComplexities.aspx. Updated: June 11, 2018. Accessed: October 1, 2018.

4. U.S. Food and Drug Administration. CLIA Categorizations. Medical Devices. https://www.fda.gov/MedicalDevices /DeviceRegulationandGuidance/IVDRegulatory Assistance/ucm393229.htm. Updated: March 22, 2018. Accessed: October 1, 2018.

5. Tille PM. *Bailey & Scott's Diagnostic Microbiolgy, Fourteenth Edition.* St. Louis, MO: Elsevier; 2017.

6. National Institutes of Health. Office of Strategic Coordination—The Common Fund. Human Microbiome Project. https://commonfund.nih.gov/hmp. Updated: April 23, 2018. Accessed: August 28, 2018.

7. Litwin CM, Litwin SE, Hill HR. Diagnostic methods for group A streptococcal infections. In: Detrick B, Schmidt JL, Hamilton RG, ed. *Manual of Molecular and Clinical Laboratory Immunology,* 8th ed. Washington, DC: ASM Press; 2006:394–403.

8. Faé KC, da Silva DD, Oshiro SE, et al. Mimicry in recognition of cardiac myosin peptides by heart-intralesional T-cell clones from rheumatic heart disease. *J Immunol.* 2006;176(9):5662–5670.

9. Parks T, Smeesters PR, Curtis N, et al. ASO titer or not? When to use streptococcal serology: a guide for linicians. *Eur J Clin Microbiol Infect Dis.* 2015;34(5):845–849.

10. Miller JM, Phillips HL, Graves RK, et al. Evaluation of the directigen group A strep test kit. *J Clin Microbiol.* 1984;20(5):846–848.

11. Gerberg MA, Spadaccini LJ, Wright LL, et al. Latex agglutination tests for rapid identification of group A streptococci directly from throat swabs. *J Pediatr.* 1984;105(5):702–705.

12. BBL Streptocard Enzyme Latex Test Kit [package insert]. Sparks, MD: Beckton Dickinson; 2016.

13. PathoDx Strep Grouping Universal Kit [package inert]. Lenexa, KY: Remel Diagnostics; 2016.

14. StrepPRO Grouping Kit [package insert]. Santa Monica, CA: Hardy Diagnostics; 2016.

15. US Food and Drug Administration. Streptococcus, group A. CLIA—Clinical Laboratory Improvement Amendments, medical devices, databases. https://www .accessdata.fda.gov/scripts/cdrh/cfdocs/cfCLIA/results .cfm. Updated: August 6, 2018. Accessed August 8, 2018.

16. Shulman ST, Bisno AL, Clegg HW, et al. Clinical practice guideline for the diagnosis and management of group A streptococcal pharyngitis: 2012 update by the Infectious Diseases Society of America. *Clin Infect Dis.* 2012;55(10):1279–1282.

17. Centers for Disease Control and Prevention. Tubercuosis (TB). Data and statistics. https://www.cdc.gov/tb/statistics /default.htm. UpdatedL June 5, 2018. Accessed: August 7, 2018.

18. Stewart RJ, Tsang CA, Pratt RH, et al. Tuberculosis—United States, 2017. *MMWR Morb Mortal Wkly Rep.* 2018;67(11):317–323.

19. Targeted tuberculin testing and treatment of latent tuberculosis infection. American Thoracic Society. *MMWR Recomm Rep.* 2000;49(RR-6):1–51.

20. Litwin CM. Immunological tests in tuberculosis. In: Detrick B, Schmidt J, Hamilton R, eds. *Manual of Molecular and Clinical Laboratory Immunology,* 8th Ed. Washington, DC: ASM Press; 2006:433–443.

21. Mazurek GH, Jereb J, Vernon A, et al. Updated guidelines for using Interferon Gamma Release Assays to detect mycobacterium tuberculosis infection—United States, 2010. *MMWR Recomm Rep.* 2010;59(RR-5):1–25.

22. QuantiFERON-TB Gold Plus (QFT-Plus) [package insert]. Germantown, MD: Qiagen; 2017.

23. T.Spot-TB [package insert]. Marlborough, MA: Oxford Immunotec; 2017.

24. GeneXpert MTB/RIF [package insert]. Sunnyvale, CA: Cepheid; 2015.

25. Mathew P, Kuo YH, Vazirani B, et al. Are three sputum acid-fast bacillus smears necessary for discontinuing tuberculosis isolation? *J Clin Microbiol.* 2002;40(9):3482–3484.

26. Swai HF, Mugusi FM, Mbwambo JK. Sputum smear negative pulmonary tuberculosis: sensitivity and specificity of diagnostic algorithm. *BMC Res Notes.* 2011;4:475.

27. Lafond RE, Lukehart SA. Biological basis for syphilis. *Clin Microbiol Rev.* 2006;19(1):29–49.

28. Henao-Martínez AF, Johnson SC. Diagnostic tests for syphilis: new tests and new algorithms. *Neurol Clin Pract.* 2014;4(2):114–122.

29. Centers for Disease Control and Prevention (CDC). Sexually transmitted disease surveillance 2016. Atlanta, GA: U.S. Department of Helath and Human Serivces; 2017. https://www.cdc.gov/std/stats16/CDC_2016_STDS _Report-for508WebSep21_2017_1644.pdf.

30. APHL Sexually Transmitted Disease Subcommittee. Suggested Reporting Language for Syphilis Serology Testing. Silver Spring, MD: Association of Public Health Laboratories; 2015.

31. BD Macro-Vue RPR Card Tests [package insert]. Sparks, MD: Beckton, Dickinson and Company; 2015.

32. Kennedy EJ, Creighton ET. Venereal disease research laboratory (VDRL) slide test. In: Larsen S, Pope V, Johnson R, Kennedy E, eds. *Syphilis: A Manual of Tests and Supplements.* 9th ed. Washington, DC: APHA Press; 1998.

33. Binnicker MJ, Jespersen DJ, Rollins LO. Direct comparison of the traditional and reverse syphilis screening algorithms in a population with a low prevalence of syphilis. *J Clin Microbiol.* 2012;50(1):148–150.

34. Centers for Disease Control and Prevention (CDC). National Notifiable diseases surveillance system, 2016 annual tables of infectious disease data. Atlanta, GA. CDC Division of Health Informatics and Surveillance, 2017. https://www.cdc.gov/nndss/infectious-tables.html. Accessed: November 16, 2017.

35. Wang G, Aguero-Rosenfeld M. Lyme disease, relapsing fever, and leptospirosis. In: Detrick B, Schmitd J, Hamilton R, eds. *Manual of Molecular and Clinical Laboratory Immunology, 8th Ed.* Washington, DC: ASM Press; 2006:419–433.

36. Wormser GP, Dattwyler RJ, Shapiro ED, et al. The clinical assessment, treatment, and prevention of Lyme disease, human granulocytic anaplasmosis, and babesiosis: clinical practice guidelines by the Infectious Diseases Society of America. *Clin Infect Dis.* 2006;43(9):1089–1134.

37. Sofia Lyme FIA [package insert]. San Diego, CA: Quidel Corportion; 2017.

38. Centers for Disease Control and Prevention. Lyme Disease. Two-tiered testing decsion tree. https://www .cdc.gov/lyme/healthcare/clinician_twotier.html. Updated: November 15, 2011. Accessed: September 27, 2018.

39. Biggs HM, Behravesh CB, Bradley KK, et al. Diagnosis and management of tickborne Rickettsial Diseases: Rocky Mountain Spotted Fever and other spotted fever group rickettsioses, ehrlichioses, and anaplasmosis—United States. *MMWR Recomm Rep.* 2016;65(2):1–44.

40. Centers for Disease Control and Prevention (CDC). Epidemiology and Statistics. Rocky Mountain Spotted Fever (RMSF). https://www.cdc.gov/rmsf/stats/index .html. Updated: August 6, 2018. Accessed: September 27, 2018.

41. U.S. Food and Drug Administration. CLIA - clinical laboratory improvement amendments. https://www .accessdata.fda.gov/scripts/cdrh/cfdocs/cfCLIA/results .cfm. Updated: October 1, 2018. Accessed: October 3, 2018.

42. Dunn B, Phadnis S. Diagnois of Helicobacter pylori infection and assessment of eradication. In: Detrick B, Schmidt J, Hamilton R, eds. *Manual of Molecular and Clinical Laboratory Immunology, 8th Ed.* Washington, DC: ASM Press; 2006:401–411.

43. Kamboj AK, Cotter TG, Oxentenko AS. Helicobacter pylori: the past, present, and future in management. *Mayo Clin Proc.* 2017;92(4):599–604.

44. H. pylori Test Cassette [package insert]. Richmond, VA: McKesson Medical-Surgical; 2015.

45. QuickVue H. pylori Test [package insert]. San Diego, CA: Quidel Corporation; 2014.

46. Acceava H. pylori [package insert]. Waltham, MA: Alere, Inc.; 2017.

47. VIDAS H. pylori IgG [package insert]. Durham, NC: bioMerieux; 2017.

48. Centers for Disease Control and Prevention (CDC). Gonorrhea. Sexually transmitted disease surveillance 2017. https://www.cdc.gov/std/stats17/gonorrhea.htm. Updated: July 24, 2018. Accessed: September 25, 2018.

49. Centers for Disease Control and Prevention (CDC). Gonococcal infections. 2015 sexually transmitted diseases treatment guidelines. https://www.cdc.gov/std/tg2015 /gonorrhea.htm. Updated: January 4, 2018. Accessed: September 25, 2018.

50. Centers for Disease Control and Prevention (CDC). Chlamydia. 2017 Sexually Transmitted Diseases Surveillance. https://www.cdc.gov/std/stats17/chlamydia .htm. Updated: July 24, 2018. Accessed: September 29, 2018.

51. Centers for Disease Control and Prevention (CDC). Recommendations for the laboratory-based detection of Chlamydia trachomatis and Neisseria gonorrhoeae—2014. *MMWR Recomm Rep.* 2014;63(RR-2):1–19.

CHAPTER 11

Fungal and Parasitic Serology and Immunodiagnostics

Barbara Spinda, MS, MLS(ASCP)CM

KEY TERMS

Acute
Aerosolization
Amoebiasis
Antibody titer
Arthroconidia
Axonemes
Blastoconidia
Blastomycosis
Candidiasis
Chromotrope
Coccidian
Coccidioidomycosis
Complement fixation
Conidia
Conidiophores
Convalescent
Cryptococcosis
Cysts
Dysjunctor cells
Endemic
Epitopes

Equimolar
Eukaryotic
Excyst
Flagella
Flagellates
Giardiasis
Granulomatous
Helminth eggs
Hemolysin
Histoplasmosis
Hybridization
Hyphae
Immunocompromised
Immunodeficient
Immunodiffusion
Larvae
Lysis
Merozoites
Microbiota
Microsporidia
Mycotic

Oocysts
Opportunistic
Phylogenetic
Postzone
Proglottids
Prozone
Pseudohyphae
Pyriform
Refractile
Saprobe
Septation
Septum
Serotypes
Sporozoites
Teleomorph
Thrush
Toxoplasmosis
Trophozoites
Unicellular
Vulvovaginitis
Zone of equivalence

▶ Fungal Infections

For many fungal infections, identification of the fungus is performed using traditional cultivation techniques. However, to ensure adequate growth and isolation, a plethora of selective and nonselective media is required, incubation temperatures are specific and outside of normal bacterial needs, and the incubation time must be extended. Inoculated media for fungus cultures are incubated aerobically at 30°C for 21 to 28 days. If a 30°C incubator is not available, incubation at 25°C is an acceptable alternative. Cultures specifically requested to screen for *Candida* spp. can be incubated in an aerobic 35 to 37°C incubator, with bacterial cultures.[1] Cultures are scanned every 2 to 3 days for growth, subcultured for isolation or macroscopic and microscopic characteristics if needed, and examined using lactophenol cotton blue for identification. This traditional method for fungus identification is often time-consuming, highly complex, and requires a class II biological safety cabinet.

Immunoassay Methods

The definitive diagnosis of many fungal infections is based on the isolation of the etiologic agent or the microscopic detection of the organism in histology or other clinical specimens.[2] These highly complex methods require a technologist with experience and knowledge of fungal agents. Even with the most experienced technologist, these methods are often insensitive and unsuccessful,

despite repeat specimen collection and cultivation. Alternative diagnostic methods are available for the diagnosis of **mycotic** diseases. Commercially available antigen and antibody immunodiagnostic assays give promise for earlier and more specific diagnosis of fungal infections.

Antibody detection methods are used for the diagnosis and monitoring of disease progression. Titers are determined from serum collected during the **acute** infection and compared with titers in serum collected weeks later (**convalescent**). A fourfold rise in **antibody titer**, or an increase of two doubling dilutions, is considered diagnostic of current infection. Diagnosis is achieved best when both specimens are tested concurrently using the same test system. Unfortunately, not all infected individuals demonstrate a rise in titer. Additionally, because of the inherent delay in testing to compare acute and convalescent specimens, the information obtained is often too late to affect therapy. An increased number of early infection serologic testing assays to identify IgM antibodies are becoming commercially available.[3]

A variety of commercial antigen and antibody immunodiagnostic assays are available, and range from rapid latex agglutination to immunodiffusion and complement fixation, to lateral flow and microtiter enzyme immunoassays (EIA). Even with recent advancements in diagnostic testing, the number of immunoassays for fungal diagnosis is not as abundant as one would expect. Many antigens used in antibody detection immunoassays carry cross-reactive **epitopes** that are shared among different fungal genera or other microorganisms. False-positive results must be ruled out by performing serologic tests with a battery of antigens.[2]

Immunodiffusion

The first immunoassays developed in the early 1940s were referred to as **immunodiffusion** assays. These assays were dependent on the visualization of antigen-antibody precipitation bands. Improvements in technology have slowly removed immunodiffusion assays from many areas of the clinical microbiology and immunology laboratories; however, the area of mycology, specifically, detection of systemic fungi, still uses immunodiffusion assays. While techniques have improved, the immunodiffusion assays are notoriously labor-intensive to set up and perform, require extensive technical expertise, and have subjective result interpretation. The approximate sensitivity for immunodiffusion assays is only 1 to 3 mg per mL, much less sensitive than chemiluminescence immunoassays, radioimmunoassays, and even enzyme immunoassays.[4]

Immunodiffusion assays detect soluble antibodies with the formation of a line of precipitation when the antibody and corresponding antigen meet. This method utilizes a porous medium, such as agarose gel, in which the antigens and antibodies are able to disperse. The double immunodiffusion method, also referred to as the Ouchterlony gel diffusion, uses small circular wells cut into an agarose plate. Specific reference antigens and antibodies are added to individual wells in a ring formation around a central well that contains the test serum. During the 18- to 24-hour incubation, the antigens and antibodies diffuse toward each other, creating a visible band of precipitation where the antigens and antibodies come together to form an insoluble lattice.[3] A precipitin line seen between the reference antigen and antibody acts as a positive control. A precipitin line between the test serum and antigen indicates a positive patient result for the respective antibody (**FIGURE 11–1**).

The biological foundation of the immunodiffusion assay is simple; however, the assay itself is easily influenced by antigen and antibody interactions. When the antigens and antibodies are **equimolar**, they easily bind and form the precipitin line expected in the assay. This is known as the zone of equivalence. On either side of the **zone of equivalence**, the **prozone** and **postzone** phenomena may be seen. The prozone phase is characteristic of too much antibody, preventing the formation of precipitate. The postzone phase is characteristic of too much antigen, allowing for some precipitation, but often not enough to detect visually. Immunodiffusion assays have specificity reaching 100%. False-negative results may be seen in individuals with antibody levels below the assay detectable limits or when the prozone or postzone phenomena are seen. In instances in which a negative result is seen and the individual presents with symptoms of fungal infection, culture is recommended.

Complement Fixation

Complement fixation is a classic method to demonstrate the presence of antibodies in a serum sample. This assay is based on the interaction of antigen-antibody immune complexes with components of the classical complement pathway (**FIGURE 11–2**). A two-step process is used in this technique to detect antibodies in serum and determine a titer. Test serum is heated at 56°C for 30 minutes. During this process, native complement components are inactivated. The treated serum is then incubated with pathogen-specific antigens to form antigen-antibody immune complexes. Purified complement is added and binds to any antigen-antibody complexes in the serum. **Hemolysin**-sensitized red blood cells (RBCs) are then added to the serum as an indicator of test results. If complement is bound to the antigen-antibody complexes, the RBCs are protected from **lysis** by complement, and pellet at the bottom of the reaction well after centrifugation. This is a positive result for antigen-antibody complexes in the test serum, and thus indicates infection with the specific pathogen. If antigen-antibody complexes are not formed because antibodies are not present in the serum, complement will remain active and cause lysis of the RBCs. A pellet will not form

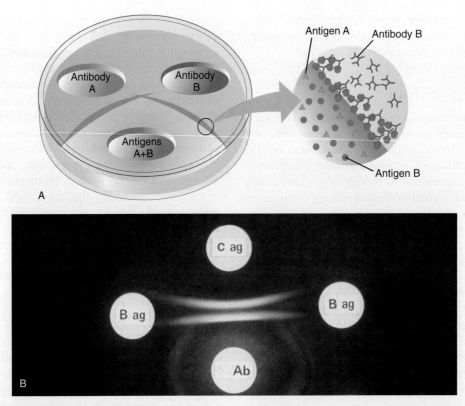

FIGURE 11-1 Double immunodiffusion technique. **(A)** Wells cut into agar contain known antibodies or antigens. When test serum is allowed to diffuse from the remaining well, a line of precipitation is seen where the antigen or antibody in the test serum meets the corresponding reference antigen or antibody. **(B)** Two lines of precipitation are shown indicating that the test serum contains antibodies corresponding to antigen C.

From Pommerville, J. C. (2017). Fundamentals of Microbiology, 11e. Jones & Bartlett Learning.

upon centrifugation and indicate that the individual does not have an active infection.[4]

New methods have replaced complement fixation for the detection of antibodies for many infectious agents. This method requires many manipulations, takes at least 48 hours to complete, and typically gives nonspecific results. Complement fixation is routinely used for the detection of antibodies to particular fungi and viruses.

▶ Candidiasis

Etiology

Yeasts of the genus *Candida* are some of the most commonly isolated fungi in the clinical microbiology laboratory. *Candida* species are eukaryotic, unicellular organisms that range in size from 2 µm to 4 µm. They typically reproduce asexually by blastoconidia formation, or budding. Budding occurs through an initial weakening of the cell wall. The cell wall pushes outward, eventually forming a bud, also called a daughter cell. The cytoplasm of the daughter cell is formed from the mother cell and stays connected until a septum is created between the two cells. Eventually, the daughter cell breaks away from the mother cell, leaving a bud scar on the mother cell[3] (FIGURE 11-3). Of the *Candida* species known to cause disease in humans, *Candida albicans* is the species seen most abundantly. The unique thing about the identification of *Candida* spp. is that unless the isolate is recovered from a sterile body site, it is generally not speciated. Yeast are found naturally in and on the human body

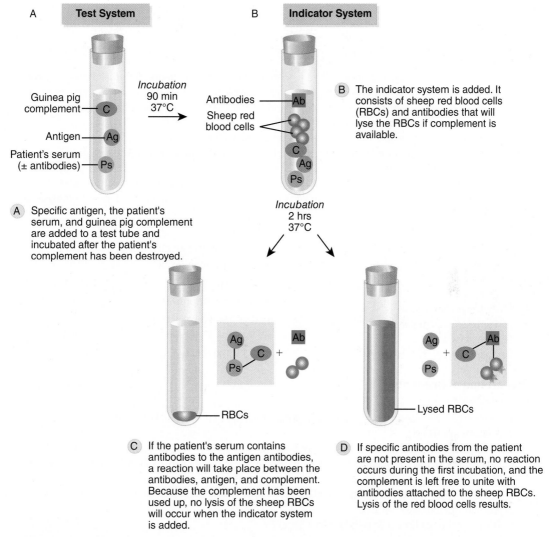

A Test System

B Indicator System

Guinea pig complement — C

Antigen — Ag

Patient's serum (± antibodies) — Ps

Incubation 90 min 37°C

Antibodies — Ab

Sheep red blood cells

C
Ag
Ps

B The indicator system is added. It consists of sheep red blood cells (RBCs) and antibodies that will lyse the RBCs if complement is available.

A Specific antigen, the patient's serum, and guinea pig complement are added to a test tube and incubated after the patient's complement has been destroyed.

Incubation 2 hrs 37°C

Ag
C
Ps
+ Ab

—RBCs

Ag
Ps
+ C
Ab

—Lysed RBCs

C If the patient's serum contains antibodies to the antigen antibodies, a reaction will take place between the antibodies, antigen, and complement. Because the complement has been used up, no lysis of the sheep RBCs will occur when the indicator system is added.

D If specific antibodies from the patient are not present in the serum, no reaction occurs during the first incubation, and the complement is left free to unite with antibodies attached to the sheep RBCs. Lysis of the red blood cells results.

FIGURE 11–2 Complement fixation tests are carried out in two stages involving **(A)** a test system. **(B)** an indicator system.

From Pommerville, J. C. (2017). Fundamentals of Microbiology, 11e. Jones & Bartlett Learning.

where they coexist with other bacteria and fungi. It is only when these yeast become overgrown or gain access to sterile locations that they are considered clinically significant.

Epidemiology and Pathogenesis

Candida species are part of the normal human **microbiota**, found on the skin and in the genital and gastrointestinal tracts. *C. albicans,* the most commonly encountered species, is the causative agent of **candidiasis**; however, simply recovering the organism in a clinical specimen does not automatically mean the patient has candidiasis. Consideration must be taken when evaluating the clinical specimen and isolate; is the isolate more abundant than other normal flora and is the specimen normally sterile? They are the most commonly encountered **opportunistic** fungal infection and a significant cause of hospital-acquired blood stream infections in the United States. Mortality rates reach 50% with

STEP-BY-STEP PROCEDURE 11–1 Sensitization of Sheep RBCS for use in Complement Fixation

Purpose: The complement fixation assay is used to identify antibodies in patients for fungal diseases such as histoplasmosis, blastomycosis, coccidioidomycosis, and aspergillosis. The following procedure represents a method for creating sensitized Sheep Red Blood Cells (SRBCs) for use in complement fixation assay when a normally commercially available reagent is unavailable.

Principle: Antibodies present in patient serum, when mixed with the corresponding antigen, will form an antigen-antibody complex that binds complement found in fresh serum. The amount of complement bound is indirectly measured using sheep red blood cells (SRBC) sensitized with anti-SRBC (hemolysin). The remaining free complement in the serum will initiate lysis of the sensitized SRBC. The presence of antibodies in the patient's serum will bind all free complement, resulting in no hemolysis of the sensitized SRBC.

Materials and Equipment:

- Washed SRBC
- Hemolysin
- Complement
- Glycerin
- Phenol (crystalline)
- Sodium diethyl barbiturate
- Sodium chloride
- Veronal-buffered saline solution
- Magnesium chloride ($MgCl_2$)
- Calcium chloride ($CaCl_2$)
- Centrifuge
- Spectrophotometer
- Electrometric pH meter
- Pipettes, 1 mL and 5mL
- 12 × 100 mm test tubes

Preparation of Reagents

Veronal-buffered saline:

1. Dissolve 83 g NaCl and 10.10g sodium diethyl barbiturate in 1,500 mL distilled water.
2. Add 34.6 mL 1N HCL.
3. In a separate container, dissolve 20.33 g $MgCl_2$ and 4.4 g $CaCl_2$ in 100 mL distilled water.
4. Pipette 5 mL of this solution into the buffered saline made in steps 1 and 2 and make up the volume to 2000 mL.
5. Keep this solution in the refrigerator until use. Dilute one part solution with four parts distilled water each time before use.
6. The pH of the solution must be between 7.3 and 7.4.

3% sheep red blood cells:

1. Centrifuge 10 mL sheep blood and discard the supernatant.
2. Wash the red blood cells at least three times with buffered saline to remove the plasma proteins.
3. Take 3.0 mL of the backed and washed red blood cells and pipette into 97 mL buffered saline. Rinse the pipette by drawing up the red cell suspension several times.

Complement:

1. Commercially available complement should be dissolved in the proper diluent, as indicated by the manufacturer.
2. Pipette 0.5mL aliquots of the complement solution into freezer-stable tubes for long-term storage. Stability should be maintained for several weeks in the freezer.
3. For the complement fixation assay, pipette 0.2 mL of the complement solution into 7.8 mL of cold, buffered saline, creating a 1:40 dilution. This dilution must be kept in the refrigerator or an ice bucket during the experiment and must be made fresh each day of use.

Stock Hemolysin Dilution:

1. Prepare glycerinized hemolysis by mixing equal volumes of hemolysin and neutral glycerol.
2. In a separate container, mix 94 mL of buffered saline with 4 mL of saline containing phenol (5% phenol crystals dissolved in 100 mL buffered saline).
3. Add 2 mL of the glycerinized hemolysin.
4. Store this standard hemolysin stock solution (1:100) in the refrigerator for up to 1 year.

Hemoglobin color standard:

1. Prepare a hemoglobin color standard curve by creating 0, 30, 50, 70, 90, and 100% lysis standards.
2. First prepare a hemoglobin solution by adding, in order, 1 mL 3% sheep red cell suspension, 7mL distilled water, mix, and then 2 mL of undiluted buffered saline.
3. Prepare a 0.3% red cell suspension by adding 1 mL 3% sheep red blood cells to 9 mL diluted buffered saline.
4. Label six tubes and prepare as follows:

% lysis	0	30	50	70	90	100
Hemoglobin solution	0 mL	0.3 mL	0. 5mL	0.7 mL	0.9 mL	1.0 mL
3% SRBC suspension	1.0 mL	0.7 mL	0.5 mL	0.3 mL	0.1 mL	0 mL

5. Mix each tube briefly.
6. Read the optical density of each tube at 541 nm to determine a calibration curve.
7. Prepare a new standard curve each day of testing.

Hemolysin Titration/ SRBC sensitization

1. Prepare a 1:1,000 dilution of the standard hemolysin by diluting 1 mL of the stock hemolysin dilution into 9 mL of buffered saline.
2. Pipette 1 mL of the 1:1,000 dilution into each of eight tubes and prepare dilutions as shown below by adding appropriate volumes of buffered saline:

Final Dilution	1:1,000 Dilution	Buffered Saline
1:1,000	1 mL	0 mL
1:2,000	1 mL	1 mL
1:3,000	1 mL	2 mL
1:4,000	1 mL	3 ml
1:5,000	1 mL	4 mL
1:6,000	1 mL	5 mL
1:7,000	1 mL	6 mL
1:8,000	1 mL	7 mL

(continues)

STEP-BY-STEP PROCEDURE 11–1 Sensitization of Sheep RBCS for use in Complement Fixation *(Continued)*

3. Take another eight tubes and transfer 0.3 mL of each dilution from 1:1,000 to 1:8,000 into the new set of test tubes.
4. Pipette 0.3 mL of the 3% SRBC suspension into each tube and mix.
5. Let the tubes stand at room temperature for 20 minutes.
6. To these sensitized cells, add 1.2 mL buffered saline and 1.2 mL of the freshly prepared 1:30 complement dilution.
7. Mix well and incubate at 37°C for 1 hour.
8. Centrifuge the tubes at 1,000× for 10 minutes and measure the optical density of the supernatant at 541 nm.
9. Use the calibration curve prepared using the hemolysin color standards to determine the proper amount of hemolysin to use in the complement fixation assay.

Complement Titration (CH$_{50}$ assay)

1. Prepare sensitized, standardized SRBC as previously described.
2. Prepare complement dilutions as follows. Titration should be completed in duplicate, at least, due to the fragile nature of complement.

Final Dilution	1:100 Dilution Complement	Buffered Saline
1:100	2.70 mL	0 mL
1:200	1.35 mL	1.35 mL
1:300	1.80 mL	0.90 mL
1:400	2.03 mL	0.67 mL
1:500	2.16 mL	0.54 mL
1:600	2.25 mL	0.45 mL

3. Add 0.3 mL sensitized SRBC to each tube, mix well, and incubate at 37°C for 1 hour.
4. Centrifuge the tubes at 1,000x for 10 minutes and measure the optical density of the supernatant at 541 nm.
5. Using log-log graph paper, determine the amount of complement required to lyse 50% of the SRBC.
6. The final dilution that lyses 50% of the SRBCs can now be used as the reagent in a complement fixation assay.

these infections.[3] Although *C. albicans* is the most commonly isolated yeast, other species such as *C. glabrata, C. parapsilosis, C. tropicalis, C. krusei,* and, more recently, *C. auris,* are increasing in their occurrence and significance to disease.

C. albicans is able to cause infection inside and outside of the body, ranging in locations from skin, mucous membranes, respiratory tract, and urogenital tract to sterile sites such as blood and meninges. **Thrush** is a frequently encountered infection

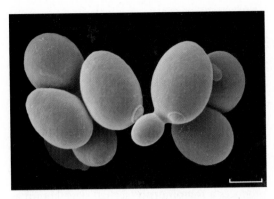

FIGURE 11–3 False-color scanning electron micrograph of budding yeast cells showing scars on the mother cell.

© SCIMAT/Science Source

of the mucous membranes in the mouth seen in newborns and immunocompromised individuals (**FIGURE 11–4**). **Vulvovaginitis** is seen in women when a change occurs in vaginal pH or microbiota, allowing an overgrowth of *Candida* spp. Indwelling catheter devices present an increase in infection possibility. Other species of *Candida* are emerging as significant agents of infection. These species are making appearances in neonatal intensive care units and oncology units.[3] Some species, such as *C. glabrata* and *C. auris*, show increased resistance to common antifungal agents, thus making treatment a challenge. In the case of the *Candida* spp., accurate identification is necessary to ensure treatment occurs timely and effectively.

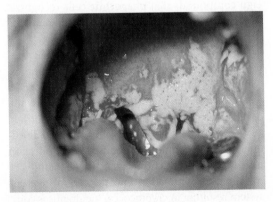

FIGURE 11–4 Severe case of oral candidiasis, also referred to as thrush.

Courtesy of CDC.

Conventional Methods

In direct microscopic examinations of clinical specimens, *Candida* spp. appear similar to many other yeasts. They form budding yeast, blastoconidia, and may produce **hyphae**. **Pseudohyphae**, or germ tubes, are seen in some clinical specimens and resemble sausage links projecting from the yeast cell with an irregular point of constriction. True hyphae, produced by *C. albicans* and *C. dublinensis,* are seen as filaments with **septation**. In Gram-stained slides, yeast appear strongly Gram-positive.

Cultivation of *Candida* spp. is simple and rapid. Colonies grow on standard mycology media as well as routine bacterial media within 2 to 3 days. Most *Candida* spp. produce colonies that are smooth and creamy with a slight matte appearance, while others may produce dry, wrinkled, dull colonies. Speciation cannot be made from macroscopic and microscopic morphology alone, although growth on cornmeal agar containing Tween 80 will give differentiating **conidia** formations.

Newer identification methods for yeast rely on yeast utilization of carbohydrates and other substances. A number of manual and automated biochemical panels are commercially available for speciation of *Candida* from culture. These assays are generally well established and routinely used in the clinical microbiology laboratory. Automated systems often identify bacterial isolates in addition to yeast isolates. Results are obtained within 24 hours and show high correlation with traditional methods for speciating routinely encountered *Candida* spp.

Immunodiagnostic Methods

Serologic identification of yeast is generally limited to the *Candida* species and *Cryptococcus neoformans.* The unique cell wall structure of yeast is a well-suited target for many immunodiagnostic assays. Several commercial kits detect (1,3) β-D-glucan, found in the cell wall of common pathogenic yeasts.[5] These rapid assays are able to determine if yeast are present in a specimen with good predictability; however, speciation does not occur. Additional testing is required to determine comprehensive identification of the organism and initiate antifungal therapy.

Genus and species-specific antigen detection methods are available for common *Candida* pathogens; however, commercially available tests are limited to blood and cerebrospinal fluid specimens. Various platforms in use utilize antigens such as D-arabinitol, α-1,2-oligomannoside, and β-1,2-oligomannan. Studies show reasonable sensitivity and specificity with these assays. Serologic assays for the detection of IgG, IgM, and IgA antibodies to *Candida* species are used in Europe, but are not approved for use in the United States.[5]

Molecular Diagnostic Methods

Molecular diagnostic methods for the detection and identification of *Candida* species have improved and become widely available over the last decade. Several commercially available peptide nucleic acid-fluorescent in situ hybridization (PNA FISH) test kits are available for detection of yeast directly from blood culture.[6] The Yeast Traffic Light PNA FISH assay targets species-specific rRNA sequences, and are able to identify *C. albicans, C. glabrata,* and *C. tropicalis* specifically or yeast species groups. Studies found excellent performance characteristics for this assay.[7]

Another recent FDA-approved assay utilizing molecular methods for detection of *Candida* spp. is the BD Max System vaginitis panel.[6] For many years, vaginitis has been diagnosed using traditional physician examination, bedside manual methods, and vaginal culture, all of which have low sensitivity and are highly subjective. The BD Max System offers users the ability to diagnose bacterial vaginosis, trichomoniasis, and candidiasis from one vaginal swab. Although speciation does not occur, the assay is able to detect the following *Candida* species: *C. albicans, C. tropicalis, C. parapsilosis, C. dublinensis, C. glabrata,* and *C. krusei.* The turnaround time of this assay for all three parameters is approximately 3 hours. When compared with in-clinic tests and clinician diagnosis, the BD Max system was more sensitive.[8] This system is categorized as moderate complexity[6] and is able to analyze multiple assays on one platform.

▶ Cryptococcosis

Etiology

The *Cryptococcus neoformans-Cryptococcus gattii* complex is divided into two species and five **serotypes**. The various serotypes have distinct differences between them, all of which produce illness in humans.[3] For the purpose of this text, *C. neoformans* will be used to describe all serotypes associated with human infections. *C. neoformans* produces a **teleomorph** (sexual) stage known as *Filobasidiella neoformans*. *C. gattii,* once believed to be a variant of *C. neoformans,* is also an agent of human illness but will not be discussed in this text, as immunodiagnostic assays do not specifically identify it.

Epidemiology and Pathogenesis

C. neoformans is widely found in nature as a **saprobe**. It is most associated with excreta of birds, particularly pigeons. The organism has a characteristic polysaccharide capsule, used to aid in initial identification. In dry conditions, the capsule collapses and protects the yeast from desiccation. It is believed to help the yeast survive passage through the intestines of the pigeon before being excreted. When the capsule is collapsed, the resulting reduction in organism size makes it ideal for **aerosolization** and deposition in alveoli. The capsule also contains foreign compounds that phagocytic cells recognize, preventing the organism from being removed through normal immune responses.

The significance of infection and clinical symptoms relies on the host immune status. Immunocompetent individuals, who become colonized with *C. neoformans* in the respiratory tract, may not develop subsequent infection. One study followed patients for as long as 6 years with no signs of infection. In the immunocompromised host, infection usually presents as a chronic or subacute pulmonary infection. Dissemination into the central nervous system resulting in cryptococcal meningitis is common in immunocompromised individuals. Those with disseminated infection may have painless skin lesions that form ulcers. Less commonly, **cryptococcosis** may manifest as endocarditis, hepatitis, renal infection, and pleural effusion. There is a strong association of cryptococcal infection with leukemia, lymphoma, and AIDS.[3]

Conventional Methods

Direct microscopic observation of *C. neoformans* in clinical specimens is traditionally performed using India ink. This rapid, inexpensive assessment tool allows the viewer to observe the polysaccharide capsule, unique to *C. neoformans*, in a clinical specimen. The round yeast are seen with thick walls and a clearing of the India ink around the organism (**FIGURE 11–5**). The capsule is also seen in unstained wet mount preparations; however, the organism is more **refractile** in appearance and may be confused with water or oil droplets to the untrained eye.

   C. neoformans is easily cultured on standard mycology media, although it is susceptible to cycloheximide. Growth is seen within 5 days and begins as a smooth, white to tan colony that is typically mucoid to creamy.[3] Colonies are often described as *Klebsiella*-like due to the large amount of polysaccharide capsule. Identification of colonies may be accomplished using the same manual and automated biochemical panels used for *Cryptococcus* species.

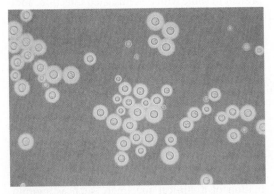

FIGURE 11–5 India ink preparation of *C. neoformans* showing a clearing where the capsule surrounds the organism amid a background of India ink.

Courtesy of Dr. Leanor Haley/CDC.

Immunodiagnostic Methods

Serologic methods for *C. neoformans* detection is of the utmost importance to initiate appropriate antifungal treatment before the individual succumbs to the illness. Serologic assays detecting the cryptococcal antigen capsular galactoxylomannan in serum and cerebrospinal fluid have been available for decades. To reduce the risk of false-positive results, serum specimens are processed to destroy interfering rheumatoid factor. These immunoassays show high sensitivity and specificity once the factor is destroyed. Methods for detecting the antigen are commercially available in a variety of latex agglutination and EIA-based, lateral flow assays.[5] It is recommended that all cerebrospinal fluids are cultured, whether results are positive or negative.

   Serologic methods are not available to detect antibodies against Cryptococcus species in clinical specimens. The time required for antibody production does not warrant the use of assays of this type. By the time antibodies are detectable, disease progresses beyond the ability for effective treatment.

Molecular Diagnostic Methods

Molecular methods are no longer used for the detection of *Cryptococcus*. The same molecular method still used for identification of systemic fungi from culture was once available for definitive identification of *C. neoformans* from cultured isolates. Advances in immunodiagnostics reduced the utility of this highly complex assay and replaced it with more cost-effective, comparable identification systems.

▸ Dimorphic Fungi

The dimorphic fungi are considered slow-growing, requiring an average of 7 to 21 days for visible growth, with some strains appearing as early as 2 to 5 days or as late as 30 days, depending on the amount of colonies present (**FIGURE 11–6**).[3] The most common dimorphic fungi in North America

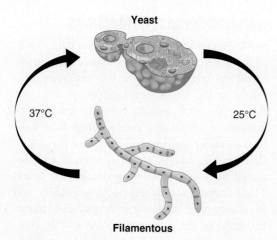

FIGURE 11–6 Dimorphic fungi convert from mold to yeast at 37°C (body temperature) and from yeast to mold at 25°C (room temperature).

are *Blastomyces dermatitidis*, *Histoplasma capsulatum*, and *Coccidioides immitis*, all of which are discussed here. The cultivation of dimorphic fungi is not only slow, it is also challenging to successfully obtain viable mold and yeast forms for definitive identification of these agents. When dimorphic fungi are suspected, cultures must be manipulated in a class II biological safety cabinet to prevent laboratory-acquired infections. Traditionally, dimorphic fungi are definitively identified by the conversion of the mold form to the tissue (yeast) form. In general, the optimal temperature for recovery of the mold form is 25°C to 30°C on standard mycology media. Conversion to the tissue form requires growth of the corresponding yeast on a blood-enriched medium that is incubated at 35°C to 37°C.

▶ Blastomycosis

Etiology

Until recently, the genus *Blastomyces* contained only one species, *B. dermatitidis*. Analysis of isolates has identified a novel species, *B. gilchristii*. Additional genotyping studies have revealed four *B. dermatitidis* strains that show an association with clinical presentation.[9]

Epidemiology and Pathogenesis

B. dermatitidis lives well in the environment, especially in moist soils and decomposing organic matter. In the United States, *B. dermatitidis* is **endemic** in the Midwest, south central, and southeastern states; it is common around the Ohio and Mississippi River valleys, the Great Lakes, and Saint Lawrence River. Infection is obtained after breathing the microscopic fungal spores in the air after activities that disturb the soil. Outbreaks of **blastomycosis** are related to occupational and recreational activities, often near streams and rivers, where exposure to moist soil and decaying vegetation occurs.[9]

Inhalation of *B. dermatitidis* conidia is the typical mode of infection. The incubation period ranges from 4 to 6 weeks.[9] Blastomycosis is seen more often in men than in women.[3] The majority of individuals who breathe in spores do not become symptomatic, while some exhibit only flu-like symptoms. Acute pulmonary blastomycosis presents nonspecifically, similar to symptoms seen with community-acquired pneumonia. Healthy individuals usually recover after 2 to 12 weeks with little to no treatment. Some individuals do not fully recover and develop chronic pulmonary disease or disseminated infection. Extrapulmonary infection is commonly seen in skin and bones; the skin is involved in >70% of cases. Lesions are seen with raised, irregular borders or ulcers present. Osteomyelitis in the spine, ribs, and long bones may present in some with disseminated infection; additionally, arthritis occurs in approximately 10% of individuals. *B. dermatitidis* is rarely an opportunistic pathogen. Individuals most effected are those with compromised immune systems. These individuals have a higher mortality rate than those who are not immunocompromised.[9]

Conventional Methods

Blastomycosis is easily diagnosed when the agent is observed in direct microscopic examination of a clinical specimen, such as sputum, bronchoalveolar lavage fluid, lung biopsies, and skin biopsies. In clinical specimens, *B. dermatitidis* appears as large, spherical yeast with thick walls (**FIGURE 11–7**). They range from 8 μm to 15 μm in

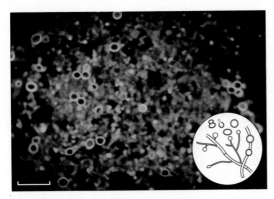

FIGURE 11–7 *B. Dermatitidis* from infected lung tissue, stained with calcofluor white under fluorescent microscopy.

Courtesy of CDC/ Dr. Leo Kaufman.

diameter and have a single bud connected to the parent cell at a broad base.[3]

Cultivation of *B. dermatitidis* requires incubation at 25°C for 5 days to 4 weeks or longer; however, growth can be seen in as little as 2 to 3 days of incubation. Enriched mycology media grows a mold form that initially appears glabrous or waxy and is off-white to white. With age, aerial hyphae are produced and turn gray to brown. On media supplemented with blood, a waxy, yeast-like appearance is typical with hyphae projecting upward from the colonies. Mold-to-yeast conversion typically takes 4 to 5 days when incubated on blood agar at 37°C. Colonies are typically waxy and wrinkled. Cultures can be identified microscopically as *B. dermatitidis* by observation of hyphae that are ropelike and delicate. Conidia are circular to **pyriform** and resemble lollipops on short **conidiophores**. When incubated at 37°C, the yeast form appears microscopically as large, thick-walled yeast cells ranging from 8 to 15 μm in diameter with bud attached at a broad base.[3]

Immunodiagnostic Methods

A search of FDA-approved, commercially available diagnostic tests for the detection and identification of *B. dermatitidis* gives only three results, all of which were approved in 1993. The Exo-Antigen test kit is a classic immunodiffusion method. This

assay is available as a single analyte plate that is able to detect direct antibodies against *B. dermatitidis* or as a panel for up to four antibodies. The identification assay detects antibodies against the "A" antigen of *Blastomyces*. When antibodies are present in the test serum, a line of precipitation is seen indicating such. Titers can be determined and correlated with disease severity. When compared with culture, the immunodiffusion test is positive for *Blastomyces* antibodies in approximately 80% of individuals. When a positive result is obtained, confirmation by complement fixation is not necessary.[10] Complement fixation reagents are available from the same manufacturer.[11] The corresponding complement fixation procedure is based on a complement fixation guide published by the Centers for Disease Control (CDC) in 1965.[12] Immunodiffusion and complement fixation assays are available through other manufacturers. In general, all serologic tests for blastomycosis lack both sensitivity and specificity[9]; however, the ability to obtain a result is much quicker and considered useful for initial screening of infection. Negative results for any serologic method do not rule out infection. All specimens for which a negative serologic result is obtained should be cultured for confirmation.

An antigen detection method for *B. dermatitidis* from direct specimens is available through MiraVista Laboratories. This quantitative sandwich EIA is available for the diagnosis of blastomycosis and monitoring treatment during infection. Specimens acceptable for testing include serum, plasma collected in EDTA, urine, CSF, bronchoalveolar lavage fluid, and other sterile body fluids. All other specimen types are rejected for analysis. The assay is able to detect antigen concentrations as low as 0.2 ng/mL. Cross-reaction is seen with *Histoplasma capsulatum*, *Paracoccidioides brasiliensis*, *Penicillium* spp, and, less frequently, *Coccidioides immitis* and *Aspergillus* spp.[13]

Molecular Diagnostic Methods

There are currently no commercially available molecular methods for the detection of fungal nucleic acids in direct clinical specimens. However, there is a rapid DNA probe test to definitively identify *Blastomyces dermatitidis* isolates from culture. The assay performs nucleic acid hybridization using a single-stranded DNA probe complementary to the RNA target of the fungus.[14] Unfortunately, this assay does require a fresh culture of the fungus for testing. While the reported sensitivity and specificity are high,[14] the time required to culture the isolate initially does not warrant this assay as an effective screening tool for disease.

Histoplasmosis

Etiology

Histoplasma capsulatum is the causative agent of **histoplasmosis**, typically referred to as simply *H. capsulatum*. Historically, it was divided into three varieties based on the geographic location or species in which disease was found. More recent **phylogenetic** studies define at least eight different clads within *H. capsulatum*. Additional phylogenetic species have been identified within the various clads.[9]

Epidemiology and Pathogenesis

Histoplasmosis is one of the most common systemic fungi infections seen in the Midwest and southern United States, including around the Mississippi River, the Ohio River Valley, and the Appalachian Mountains. Infections are seen when inhalation of aerosolized conidia or small hyphal fragments occurs. Numerous infections are reported in individuals who work in or clean old chicken coops or areas where starlings or similar birds have roosted. Birds are not colonized or infected due to their high body temperature. Fungi are released in droppings.[9] Infections are common in spelunkers (cave explorers) who are routinely exposed to aerosolized organisms from bat guano in caves. It is estimated that 500,000 individuals are infected with *H. capsulatum* annually in the United States. The severity of disease is directly related to the inoculum size and the immune status of the host.[3]

Infections with *H. capsulatum* begin in the lungs and eventually invade the reticuloendothelial system. Approximately 95% of infections are asymptomatic or self-limiting. Chronic primary infections do occur, which commonly produce chronic, **granulomatous** infections. Disease can be disseminated throughout the body, primarily through the lymph nodes, liver, spleen, and bone marrow. Infections may occur in the kidneys and meninges, although not as commonly. In an immunocompetent host, infection typically resolves. It is in the immunocompromised host in which progressive disease is found more often.[3]

Conventional Methods

H. capsulatum is often missed when respiratory tract specimens are examined directly. It requires a perceptive technologist to detect the organism in blood or bone marrow when stained with Wright or Giemsa. The tiny oval yeast cells are found intracellularly in mononuclear cells.[3] *H. capsulatum* yeast cells can also be seen in tissue section when stained with Gomori's methylene silver or periodic acid Schiff.[9]

The organisms is easy to culture from clinical specimens; however, bacteria and other rapid growing molds also easily overgrow it. *H. capsulatum* is a slow-growing mold, requiring at least 2 to 4 weeks for colonies to appear. When grown on standard mycology media, colonies are white and fluffy and turn brown to buff with age. Tufts of hyphae, similar to those seen in *B. dermatitidis*, project upward from colonies. Differentiation by colony morphology alone cannot be made between *H. capsulatum* and *B. dermatitidis*. Identification is made by observing colonies microscopically. Hyphae are thin and often intertwined to form ropelike strands. Large macroconidia, produced on conidiophores, are spherical or pyriform and become rough or tuberculate with age (Figure 11–7).[3] Conversion to the yeast phase is difficult and not recommended.

Immunodiagnostic Methods

Serologic tests are most useful for diagnosis of individuals with chronic pulmonary or disseminated histoplasmosis. Detection of antibodies against

H. capsulatum can be accomplished using the same immunodiffusion assay described for *B. dermatitidis*. The assay can detect antibodies to two antigens: "M" and "H." The anti-"M" antibodies appear first in acute pulmonary histoplasmosis and are the basis for clinical diagnosis. The anti-"H" antibodies occur later and less frequently; their appearance is suggestive of extrapulmonary dissemination. Antibodies to "H" antigen are rarely seen without antibodies to "M" antigens. When both antibodies are present, two lines of precipitation are seen. When compared with culture, the immunodiffusion assay is positive in approximately 85 to 94% of sera from histoplasmosis patients. Use of immunodiffusion and complement fixation is effective for specific diagnosis of histoplasmosis.[10] Complement fixation reagents are available from the same manufacturer.[11] The corresponding complement fixation procedure is based on complement fixation guide published by the CDC in 1965.[12] Recent studies have examined the use of various enzyme immunoassays for antigen detection and the use of the cell wall protein (1,3)-β-D-glucan.[15-18] None of these is commercially available for use in the clinical laboratory.

Two immunoassays are currently available for the detection of *H. capsulatum* antigens. MiraVista Laboratories offer an *H. capsulatum* antigen detection method for direct specimens. This quantitative sandwich EIA is available for the diagnosis of histoplasmosis and monitoring treatment during infection. Specimens acceptable for testing include serum, plasma collected in EDTA, urine, CSF, bronchoalveolar lavage fluid, and other sterile body fluids. All other specimen types are rejected for analysis. The assay is able to detect antigen concentrations as low as 0.4 ng/mL. Cross-reaction is seen with *Blastomyces capsulatum*, *Paracoccidioides brasiliensis*, *Penicillium* spp, and, less frequently, *Coccidioides immitis* and *Aspergillus* spp.[19] A well-known single sandwich EIA is commercially available for the detection of *H. capsulatum* antigens in urine specimens only. This microplate assay utilizes rabbit anti-*Histoplasma* IgG antibodies to capture antigens. Results are read and interpreted using a microplate reader at 450 nm. The test is categorized as high complexity. When compared with culture, the assay demonstrates 80.9% sensitivity and 98.7% specificity.[20]

Molecular Diagnostic Methods

There are currently no commercially available molecular methods for the detection of fungal nucleic acids in direct clinical specimens. However, there is a rapid DNA probe test to definitively identify *Histoplasma capsulatum* isolates from culture. The assay performs nucleic acid hybridization using a single stranded DNA probe complementary to the RNA target of the fungus.[21] Unfortunately, this assay does require a fresh culture of the fungus for testing. While the reported sensitivity and specificity are excellent,[21] the time required to culture the isolate initially does not warrant this assay as an effective screening tool for disease.

▶ Coccidioidomycosis

Etiology

There are two recognized species within the genus *Coccidoides*: *C. immitis* and *C. posadasii*. Previously known only as *C. immitis*, this species is now restricted to isolates from California. *C. posadasii* has been proposed for all other isolate belonging to the genus. Some studies show evidence of **hybridization** and genetic interchange between these two species.[9]

Epidemiology and Pathogenesis

Coccidioides species are soil-inhabiting fungi found in the Western Hemisphere in desert regions. In the United States, it is endemic to the Desert Southwest, including central and southern California, southern Arizona, southern New Mexico, parts of Utah, and western Texas. Fungal infections are endemic into northern Mexico and parts of Central and South America.[9] Coccidioidomycosis, also referred to as Valley Fever, is acquired by inhalation of infective

arthroconidia. Environmental exposure is the main risk factor for acquiring infection. Activities that disturb contaminated soil and create dust produce great numbers of infection. These activities include construction, landscaping, farming, and archaeology excavation. Natural disasters such as earthquakes and windstorms create dust clouds and are associated with an increased risk of infection. Large outbreaks have resulted from such natural events. It is not considered contagious; however, occasional transmission has occurred via contaminated fomites and through organ transplant.[9]

More than half of individuals with **coccidioidomycosis** are asymptomatic or have self-limiting respiratory infections. Symptoms are similar to those seen in other community-acquired pneumonias, and include cough, fever, chills, and fatigue. Less than 3% become seriously ill. Dissemination extends to visceral organs, meninges, bone, skin, lymph nodes, and subcutaneous tissues. Dissemination is most common in dark skinned individuals as well as pregnant women.[9] Laboratory-acquired infections with *Coccidioides* spp. are of concern. Fungal cultures and environmental material known to contain arthroconidia should be handled within a class II biological safety cabinet using biosafety level (BLS) 3 practices. Disease is almost always fatal if not treated.

Conventional Methods

Coccidioides spp. are seen microscopically in sputum and other body fluids. They appear as nonbudding, thick-walled spherules that contain granular material or numerous small, nonbudding endospores. They range in size from 20 μm to 200 μm. Endospores are released by rupture of the spherule wall, resulting in empty and "ghost" spherules. Small, immature spherules may be confused with *Histoplasma capsulatum* and *Blastomyces dermatitidis*. When two endospores or immature spherules are seen next to one another, they may appear as a budding yeast.

Isolates of *Coccidioides* spp. grow on routine mycology media, displaying variation in colony morphology. Growth takes anywhere from 3 to 21 days. Macroscopic morphology ranges from moist, glabrous, and grayish to abundant, fluffy, and white. With age, colonies may become tan and even red. Colonies are often delicate due to aerial hyphae. In endemic areas, white fluffy colonies should be opened and manipulated only within a class II BSC using BSL-3 practices, as *Coccidioides* is considered the most infectious of all fungi.

Microscopically, *Coccidioides* show small, septate hyphae seen branching at right angles. As the culture ages, arthroconidia form that are rectangular or barrel-shaped. They are larger than the hyphae from which they come, and are separated by nonviable cells, called **dysjunctor cells**. Viable and nonviable arthroconidia alternate through the length of the hyphae (**FIGURE 11–8**). It is important to definitively identify any suspect colonies as *Coccidioides* because other nonvirulent fungi appear similar macroscopically and microscopically.

Immunodiagnostic Methods

Although other methods are available, such as EIA and latex agglutination, the combination of immunodiffusion and complement fixation is considered the best serologic method for detection of

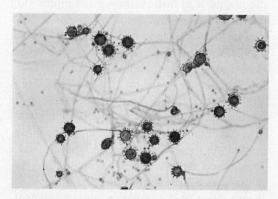

FIGURE 11–8 *H. capsulatum* macroconidia produced from hyphal tips.

Courtesy of Dr. Libero Ajello/CDC.

coccidioidomycosis. The identification assay detects antibodies to two *Coccidioides* antigens, IDTP and IDCF. IDTP antibodies are seen during primary acute infection and belong to the IgM class; IDCF antibodies are identified during the chronic, disseminated phase and are primarily IgG antibodies. When an antibody is present in the test serum, a line of precipitation is seen indicating such. If both antibodies are present in the test serum, two separate lines of precipitation are seen. While visualization of a precipitin line is presumptive for the diagnosis of *Coccidioides*, confirmation must be performed, as individuals often produce detectable antibodies for up to 1 year after recovery from active disease. Cross-reactivity is seen in patients with other systemic fungi, especially *H.* capsulatum. False positive results may be seen in those with cystic fibrosis.[10] Complement fixation reagents are available from the same manufacturer.[11] The corresponding complement fixation procedure is based on the complement fixation guide published by the Centers for Disease Control (CDC) in 1965.[12]

Assays are available for the detection of *Coccidioides* antigens. MiraVista Laboratories offer a *C. immitis* antigen detection method for direct specimens. This quantitative sandwich EIA is available for the diagnosis of coccidioidomycosis and monitoring treatment during infection. Specimens acceptable for testing include serum, plasma collected in EDTA, urine, CSF, broncho-alveolar lavage fluid, and other sterile body fluids. All other specimen types are rejected for analysis. The assay is able to detect antigen concentrations as low as 0.7 ng/mL. Cross-reaction is seen with *Blastomyces capsulatum, Paracoccidioides brasiliensis,* and *Histoplasma capsulatum.*[22]

Molecular Diagnostic Methods

Molecular methods for direct detection of *Coccidioides* in patient specimens were not available until recently. At the end of 2017, the FDA cleared a high-complexity, rapid-detection immunoassay, DxNA's GeneStat.MDx *Coccidioides* test performed on the GeneSTAT System. This system is able to

definitively diagnose both species of *Coccidioides* directly from patient specimens.[23] This multi-facility collaboration appears to be a promising detection method for coccidioidomycosis diagnosis.

Additionally, a rapid DNA probe test to identify *Coccidioides immitis* isolates from culture is commercially available. The assay performs nucleic acid hybridization using a single-stranded DNA probe complementary to the RNA target of the fungus.[24] This assay requires a fresh culture of the fungus for testing. While the reported sensitivity and specificity are high,[24] the time required to culture the isolate initially does not warrant this assay as an effective screening tool for disease.

▶ Parasitic Infections

Parasitic infections are found throughout the world. Although they are typically associated with tropical climates, many parasites that infect humans are distributed with some frequency in temperate zones. Additionally, an increase in world travel over the last decades has led to individuals arriving to their home country requiring medical attention for parasitic diseases that were once considered unlikely. An increase in the number of **immunocompromised** and **immunodeficient** patients has also lead to an increase in the need for parasite-detection methods.

Identification of parasites traditionally requires the observation of the parasite itself or its eggs in the specimen submitted. Parasites are capable of infecting humans and causing disease via numerous routes. Specimens submitted to the laboratory for parasite examination include, but are not limited to, feces, blood, body fluids, tissue, respiratory specimens, and urine. Challenges exist throughout the entire process of parasite identification from specimen collection to specimen processing, to the physical evaluation of suspected parasites. The field of parasitology is generally considered a specialized area within the clinical laboratory, and one of the areas in which a decrease in skilled technologists is observed. The ova and parasite examination is a manual method that is widely considered the method of choice for identifying intestinal parasites. This method is time consuming and technical in nature. While a comprehensive ova and parasite examination will increase the probability of identifying any parasite that the individual may harbor, the variety of parasites normally seen in the United States is quite small. Rapid immunodiagnostic methods are now available to diagnose the most often seen parasitic infections. To fully appreciate the availability of these immunodiagnostic methods, one must first become familiar with the comprehensive ova and parasite examination.

▶ Ova and Parasite Examination

The ova and parasite examination is the gold standard for identifying parasites in fecal specimens. Specimens should be collected and transported to the laboratory as soon as possible. Traditionally, three specimens, collected over 7 to 10 days, were recommended for examination before ruling out intestinal parasites. Recent updates from the Infectious Disease Society of America (ISDA) offer a more cost-effective option for testing. A second specimen is examined only when the first one is negative and the patient remains symptomatic, and a third one is examined if symptoms continue with negative test results.[25] Fresh specimens immediately submitted to the laboratory are examined by wet-mount preparations for viable, moving organisms. If any delay occurs before processing, the specimen must be preserved appropriately. There are a number of commercially available stool preservatives. Conventional preservation methods include a two-vial system that utilizes one vial with 10% formalin and one vial with polyvinyl alcohol (PVA). Ten percent formalin is considered an all-purpose fixative; however, it is not suitable for permanent slides stained with trichrome. PVA is a good preservative of morphology of protozoan **trophozoites** and **cysts**; however, it is inadequate for preserving

the morphology of **helminth eggs** and **larvae**, **coccidian**, and **microsporidia**. This two-vial system requires twice the amount of specimen, two processing steps, and twice the amount of reagent. In response to streamlining needs, a single-vial system is now available. This single vial contains sodium acetate-acetic acid-formalin (SAF), which is suitable for concentration techniques and permanently stained slides with trichrome, safranin, acid fast, and **chromotrope** stains. SAF is also compatible with many immunodiagnostic assays.

The ova and parasite examination begins with inspecting the specimen macroscopically for worms, **proglottids**, blood, and mucous. Any parasites or fragments seen must be removed and identified separately from the processed specimen. Routine microscopic examination of fecal specimens for ova and parasites consists of two distinct procedures: fecal concentration with wet mount preparation, and permanently stained fecal smear. The concentration procedure separates parasite from fecal debris, increasing the chance of detecting parasitic organisms. The sedimentation technique is the most commonly used fecal concertation method in the clinical laboratory. Specimens processed for fecal concentration are preserved in 10% formalin or SAF. Approximately 3 to 5mL of preserved specimen is mixed with 8 mL of normal saline and "washed" by centrifugation. After decanting the saline, the remaining fecal pellet is mixed with formalin and ethyl acetate. Centrifugation leaves four distinct layers: ethyl acetate, fecal debris, formalin, and the sediment containing parasites. The fecal debris is removed and the ethyl acetate and formalin are decanted. The remaining sediment is mixed with a small amount of formalin for preservation. This solution is then placed on a slide, mixed with a drop of iodine, cover slipped, and scanned under $10\times$ objective for protozoan trophozoites, cysts, **oocysts**, and helminth eggs. Coverslips may be sealed for preservation; however, preserved wet mounts do not retain stability for as long as permanently stained slides.

The second procedure in the ova and parasite examination is the permanently stained fecal smear. Specimens used for creation of permanent slides are preserved in PVA or SAF. If a specimen is preserved in SAF, the permanent slide(s) should be made prior to performing the fecal concentration. Slides are made by placing two to three drops of the specimen on a slide, and a wooden applicator stick is used to spread the specimen evenly with a rolling motion or an up-and-down dabbing motion. The slide is air dried completely before staining. The most commonly used stain is a trichrome stain, which requires the slide to be passed through a series of reagents beginning with ethanol, then the trichrome stain solution, acidified ethanol, 100% ethanol, and finally xylene or toluene. The slide can be permanently sealed using a mounting medium and coverslip for preservation. Modified iron-hematoxylin stain, modified acid-fast stain, and calcofluor white stain are all suitable for use with prepared smears; refer to the reagent for preservative compatibility.

All specimens, whether concentrated and stained with iodine, permanently made and stained with trichrome, or blood smears stained with Wright-Giemsa, are scanned under 10× objective and examined closer for morphology under 40× objective: 100× and 400× total magnification, respectively. Blood smears for malaria and microfilaria are examined for morphology under 100× objective, 1000× total magnification.

Cryptosporidium
Etiology

Cryptosporidium spp. are intracellular parasites of the phylum Apicomplexa, also known as sporozoa. These parasites primarily infect the epithelial cells of the stomach, intestine, and biliary ducts. There are more than 20 different species of *Cryptosporidium*, two of which infect humans. Once only known as *C. parvum,* the *Cryptsporidium* species thought to primarily infect humans, are now classified into two species: *C. parvum,* infecting mammals including humans; and *C. hominis,* primarily infecting humans. Differentiation between these two species cannot be performed based on oocyst morphology alone.[3] For the purpose of this chapter, the human infecting *Cryptosporidium* spp. will be referred to as *Cryptosporidium* spp.

Cryptosporidium oocysts are small, measuring just 4 μm to 6 μm in diameter. Infection begins with ingestion of these oocysts. In response to contact with gastric and duodenal fluids, each oocyst releases four **sporozoites**. These sporozoites invade duodenal epithelial cells and develop into trophozoites. Here, the trophozoites undergo a few generations of asexual amplification, known as merogony. This results in the formation of different meronts, each containing 4 to 8 **merozoites**. The merozoites then differentiate by gametogony into sexually distinct stages. This process ultimately forms new oocysts in the epithelial cells through a process called sporogony. Of the newly formed oocysts, approximately 20% are thin-walled and may **excyst** in the digestive tract causing autoinfection and the formation of new cells; the remaining 80% are excreted into the environment.[3] Oocysts of *Cryptosporidium* spp. are environmentally durable, resistant to low temperatures, high salinity, and most disinfectants, including bleach.

Epidemiology and Pathogenesis

Infections with *C. parvum* occur worldwide and are not limited to tropical climates or areas with sanitation challenges, as many other parasites are. It is estimated that *Cryptosporidium* spp. cause over 64 million illnesses annually.[26] Cryptosporidiosis is acquired through several routes, such as direct contact with infected people or consumption of infected food or water. Children under the age of 5 years are primarily infected in developing countries where hygiene and sanitation practices are not sufficient. In developed countries, infections are seen in older children due to later exposure to environmental conditions. Infections are also seen in the elderly where transmission occurs from person to person in nursing homes. In the general public, sporadic infections occur when individuals consume infected food or water. Cryptosporidiosis is common in individuals who are immunocompromised, such as those with AIDS, primary immunodeficiency, cancer, and transplant patients.[3]

When outbreaks of cryptosporidiosis are seen in developed countries, typically there is a source that explains the presence of the parasites. For example, in 1993, a waterborne outbreak of cryptosporidiosis occurred in Milwaukee, Wisconsin. This was the largest outbreak of cryptosporidiosis from a contaminated public water source reported in the United States.[27] An estimated 419,000 residents of the greater Milwaukee area became ill, 26% of the population at the time.[28] The outbreak resulted when an ineffective filtration process did not adequately remove *Cryptosporidium* oocysts from the one of two municipal water treatment plants. The total cost of illness associated with this outbreak was approximately $96.2 million; $31.7 million in direct medical costs and $64.6 million in lost productivity.[27] Information obtained from this outbreak identified the ineffectiveness of chlorine bleach to remove *Cryptosporidium* oocysts and the need for filtration systems with smaller pores.

Conventional Methods

Using traditional ova and parasite procedures, the oocysts of *Cryptosporidium* become challenging to see. They are small and are easily misidentified as yeast cells in wet mount preparations. On occasion, sporozoites are seen inside the oocyst, but that is rare. When stained with trichrome, results are variable and the oocysts often appear as "ghost" cells. Yeast pick up trichrome stain better than oocyts, directing the observer's eyes to them and away from oocysts in the slide (**FIGURE 11-9**).[29] Modified acid-fast stain is the method of choice when cryptosporidiosis is suspected. Oocysts are considered partially acid-fast and pick up this primary stain more sufficiently than the non–acid-fast trichrome stain. Oocysts stained magenta stand out against the blue-green background, and are more apparent than in a trichrome-stained slide (**FIGURE 11-10**). When the technologist does not know that cryptosporidiosis is suspected, specimens are not initially stained with a modified acid-fast and may be easily missed by the inexperienced eye.

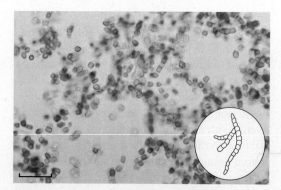

FIGURE 11-9 Large barrel-shaped arthroconidia of *C. immitis.*
Courtesy of CDC/ Lucille Georg.

Immunodiagnostic Methods

Immunodiagnostic methods for the detection of *Cryptosporidium* oocysts in fecal specimens were FDA-approved for use in the mid-1990s. The first assays employed spectrophotometric or visual detection methods and were all considered high-complexity testing. Since then, testing

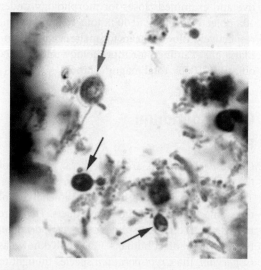

FIGURE 11-10 Ova and parasite examination of fecal specimen, stained with trichrome. *Cryptosporidium* spp. oocysts (red arrow) may be detected but should be confirmed by better methods. Yeast (blue arrows) take trichrome stain more sufficiently and stain darker than oocysts.

Courtesy of Centers for Disease Control and Prevention. Cryptosporidiosis. DPDx – Laboratory Identification of Parasites of Public Health Concern. Accessed at https://www.cdc.gov/dpdx/cryptosporidiosis/index.html

capabilities have improved and turnaround times have decreased. Rapid chromatographic immunoassays that detect *Cryptosporidium* utilize sample wicking to move the specimen along a membrane containing capture antibody stripes. If present, immune complexes on the surface of the oocysts combine with the antibodies attached to the membrane, resulting in a visible line to indicate the presence of oocysts.[30–33] These rapid assays produce results in as little as 15 minutes[30,31,33] to as long as 30 minutes.[32] Specimens submitted for testing may range from fresh stool to those preserved with Cary-Blair, 10% formalin, or SAF. PVA is not compatible with many rapid immunodiagnostic methods.[30,31,33] While the technical time and knowledge required for an individual to perform these assays is minimal, and reminiscent of many CLIA-waived rapid assays, these methods are categorized as moderate complexity under CLIA designation.[34] The rapid assays are simple to interpret. Although each assay has unique aesthetic characteristics, each must contain an internal control that indicates the assay was performed correctly, as well as test result indicators for each analyte tested. Performance characteristics of rapid Cryptosporidium immunoassays, when compared with microscopy, show sensitivities ranging from 96 to 100%[30–33] and specificities ranging from 98 to 100%.[30,31,33] Rapid immunodiagnostic methods for *Cryptosporidium* spp. are available in a single-analyte format as well as a multi-analyte format, combined with *Giardia duodenalis* and even *Entamoeba histolytica/dispar.*

Solid-phase enzyme immunoassays (EIA) are available for detection of *Cryptosporidium* oocysts in fecal specimens. These EIA methods employ monoclonal antibodies to *Cryptosporidium* spp. specific oocyst-surface antigens. Similar to the rapid immunodiagnostic tests, specimens approved for testing include fresh or frozen stool, and those preserved in Cary-Blair, 10% formalin, or SAF. PVA is not compatible.[35,36] Higher level technical knowledge and skills are required for the rapid immunoassays; therefore, the EIA methods are categorized as high complexity under CLIA designation.[34] These assays require multiple reagents and wash steps during the test performance. The entire process takes from 2 to 3 hours to complete, depending on the number of specimens tested. Results must be read and interpreted using a microplate reader capable of measuring at 450 nm. Controls must also be tested with each batch of patient sample,[35,36] leading to a batched testing protocol for many laboratories. Performance characteristics, when compared with microscopy, are reported with sensitivities of 93 to 99% and specificities of 99 to 100%.[10,11] These assays are often available in single-analyte and multi-analyte forms, as seen with the rapid immunoassays.

Microscopy-based direct immunofluorescent (DFA) methods are used in some laboratories; however, these immunoassays require a fluorescent microscope for the detection and interpretation of results. FITC-labeled monoclonal antibodies directed against *Cryptosporidium* oocysts are used. After multiple incubation and wash steps, slides are cover slipped with mounting media and examined under a fluorescent microscope equipped with a FITC filter system (**FIGURE 11–11**). Specimens should be preserved

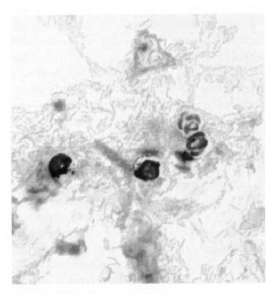

FIGURE 11–11 Modified acid-fast stain of fecal specimen. *Cryptosporidium* spp. oocysts stain magenta against a blue-green background. Sporozoites may be seen inside oocysts.

in 10% formalin or SAF. Fresh specimens and those preserved in PVA are not appropriate for DFA methods. As with the EIA methods, controls must be tested with each batch of patients. When compared with acid-fast staining, the reported sensitivity and specificity for identification of *Cryptosporidium* oocysts are 92% and 85%, respectively.[37] Due to the technical nature of these assays, they are categorized by CLIA as high complexity.[34]

At this time, assays for the detection of *Cryptosporidium*-specific antibodies in serum are not recommended due to a lack of sensitivity and specificity. Serologic tests for *Cryptosporidium*-specific antibodies are limited to reference laboratories and state and national laboratories. They should be used only for epidemiologic purposes.[38]

Molecular Methods

Molecular methods for the detection and speciation of *Cryptosporidium* spp. are not commonly used in the clinical laboratory. Testing is available through most commercial reference laboratories and the CDC. Specimens for most tests require fresh specimens or ones preserved in PVA.[38]

In 2013, the first molecular platform was approved by the FDA to simultaneously detect multiple gastrointestinal infectious agents, including *Cryptosporidium* spp. More recently, the Biofire FilmArray gastrointestinal panel from BioFire Diagnostics offered an FDA-approved molecular method for the detection of 22 targets of gastrointestinal infection, including bacteria, viruses, and parasites. *Cryptosporidium* spp. is included as one of the four parasites detected. The FilmArray performs traditional nucleic acid purification using chemical and bead methods, two rounds of polymerase chain reaction (PCR), with the first round including reverse transcription, and DNA melting analysis. The FilmArray software interprets results. Specimens must be collected in Cary Blair transport media,[39] which requires a separate specimen if traditional ova and parasite tests are required. This high complexity

test[40] requires a well-trained, knowledgeable technologist to perform the test and obtain accurate results. The panel contains two assays for the detection of *Cryptosporidium* spp. It is able to detect approximately 23 different species of *Cryptosporidium*, including *C. hominis* and *C. parvum*, the most common in human infections, as well as several less-common species. The assay does not differentiate species; results are reported as: *Cryptosporidium* detected. When compared with PCR with bi-directional sequencing, performance characteristics for the detection of *Cryptosporidium* in clinical specimens are as follows: 81 to 100% positive predictive value (PPV) and 99.2 to 99.9% negative predictive value (NPV).[39]

With the immunodiagnostic methods available to detect *Cryptosporidium* spp., a negative result does not indicate an absence of infection. As with all immunodiagnostic methods, if the specimen contains parasites below the lower limit of detection, or if the specimen is not preserved or processed appropriately, a false-negative result may be seen.

▶ Giardia

Etiology

Giardia dudenalis, formerly *G. lamblia*, is the most common cause of intestinal infections worldwide. It is estimated to cause more than 280 million diarrheal infections annually.[41] *G. duodenalis* is a single-cell protozoa found in the division Mastigophora, or **flagellates**. Flagellates have specialized locomotor organelles that are long, thin, cytoplasmic extensions known as **flagella**. These flagella allow the parasite to move easily throughout the intestinal tract.

The life cycle of *G. duodenalis* includes both a trophozoite form and a cyst form. Trophozoites divide by fission, producing two daughter trophozoites. The trophozoites are most often found in the crypts of the duodenum where they attach by means of a ventral disk to the epithelium of duodenal villi. This attachment is strong enough that an impression print remains when the organism detaches from the epithelium. Epithelial cells slough from the tip of the villi every 72 hours, at which time *G. duodenalis* detach from the villi. Trophozoites may reattach at another location or are excreted. The formation of cysts takes place as the trophozoites move through the jejunum after exposure to biliary secretions. Trophozoites retract their flagella into the **axonemes**. The cytoplasm becomes condensed and the cyst wall is secreted. The internal structure doubles as the cyst matures. When excystation occurs in the duodenum or culture medium, the cytoplasm divides, resulting in two trophozoites.[3]

Epidemiology and Pathogenesis

Infections with *Giardia duodenalis* occur after ingestion of viable cysts. Cysts may be encountered through contaminated food or water, or from intimate contact with an infected individual via fecal-oral routes. **Giardiasis** is found more frequently in children or in groups living in close quarters. Outbreaks have also been associated with poor sanitation or sanitation breakdowns. Occupations with exposure to sewage, such as sanitation workers and irrigation workers, correlate with a higher risk of exposure to the parasite and, therefore, increased cases of giardiasis are seen in this population. Cases of giardiasis are more prevalent in warmer climates;[29] however, some evidence suggests an association with cooler, wetter months.[3] While these data are limited, they suggest an environmental condition that is advantageous to the survival of cysts.

Giardiasis typically has an incubation period ranging from 12 to 20 days with disease lasting from 1 to 3 weeks. However, the infection is not always recognized as giardiasis because it often mimics acute viral enteritis, bacillary dysentery, food poisoning, acute intestinal **amoebiasis**, and even traveler's diarrhea caused by nontoxigenic *Escherichia coli*. Individuals may also have an asymptomatic infection where the trophozoites feed on intestinal mucous secretions but do not penetrate the mucosa. Parasites found in the crypts of the duodenal mucosa may reach high numbers but do not cause a pathological condition.[3]

More recognizable are the symptoms of acute intestinal disease. Symptomatic patients present with nausea, anorexia, malaise, low-grade fever and chills. Individuals often have sudden onset of explosive, watery, foul-smelling diarrhea. Other symptoms may include epigastric pain, flatulence, and increased amounts of fat and mucous in diarrhea, with an absence of blood[3] typically seen in other diarrhea-causing diseases. These symptoms often lead to weight loss. Acute diarrhea, associated with giardiasis, is often a major cause of death in young children in developing countries. An extensive meta-analysis showed no statistical evidence of an association between acute diarrhea and *G. duodenalis* parasite load in children over the age of 5 years. The study did suggest that giardiasis in infancy (<1 year old) has higher prevalence of acute diarrhea when compared with *G. duodenalis* parasite load in older children.[42]

Chronic or subacute disease often follows the acute intestinal disease. Individuals experience recurrent, brief episodes of loose, foul-smelling stools, increased distension, and foul flatulence. Between these episodes, the individual may have normal stools or even constipation. Belching may occur with a taste of rotten eggs. Chronic disease presents similarly to other conditions and must be differentiated from amoebiasis, other intestinal parasites including *Dientamoeba fragilis, Cryptosporidium* spp., *Cyclospora cayetanesis,* and *Strongyloides stercoralis,* inflammatory bowel diseases, and irritable colon. Symptoms of chronic disease, such as upper intestinal discomfort, heartburn, and belching, require differentiation from duodenal ulcer, hiatal hernia, gallbladder disease, and pancreatic disease.[3] The same meta-analysis that examined the association with acute diarrhea and *G. duodenalis* showed a strong association between persistent diarrhea and *G. duodenalis* parasite load in children of all ages.[42]

Conventional Methods

The traditional method for identification of *Giardia duodenalis* in fecal specimens is the ova and parasite examination. As an intestinal parasite, the specimen of choice is feces; however, multiple fecal specimens are needed to ensure identification of the parasites. The organism is securely attached to the duodenal mucosa and tends to be passed in a cyclic fashion. It may take up to six specimens, collected over multiple days, to observe the parasites.[3] The Entero-Test capsule is available to help recover the parasites. *G. duodenalis* may also be recovered from duodenal aspirates and bronchoalveolar lavage fluid.

The cyst and trophozoite forms of *G. duodenalis* are recoverable in fresh fecal specimens. Cysts are seen in both iodine-stained, wet-mount preparations and fixed slides stained with trichrome. The cysts of *G. duodenalis* are oval or elliptical, and measure 8 to 19 μm. Nuclei and fibrils are noticeable in both specimen preparations. Mature cysts have four nuclei, while immature cysts have two nuclei. The location and visibility of the nuclei and fibrils sometimes result in a cyst with the appearance of a smiling face. The trophozoites are also visible in both iodine-stained, wet-mount preparations and fixed slides stained with trichrome; however the trichrome slides are better preparation for visualizing this form. Trophozoites are pear- or balloon-shaped and measure 10 to 20 μm in length. In a trichrome-stained slide, the two large nuclei are usually visible, along with the ventral disk used to attach to the duodenal mucosa, median bodies, and up to eight flagella (**FIGURE 11−12**).[29] The overall shape of *G. duodenalis* trophozoites may be seen in a wet mount, but the internal structures are often too faint to observe. In a fresh specimen, forward movement may be observed if the trophozoites are still viable.

Immunodiagnostic Methods

The advent of immunodiagnostic methods for detection of *G. duodenalis* in fecal specimens has greatly increased the sensitivity of detection and reduced the time number of specimens needed to do so. Immunodiagnostic methods for the detection of *Giardia* cysts and trophozoites generally mirror those of *Cryptosporidium* oocysts; FDA-approved immunodiagnostic methods became available for use in the mid-1990s. The first group of assays employed spectrophotometric or

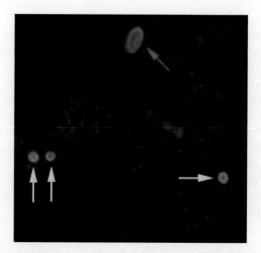

FIGURE 11−12 Oocysts of *Cryptosporidium* spp. (yellow arrows) and trophozoites of *Giardia duodenalis* (red arrow) stained with labeled immunofluorescent antibodies.

Courtesy of Centers for Disease Control and Prevention. Cryptosporidiosis. DPDx − Laboratory Identification of Parasites of Public Health Concern. Accessed at https://www.cdc.gov/dpdx/cryptosporidiosis/index.html

visual detection methods, and all were considered high complexity testing. As with many immunodiagnostic methods for parasitology, testing capabilities have improved and turnaround times have decreased. Rapid chromatographic immunoassays that detect *Giardia* utilize sample wicking to move the specimen along a membrane containing capture antibody stripes. If *Giardia* cysts or trophozoites are present, anti-*Giardia*-specific antibodies in the immunoassay will capture the parasite by binding with target antigens on its surface, resulting in a visible line to indicate the presence of parasites in the specimen.[30-33] These rapid assays produce results in as little as 15 minutes[30,31,33] to as long as 30 minutes.[32] Specimens submitted for testing may range from fresh stool to those preserved with Cary-Blair, 10% formalin, or SAF. PVA is not compatible with many rapid immunodiagnostic methods.[30,31,33] Despite the minimal technical time and knowledge required for an individual to perform these assays, they are categorized as moderate complexity under CLIA designation.[43] The rapid assays are simple to interpret. Although each assay has unique aesthetic characteristics, each must contain an internal control that indicates the assay was performed correctly, as well as test result indicators for each analyte tested. Performance characteristics of rapid *Giardia* immunoassays, when compared with microscopy, show sensitivities ranging from 89 to 100%[30–33] and specificities ranging from 97 to 100%.[30,31,33] Rapid immunodiagnostic methods for *Giardia* spp. are available in a single analyte format as well as a multi-analyte format, combined with *Cryptosporidium* spp. and *Entamoeba histolytica/dispar.*

As seen with *Cryptosporidium*, EIAs are available for detection of *Giardia* cysts and trophozoites in fecal specimens. These EIA methods employ monoclonal antibodies to cell-surface antigens of *Giardia* spp. Similar to the rapid immunodiagnostic tests, specimens approved for testing include fresh or frozen stool, and those preserved in Cary-Blair, 10% formalin, or SAF. PVA is not compatible.[35,36] Higher level knowledge and skills are required for the rapid immunoassays; therefore, the EIA methods are categorized as high complexity under CLIA designation.[43] These assays require multiple reagents and wash steps during test performance. The entire process takes from 2 to 3 hours to complete, depending on the number of specimens tested. Results must be read and interpreted using a microplate reader capable of measuring at 450 nm. Controls must also be tested with each batch of patient sample,[35,36] leading to a batched testing protocol for many laboratories. Performance characteristics, when compared with microscopy, are reported with sensitivities of 94 to 99% and specificities of 95 to 100%.[10,11] These assays are often available in single-analyte and multi-analyte forms, as seen with the rapid immunoassays.

Microscopy-based direct immunofluorescent (DFA) methods are used in some laboratories; however, these immunoassays require a fluorescent microscope for the detection and interpretation of results. FITC-labeled monoclonal antibodies directed against *Giardia* cyst cell-wall antigens are used. After multiple incubation and wash steps, slides are cover slipped with mounting media and examined under a fluorescent microscope equipped with a FITC

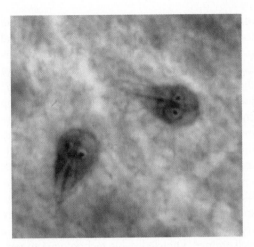

FIGURE 11–13 Trophozoite of *G. duodenalis* with Kohn stain. Two large nuclei, ventral disk, median bodies, and flagella may be seen.

Courtesy of Centers for Disease Control and Prevention. Giardiasis. DPDx – Laboratory Identification of Parasites of Public Health Concern. Accessed at https://www.cdc.gov/dpdx/giardiasis/index.html

filter system (**FIGURE 11–13**). Specimens should be preserved in 10% formalin or SAF. Fresh specimens and those preserved in PVA are not appropriate for DFA methods. As with the EIA methods, controls must be tested with each batch of patients. When compared to traditional concentration methods and stained with iodine, the reported sensitivity and specificity for identification of *Giardia* cysts are 95% and 100%, respectively.[37] Due to the technical nature of these assays, they are categorized by CLIA as high complexity.[43]

Molecular Methods

Molecular methods for the detection and speciation of *Cryptosporidium* spp. are not commonly used in the clinical laboratory. Testing is available through most commercial reference laboratories and the CDC. Specimens for most tests require fresh specimens or ones preserved in PVA.[38]

In 2013, the first molecular platform approved by the FDA to simultaneously detect multiple gastrointestinal infectious agents, including *Giardia duodenalis*. More recently, the BioFire FilmArray gastrointestinal panel from BioFire Diagnostics offered an FDA-approved molecular method for the detection of 22 targets of gastrointestinal infection, including bacteria, viruses, and parasites. *Giardia duodenalis* is included as one of the four parasites detected. The FilmArray performs traditional nucleic-acid purification using chemical and bead methods, two rounds of polymerase chain reaction (PCR), with the first round including reverse transcription, and DNA melting analysis. The FilmArray software interprets results. Specimens must be collected in Cary-Blair transport media,[39] which requires a separate specimen if traditional ova and parasite tests are required. This high-complexity test[40] requires a well-trained, knowledgeable technologist to perform the test and obtain accurate results. The panel contains a single assay for the detection of *Giardia duodenalis,* as this is the only species to cause infections in humans. When compared with PCR with bidirectional sequencing, performance characteristics for the detection of *Giardia duodenalis* in clinical specimens are as follows: 83.2 to 100% positive predictive value (PPV) and 99.1 to 99.8% negative predictive value (NPV).[39]

With the immunodiagnostic methods available to detect *Giardia duodenalis*, a negative result does not indicate an absence of infection. As with all immunodiagnostic methods, if the specimen contains parasites below the lower limit of detection, or if the specimen is not preserved or processed appropriately, a false-negative result may be seen.

▶ Toxoplasmosis

Etiology

Toxoplasma gondii are protozoan parasites that infect humans and cause a disease known as **toxoplasmosis**. Cats are the only known definitive host of *T. gondii* sexual stages. *T. gondii* oocysts are most often acquired through exposure of feces from infected cats of the family *Felidae*. They serve as the main reservoir for human infections. Cats shed noninfective oocysts, which become infective 1 to 5 days after excretion. Oocysts are resistant to disinfectants, freezing

and drying, and can survive in the environment for several months to more than a year.[3] Oocysts are then transmitted to humans through direct ingestion of infected food or water or through exposure to feline feces.[44]

T. gondii has three infectious stages: tachyzoites, bradyzoites, and sporozoites. Tachyzoites are found in blood specimens and therefore are best identified using Giemsa-stained smears of EDTA collected blood. They are crescent-shaped and 2 to 3 μm wide by 4 to 8 μm long with one end more rounded than the other. The nucleus is large and is seen near the more rounded end.[44] Tachyzoites are seen in early, more acute phases of infection and multiply rapidly in any cell of the intermediate host, including many animals and humans, and the nonintestinal epithelial cells of the definitive host, the cat.[3]

Tachyzoites develop into bradyzoites. Bradyzoites are found within tissue cysts and multiply slowly. Cysts may contain few to hundreds of bradyzoites[3] and usually range from 5 to 50 μm in diameter,[44] with some cysts found intramuscularly reaching 100 μm in size.[3] Cysts are commonly seen in brain, eye, skeletal, and cardiac muscle; visceral organs such as lung, liver, and kidneys may contain cysts. Cysts form in chronic infection and are strongly positive by periodic acid Schiff stain (PAS). In acute phases, clusters of tachyzoites may resemble bradyzoite cysts, but they are not PAS positive.[3]

Sporozoites are found in the feces of cats and not seen in human infections.

Epidemiology and Pathogenesis

Toxoplasmosis is one of the most common human infections throughout the world. In some populations, more than 60% of individuals have been infected with *T. gondii*. In the United States, it is estimated that at least 11% of individuals 6 years of age or older have been infected. Transmission from person to person is rarely seen, and then only in cases of mother-to-child, blood transfusion, or organ transplant. Humans typically become infected either by a foodborne route or zoonotic transmission.[45] As tachyzoites grow, they begin to invade adjacent cells, creating more lesions. Formed cysts are able to disseminate through the lymphatic system and the bloodstream to other tissues.[3] Foodborne transmission occurs when humans eat tissue cysts containing bradyzoites from undercooked or contaminated pork, lamb, venison, or shellfish. Unpasteurized goat milk may contain tachyzoites that are transmitted to humans when consumed.[45]

Cats, as the only known definitive host, play an important role in transmission of *T. gondii* to humans. Cats become infected upon eating rodents, birds, or small animals that harbor the parasite. It is important to note that cats are not naturally infected with *T. gondii*. Domestic cats that remain indoors and do not have the opportunity to catch and consume infected animals will not become a source for toxoplasmosis. Domestic cats that are allowed outside have a greater probability of becoming infected and transmitting *T. gondii* to humans. Infection can occur through accidental ingestion of oocysts while cleaning a litter box, accidental ingestion after touching anything that came in contact with cat feces, accidental ingestion of oocysts in contaminated soil, or drinking contaminated water.[45]

When seen in an immunocompetent individual, toxoplasmosis is generally asymptomatic during acute infection. Only 10 to 20% of individuals may develop cervical lymphadenopathy and a flu-like illness. Symptoms often resolve within weeks to months and are self-limiting at most; many describe illness as nothing more than a common cold. Immunocompromised individuals, such as those with AIDS, Hodgkin disease, non-Hodgkin lymphomas, leukemias, tumors, and organ transplants can have severe complications. More than half of these patients with toxoplasmosis show altered mental state, motor impairment, seizures, and other neurologic problems. Reactivation of latent toxoplasmosis or acute primary infection may occur from transplanted organs received from donors previously exposed to *T. gondii*.[3]

Congenital infections, especially during the first and second trimester, can be severe. Studies suggest that oocysts are the predominant route of transmission of *T. gondii* in pregnant women in the United States.[46] Symptoms are seen at birth or soon after, and may include retinochoroiditis, cerebral calcification, hydrocephalus, or microcephaly. As prevention of congenital toxoplasmosis, pregnant women are advised to refrain from contact with feline feces or any source that may be contaminated with feline feces. If infection is suspected in the mother, accurate diagnosis and treatment is imperative to reduce the severity of disease in the infant.[3]

Conventional Methods

T. gondii parasites are not seen in fecal specimens; therefore, traditional ova and parasite examination for parasites is not appropriate for toxoplasmosis infections. Tachyzoites and bradyzoites of *T. gondii* may be seen in a variety of tissues, the buffy coat of EDTA collected blood, cerebrospinal fluid, and even bronchoalveolar lavage fluid. However, specimens must be collected appropriately, processed, and identified using Giemsa-stained slides. These methods are highly complex in technique and rarely performed in the clinical laboratory. Tissue biopsies may be processed in the histology laboratory and examined by pathologists for diagnosis.

Immunodiagnostic Methods

There are four groups of people in which it is critical to diagnose toxoplasmosis: pregnant women with infection during gestation, congenitally infected newborns, individuals with chorioretinitis, and the immunocompromised. Interpreting serologic results for IgG and IgM antibodies for individuals greater than 1 year of age follows an algorithm that can be found at the CDC DPDx resource for toxoplasmosis.[44]

The most common methods for the diagnosis of toxoplasmosis are serologic assays for *T. gondii*-specific antibodies. Serologic identification of toxoplasmosis began in 1941 when Sabin and Feldman discovered that the parasites could be stained with methylene blue in serum specimens.[47] Since then, many different serologic methods have been used in clinical laboratories for *T. gondii* antibody detection. The EIA, ELISA, and IFA methods used for detecting antibodies are well described and have been used for decades.[48] These moderate and high-complexity assays detect both IgG and IgM antibodies against *T. gondii* and are available as both manual and automated test kits. Immunoassays are now widely available on large analyzers and as part of panels to detect congenital infections.[49]

Molecular Methods

Molecular methods are not available for the detection or identification of *T. gondii* in clinical specimens.

CASE STUDY

A 27-year-old male came to the emergency room complaining of fever, headache, neck pain, nausea, and vomiting for several weeks. Prior to these symptoms, the patient experienced a lower-respiratory infection that lasted for approximately 1 week. The patient informed the physician that he has been HIV-positive for 5 years. The physician collected blood cultures and CSF. Specimens were sent to the laboratory for testing. Analysis of the CSF showed white blood cells in normal range, with a predominance of lymphocytes, elevated protein, and low glucose. CSF sent to microbiology was plated and incubated according to protocol. A Gram stain was not ordered or performed. Two days later, the CSF culture grew creamy white yeast-like colonies. Gram stain of the growth demonstrated perfectly round microorganisms that did not bud, as seen with Candida species.

Critical Thinking Questions
1. What is the likely identification of this microorganism?
2. What should have been performed upon receiving this specimen in the microbiology laboratory?
3. What serologic methods could have been used to diagnose this patient quicker than waiting for growth of the yeast?

▶ References

1. McGowan KL. Specimen collection, transportation, and processing: mycology. In: Jorgensen JH, Pfaller MA, Carroll KC, et al., eds. *Manual of Clinical Microbiology, Eleventh Edition*. Washington, DC: ASM Press; 2015: 1944–1954.

2. Lindsley MD, Warnock DW, Morrison CJ. Serological and molecular diagnosis of fungal infections. In: *Manual of Molecular and Clinical Laboratory Immunology, 7th Edition*. American Society of Microbiology; 2006:569–605. doi:10.1128/9781555815905.ch66

3. Tille PM. *Bailey & Scott's Diagnostic Microbiolgy, Fourteenth Edition*. St. Louis, MO: Elsevier; 2017.

4. Theel ES, Carpenter AB, Binnicker MJ. Immunoassays for diagnosis of infectious diseases. In: Jorgensen JH, Pfaller MA, Carroll KC, et al., eds. *Manual of Clinical Microbiology, Eleventh Edition*. Washington, DC: ASM Press; 2015:91–105.

5. Howell SA, Hazen KC, Brandt ME. Candida, Cryptococcus, and other yeast of medical importance. In: Pfaller MA, Carroll KC, Landry ML, Funke G, Richter SS, Warnock DW, eds. *Manual of Clinical Microbiology, Eleventh Edition*. Washington, DC: ASM Press; 2015:1984–2014.

6. CLIA—Clinical Laboratory Improvement Amendments. https://www.accessdata.fda.gov/scripts/cdrh/cfdocs/cfCLIA/results.cfm?start_search=1&Test_System_Name=&Qualifier=&Analyte_Name=candida&Document_Number=&Clia_Analyte_Specialty=&Clia_Complexity=&Effective_Date_FROM=&Effective_Date_TO=01%2F01%2F2019&Exempt_510k=&Sort Column=ded&PAGENUM=50. Accessed January 1, 2019.

7. Hall L, Le Febre KM, Deml SM, Wohlfiel SL, Wengenack NL. Evaluation of the yeast traffic light PNA FISH probes for identification of Candida species from positive blood cultures. *J Clin Microbiol*. 2012;50(4):1446–1448.

8. Schwebke JR, Gaydos CA, Nyirjesy P, Paradis S, Kodsi S, Cooper CK. Diagnostic performance of a molecular test versus clinician assessment of vaginitis. *J Clin Microbiol*. 2018;56(6):e00252–e002518.

9. Thompson III GR, Gomez BL. Histoplasma, blastomyces, coccidioides, and other dimorphic fungi causing systemic mycoses. In: Jorgensen JH, Pfaller MA, Carroll KC, et al., eds. *Manual of Clinical Microbiology, Eleventh Edition.* Washington, DC: ASM Press; 2015:2109–2127.

10. IMMY. Fungal antigens, positive controls, and immunodiffusion plates for use in the immunodiffusion (ID) test [package insert]. Norman, OK: IMMY, Inc., 2016.

11. CF Fungal Antigens and Positive Controls [package insert]. Norman, OK: IMMY, Inc.; 2016.

12. Diagnostic Micro-complement Fixation Procedure Manual. Norman, OK: Immuno-Mycologics, Inc.; 2010.

13. MiraVista. Blastomyces quantitative EIA test diagnostic. https://miravistalabs.com/medical-fungal-infection -testing/antigen-detection/blastomyces-dermatitidis -quantitative-eia-test/. Accessed December 28, 2018.

14. AccuProbe Blastomyces dermatitidis Culture Identification Test [package insert]. San Diego, CA: Hologic, Inc.; 2016.

15. Scheel CM, Samayoa B, Herrera A, et al. Development and evaluation of an enzyme-linked immunosorbent assay to detect Histoplasma capsulatum antigenuria in immunocompromised patients. *Clin Vaccine Immunol.* 2009;16(6):852–858.

16. Cloud JL, Bauman SK, Neary BP, et al. Performance characteristics of a polyclonal enzyme immunoassay for the quantitation of *Histoplasma* antigen in human urine samples. *Am J Clin Pathol.* 2007;128(1):18–22.

17. Theel ES, Jespersen DJ, Harring J, Mandrekar J, et al. Evaluation of an enzyme immunoassay for detection of Histoplasma capsulatum antigen from urine specimens. *J Clin Microbiol.* 2013;51(11):3555–3559.

18. Girouard G, Lachance C, Pelletier R. Observations on (1–3)-beta-D-glucan detection as a diagnostic tool in endemic mycosis caused by Histoplasma or Blastomyces. *J Med Microbiol.* 2007;56(pt 7):1001–1002.

19. MiraVista Diagnostics. Histoplasma Quantitative EIA Test. https://miravistalabs.com/medical-fungal-infection -testing/antigen-detection/histoplasma-quantitative -eia-test/. Accessed December 28, 2018.

20. Alpha Histoplasma EIA Test Kit [package insert]. Norman, OK: IMMY, Inc.; 2018.

21. AccuProbe Histoplasma capsulatum Culture Identifi- cation Test [package insert]. San Diego, CA: Hologic, Inc.; 2016.

22. MiraVista Laboratories. Coccidioides Quantitative EIA Test. https://miravistalabs.com/medical-fungal-infection -testing/antigen-detection/coccidioides-quantitative-eia -test/. Accessed December 28, 2018.

23. Yozwiak S. DxNA LLC receives a de novo regulatory clearance by the FDA for the GeneSTAT.MDx™ Coccidioides Test on the GeneSTAT® Analyzer — the only FDA cleared molecular test for Valley Fever. https:// www.tgen.org/news/2017/december/06/tgen-technology -results-in-new-fast-accurate-valley-fever-test/. Published 2017. Accessed January 1, 2019.

24. AccuProbe Coccidioides immitis Culture Identification Test [package inert]. San Diego, CA: Hologic, Inc.; 2016.

25. Miller JM, Binnicker MJ, Campbell S, et al. A guide to utilization of the Microbiology Laboratory for Diagnosis of Infectious Diseases: 2018 update by the Infectious Diseases Society of America and the American Society for Microbiology. *Clin Infect Dis.* 2018;67(6):813–816.

26. Torgerson PR, Devleesschauwer B, Praet N, et al. World Health Organization estimates of the global and regional disease burden of 11 foodborne parasitic diseases, 2010: a data synthesis. *PLoS Med.* 2015;12(12):e1001920.

27. Corso PS, Kramer MH, Blair KA, et al. Costs of illness in the 1993 waterborne *Cryptosporidium* outbreak, Milwaukee, Wisconsin. *Emerg Infect Dis.* 2003;9(4):426–431.

28. Mac Kenzie WR, Hoxie NJ, Proctor ME, et al. A massive outbreak in Milwaukee of Cryptosporidium infection transmitted through the public water supply. *N Engl J Med.* 1994;331(3):161–167.

29. Centers for Disease Control and Prevention (CDC). DPDx - Laboratory identification of parasites of public health concern: Giardiasis. https://www.cdc.gov/dpdx/giardiasis /index.html. Accessed December 11, 2018.

30. Giardia/Cryptosporidium Quick Chek [package insert]. Blacksburg, VA: TechLab, Inc.; 2013.

31. Xpect Giardia/Cryptosporidium [package insert]. Lenexa, KY: Remel, Inc.; 2011.

32. Cardinal Health. Crypto Giardia Rapid Test. Available at: https://www.cardinalhealth.com/en/product-solutions /medical/laboratory-products/poc-infectious-diseases /rapid-test-kits/crypto-giardia-rapid-test.html" https://www .cardinalhealth.com/en/product-solutions/medical /laboratory-products/poc-infectious-diseases/rapid -test-kits/crypto-giardia-rapid-test.html. Published 2015. Accessed December 18, 2018.

33. ImmunoCard STAT! Crypto/Giardia Rapid Assay [package insert]. Cincinnati, OH: Meridian Bioscience, Inc.; 2015.

34. Clinical Laboratory Improvement Amendments (CLIA). https://www.accessdata.fda.gov/scripts/cdrh/cfdocs /cfCLIA/results.cfm?start_search=1&Test_System _Name=&Qualifier=&Analyte_Name=cryptosporidium &Document_Number=&Clia_Analyte_Specialty =&Clia_Complexity=&Effective_Date _FROM=&Effective_Date_TO=12%2F16%2F2018 &Exempt_510k=&SortColumn=ded&PAGENUM =100. Accessed December 18, 2018.

35. ProSpecT Giardia/Cryptosporidium Microplate Assay [package insert]. Basingstoke Hants, UK: Oxoid Ltd.; 2013.

36. Colpan A. Techlab Giardia Cryptosporidium Check. 2018;65:129–132.

37. Merifluor Cryptosporidium/Giardia [package insert]. Cincinnati, OH: Meridian Bioscience, Inc.; 2016.

38. Wilkins PP, Nutman TB. Immunological and molecular approaches for the diagnosis of parasitic infections. In: Detrick B, Schmidt J, Hamilton R, eds. *Manual of Molecular and Clinical Laboratory Immunology, 8th Ed.* Washington, DC: ASM Press; 2006:486–502.

39. FilmArray® Gastrointestinal (GI) Panel Instruction Booklet.

40. Clinical Laboratory Improvement Amendments (CLIA). https://www.accessdata.fda.gov/scripts/cdrh/cfdocs/cfCLIA/results.cfm?start_search=1&Test_System_Name=filmarray&Qualifier=&Analyte_Name=&Document_Number=&Clia_Analyte_Specialty=&Clia_Complexity=&Effective_Date_FROM=&Effective_Date_TO=12%2F19%2F2018&Exempt_510k=&SortColumn=ded&PAGENUM=500. Accessed December 20, 2018.

41. Einarsson E, Ma'ayeh S, Svärd SG. An up-date on Giardia and giardiasis. *Curr Opin Microbiol.* 2016;34:47–52.

42. Muhsen K, Levine MM. A systematic review and meta-analysis of the association between Giardia lamblia and endemic pediatric diarrhea in developing countries. *Clin Infect Dis.* 2012;55(suppl 4):S271–S293.

43. Clinical Laboratory Improvement Amendments (CLIA). https://www.accessdata.fda.gov/scripts/cdrh/cfdocs/cfCLIA/results.cfm?start_search=1&Test_System_Name=&Qualifier=&Analyte_Name=giardia&Document_Number=&Clia_Analyte_Specialty=&Clia_Complexity=&Effective_Date_FROM=&Effective_Date_TO=12%2F12%2F2018&Exempt_5. Accessed December 12, 2018.

44. Centers for Disease Control and Prevention (CDC). Toxoplasmosis. https://www.cdc.gov/dpdx/toxoplasmosis/index.html. Accessed December 26, 2018.

45. Centers for Disease Control and Prevention (CDC). Toxoplasmosis: epidemiology & Risk Factors. 2018. https://www.cdc.gov/parasites/toxoplasmosis/epi.html. Accessed December 26, 2018.

46. Maldonado YA, Read JS, Committee on Infectious Diseases. Diagnosis, treatment, and prevention of congenital toxoplasmosis in the United States. *Pediatrics.* 2017;139(2):e20163860.

47. Sabin AB, Feldman HA. Dyes as microchemical indicators of a new immunity phenomenon affecting a protozoon parasite (toxoplasma). *Science.* 1948;108(2815):660–663.

48. McAuley JB, Jones JL, Singh K. Toxoplasma. In: Pfaller MA, Carroll KC, Landry ML, Funke G, Richter SS, Warnock DW, eds. *Manual of Clinical Microbiology, Eleventh Edition.* Washington, DC: ASM Press; 2015:2373–2386.

49. Clinical Laboratory Improvement Amendments (CLIA). https://www.accessdata.fda.gov/scripts/cdrh/cfdocs/cfCLIA/results.cfm?start_search=1&Test_System_Name=&Qualifier=&Analyte_Name=toxoplasma&Document_Number=&Clia_Analyte_Specialty=&Clia_Complexity=&Effective_Date_FROM=&Effective_Date_TO=01%2F01%2F2019&Exempt_510k=&SortColumn=ded&PAGENUM=500. Accessed January 1, 2019.

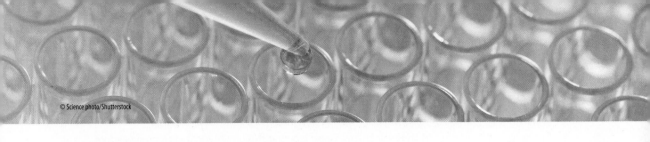

CHAPTER 12

Blood Bank Serology and Immunotyping for Transfusion and Transplant Medicine

Ian Clift, PhD, MLS(ASCP)CM

KEY TERMS

Acute hemolytic transfusion reaction (AHTR)
Agglutinogen
Amorph
Antiglobulin
Bombay Phenotype
Complement-dependent microcytoxicity (CDC)

Delayed hemolytic transfusion reaction (DHTR)
Febrile nonhemolytic transfusion reaction (FNHTR)
Graft-versus host disease (GVHD)
Hemagglutination
Hemolytic disease of the fetus and newborn (HDFN)

Hemolytic transfusion reactions (HTR)
Human leukocyte antigens (HLA)
Immunodominant sugar
Transfusion-associated circulatory overload (TACO)
Transfusion-related acute lung injury (TRALI)

LEARNING OBJECTIVES

Upon completion of this chapter, the reader should be able to:

1. Correlate serological findings with clinical characteristics.
2. Review regulatory oversight for blood bank serology.
3. Explain how the H gene is required for ABO blood group determinations.

(continues)

(Continued)

4. Review and diagram the antigenic structure of the H, A, and B immunodominant sugars.
5. Compare and contrast the Fisher-Race and Wiener terminologies for the Rh blood group.
6. Distinguish the purpose and antigenic source for each pretransfusion serological testing procedure.
7. Describe the International Society of Blood Transfusion Numeric Terminology for group and antigen.
8. Review the common forms of testing for ABO and Rh groups.
9. Explain the clinical utility of the Coomb's Antiglobulin Tests.
10. Provide rationale for performing an antibody screen and antibody identification.
11. Define the components used in a cross-match procedure.
12. Examine the major transfusion reactions and define them based on clinical presentation and laboratory results.
13. Compare and contrast transfusion and transplant serological testing.

▶ Fundamentals of Blood-Bank Immunology

ABO and Rh blood typing is one of the most commonly performed serological immunoassays. Red blood cells are a significant source of antigens detected by the body's immune system. Unlike many systems, ABO antibodies are formed without prior exposure to foreign antigens. It is, therefore, important that the A and B antigens found on the surface of donor cells do not conflict with the antibodies found in the patient's serum. The primary function of the clinical blood bank and transfusion centers is to insure that blood products used in patient therapy do not pose an additional risk to the patient through the introduction of foreign antigenic targets. The reagents found in the blood banking laboratory are both antigens and antibodies, depending on the target of the investigation.

Transfusions of blood were performed without serological testing up until the 19th century, which led to many unexplainable deaths. However, early in the 20th century, a scientist name Karl Landsteiner performed crucial experiments that revolutionized our understanding of blood-type specification with his elucidation of the A and B red blood cell antigens. These and further discoveries formed the foundation of contemporary pretransfusion screening and crossmatching, also

referred to as compatibility testing, commonly performed in the immunohematology/blood bank laboratory.

Erythrocyte, or red blood cell (RBC) markers, are often the immunological target of blood-bank serology testing. Blood collected for use in donor populations is regulated in the United States by the US Food and Drug Administration (FDA), which mandates the use of special containers such as sterile, pyrogen-free blood bags with specific lot number identification as well as a specific quantity of anticoagulant. For example, a 500-mL blood bag contains 63 mLs of anticoagulant. Along with acid citrate dextrose (ACD), used most often in tube draws and apheresis, citrate phosphate dextrose (CPD), citrate phosphate dextrose adenine (CPDA-1), and adenine-saline are all used as anticoagulants for whole blood to ensure longer shelf life; specifically 21, 35, and 42 days, respectively, when kept in a monitored refrigerated unit.

This chapter focuses on the examination of RBC surface markers that can have adverse effects on blood transfusions and transplants. However, serological examination of donor units is not only relegated to RBC surface markers but also for the presence of infectious disease exposure. While not covered here, an assessment of infectious disease serology, found elsewhere, will review the ways and means by which this is accomplished in blood-bank specimens as well.

▶ General Transfusion Medicine Laboratory Operations

The transfusion services department is often divided into two units. The donor collection unit, sometimes completely separate from the hospital and other laboratory operations, which includes a large number of phlebotomists and a smaller number of specimen testing and processing personnel; and the hospital blood bank, which typically performs patient blood typing, screening, cross-matching, and unit processing. Immunodiagnostic testing is only one component of the functions of all blood bank personnel, as the field is heavily regulated in most developed countries.

In general, donor units are solicited from the general population of healthy individuals, who must complete both a medical history questionnaire[1] and physical examination used to rule out donations from potentially risky populations through temporary, indefinite, and permanent deferrals. Units collected are further tested for communicable diseases and for the major natural blood group antigens, specifically, the ABO and Rh blood group antigens. Erythrocytes can be separated from the whole blood through a differential centrifugation process that can also separate out platelets and plasma through variations in the centrifugation spin time and speed. In the blood bank, centrifugation can separate out the plasma and leave behind packed red cells. Apheresis can be used to spin out and remove the plasma and directly return the red cells to the patient. Other methods of separation can also be used to remove leukocytes, white blood cells, which can minimize the transmission of diseases such as cytomegalovirus (CMV), which reside in leukocytes. However, normal serological testing of erythrocyte antigens occurs within a typically anticoagulated whole blood unit. This information is then stored in association with the unit for later compatibility testing during the practice of transfusion and during the investigation of any later transfusion reactions.

The hospital blood bank primarily performs a process known as pretranfusion testing, which includes a series of serological and immunological testing on patient and donor units to ensure compatibility. Like the collection of donor blood for transfusion, the testing and distribution of donor units to patients is heavily regulated to reduce the occurrence of disease and transfusion-related reactions. Erythrocytes in whole blood are screened for the common blood type antigens A, B, and D (Rh factor) as part of pretransfusion testing. Typically, this patient sample comes from a venous blood draw in a heparin or EDTA tube during routine phlebotomy.

A deeper assessment of nondiagnostic blood bank practices is beyond the scope of this chapter. In addition to an understanding of red-cell immunodiagnostics, compliance with institutional policies, regional regulations, and aspects of blood and tissue storage, i.e., blood and tissue banking and distribution, it is important for anyone interested in working in the field of immunohematology.

Transfusion Services Operating Procedures

Like all other areas of the clinical laboratory, standard operating procedures have been established in the blood bank to conform to the standards, regulations, and guidelines of the overarching laboratory regulatory organizations as well as to conform to institutional policy for safety and quality control. Therefore, the blood bank procedures provided within this chapter are meant only as a guideline to theory and operation, not as prescriptive of all practices.

Regulators

The performance of pretransfusion testing and the control of blood units and products are the most regulated processes of the clinical laboratory. While a cursory examination of some of the regulatory bodies with oversight of blood-bank operations are provided below, the primary focus of this chapter is the serological and immunological methods and definitions used in performing transfusion testing. The reader is encouraged to examine more thorough texts about the performance and regulation of blood-bank operations found elsewhere, including those at the organizational websites for the following regulatory organizations.

FDA

The US Food and Drug Administration (FDA) regulates units of blood used for transfusion services. The FDA has input into the regulations regarding donor screening and recruitment as outlined in the *Code of Federal Regulations* (CFR). A branch of the FDA called the Center for Biologics Evaluation and Research (CBER) was formed in 1988 to regulate the collection of blood and blood components, which are considered both a biologic and a drug in the United States. CBER regulates all pharmaceuticals derived from blood and blood components. The FDA has oversight for the licensing of blood collection and processing centers.

AABB

Established in 1947, the American Association of Blood Banks (AABB) is an international association that provides guidelines and standards for the operation of blood centers, transfusion, and transplant services. It provides inspection services for their members who meet the requirements of the US Center for Medicare and Medicaid (CMS) and CLIA '88 (Clinical Laboratory Improvement Amendments of 1988). It provides two essential resources for immunohematology specialists; the *AABB Standards for Blood Banks and Transfusion Services* and the *AABB Technical Manual*.

European Commission

After the establishment of the European Union (EU), the European Commission now has oversite of many of the aspects of what it terms "substances of human origin," including blood and blood products, although several directives focus on coordinating the blood transfusion policies in the member states.[2] Two important measures are

the addition of nonremuneration and the ban on financial gain, which emulates US policy. Currently, however, the policies are still being structured and rely on the WHO guidelines and prior policies from the member states.

WHO

The World Health Organization (WHO), as part of the United Nations, provides guidelines to countries attempting to develop blood transfusion safety and management policies in member states. Aimed at the Ministries of Health, the WHO advises countries to develop a National Blood System, which includes the development of offices within the state to coordinate blood collection and testing activities, and to facilitate safe collection and distribution practices in both blood transfusion services and hospital blood banks.[3]

▶ Blood Group Genetics

Although the original categorizations of blood-group antigens were derived from the structural homology of these antigens as recognized by known antibodies as well as their concurrence in individual donors/patients, subsequent examinations have found many of them occur as a result of genetic homology as well. Specifically, the blood groups have been classified by their association with alleles of a single gene locus or as a result of extremely homologous genes with limited crossover. While the focus of this text is on the antigenic-antibody interactions important for detection and reactions, a significant body of literature has been dedicated to elucidating the genetic underpinnings of antigenic crossover and expression. Genetic crossover and mutation account for a significant number of the variant forms of antigens expressed within these blood groups, and are responsible for rare transfusion reactions in which crossmatching with compatibility screens have already been performed. While genetic passage of specific blood groups defined in this chapter has been eluded to during a later discussion of these blood groups, two of the major blood groups will be critically examined: ABO and Rh are discussed here, due to their importance in prevention of therapy-mediated complications.

The inheritance of the ABO blood group was first theorized in 1924 by the mathematician Felix Bernstein and follows a simple Mendelian inheritance pattern. That is, the ABO blood type is a result of gene alleles that compete for a single position in the genetic code. Specifically, one position on chromosome 9 contains an *A, B,* or *O* gene, with both the *A* and *B* gene coding for an antigen and the *O* gene leading to no antigen; a term known as **amorph**. The *O* gene is, therefore, autosomal recessive, i.e., only phenotypic (presenting) in the absence of both A and B. If an individual presents with one *A* gene allele and one *O* allele, he or she will phenotype as A, as will an individual with two A alleles. However, the surface levels of this antigen are higher. Only individuals with one *A* allele and one *B* allele present as AB phenotypically.

In addition to the A and B antigens, a precursor antigen known as the H antigen, is genetically required for A and B antigenic expression. Expression of the H antigen is required for expression of A or B antigens. Genetically, an individual is either *HH* or *Hh*. Rarely will an individual be *hh*, which leads to a lack of H antigen expression and a subsequent lack of A or B antigenic expression despite the genetic presence of the trait. This phenotype has been clinically termed the **Bombay Phenotype**. The *H* gene codes for a glycosyltransferase called α-2-L-fucosyltransferase, which transfers the sugar L-fucose to a terminal galactose of a type-2 oligosaccharide chain. This **immunodominant sugar** is then recognized by specific antibodies and is defined as the H antigen. Without L-fucose, additional sugars cannot bind (**FIGURE 12–1**). The gene for A codes for the glycosyltransferase α-3-N-acetylgalactosaminyltransferase, and the gene for B codes for α-3-D-galactosyltranferase. These gycosyltranferases lead to the attachment of N-acetyl-D-galactosamine or D-galactose to L-fucose, which are recognized by the A or B

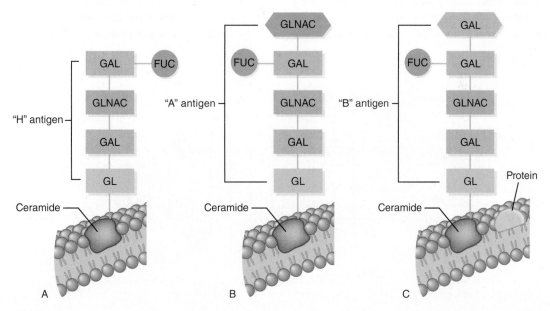

FIGURE 12–1 Sugar structure of the immunogenic H, A, and B antigens on red cells. All red cell antigens identifiable in the ABO group are defined by a sugar chain attached to the lipid ceramide; the addition of the sugar molecule N-acetylgalactosamine (GALNAC) or D-Galactose (GAL) converts the H antigen to either A or B, respectively. **(A)** The H antigen is detected by the immunodominant L-fucose sugar. **(B)** The A antigen is detected via the N-acetylgalactosamine sugar. **(C)** The B antigen is identified by the immunodominent D-galactose sugar molecule.

antibodies, respectively. Hence, lack of *H* gene leads to a lack of expression of A and B antigens. In the case of the O "phenotype," there is no detectable surface antigen; this occurs only if two nonfunctional genes at the A/B locus are inherited. In addition to specific A and B antigens that may be present, the precursor antigen for both, known as the H antigen, may also be detectable, specifically in early childhood as the A and B antigens do not fully develop until age 2 to 4.

As cell-surface glycoprotein antigens, the H antigen has a terminal L-fucose sugar moiety that functions in "H" antibody specificity. The A antigen has the additional sugar moiety N-acetylgalactosamine attached above L-fucose, which becomes immunodominant, i.e., responsible for "A" specific antibodies; the B antigen has the immunodominant D-galactose terminally. In all cases, it is the terminal sugar moiety that is the target for antibody specificity.

The genetic elucidation of antigens in the Rh system has undergone many turns based on varying theories regarding the allelic structure of the underlying genes. These theories, long accepted in many circles, have been applied to the various terminologies still employed in the labelling and discussion of reagents sold for blood bank analysis. Two terminologies with a continued influence on the Rh system are the Fisher-Race: DCE system and the Wiener: Rh-hr system. Fisher and Race suggested that there are three genes; *D/d*, *C/c*, and *E/e*. It is now considered that the *d* allele represents only the absence of *D*; however, antigens were identified for *c* and *e* (verbalized as "little c" and "little e"). In contrast, Wiener suggested that there is only one factor, **agglutinogen** (agglutinating antigen), in which antibodies bind to different epitopes. He called this the Rh factor with multiple subvariants (with the "hr" nomenclature) of this factor being recognized by different antibodies. It was subsequently determined that neither of these theories was exactly correct. Instead, it has now been well established that the Rh blood group system is a product of two closely related genes on chromosome 1 that codes for similarly structured transmembrane proteins. Specifically, one of these genes, *RHD*, codes for a protein called RhD, and the other, *RHCE*, codes for a series of proteins called RhCe, RhcE, Rhce, or RhCE, where C or c and E or e complete for the same extracellular locations on a single protein (**FIGURE 12–2**).

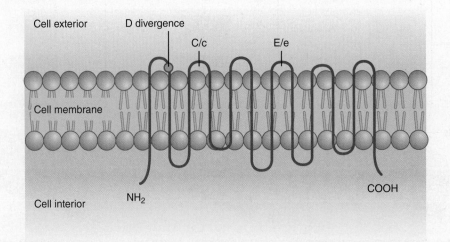

FIGURE 12–2 The protein structure of Rh gene products. All five Rh antigenic types are expressed in a similar protein structure within the cell membrane based on two genes: *RHD* and *RHCE*. This figure denotes the location in which the D protein product diverges from that of C/c and E/e. The regions denoted C/c and E/e are responsible for serological differences in detecting C/c and E/e.

The long usage of these nomenclatures and the similarity of the actual system have allowed both terminologies to continue in practice. Currently, the system is described as the Rh system, while the antigens are said to bind to D, C, c, E, or e antigens. When referenced alone, the D antigen is often also called the Rh factor and is reported as (+) or (−) in pretransfusion and blood donor testing.

In addition to the major gene variants described above, both the ABO and Rh blood group systems have been extensively divided phenotypically, i.e., through antibody identification, as a result of subtle genetic variations, which may affect responses to therapy and have other clinical implications. An in-depth examination of these variants is beyond the scope of this book.

Although much is known about the genetic underpinnings of these blood-group antigens, current practice is still rooted in the usage of antigen-antibody based serological testing. However, the 21st century may see an increase in blood-group genotyping analysis in clinical practice, including the use of gene arrays and SNP analysis where proof of principle has already been shown.[4] The challenges for RBC genotyping, including surface-marker profiling, in regular clinical practice are the lack of closed systems and a cost barrier for low- to mid-sized hospital labs.[5]

▶ Pretransfusion Testing

Karl Landsteiner's discoveries of the ABO system formed the foundation of contemporary pretransfusion screening and crossmatching, also referred to as compatibility testing. Most blood-bank laboratories follow a protocol which includes a physician's request to perform testing and prepare components. In the United States, strict guidelines are provided through FDA regulations and *AABB standards,* including the receipt of an acceptable blood specimen that then has ABO blood group and RH typing performed, including an antibody screen to identify unexpected antibodies, as well as a review of the records of previous blood type and screens. This is followed by a section of potential in-stock blood units for transfusion, which are then tested for compatibility through standard serological crossmatch testing. If acceptable in-stock units cannot be determined compatible, a request for units from regional blood centers is performed.

Pretransfusion testing begins with the identification and collection of a patient specimen for testing, following all internally established guidelines with effort made to avoid specimen hemolysis (blood lysis) at the time of collection, as hemolysis can be an indicator of antigen-antibody reaction during the testing

Pretransfusion Testing

Procedure	Purpose	Source of Antigen
ABO/Rh typing	Detects A, B, and D	Patient's RBCs
Antigen typing	Detects antigens of other blood-group systems	Patient's RBCs or donor RBCs
Antibody screening	Detects antibodies with specificity of RBC antigens	Commercial screening cells
Antibody identification	Identifies the specificity of RBC antibodies	Commercial panel cells
Crossmatch	Determines serologic compatibility between donor and patient before transfusion	Donor RBCs

phase. Either serum or plasma can be used for pretransfusion testing; however, the presence of clotting factors in plasma may lead to fibrin clot formation, which should not be confused with agglutination. Donor samples tested for compatibility with a transfusion patient are typically collected at the same time as the full donor unit is collected.

Per AABB guidelines, a donor unit is both tested by the blood donor center and at the transfusing facility to confirm ABO on all units and Rh typing on all Rh (−) negative units.[6] A patient specimen can be tested in advance or at the same time as a donor crossmatch for ABO, Rh, and antibody screen. In all cases, reagents must be in-date (i.e., not expired) for the data to be considered clinically acceptable. Patient specimens must undergo ABO grouping, Rh typing, and antibody screening prior to transfusion. The results of these assays, whose procedures are described in a later section, determine the selection of a donor unit in which ABO and Rh testing have already been performed, both by the donor center and verified by the transfusing center. A final check called crossmatch testing is then performed in which the patient's serum is tested against the donor RBCs through the antiglobulin phase; this is described in greater detail below. However, many blood-bank centers have opted to eliminate the serological crossmatch and have instead instituted an electronic crossmatch, which compares the patient's results to the electronic record for the donor unit.

Blood bank reactions, i.e., ABO groupings, Rh typing, antibody screening, and crossmatching, are determined through the examination of graded agglutination responses. While some of the primary tests performed in the typing of blood require only a room temperature interaction, later screening tests are also performed at 37° Celsius (physiological temperature) and what is known as the **antiglobulin** (AG) phase (Coombs antiglobulin test). The term **hemagglutination** was derived to indicate the interaction of antibodies with red blood cells to form a visible agglutination response (**FIGURE 12–3**). Positive agglutination responses indicate the

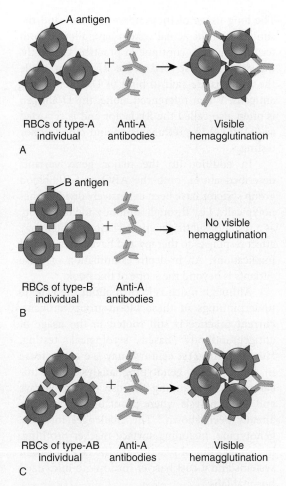

FIGURE 12–3 Anti-A Antibody hemagglutination reactions to red-cell Antigens. Anti-A antibody will respond to both red cells with an A phenotype or AB phenotype, leading to an agglutination response known as hemagglutination.

occurrence of an antigen-antibody interaction. The grading of the agglutination provides for a relative indication of the amount of antibodies or antigens present. Suspended cells are combined with patient or reagent antibodies and viewed under an agglutination lamp (**FIGURE 12–4**). Conversely, patient serum is added to donor or reagent red cells and viewed similarly. Gentle shaking is used to suspend the cells.

In general, manual techniques, including traditional tube and slide methods, are losing

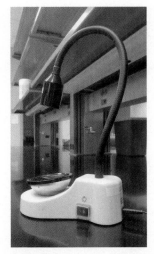

A

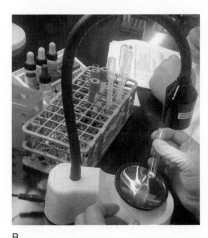

B

FIGURE 12–4 **(A)** Agglutination lamp, **(B)** agglutination lamp in use.

Courtesy of Ian Clift.

ground to more automated approaches, including the popular gel column agglutination technology (CAT) or gel method, including the ID-MTS gel cards produced by Ortho-Clinical Diagnostics. Manual approaches still account for a large proportion of testing and continue to garner commercial support in product development based on recently introduced centrifuges that can spin either gel cards or tubes.[7] Manual methods also provide the most guidance for training

purposes and are, therefore, used for explanatory purposes herein. Advanced techniques such as CAT and others such as Solid Phase Red Cell Adherence (SPRCA) assays, and erythrocyte-magnetized technique (EMT) may lead to more reproducible and precise results,[8] but are simpler for the technologist/scientist to perform by comparison.

▶ International Society of Blood Transfusion Numeric Terminology

The International Society of Blood Transfusion (ISBT: www.isbtweb.org) is a scientific society founded in 1935 by transfusion medicine professionals with the goal of improving the safety of blood transfusion through increased knowledge. In 1980, in order to facilitate the conversion of information into computer storage systems, the ISBT developed the Working Party on Terminology for Red Cell Antigens, which created a six-digit code to define the various surface antigens examined clinically in transfusion medicine. While the terminology was never intended to replace traditional nomenclature, it has facilitated and simplified the naming of new members introduced into the various blood system groups. Each blood system group was given a three-digit number, e.g., 001 for the ABO blood group system and 004 for the Rh system, which was followed by a three-digit code for the specific antigen. In the ISBT system, the Lewis antigen Le^a is called 007001, where 007 indicates the Lewis system (symbol: LE) and 001 indicates Le^a. While details for each group of antigens are beyond the scope of this text, a later section will examine some important members of these other blood system groups. This is the most common terminology system employed in blood-bank facilities today. More extensive discussions of the ABO and Rh systems are provided below in correlation with their commonly performed serological testing in the blood bank laboratory.

List of Blood Groups With ISBT Codes

ISBT No.	System Name	System Symbol	CD Number
001	ABO	ABO	
002	MNS	MNS	CD235a, CD235b
003	P1PK	P1PK	CD77
004	RhRH	RHD	CD240
005	Lutheran	LU	CD239
006	Kell	KEL	CD238
007	Lewis	LE	
008	Duffy	FY	CD234
009	Kidd	JK	
010	Diego	DI	CD233
011	Yt	YT	
012	Xg	XG	CD99
013	Scianna	SC	
014	Dombrock	DO	CD297
015	Colton	CO	
016	Landsteiner-Wiener	LW	CD242
017	Chido/Rodgers	CH/RG	
018	H	H	CD173

Adapted from international Society of Blood Transfusion (ISBT) Table of blood group systems v6.0 6th August 2019. Retrieved from: http://www.isbtweb.orslfileadmin /user upload/Red Cell Terminology and Immunogenetics/Table of blood group systems v6.0 5th August 2019.pdf

▶ ABO Blood Grouping

The source of antigens in ABO blood group testing is the patient's RBCs. The ABO system is the most important blood group for screening in transfusion practice, as the ABO system is the only one in which antibodies occur naturally without prior exposure to antigens on RBCs. These are typically IgM in nature, can produce strong direct agglutination reactions during testing, and can cause rapid hemolysis of blood when the wrong ABO group is transfused. Although the source of nature ABO antibodies in humans serum is still debated, some have speculated that bacteria and other substances may mimic A and B antigens, leading to anti-A and anti-B antibodies.

The ABO blood group genes are inherited from the father and the mother in a Mendelian fashion, which then present as the ABO antigens on the surface of red cells. While phenotypes vary depending on ethnicity, the number of donors with either A, B, or both on the surface of their RBCs is approximately 50%, making them an important factor in blood-cell acceptance or rejection. In those of western European descent, approximately 46% have the A antigen on their cell surface, while 14% have the B antigen on their cell surface. There is a 10% increasein the incidence of B antigen in individuals of African descent, while the highest percentage of individuals with neither antigen (phenotypically O) is in the Native-American population—estimated as high as 79%. Depending on both the ethnicity and the locality of the population, variations in percentages may be noted.

Procedure

In general, the reference to ABO grouping in the blood-bank laboratory refers to two specific types of testing for ABO blood-group antigens.

Specifically, these are known as forward grouping—the testing of RBCs for the presence of the A and B antigen, and reverse grouping—the testing of serum or plasma for the presence of anti-A and anti-B antibodies. Modifications to these traditionally manual assays include the use of 96-well microplate testing in larger blood-bank facilities, and the use of commercially available gel card technologies. Molecular testing of RBCs for the underlying genes has also gained favor.

Forward grouping, also known as forward typing, is performed using commercially available antibodies, specifically anti-A, anti-B, and sometimes anti-A,B, which is used to confirm purported O-positive blood; reverse grouping is performed using commercially available RBC populations of known antigen type, i.e., A, B, or O. Testing is traditionally performed at room temperature using either a manual or automated technique. Manual approaches include both a slide and tube method.

In the slide method, one drop of the reagent anti-serum is added to a similar volume of 20% to 30% suspension of specimen RBCs in saline (or other solution) on a glass slide and mixed with an applicator stick. This can be a patient or a donor specimen. Tube typing, the other classic method, is performed similarly, but in a 10 × 75-mm or 12 × 75-mm glass tube and uses a 2 to 5% solution of RBCs in saline (or other solution) and is mixed by centrifugation. The centrifuges used in the blood

Estimated ABO Phenotypic Distribution in Us Ethnic Groups					
Phenotype	**White (Non-Hispanic)**	**Hispanic**	**Black (Non-Hispanic)**	**Asian**	**Native American**
O	45.2	56.5	50.2	39.8	54.6
A	39.7	31.1	25.8	27.8	35
B	10.9	9.9	19.7	25.4	7.9
AB	4.1	2.5	4.3	7.1	2.5

Data from Garratty[10] G, Glynn SA, McEntire R, Retrovirus Epidemiology Donor S. ABO and Rh(D) phenotype frequencies of different racial/ethnic groups in the United States. *Transfusion*. 2004;44(5):703–706.

bank for this purpose run at a relatively low RPM and are sold commercially as serofuges. In both cases, agglutination can be seen as a clumping of cells (hemagglutination) that can be seen macroscopically. A gentle shaking of the tube has been used to further analyze the hemagglutination observed for grading on a scale of 1 to 4 with 4+ indicating the strongest reaction (**FIGURE 12–5A** and **FIGURE 12–5B**). Weaker reactions should be suspect and may be the result of rouleax, missing isoagglutinins, or unidentified cold reactive

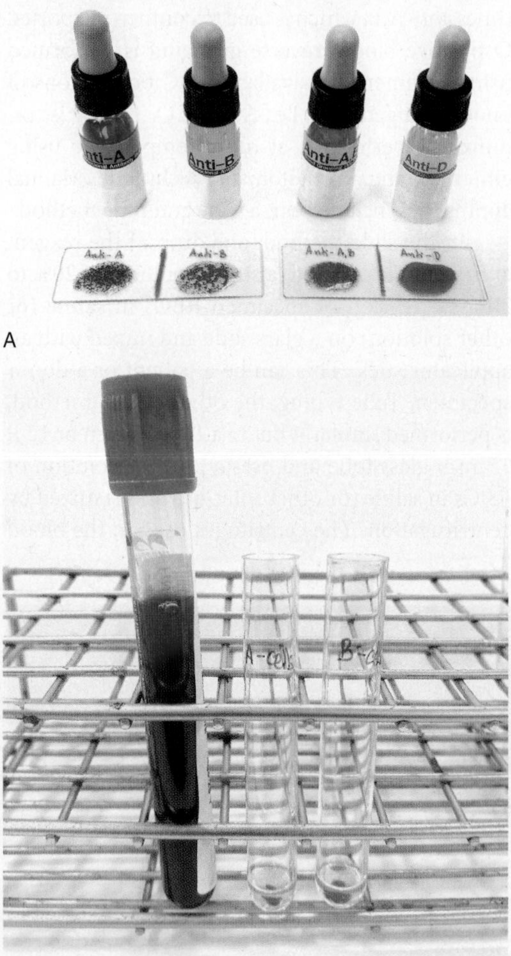

A

B

FIGURE 12–5 Red cell ABO testing by slide and tube method. **(A)** Slide method. **(B)** Tube method.

© Sunisa Butphet/Shutterstock

antibodies. A similar grading can be seen in other forms of testing as well, including the popular gel method.

Clinical Utility

The primary value of most ABO testing is in preventing transfusion-related events from occurring. ABO antibodies against blood surface antigens are some of the few naturally occurring antibodies; that is, they require no prior exposure to the antigen to be present. However, it is now thought that they occur as a result of some ABO-like antigens ubiquitous in the environment to which the individual was exposed. Regardless of their origins, they have historically been the leading cause of life-threatening situations in first-time transfusion patients, and ABO incompatibility is considered the leading cause of intravascular **hemolytic transfusion reactions (HTR)**. Intravascular hemolysis is the most severe reaction to foreign bodies. The donor RBCs are destroyed by complement inside the vascular space, hemoglobin is release and excreted in the urine, increased bilirubin causes jaundice, and the massive activation of complement causes shock and uncontrollable clotting. A list of common transfusion reactions is provided later in this chapter but includes HTR and more specific injuries such as transfusion-related acute lung injury (TRALI) and transfusion-associated circulatory overload (TACO).

In some cases, identification of the ABO group is only the first step. For cases where organ transplant is required, ABO testing may also be accompanied by antibody titers. The monitoring of these titers is of the most relevance in transplant situations where incompatible organs, i.e., the kidney, may be the only choice in patient survival, and a careful monitoring of these titers is useful in therapy for successful engraftment.[11,12] In most cases, the immune reaction to ABO incompatibility occurs as a result of IgM antibodies; however, IgG antibodies may also play a role.[12] Both A and B antigen-specific IgM and IgG antibodies have been found to be stronger in type O individuals.[12] Immunosuppressive therapies can be used to reduce the titers of antibodies.

Rh D Typing

The positive (+) or negative (−) indication found at the end of the traditionally reported blood type; i.e., B+, indicates the presence or absence of the Rh1 or D antigen. It is the second most important blood group tested in terms of transfusion. In common dialog, reference to the Rh antigen is synonymous with the D antigen, but in the International Society of Blood Transfusion Committee (ISBT) terminology, the D antigen is called Rh1 (or more precisely, 004001 with 004 indicating the Rh blood group and 001 indicating the specific D antigen). The four next most common Rh antigens are called RH2, C; Rh3, E; Rh4, c; and Rh5, e. While ISBT terminology is difficult during common oral dialog, the terminology is often used in computer coding, for example, a −1 means the absence of D and a 1 means the presence of D. This terminology was used by Rosenfeld and coworkers to develop a phenotypic code for the five most common Rh antigens, called the Rosenfeld Phenotype; for example, Rh:1, −2, −3, 4, 5 indicated D positive, C negative, E negative, c positive, and e positive. Roughly 60 Rh antigens have been documented and coded using the ISBT system, some with alternate names. However, clinical Rh typing typically consists only of testing for the D antigen or, at most, the top five most prevalent antigens as discussed above, which are deemed the most important for transfusion responses. Similar to ABO grouping, Rh typing is performed by examining antigens from the patient's RBCs, while the antibody is typically a commercially purchased anti-D. Commercial packs of all of the five major Rh antigens are readily available from numerous diagnostic medical supply companies.

Procedure

Similar to other RBC-based serological assays, the performance of traditional Rh typing can occur via a slide or tube method, and has been semi-automated via the use of microplate and gel testing methods. Furthermore, the Rh typing performed in most blood-bank facilities is a test for the presence of only the D antigen on RBCs. Therefore, unlike ABO grouping, no reverse type is attempted at this phase. A 3% to 6% suspension of RBCs in blood-bank saline is prepared, and a drop of anti-D reagent is added. In the tube method, the mixture is centrifuged, resuspended, and observed macroscopically for agglutination. The observation is graded and documented. This is often performed at the same time as AB grouping. Therefore, if tests are positive for A, B, and D, an Rh control serum, containing only 6% albumin, is tested and should be negative before reporting the result. This is to ensure that spontaneous, or auto-agglutination, has not led to a false-positive result.

The slide method often uses a higher concentration of RBCs, from 30% to up to 60%, depending on standard operating procedure (SOP). Other tests such as weak-D testing, examination of a weaker than normal D antigen caused by mutations in the *RHD* gene, and other causes is typically not performed at this stage. C, E, c, and e antigen testing is similarly not performed at this stage but is performed later during the antibody screen.

Clinical Utility

Rh D testing is one of the most important antigenic tests performed prior to transfusion. Due to increased vigilance in the clinical setting, the cases of hemolysis and other transfusion-related diseases resulting from D incompatibility have become extremely rare events. Nevertheless, contemporary cases of hemolysis due to D-incompatibility in the case of ABO compatible blood transfusion have been reported. Furthermore, D-incompatibility has been the cause of hemolysis in cases of transplant, such as liver transplant,[13] as well.

The D antigen is also the primary cause of **hemolytic disease of the fetus and newborn (HDFN)**, and therefore, in addition to its testing in the transfusion setting, the D antigen is also closely monitored in all pregnant and expecting mothers in modern healthcare systems. In Caucasians and individuals of European descent, the D negative phenotype is found

STEP-BY-STEP PROCEDURE 12–1   Tube Typing for D

1. Label two glass 10 or 12 × 75-mm test tubes with "D" or "Control."
2. Wash specimen RBCs in blood-bank saline (0.9% w/v saline).
3. Dilute RBCs to 2 to 5% in blood-bank saline.
4. Add one drop of anti-D to the tube marked "D."
5. Add one drop of 6% albumin (or Rh control solution) to the tube marked "Control."
6. Centrifuge for 30 seconds at 3,000 RPM in a serofuge.
7. Manually shake to resuspend the cell button while watching for any agglutination macroscopically. Be sure to resuspend completely before marking your observation. If there is agglutination in the "Control," the test is invalid.
8. Record the agglutination score as 4+, 3+, 2+, 1+, w+, or negative 0.

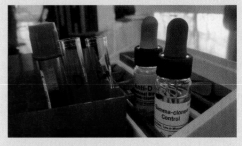

Reagents and Tube Setup.

Courtesy of Ian Clift.

in approximately 15% of the population and is considered even rarer in other populations. HDFN is caused by the destruction of RBC's in the unborn fetus via the passage of IgG antibodies produced by the mother. Specifically, mothers who are found to be Rh (D) negative may produce antibodies that attack their unborn fetus if the fetus is Rh (D) positive. This traditionally occurs only to the second child as the mother must first be immunized to the D antigen during the first pregnancy. However, a prior transfusion of Rh (D) positive blood can lead to a prior immunization. The majority of effort has focused on prevention through routine type and screen procedures on all pregnant mothers during their first prenatal visit. If the mother is Rh (D) negative and does not have the presence of a preexisting anti-D, she is a candidate for RhIG therapy. By administering the anti-D antibody during the mixing of maternal and fetal blood, active immunization has been shown to be prevented. This is thought to occur by coating the fetal blood, which targets it for removal via macrophages. However, the true mechanism is still uncertain.

The presence of other members of the Rh blood group family is also detected through the performance of the antibody screening process, as these can also have clinical implications.

▶ Coombs Antiglobulin Tests

The antibody screen, described in more detail below, requires a deeper understanding of one of the oldest used pretransfusion diagnostic tests, called the Coombs test (or the Antiglobulin Test). It was first described in humans in 1945, when Robin Coombs, immunologist, and colleagues detected weak and nonagglutinating Rh antibodies in serum; the Coombs test and Coombs reagents continue to play a role in weak Rh identification as well as identification of other blood-group antigens such as the Kell antibodies. The Coombs test is based on the observation that antihuman globulins (AHGs) from immunized nonhumans will bind to human immunoglobulins and complement components. The Coombs procedure consisted of the injection of human serum into rabbits to produce antihuman serum. After absorption to remove nonspecific antibodies, the serum was still capable of binding to RBCs that had been previously sensitized to (i.e., exposed to and associated with) immunoglobulins. In other instances, the same principles have been applied to the development of labeled secondary complexes of all organism types. In the specific Coombs case, AHGs might be otherwise known as rabbit-antihuman antibodies. However, the principle of agglutinating RBCs using these antibodies was first described by Moreschi, based on Coombs research, to agglutinate rabbit RBCs using goat-antirabbit antibodies. As in most cases when a foreign substance enters the blood stream or body, the immune system of that organism produces antibodies against it. Thus is the case when human serum or isolated human complement or IgG is introduced to another animal. Injection of these products into animals such as rabbits and murine organisms has been the classic source of AHG. However, more advanced techniques utilize the hybridization of sensitizing animal splenic cells with myeloma cells to produce hybridomas.

Most commercially defined AHG reagents bind either to IgG or to C3b of the complement cascade. Certain polyclonal antibodies bind to both, while monoclonal antibodies have been formed to bind to either and/or IgG chains specifically. Additional polyclonals have been produced that bind to other components of the complement cascade, such as C3d and C4b.

Clinical Utility

The primary usage of the direct and indirect Coombs test (direct and indirect antiglobulin test) is in the detection of in vivo sensitization of RBCs with IgG or complement components. The three primary clinical conditions in which the direct antiglobulin test (DAT) is indicated are the hemolytic disease of the newborn (HDN), hemolytic transfusion reaction (HTR), and autoimmune and drug-induced hemolytic anemia (AIHA). It is not commonly performed in routine pretransfusion testing. Furthermore, the AABB Technical Manual suggests that a positive DAT test alone is not diagnostic, and evidence indicates that in most situations the DAT is inefficient. More valuable clinically is the indirect antiglobulin test (IAT), which is used in the detection of incompletely agglutinating (or nonagglutinating) antibodies to potential donors, during cell screening, during the determination of RBC phenotype using known antisera, and in the titration of incomplete antibodies. It is commonly performed during the antibody screening and identification steps of pretransfusion compatibility examinations, after the performance of the immediate spin (IS) and 37°C agglutination steps. Therefore, the clinical utility of this assay is primarily seen in the blood bank/transfusion laboratory. However, the DAT and IAT may find other clinical utilities in non-RBC analysis of cells and tissues when antibody screening or identification is needed.

Modifications to the AHG tests have made their usage more robust. Specifically, several additions to the test solution, such as the rouleux-forming polybrene reagent, allow the ionic barriers to be reduced to agglutination. With this technique, a low-ionic strength solution (LISS) containing polybrene is added to form agglutination, which is followed by a high-ionic strength solution to reverse agglutination. In this case, where antibodies are present, the reversal will not occur. Likewise, labeled AHG reagents, such as the enzyme-linked antiglobulin test, have been designed in which an enzyme is attached the AHG reagents. Washing away excess antibody and adding a substrate means that bound antibody can be measured colorimetrically. Finally, these techniques have been partially automated via the use of solid phase and gel technologies. Companies such as Ortho-Clinical Diagnostics have produced reagents for their ID-MTS gel cards that can be used to perform both the DAT and IAT assays. Furthermore, the conventional tube technique has been losing favor with technologists who prefer the sensitivity and reduced steps used by the gel technique. Like many other technological advances in the clinical laboratory, advances to the test methodology have reduced the time and specialized training required to perform this assay.

STEP-BY-STEP PROCEDURE 12–2 DAT and IAT Procedures

Direct Antiglobulin Test (DAT)

1. Place one to two drops of a 3% to 5% v/v suspension of the cells to be tested into two properly labeled glass 10-mm or 12-mm × 75-mm test tubes (antihuman globulin [AHG] and control tube).
2. Wash the cells at least three times with the tubes full of saline, decant the saline between washes, and resuspend the cells between washes. (Cord blood cells are washed six times.)
3. Decant the saline completely following the last wash.
4. Add two drops of anti-IgG, –C3d (polyspecific) reagent to the tube labeled AHG, and two drops of saline to the control tube and mix well. Monoclonal anti-IgG may be used in the test procedure if the specimen is a cord blood or if the initial polyspecific AHG was positive.
5. Centrifuge immediately at 500 relative centrifugal force (RCF) for 15 to 20 seconds.
6. Completely resuspend the cell pellet by gently tipping and rolling the tube.
7. Read and score agglutination macroscopically with the aid of an agglutination lamp.
8. If the polyspecific immediate spin is negative, incubate the AHG and control tubes at room temperature for 5 minutes and repeat steps 5 through 7.
9. Confirm negative tests by adding one drop of IgG-coated cells (check cells) to each tube. Then immediately repeat steps 5 through 7. If the appropriate test tubes do not give a positive reaction after the addition of Coombs control cells and recentrifugation, THE COMPLETE TEST MUST BE REPEATED.
10. If the polyspecific AHG tube is positive at immediate and/or room temperature (RT) incubation phase, it is recommended that you repeat steps 4 through 9 replacing polyspecific AHG reagent with monospecific anti-IgG and monospecific anti-C3b (the RT incubation phase is not required for direct antiglobulin test [DAT] using monoclonal anti-IgG).

Indirect Antiglobulin Test (IAT)

1. Using a labeled glass 10-mm or 12-mm × 75-mm test tube, place two to four drops of test serum and one drop of a washed 3% v/v suspension of reagent RBCs.
2. Mix the cell suspension and centrifuge the tube at 500 relative centrifugal force (RCF) for 15 to 20 seconds.
3. Examine for hemolysis and record if present. *Most often, antibodies capable of producing hemolysis have specificity in the ABO, P, Lewis, Kidd, or Vel blood group systems. Hemolysis may be caused by bacterial contamination as well.*
4. Completely resuspend the cell pellet by tapping the tube. Read and score agglutination macroscopically with the aid of an agglutination lamp.
5. Incubate for 30 to 60 minutes in a 37°C water or dry bath.
6. Examine for hemolysis and record if present.
7. Centrifuge the tube at 500 RCF for 15 to 20 seconds.
8. After centrifugation, completely resuspend the cell pellet by gently tapping and rolling the tube. Read and score agglutination macroscopically with the aid of an agglutination lamp.
9. Wash the cells at least three times with saline and ensure that all saline is completely decanted following the final wash.
10. Add one to two drops of antihuman globulin (AHG), as recommended by the manufacturer, and mix.
11. Repeat steps 2 and 3.
12. Add one drop of IgG-coated RBCs (check cells) to all negative tubes from above.
13. Mix the cell suspension and centrifuge the tube at 500 RCF for 15 to 20 seconds.
14. After centrifugation, completely resuspend the cell pellet by tapping the tube. Read and score agglutination macroscopically with the aid of an agglutination lamp.

If the appropriate test tubes do NOT give a positive reaction after addition of IgG-coated RBCs and recentrifugation, THE COMPLETE TEST MUST BE REPEATED.

▶ Antibody Screening

The purpose of the antibody screen is to detect antibodies found in the patient's serum that have potential clinical significance during transfusion. This is performed through the purchase of a set of screening RBC cells: A and B negative, which are each tested against the patient's serum. The screening sets, traditionally two or three reagent cell sets, must contain antigenic expression of D, C, c, E, e, Kell, k, Le[a], Ke[b], Jk[a], Jk[b], Fy[a], Fy[b], P1, M, N, S, and s antigens (described in a later section in more detail). Cells are scored as either reactive or nonreactive. Antigenic targets are eliminated through this process and narrowed to a smaller subset, which can be further identified using the antibody identification methods described below. The goal of antibody screening is to improve the sensitivity and specificity of detection, specifically controlling the first stage of agglutination, and certain additional aspects of the second stage of agglutination. The stages of agglutination tested during the antibody screen are room temperature or immediate spin (IS), 37°C and antiglobulin phase. A negative antibody screen is the end of the type and screen procedure of pretransfusion testing, unless a donor crossmatch is ordered or incorporated into the SOP. However, a positive antibody screen triggers antibody identification (antibody ID).

Procedure: Tube Method

One of the oldest testing methods for antibody screening is the tube test method. In the most primitive form, this test takes the form of adding serum (two drops) to a cell-saline solution. This test is easy to perform and low in cost but has poor sensitivity, particularly with shorter incubation times; thus, its usage in clinical labs has steadily decreased since the 1960s with the advent of more improved methods. However, improvements to this method, including the use of BSA, have increased sensitivity but still require longer incubation times. This conflicts with the sometimes-rapid turnaround time necessary for STAT blood unit transfusion.[14] Other attempted improvements used in the diagnostic laboratory include increasing the serum-to-cell ratio (four to eight drops), adding potentiators such as low ionic-strength saline (LISS) RBC suspensions and other LISS-additive methods, as well as the addition of an additive such as polybrene (i.e., heamethrine bromide) and PEG (polyethylene glycol).[15]

In general, the tube method is performed by combining either patient serum or plasma with the appropriate RBCs, most commonly, O type screening cells provided commercially as well as the donor's own cells for an auto control (additionally, the donor's cells can be added for antibody cross-matching). Three types of screens are potentially performed to account for all potential antibody-antigen agglutinations. An immediate spin procedure is performed if IgM antibodies are suspected but is often omitted as IgM responses are considered nuisance antibodies. A LISS or other potentiating solution can then be added. This is followed by a required incubation phase at 37°C for at least 10 minutes or considerably longer. Tubes are then centrifuged and examined. However, an additional Coombs phase testing can be performed in which antihuman globulin (AHG) is added after three cell washes and saline removal. Cells are mixed and centrifuged and read for agglutination. All negative results should have Coombs control cells added to confirm the negative response. All reactions detected during this final phase are from IgG antibodies and considered clinically significant. Like the prior assays performed in the blood-bank laboratory, the manual tube method has been modified by commercial manufacturers to be completed using a gel method as well.

Clinical Utility

Although the first stage of pretransfusion testing is to examine the most common culprits for transfusion-related reactions, the clinical utility of the antibody screen is to examine the possibility of additional antibodies in the patient that may lead to complications. Only a small percentage of the population has additional detectable RBC antibodies; however, this number is greatly increased in certain populations including repeat transfusion recipients and is required by the AABB in the testing of both the patient and the donor. The screening of patients is typically followed by antibody identification and verification, as well as the selection of donor units that are negative for the identified antigen. Donor units that have detectable antibodies may undergo additional filtration to remove plasma in order to reduce the possibility of a reaction in the recipient.

▶ Antibody Identification and Other Red Cell Antigens

Although more than 600 antigens have been described on the surface of red cells, a shorter list of antigens is commonly tested during the antibody screening procedures performed in the clinical blood bank. Specifically, the antibody screening sets contain antigenic expression of D, C, c, E, e, Kell, k, Le^a, Ke^b, Jk^a, Jk^b, Fy^a, Fy^b, P1, M, N, S, and s antigens, and occasionally include a bonus cell with a very rare antigen (**FIGURE 12–6**). Similar to the two and three reagent cell screening sets provided by commercial manufactures, more complete sets of 10 to 12 reagent cells are used for antibody identification. Testing with these sets allows the blood bank technologist to isolate and identify potential transfusion-reaction causing antibodies in the patient's serum/plasma. Additionally, single antibodies for the majority of clinically relevant antigens, e.g., anti-Le^a, are commercially available for use in compatibility testing.

PANOCELL -10
Master List

IMMUCOR, INC. Norcross, GA 30071 USA
US LICENSE NO: 886
LOT NO: 23732
EXPIRES: 2019/08/16

NAME _____
NO. _____
INSTITUTION _____
BLOOD GROUP _____
ANTIBODY IDENTITY _____
TECH _____ DATE _____

VIAL	Special Type	Donor	D	C	c	E	e	Cʷ	K	k	Kpᵃ	Kpᵇ	Jsᵃ	Jsᵇ	Fyᵃ	Fyᵇ	Jkᵃ	Jkᵇ	Leᵃ	Leᵇ	P₁	M	N	S	s	Luᵃ	Luᵇ	Xgᵃ	
1	Co(b+)	R1R1 B9492	+	+	0	0	+	0	0	+	0	+	0	+	0	+	0	+	0	+	0	+	+	+	0	0	+	+	1
2		R1wR1 B2599	+	+	0	0	+	+	+	+	0	+	0	+	0	+	+	+	0	0	0	0	+	0	+	+	+	+	2
3		R2R2 C6551	+	0	+	+	0	0	0	+	0	+	0	+	+	0	0	+	0	+	+	0	+	0	+	0	+	+	3
4	V+, VS+, U-	Ror D1133	+	0	+	0	+	0	0	+	0	+	0	+	0	0	+	0	0	+	+	0	+	0	0	0	+	+	4
5		r'r E1102	0	+	+	0	+	0	0	+	0	+	0	+	+	+	0	+	0	+	+	0	+	+	+	+	+	+	5
6		r"r F621	0	0	+	+	+	0	0	+	0	+	0	+	+	0	0	+	0	+	+	+	+	+	+	0	+	+	6
7		rr G1782	0	0	+	0	+	0	+	+	0	+	0	+	0	+	+	0	0	+	+	+	0	0	+	0	+	0	7
8	Bg(a+)	rr H177	0	0	+	0	+	0	0	+	0	+	0	+	+	0	+	+	+	0	0	+	0	0	+	+	+	0	8
9		rr N4642	0	0	+	0	+	0	0	+	+	+	0	+	0	+	0	+	0	+	+	0	+	0	+	0	+	0	9
10		rr G1547	0	0	+	0	+	0	+	+	0	+	0	+	0	+	0	+	+	+	+	+	+	0	0	0	+	+	10
TC	I-, Yt(b+)	R1R1 B3715	+	+	0	0	+	0	0	+	0	+	0	+	+	0	+	+	0	0	+	+	0	+	0	0	+	+	TC
		Patient's Cells																											PC

Direct Antiglobulin Test		Eluate Result	
	Poly	IgG	C3
LOT			
RESULT			

NOTES:
An antigen designated with a 'w' represent a weakened expression of the antigen that may or may not react with all examples of the corresponding antibody.

TC: In most individuals, the amount of i antigen present on red blood cells gradually decreases during the first 18 months of age, while the amount of I antigen increases. In rare individuals, this transition does not occur and the i phenotype persists on the adult red blood cells. Trace amounts of I antigen may be detected on cord blood cells and i adult cells with potent examples of anti- I . The frequency of i adult cells is approximately 1 in 4400 samples tested. The Ii antigens are closely associated with ABH, Lewis, and P, often forming compound antigens, e.g. IA, IH, iH , etc. Additional information may be found in Blood Groups: P, I , Sd ᵃ and Pr, published in 1991 by the American Association of Blood Banks.

PATIENT'S SERUM TEST RESULTS / TEST METHODS

PATIENT'S SERUM / PANOSCREEN LOT: I, II, III
REVERSE GROUPING CELLS: A1, A2, B

* Indicates those antigens whose presence or absence may have been determined using only a single example of a specific antibody.

410-18

FIGURE 12–6 Example antibody identification panel for blood bank. Patient serum is tested in various conditions: immediate spin, 37oC, IAT and others, against each cell in the panel and the results recorded. Process of elimination based on the known antigens for each cell is used to narrow down potential antibodies in the patient.

Courtesy of Immucor, Inc.

Blood group systems are defined as one or more antigens that are controlled by a single-gene locus, or two closely-linked homologous genes. These are generally considered important for their roles in transfusion-related events and reactions, including hemolytic disease of the fetus and newborn (HDFN), HTR, TRALI, and TACO. Specifically, and in addition to the ABO blood group, antibodies against the P, Lewis, and Vel blood group systems have been shown to produce hemolysis and are carefully reviewed. While the list of other blood groups is quite extensive, a few examples are provided here.

The MNS blood group (002) antibodies against M and N were among the earliest antibodies discovered by Landsteiner and his colleague Levine in the sera of rabbits. Later additions to the group were the antigens S and s. When found in the patient sera, an anti-M antigen, for example, can react at room temperature and 37°C; however, it is considered clinically significant only when reactive at 37°C.

The most clinically important members of the Kell (006) blood-group system are K, named for a Mrs. Kelleher in which it was first described. Others in the system were named for the individuals in whom they were found as well, such as Js^a after the producer of the antibody John Sutter. This group also contains the k antigen found in the antibody screen. Only later were they connected through genetics and grouped accordingly, as well as given an IBST number. The K antigen is the most immunogenic antigen after ABO and Rh, and is the cause of HDFN and immediate and delayed HTRs.

Another clinically important antigen is Le^a of the Lewis (007) blood-group system. The system now contains six antigens; the two main ones are Le^a and Le^b. The antibody is typically reactive at room temperature and not at 37°C. While Lewis antibodies are rarely involved in HDFN or HTRs because they are usually IgM (thus, do not cross the placenta) and do not react with RBCs at physiological temperatures. They are common antibodies that should be ruled out during testing.

Two other groups that commonly examine the blood-bank laboratory are the Duffy (008) and Kidd (009) systems. The most important members of these systems are Fy^a and Fy^b in Duffy and Jk^a and Jk^b in Kidd. Both the Duffy antibodies and Kidd antibodies have been seen in patients with a history of transfusion or childbirth and can lead to HTR and HDFN.

While this is not an exhaustive list of antibodies that lead to transfusion and hemolytic reactions, it illustrates the necessity for the detailed investigation and diagnosis of patient and donor phenotypes in the blood-bank laboratory.

Antiglobulin Crossmatch

In a final safety check, the patient's serum is used against the donor's RBCs to determine compatibility between the two before the donor's cells are administered during transfusion, a process known as an antiglobulin crossmatch. This is typically performed via the immediate spin (IS) and indirect antiglobulin test (IAT) methods described previously in relation to ABO, Rh, and antibody screening steps. Briefly, the IS crossmatch is performed by mixing a 3 to 5% suspension of donor RBCs with patient serum and spinning at low RPM. The cell button is dislodged and assessed for the presence of agglutination or hemolysis. The lack of these two markers is considered acceptable for transfusion. However, if a patient has a history of significant antibodies, or a previously positive crossmatch, an IAT crossmatch will be performed. The donor cells, are mixed with the patient serum in an enhancement media and incubated at 37°C, followed by the antiglobulin phase, i.e., the addition of an antihuman globulin to amplify crossreactivity. A negative hemolysis or agglutination response is considered acceptable for transfusion. A positive response at either phase is considered incompatible for transfusion; however, additional information may be collected to verify the positive result. Due to the wide accessibility and reliability of stored data, many facilities have moved away from the physical crossmatch toward a computerized or virtual crossmatch.

Other Immunodiagnostic Testing in Immunohematology

All donated blood units must not only be tested for ABO and Rh typing, but also for several viral infection indicators. Specifically, all units are tested for hepatitis B surface antigen (HBsAg), hepatitis B core antigen (HBcAg), hepatitis C virus antibody (anti-HCV), syphilis, HIV antigen, HTLV-I, and HTLV-II antigens. Most of these infections are commonly detected through immunodiagnostic methods that are discussed elsewhere in this text; however, some of these tests are being replaced with alternative detection methods, such as nucleic acid tests (NAT) for HIV and HCV.

In addition, an increasing number of blood-bank and transfusion laboratories are beginning to perform testing for human leukocyte antigen (HLA), also known as the human major histocompatibility complex (MHC) antigens, which have been shown to have a significance in a small number of transfusion reactions, specifically transfusion-related acute lung injury (TRALI), and are gaining significance for what is called histocompatibility testing prior to transplantation. Finally, a series of other tests are performed in specific cases within the immunohematology department or transfusion lab. The Leukoagglutinin Test is performed on the donor's plasma to look for agglutinating antibodies toward white blood cells that could cause transfusion-related febrile reactions. The platelet antibody detection test looks for antibodies to antigens on the surface of platelets that may derive from two sources, prior transfusion of platelets and autoantibodies, such as those occurring in idiopathic thrombocytopenic purpura. Immunohematologists perform the qualitative rosette test performed on postpartum mothers to assess anti-Rh antibody formation after a fetomaternal bleed of an Rh-positive fetus into an Rh-negative mother. When few or no rosettes are formed, it means little to no fetal blood made it to the mother's circulation; however, a positive test must be confirmed with the quantitative Kleihauer-Betke stain for fetal hemoglobin, which allows the physician to determine how many doses of RhIG to administer to the mother.

Transfusion vs Transplant: Similarities and Differences

One major benefit derived from the long history of transfusion testing is that it elucidated many of the critical concerns that may arise in the organ transplant field, especially in the area of infectious-disease transfer and immunological compatibility between host and recipient. Therefore, it is of some benefit to discuss common transfusion reactions with an eye toward potential similarities and differences from transplant serology.

Common Transfusion Reactions

Transfusion reactions are caused by two major sources, 1) is infection related to the passage of infectious agents, such as viruses and bacteria from the donor to the recipient, and 2) are immune responses resulting from the delivery of incompatible donor units. The preceding discussion has focused exclusively on the latter of these two sources of transfusion reactions, while the first source is more exhaustively examined in chapters focused on bacterial and viral detection. Nevertheless, the infectious sources of transfusion reactions are an important part of the blood bank practice and a major reason for many of the preliminary questionnaires and much of the testing done on donor units. Units found to be infectious are discarded, and donors are deferred temporarily or permanently as a result of prior exposures or from the answers provided in the predonation questionnaires. Virus such as HIV, HBV, HCV, HTLV, and WNV are tested for in the serum and blood of all donors in the

United States, as they can lead to what is known as transfusion-transmitted diseases. Bacterial contaminants, such as *Staphylococcus, Yersinia,* and *Escherichia* species can be a major source of transfusion-related sepsis, often as a result of platelet transfusion, which has a higher incidence of bacterial transfer due to its room-temperature storage requirements. Many other microorganisms can be transmitted through transfusion, but not all are tested for routinely and should be considered in the post-transfusion, follow-up if clinically indicated.

RBC surface factors, such as ABO, Rh, and others, are the primary sources of most immune-mediated transfusion-related reactions. These are also typically defined by their timing as "acute," if occurring within the first 24 hours of transfusion, or "delayed," if occurring after 24 hours. However, some reactions such as the **febrile nonhemolytic transfusion reaction (FNHTR)**, seen as an increase in body temperature above 1°C with accompanying chills, nausea, and tachycardia, may be caused by WBC pyrogens or cytokines, not RBC interactions. FNHTR is typically self-limiting and does not usually require intervention. Others such as **acute hemolytic transfusion reaction (AHTR)** may have either an immune or nonimmune etiology. In the immune-mediated mechanism previously formed, IgM or IgG bind the donor RBCs and immune complexes are formed, activating the complement cascade leading to red cell lysis. When AHTR is suspected, the transfusion is immediately stopped and clerical verification of compatibility is performed between donor and patient. A specimen is collected and DAT testing is performed. A negative DAT does not rule out an immune response, and typically all pretransfusion testing is repeated on the posttransfusion specimen.

In contrast to AHTR, **delayed hemolytic transfusion reaction (DHTR)**, also known as delayed serologic transfusion reaction (DSTR) if hemolysis does not occur, is typically defined as being caused by the formation of a "new" RBC antibody within the patient. These reactions occur days to weeks after the transfusion. Coated RBCs are removed from the vasculature by the endothelial system. In some cases, jaundice or unexplained fever may occur, but DHTR/DSTR is often nonsymptomatic and may be discovered only on repeat serological testing. However, DHTR can sometimes lead to severe or life-threatening hemolysis and therefore, the blood bank physician should be notified of all suspected cases.

Transfusion-related acute lung injury (TRALI) is an acute transfusion reaction that presents with respiratory distress and sever hypoxia, typically within the first 6 hours of transfusion. It is identifiable via radiographic imaging, which shows bilateral edema via interstitial infiltrates, similar to what is seen in acute respiratory distress syndrome (ARDS) but following transfusion. The immune-mediated pathway is thought to occur as a result of antibodies against human leukocyte antigens (HLAs) or, alternatively, human neutrophil antigens (HNAs). HLAs, although not routinely tested in transfusion practice, are a common source of reaction to transplant and are tested more commonly in that context. A genetic pre-disposition to TRALI is thought to account for the nonimmune pathway to injury. Plasma units can be used to decrease the potential of TRALI. Donors implicated in cases of TRALI are often excluded from further donation. Treatment for TRALI is usually through supportive therapy similar to that for other patients with permeability edema; i.e., ventilation and oxygen.

One final commonly encountered transfusion reaction, which is often difficult to distinguish from TRALI, is **transfusion-associated circulatory overload (TACO)**. Although some distinctive signs exist, the simultaneous occurrence of both can make differentiation difficult. TACO presents with respiratory distress, hypoxemia, and associated headache, chest tightness, coughing, and jugular vein distention. TACO is thought to result from an expansion in the intravascular volume and creates a heightened risk in patients with pre-existing heart, lung, or kidney failure. Reducing the rate of transfusion may decrease the risk of TACO. Treatment consists of sitting the patient up, starting diuresis, and applying additional oxygen.

Transplant Serology

Human organ, tissue, and bone-marrow transplant has been a possibility for much less time than transfusion; therefore, a good percentage of

Infectious Disease Serological Testing Performed in all Transplant vs all Transfusion Donors		
Infectious Disease Testing	**Transplant Donors[18]**	**Transfusion Donors[19]**
Cytomegalovirus (CMV) IgG	+	+
Herpes simplex virus (HSV) IgG	+	+
Varicella-zoster virus (VZV) IgG	+	+
Epstein-Barr virus (EBV) (VCA IgG)	+	+
Human immunodeficiency virus (HIV-1 and -2 immunoassay)	+	+ *Antibodies and HIV-1 viral load*
Hepatitis B virus: HBsAg, HBsAb, HBcAb	+	+ *Antibodies, antigens, and occasional viral load*
Hepatitis C virus (HCV) IgM, IgG	+	+ *Antibodies and viral load*
Treponema pallidum (Venereal Disease Research Laboratory [VDRL] or rapid plasma regain [RPR])	+	+
Toxoplasma gondii (in heart transplant candidates) IgG	+	+
Measles, mumps, and rubella	+	–
West Nile virus antibodies	–	+
Serum Aspergillus galactomannan antigen	–	+
HTLV-1, -2 antibodies	–	+

Modified from Fishman, J. A., Marr, K. A., & Thorner, A. R. (March 2015). Evaluation for infection before solid organ transplantation. UpToDate.

the best practices for transplantation have come from our understanding of transfusion. Like pretransfusion testing, the ABO and Rh blood groups are also carefully monitored during pretransplant testing. However, the donor and recipient systems are now interacting at more than just the RBC and, to a lesser extent, WBC level.

Like blood-donor screening, transplant donors undergo a similar screening process with the goals of disqualifying both the donor and/or recipient for safety, detecting potential infectious agents, defining the risk of infection, and implementing interventions when possible.[16] Unlike blood donations, organ donations may arrive from either living or deceased individuals in both cases, infectious disease, nucleic acid testing (NAT), and serological tests are performed. Infectious viral disease serology testing recommendations are more robust than required transfusion testing requirements, specifically for known tissue dormant herpes viruses such as cytomegalovirus (CMV) and Epstein-Barr virus (EBV).[17]

The major difference between immunological testing prior to transfusion (pretransfusion testing) and pretransplant testing is the examination of the **human leukocyte antigens (HLA)**, commonly referred to as the major histocompatibility complex (MHC) antigens in other animal species. The MHC antigens are composed of class I and II proteins, which are crucial in the acceptance of transplantation. In humans, class I proteins consist of HLA-A, HLA-B, and HLA-C, and class II proteins consists of HLA-DR, HLA-DQ, and HLA-DP. These proteins are encoded by closely linked genes located on the short arm of chromosome six within the MHC region. HLA genes are inherited as haplotypes, where the offspring receives one maternal and one paternal haplotype in a Mendelian dominant manner.[20] These molecules play an important role in immune signaling through the presentation of foreign antigens to T lymphocytes. Specifically, cytotoxic T cells interact with class I MCH through their CD8 surface molecules, and helper T cells interact with class II MHCs through their CD4 surface molecules. They continue to play an integral role in transplant acceptance,

especially in bone marrow transplants where it can greatly increase a recipient's 5-year survival rate.[21] In the United States, the American Society for Histocompatibility and Immunogenetics (ASHI) has provided guidelines for the operation of clinical HLA testing facilities in support of solid-organ and stem-cell transplant. While these laboratories may take on a variety of roles in which HLA testing is important, including platelet transfusion screening, bone-marrow screening, and solid-organ support, all centers perform HLA typing and screening via either serological or genetic methods. HLA typing and crossmatching is a cornerstone for bone marrow, cord blood, and solid organ transplant risk mitigation.[21-23] Although sometimes controversial, it has been shown that both HLA class I and class II play a role in graft rejection.[24,25] Indeed, HLA matching greatly reduces the risk of **graft-versus host disease (GVHD)** and transplant rejection. GVHD, when the donated bone marrow or stem cells attack the recipient, and organ rejection are mediated by alloimmune T cells, which respond to HLA antigens differently from other antigens to pathogens or self. Specifically, T cells react directly to alloantigens normally shown on antigen-presenting cells (APCs) in complex with HLAs, but do not recognize mismatched HLA types that have been strongly correlated with the rates of rejection and disease. Despite this fact, many organ transplants are still conducted with some level of HLA mismatching and work is being performed to indicate which HLA mismatches are most permissive to transplant.[26]

▶ **Transplant-specific Testing**

In addition to serological tests for infectious disease and RBC markers such as ABO and Rh, the most important markers identified for transplant compatibility and acceptance are the HLA marker profiles of the donor and recipient. These testing methodologies include both genetic tests, DNA-based typing, and the more-pervasive, antibody-based methods, including cell-based assays, such as flow cytometric and anti-human globulin lymphotoxicity, and solid-phase immunoassays, including ELISA assays and others.[23] Although serology is considered the most widely used method for HLA testing in the clinical setting, its challenges include crossreactivity, antisera availability issues, and decreased surface expression of HLA antigens, which can be overcome by genetic testing.[27] In this section, we will review several serological test methods still in common clinical practice: the **complement-dependent microcytotoxicity (CDC)** technique, the solid-phase ELISA test, and the HLA crossmatch.

The CDC Test

The CDC test, also known as the lymphocyte cytotoxicity test (LCT),[23] is used both for serological typing of HLA and for antibody screening and characterization (**FIGURE 12–7**). The difference is in the source of the serum and the cells. The method can be used to classify either a recipient or donor HLA class I and class II molecules by isolation of T and B cells from the blood; T cells interact with class II molecules while B cells interact with class I. Serum is provided commercially from mostly alloimmunized, multiparous women. However, since these sera tend to be low titer, monoclonal antibodies from immunized mice have been used since the 1990s as well. Commercial typing trays with the various HLA antibodies can be purchased and have been developed for specific ethnic populations, such as Black and Asian, due to the variation in HLA types found in differing ethnic groups. In contrast to the HLA typing technique, testing for HLA antibodies in the donor's serum is also performed by using HLA-typed frozen reagent cells. By a combination of these techniques, both the recipient and donor can be typed and screened for surface antigens as well as pre-existing HLA antibodies. While the CDC test has been considered the gold standard for decades, it is being replaced slowly with solid-phase assays, such as the ELISA and flow cytometric analysis. For example, lymphocytes

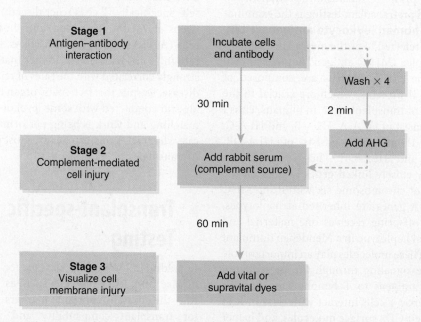

FIGURE 12–7 The basic steps of the complement-dependent microlymphocytotoxicity assay (CDC). A variation known as the antiglobulin-augmented CDC are also shown as noted between steps 1 and 2.

Modified from Eva D Quinley. Immunohematology, Lippincott Williams & Wilkins, 2010.

pooled from random donors have been used to screen for pre-existing HLA antibodies using both ELISA and flow cytometry.[25] In addition, genetic testing, such as sequence-specific primer DNA-typing, has been on the increase as it tends to be more sensitive to serological ambiguity.[21]

HLA ELISA

Solid-phase immunoassay technologies including flow cytometric assays, Luminex microbead assays, and ELISA have been used with success for HLA antibody testing. In the ELISA assay for HLA, the HLA antigens are bound to a microtiter well, and antibodies from the patient's serum are detected through an enzyme-conjugated substrate. The usage of purified HLA antigens increases the specificity of this assay.

HLA Crossmatch

A positive HLA crossmatch is a counter indication for both kidney and pancreas transplant. It is commonly performed as the antihuman globulin CDC (AHG-CDC) in many facilities. Performance of this assay is similar to the Coombs antiglobulin testing previously described, except that the cells tested are T and B lymphocytes. However, several large-scale centers have moved toward the computerized crossmatch or rely on a flow crossmatch in transplant testing.[28]

CASE STUDY

A Comparison of Tube and Column Methods for Antibody Titer

This case is adapted from Park et al., *Ann Lab Med*. 2014.[12]

It is critical to monitor ABO antibody titers in multiple-clinical situations, specifically during blood-bank transfusions and transplantations. One hundred and eighty healthy adults who underwent a normal medical examination were selected based on their blood group, 60 A, 60 B, and 60 O, to study the sensitivity of three commonly used serum agglutination assays used to determine antibody titer.

Method 1

The Immediate spin (IS) tube method was performed by preparing serial dilutions of serum in saline into 10 separate tubes. Each tube received a 3% saline-suspension of group A or B RBCs. After incubation and centrifugation, results were visually determined and confirmed by at least two other technical personnel.

Method 2

The anti-Human IgG (AHG) method (EMD Millipore) was performed on the same tubes by incubating the tubes at 37°C for 30 minutes and washing with normal saline three times. 100 µl of polyspecific AHG was added to the tubes and they were centrifuged for 15 seconds at 1,000 g. Tubes were interpreted visually as above.

Method 3

A column agglutination technique (CAT) was performed with and without dithiothreitol (DTT); this thiol agent has been used to distinguish between IgM and IgG by dissolving IgM disulfide bonds. Ten tubes were labeled and serial dilutions were performed in phosphate-buffered saline (PBS). Dilutions were incubated at 37°C for 45 minutes using a commercially available direct agglutination test (DAT) (or Coombs) card (LISS/Coombs, Bio-Rad).

Results and Discussion

The median values of anti-B titers in Group A blood and anti-A titers in Group B blood were 16 by IS and 8 by AHG for both. Titers were not significantly different when AHG was compared to CAT without DTT when anti-B

(continues)

CASE STUDY (Continued)

was placed in Group A blood and vice versa. However, titers were significantly higher for anti-A and anti-B titers by CAT without DTT when placed in type O blood; 32 vs 128 for anti-A and 32 vs 256 for anti-B. In all cases, CAT titers were higher without DTT than with DTT when compared. Due to the significant increase in detection titer, CAT tested with and without DTT was considered far more sensitive than the IS and AHG methods. The usage of this more sensitive method could reduce the number of transfusion-related deaths and injuries. However, the cost of this system is higher than the classical tube methods.

Critical Thinking Questions

1. When considering agglutination methods for determining titer, what factors are important in the sensitivity?
2. What specificity factors are important?

Distribution of ABO Antibody Titers According to Titration Methods

Blood Group Antibodies (N of Samples)	Median (Interquartile Range) of Antibody Titer for Each Method			
	IS Tube	AHG Tube	CAT without DTT	CAT with DTT
Anti-B in blood group A (60)	16 (2-256)	8 (1-512)	8 (1-64)	2 (1-16)
Anti-A in blood group B (60)	16 (2-128)	8 (2-64)	8 (1-256)	4 (1-128)
Anti-B in blood group O (60)	16 (4-128)	32 (4-256)	128 (8-2,048)	64 (2-1,024)
Anti-A in blood group O (60)	16 (4-128)	32 (8-256)	256 (16-2,048)	128 (16-2,048)

Abbreviations: IS, immediate spin; AHG, anti-human globulin; CAT, column agglutination technique; DTT, dithiothreitol.

Park ES, Jo KI, Shin JW, et al. Comparison of total and IgG ABO antibody titers in healthy individuals by using tube and column agglutination techniques. *Ann Lab Med.* 2014;34(3):223–229. Used with Permission from Korean Society for Laboratory Medicine.

▶ References

1. Blood Donor History Questionnaires. 2018; http://www.aabb.org/tm/questionnaires/Pages/dhqaabb.aspx. Accessed 9/26/2018, 2018.
2. Petrini C. Evaluation of EU legislation on blood: a bioethical point of view. *J Blood Med.* 2017;8:193–198.
3. World Health Organization. Developing a National Blood System. http://www.who.int/bloodsafety/en/
4. Avent ND. Large-scale blood group genotyping: clinical implications. *Br J Haematol.* 2009;144(1):3–13.
5. Rhamy J. Challenges to RBC Genotyping. *MedicalLab Management.* 2015;4(16).
6. American Association of Blood Banks. *Standards for blood banks and transfusion services.* 31st ed. Bethesda, Md.: American Association of Blood Banks; 2018.
7. IH-centrifuge L. In: Bio-Rad Laboratories I, ed: Bio-Rad Laboratories, Inc.; 2018.
8. Bajpai M, Kaur R, Gupta E. Automation in immunohematology. *Asian J Transfus Sci.* 2012;6(2):140–144.
9. International Society of Blood Transfusion. Table of blood group systems v5.1_180207. http://www.isbtweb.org.
10. Garratty G, Glynn SA, McEntire R, Retrovirus epidemiology donor S. ABO and Rh(D) phenotype frequencies of different racial/ethnic groups in the United States. *Transfusion.* 2004;44(5):703–706.
11. Bhangale A, Pathak A, Pawar S, et al. Comparison of antibody titers using conventional tube technique versus column agglutination technique in ABO blood group incompatible renal transplant. *Asian J Transfus Sci.* 2017;11(2):131–134.

12. Park ES, Jo KI, Shin JW, et al. Comparison of total and IgG ABO antibody titers in healthy individuals by using tube and column agglutination techniques. *Ann Lab Med.* 2014;34(3):223–229.

13. Fung MK, Sheikh H, Eghtesad B, et al. Severe hemolysis resulting from D incompatibility in a case of ABO-identical liver transplant. *Transfusion.* 2004;44(11): 1635–1639.

14. Casina TS. In search of the Holy Grail: comparison of antibody screening methods. *Immunohematology.* 2006;22(4):196–202.

15. Garratty G. Advances in red blood cell immunology 1960 to 2009. *Transfusion.* 2010;50(3):526–535.

16. Fischer SA, Avery RK, AST Infectious Disease Community of Practice. Screening of donor and recipient prior to solid organ transplantation. *Am J Transplant.* 2009;9(suppl 4): S7–S18.

17. Len O, Garzoni C, Lumbreras C, et al. Recommendations for screening of donor and recipient prior to solid organ transplantation and to minimize transmission of donor-derived infections. *Clin Microbiol Infect.* 2014;20(suppl 7): 10–18.

18. Fishman JA, Blumberg EA, Bond S. Evaluation for infection before solid organ transplantation. Wolters Kluwer; 2018. https://www.uptodate.com/contents/evaluation-for-infection-before-solid-organ-transplantation. Accessed 3/2/2019.

19. Wingard JR, Kauffman CA, Thorner AR. Evaluation for infection before hematopoietic cell transplantation. Wolters Kluwer; 2018. https://www.uptodate.com/contents/evaluation-for-infection-before-hematopoietic-cell-transplantation. Accessed 3/2/2019.

20. Dixit S, Baganizi DR, Sahu R, et al. Immunological challenges associated with artificial skin grafts: available solutions and stem cells in future design of synthetic skin. *J Biol Eng.* 2017;11:49.

21. Tipu HN, Bashir MM, Noman M. Identification of HLA class I misreads/dropouts using serological typing, in comparison with DNA-based typing. *Iran J Allergy Asthma Immunol.* 2016;15(5):420–425.

22. Yoder MC. Cord blood banking and transplantation: advances and controversies. *Curr Opin Pediatr.* 2014;26(2):163–168.

23. Yoshihara S, Taniguchi K, Ogawa H, et al. The role of HLA antibodies in allogeneic SCT: is the 'type-and-screen' strategy necessary not only for blood type but also for HLA? *Bone Marrow Transplant.* 2012;47(12): 1499–1506.

24. Won DI, Jung HD, Jung OJ, et al. Flow cytometry PRA using lymphocyte pools from random donors. *Cytometry B Clin Cytom.* 2007;72(4):256–264.

25. Won DI. Flow cytometry PRA using pooled lymphocytes for both HLA class I and II antibodies *Lab Medicine.* 2011;42(1):17–24.

26. DeWolf S, Sykes M. Alloimmune T cells in transplantation. *J Clin Invest.* 2017;127(7):2473–2481.

27. Dhurandhar PS, Halankar AR, Joshi BR. Pre and post transplant immunological evaluation for a long successful graft survival. *Int J Hum Genet.* 2012;12(1):63–67.

28. Parsons RF, Locke JE, Redfield RR 3rd, et al. Kidney transplantation of highly sensitized recipients under the new kidney allocation system: a reflection from five different transplant centers across the United States. *Hum Immunol.* 2017;78(1):30–36.

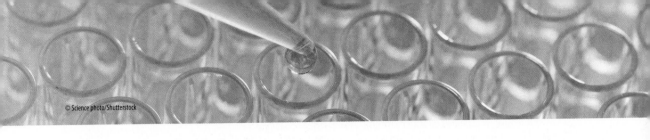

© Science photo/Shutterstock

CHAPTER 13

Autoimmunity: Diseases and Testing

Andrew McKeon, MD, D(ABMLI)

KEY TERMS

Addison disease
Anti-nuclear antibodies (ANAS)
Antiphospholipid syndrome
Celiac sprue
Citrullinated peptides
Double-stranded dna (DSDNA)
Encephalopathy
Gad65
Goodpasture's disease
Human embryonic kidney
   (HEK-293)
Human epithelial type 2
   (HEP-2) cell
Hypophysitis

Immune thrombocytopenia (ITP)
Inflammatory bowel disease (IBD)
Mixed connective-tissue disease
   (MCTD)
Multiple sclerosis (MS)
Myasthenia gravis
Myelin oligodendrocyte
   glycoprotein (MOG)
Myelopathy
Neuromyelitis optica (NMO)
Neuropathy
Oligoclonal banding (OCB)
Optic neuritis
Pemphigoid

Pemphigus
Pernicious anemia
Retinopathy
Rheumatoid arthritis
Scleroderma
Sjogren syndrome
Systemic lupus erythematosus
   (SLE)
Thyroid disease
Thyroid peroxidase (TPO)
Toll-like receptors (TLRS)
Type 1 diabetes mellitus
Uveitis

LEARNING OBJECTIVES

Upon completion of this chapter, the reader should be able to:

1. Classify the underlying phenomenon that produces autoimmunity.
2. Compare the loss of tolerance with incidence of autoimmunity.
3. Evaluate the use of antibody markers in autoimmune disease correlation.
4. Review sensitivity, specificity, and predicative values in autoimmune disease diagnostics.

(continues)

▶ Fundamentals

Autoimmunity results from a breakdown in one or more mechanisms facilitating the immune system to distinguish self from foreign antigens. Autoimmune disorders collectively are common (prevalence of 7 to 9% in the general population), although a number of individual diseases are rare. Among the most common are autoimmune **thyroid disease**, **type 1 diabetes mellitus** and **rheumatoid arthritis**. Some are systemic autoimmune diseases such as **systemic lupus erythematosus (SLE)**, while other diseases are organ-specific such as autoimmune thyroid disease.

Regarding predisposing genetic factors, certain major histocompatibility complex (MHC) haplotypes have the strongest associations and are encountered across most autoimmune diseases, such as type 1 diabetes and autoimmune thyroid disease. Rare monogenic autoimmune diseases have also been identified. For example, patients with mutations in *AIRE* or *FOXP3* have malfunctioning T regulatory cells, thus, removing a check on autoimmunity.

Components of the immune system critical to initiating cellular and organ damage in autoimmune disease include immunoglobulins, known as antibodies and cytotoxic T lymphocytes. Antibodies, although not always pathogenic, are always antigen-specific, and are physically and chemically robust molecules. For those reasons, the detection of antibodies in patient specimens (usually serum) is the mainstay of laboratory-based diagnostics for autoimmune disease.

Since the discovery of the clinical benefit from immune suppressing corticosteroids in rheumatoid arthritis in the 1950s at the Mayo Clinic, it has been recognized that early treatment of many of these diseases can bring about remission and prevent irreversible organ damage. Over the last 60 years, a diverse array of immune-suppressing drugs have been developed for clinical use, often to supplement or replace corticosteroids, which have many long-term side effects. Some of those drugs have broad effects on the immune system, while others are directed at specific molecules in the immune system.

In this chapter, the clinical and laboratory approach to the diagnosis of autoimmune diseases will be discussed. A detailed description of testing methodologies will be discussed, using certain autoimmune disease tests as examples. The importance of testing algorithms will also be discussed. Thereafter, each disease and pertinent biomarkers will be presented.

Tolerance and Autoimmunity

Tolerance encapsulates a variety of built-in mechanisms in the adaptive immune system to prevent autoimmunity.[1] These mechanisms are largely localized centrally at the point of origin of lymphocytes: in the thymus, for T lymphocytes; and in the fetal liver and bone marrow, for B lymphocytes. During differentiation, autoreactive T-cell precursors and B-cell precursors are eliminated by "positive selection" in the thymic cortex and bone marrow, respectively. Autoreactive T cells are deleted or differentiate into FOXP3+ T regulatory cells, under the control of autoimmune regulator (AIRE), while autoreactive B cells are deleted or their receptors are edited. Mutations in both of those molecules are known to cause rare forms of monogenic autoimmune disease. Those lymphocyte precursors with low self-avidity are exported to the periphery.

Because central tolerance is not foolproof, some autoreactive T and B cells escape these mechanisms and are exported to the periphery. The generation of autoreactive B cells and autoantibodies can also occur at the periphery by somatic hypermutation. The exported cells are normally controlled by peripheral tolerance mechanisms. These mechanisms include inhibitory molecules (such as CTLA-4 and PD-1 expressed on T cells), anergy (functional unresponsiveness, due to absence of costimulatory signals between T-cell and antigen-presenting cell), ignorance (a lack of knowledge of autoreactive lymphocytes of self-antigen sequestered behind anatomical barriers such as the blood-brain barrier), and suppression by T regulatory cells.

Autoimmune diseases are thought to be multifactorial, requiring contribution of both genetic and environmental factors. In genetically predisposed organisms, tissue damage, inflammation, and presentation of new self-antigens or microbial mimics might elicit a break in tolerance and autoimmunity. The initial trigger for both systemic and organ-specific autoimmune disorders involves the recognition of self or foreign molecules, especially nucleic acids, by **toll-like receptors (TLRs)** in the innate immune system. TLRs recognize foreign and self-nucleic acids. Examples include TLR3 for double-stranded RNA, TLR7 and TLR8 for single-stranded RNA, and TLR9 for DNA. After recognizing specific ligands, these TLRs initiate a signaling cascade, which results in the activation of several transcription factors (including nuclear factor kappa-light-chain-enhancer of activated B cells[NF-κB]), which promote cell activation and the production of pro-inflammatory mediators, such as type I interferons (IFN-α and IFN-β) and cytokines, and engagement of previously quiescent autoreactive T cells and B cells.

Causes of Autoimmunity

There is no single factor causing the development of autoimmunity. Determinants influencing the break in immune tolerance include genetic background, sex, age, and exogenous factors.[1]

Autoimmunity commonly runs in families, although there may be different manifestations in different individuals. For example, a patient diagnosed with pernicious anemia, when questioned, would commonly disclose a history of thyroid autoimmunity in a parent and siblings. Also, autoimmune diseases tend to cluster in individuals. For example, patients with pernicious anemia have a higher probability of developing autoimmune thyroid diseases than age- and sex-matched control subjects from the general population. The presence of certain HLA haplotypes also influences the occurrence of autoimmunity to a greater or lesser degree, depending on the disease. For example, HLA-DQ2 and DQ8, although common in the general population and weakly predictive of a diagnosis of celiac disease, have high negative predictive values for that diagnosis. In other words, patients without HLA-DQ2 or DQ8 almost never develop celiac disease. In contrast, HLA-DR4 is known to be a risk factor for multiple sclerosis (MS) in population-based studies only. The presence or absence of this molecule in no way confirms or refutes an MS diagnosis in an individual patient.

Autoimmune diseases, in general, are more common in women. Some diseases have a strong predilection for women and girls. For example, in **neuromyelitis optica (NMO)**, a rare inflammatory disease that mimics MS, the ratio of affected women to men is 9:1. In contrast, paraneoplastic neurological disorders related to small cell lung carcinoma (and hence, smoking) are more common in men. Although autoimmune disorders can occur across the age range, autoimmunity occurs most commonly in the 7th and 8th decades, at a time when the immune system is becoming senescent. Consistent with this observation, autoantibodies are more frequently detected in elderly people in general.

Exogenous factors have a role that is increasingly recognized. Specific cancer types are known to trigger the production of specific IgG antibodies in patients with paraneoplastic neurological disorders. For example, a woman with incoordination due to an autoimmune disease affecting the cerebellum, who has Yo antibody detected, almost always will have breast or gynecological cancer diagnosed subsequently. Exposure to certain infectious agents is recognized as an important risk factor for specific autoimmune diseases. Examples include campylobacter (in an inflammatory peripheral neuropathy known as Guillain-Barre syndrome) and herpes simplex virus (in N-methyl-D-aspartate [NMDA] receptor encephalitis). Hydralazine hydrochloride and procainamide hydrochloride can cause drug-induced lupus.

Role of Antibody Testing in the Broader Clinical Context

Immunoglobulins, the major components of antibodies and several immune cell surface receptors, can act not only as biomarkers in autoimmune disease, but can also be causal of autoimmunity, and are sometimes important in both clinical contexts.

Intracellular antigens are not accessible to immune attack *in situ,* but peptides derived from intracellular proteins are displayed on upregulated MHC class-I molecules and are then accessible to peptide-specific cytotoxic T cells.[2] Antibodies targeting these intracellular antigens are detected in both serum and CSF but are not pathogenic. In clinical practice, these antibodies serve as diagnostic markers of a T-cell predominant effector process. An example is a brain disease known as "paraneoplastic cerebellar degeneration," which occurs in women with a neurological disorder triggered by an immune response against cancer. These women are seropositive for Purkinje cell cytoplasmic antibody-type 1 (PCA-1, also known as "anti-Yo"). This autoantibody predicts with 90% certainty the presence of adenocarcinoma of ovary, uterus, fallopian tube, peritoneum, or breast. The target antigen is cytoplasmic (cerebellar degeneration-related protein 2 [CDR2]) and, therefore, inaccessible in intact cells to the circulating antibody, the depletion of which does not lead to neurological recovery. Afflicted patients die more often from complications of the neurological disorder than from metastatic cancer.

In contrast, IgGs targeting neural cell surface receptors and channels do have a pathogenic role in causing paraneoplastic disorders affecting the CNS. The response to antibody-depleting therapies is usually excellent. For example, patients with antibodies targeting the ionotropic glutamate receptor (NR1 subunit of N-methyl D-aspartate [NMDA] receptor, often associated with ovarian teratoma) present with encephalopathy. This generally improves or remits with antigen source (teratoma) removal and immunotherapies targeted at removing antibody or reducing its production.

▶ Antibodies: Pertinence to Autoimmune Diseases

Antibody testing is mostly a qualitative science. That is to say, distinguishing positive from negative for the purposes of aiding in or confirming a diagnosis is the most important task.

Under certain circumstances, the quantitative value of the antibody may be pertinent. This may be obtained by performing doubling dilutions, within an ELISA or indirect immunofluorescence format, to obtain a titer (highest dilution at which antibody is still detectable), or by a quantitation of antibody in nmol or pmol per liter using an immunoprecipitation assay. Semi-quantitative data in international units per milliliter (IU/mL) may be obtained from ELISA.

Antibody values may be used to estimate the positive predictive value for the disease in question (which might be lower for low antibody values, and higher for higher for high antibody values). **GAD65** antibody testing exemplifies the occasional utility of interpreting the antibody value. By immunoprecipitation in the author's laboratory, any value greater than 0.02 nmol/L is considered a positive result. However, further interpretation may be required on the basis of the clinical scenario and antibody value. Patients with GAD65 autoimmune neurological disorders tend to have values greater than 20 nmol/L (usually hundreds of nmol/L), while patients with type 1 diabetes, thyroid disease, or pernicious anemia alone, usually have values between 0.03 and 2.00 nmol/L.

Sometimes, antibody values are determined sequentially over time as a measure of clinical state and response to therapy. However, in this author's experience, antibodies tend to decrease in concentration or become undetectable in the context of immune suppression, regardless of clinical outcome. Thus, measuring outcomes from treatment should be based on nonserological clinical or paraclinical measures.

Measuring for specific isotypes and subclasses may also be pertinent. For example, although the IgG isotype is most commonly measured, for gastrointestinal diseases, such as celiac disease, measuring tissue transglutaminase IgA (predominant in mucosal tracts) is more sensitive and specific. Although subclasses 1 through 4 tend to be detected in most patients with most disease states, specific subclasses can sometimes be pertinent. For example, **myelin oligodendrocyte glycoprotein (MOG)** antibody is commonly detected nonspecifically in patients with diverse CNS diseases. However, MOG-IgG1 is highly specific for a spectrum of steroid-responsive inflammatory CNS diseases.[3] In contrast, MuSK-IgG4 is the most abundant subclass detected in patients with MuSK myasthenia gravis.

Sensitivity, Specificity, and Predictive Values

Sensitivity refers to the chances (in percent) of a test being positive when the disease is present (number of patients with disease who test positive, divided by the number of patients with disease tested, multiplied by 100). Specificity refers to the chances (in percent) of a test being negative when the disease is absent (number of patients without disease who test negative, divided by the number of patients without disease tested, multiplied by 100). Positive predictive value refers to the chances (in percent) of the disease being present when a test is positive (number of patients with disease who are test positive, divided by the number of patients who test positive, multiplied by 100). Negative predictive value refers to the chances (in percent) of the disease being absent when the test is negative (number of patients without disease who test negative, divided by the number of patients who test negative, multiplied by 100).

An example of a test with low sensitivity and high specificity is CSF testing for NMDA receptor-IgG in patients with encephalitis. Although this IgG marker is only found in CSF of 7% of patients with suspected autoimmune encephalitis (low sensitivity), when detected in the CSF of an encephalitic patients, it is diagnostic of autoimmune encephalitis (high specificity).

An example of a test with low sensitivity and specificity is serum testing for NMDA receptor IgG. This antibody may be detected in serum only (where CSF testing is negative) among patients without autoimmune encephalitis (low specificity). Also, testing for NMDA receptor IgG in serum in patients with NMDA receptor encephalitis (and CSF antibody positive) is negative 50% of the time (low sensitivity).

An example of a test with low specificity but high negative predictive value is HLA-DQ2/DQ8 testing in patients suspected to have celiac disease. Although this haplotype is common in the general population (low specificity), the absence of this finding is highly reassuring for the patient who does not have celiac disease (high negative predictive value).

Testing Algorithms: Single Tests, Profiles, Reflexes

Where several tests with complementary clinical utility for the same disease or syndrome have been developed, expert laboratorians may arrange testing as an algorithm or cascade to maximize diagnostic sensitivity, specificity, and predictive values. In addition to one or more screening serological tests, reflex tests may be built in for the purpose of confirming or refuting a diagnosis. Examples include a celiac disease cascade, pernicious anemia cascade, thyroid function cascade, paraneoplastic evaluation, and autoimmune encephalopathy evaluation (**FIGURE 13–1**).

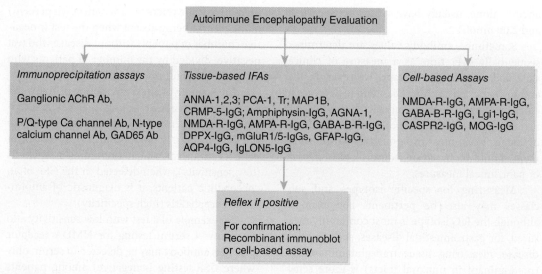

FIGURE 13-1 Example algorithm for serological diagnosis of autoimmune encephalopathy.

Testing Modalities with Examples

Details regarding testing for autoantibodies are discussed herein, using specific autoimmune diseases as examples. Principles of common immunoassays are outlined in **FIGURE 13-2**. Pathologists may separate these assays by their methodology or by their modality, either cell-based or tissue based.

Immunofluorescence, Direct and Indirect: Cell-Based and Tissue-Based

Immunofluorescence assays, both direct and indirect methods (**FIGURE 13-3**), are constructed as both cell- and tissue-based assays for autoimmune disease indications. **Anti-nuclear antibodies (ANAs)** are sensitively and specifically detected in a **human epithelial type 2 (HEp-2) cell** line by an indirect immunofluorescent technique (**FIGURE 13-4, A-D**).[4] Slides are prepared by using a HEp-2 cell line as substrate. IgG antibodies in serum specimens are detected after incubation with the slides and the addition of a fluorescein isothiocyante (FITC)-labeled antihuman

IgG reagent. All patient specimens are initially screened at 1:80 and then read using indirect immunofluorescence. High-volume laboratories may benefit from the use of an automated "ANA reader." Positive results may be reflexed to dsDNA and extractable nuclear antigen (e.g., SS-A) antibody testing.

For autoimmune neurological disorders, cell-based assays utilizing HEK293 cell line transfected with the cDNA for plasma membrane protein antigen of interest have the potential to provide screening that is both sensitive and specific, or can serve as confirmatory testing (**FIGURE 13-4 E-F**).[5] For example, NMDA receptor specificity may be confirmed by cell-based assay utilizing cDNA for the GluN1 subunit of the NMDA receptor (expressed with or without the GluN2 subunit). Commercially available slides are fixed with 1% formalin and are readily stored at 4°C. The sera (1:10 dilution) or CSF (neat) are incubated with the transfected cells. Cells are then washed and exposed to FITC-conjugated goat antihuman IgG. It is also possible to do a "live" cell assay, whereby the cells are fixed only after labeling with patient IgG and anti-human IgG secondary antibody. The principal advantage of this method is the ability to detect IgGs reactive with extracellular domains of the antigen of interest,

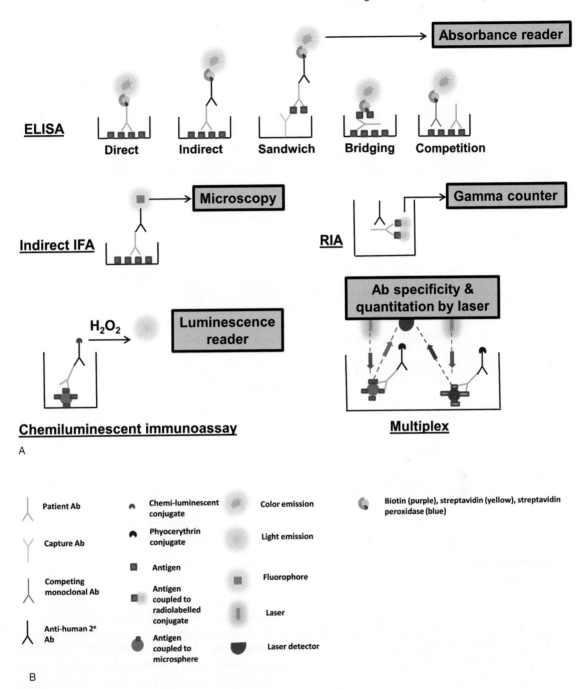

FIGURE 13–2 Principles underlying some commonly used immunoassays.

Courtesy of Andrew McKeon MD.

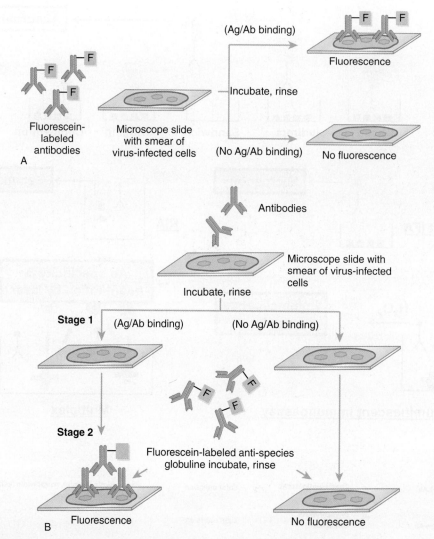

FIGURE 13-3 **(A)** Direct Immunofluorescence. **(B)** Indirect Immunofluorescence.

Courtesy of Diane Leland, PhD, Professor Emeritus, Indiana University School of Medicine.

which implies potential antibody pathogenicity. The principal disadvantage is the technical difficulties encountered with this method (setup on cover slips, keeping cells alive on slides).

Live Cell-Based Flow Cytometry

Another method of evaluating live cells, which avoids the technical difficulties of IFA-based live cell assays, is flow cytometry.[6] An example of a methodology for aquaporin-4 (AQP4)-IgG,

a biomarker for neuromyelitis optica, detection by flow cytometry, is discussed below. **Human embryonic kidney (HEK-293)** cells are transfected using plasmid DNA (pIRES2- green fluorescent protein [GFP]/human AQP4, either M1 or M23 AQP4-4 isoform). Cells are cultured for an additional 36 hours post-transfection and are lifted by being exposed for 2 minutes at room temperature to 0.25% trypsin/ EDTA. Subsequent steps are at 4°C, to avoid physiologic effects of bound IgG. Washed cells are suspended

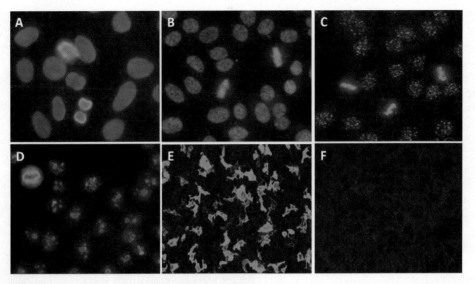

FIGURE 13–4 Cell-based assays: antinuclear antibody patterns, and neural antigen specific. A–D demonstrated ANA staining of HEp-2 cells that are homogenous **(A)**, Speckled **(B)**, Centromeric **(C)** or nucleolar **(D)**. **(E)** HEK293 cells expressing IgLON5 are reactive with the serum of a patient with autoimmune encephalopathy. **(F)** Mock transfected cells are nonreactive.

Panels A-D obtained from Autoantibody Standardization Committee Inc. (parent committee of ICAP) with permission. Panels E-F, Courtesy of Andrew McKeon MD.

in phosphate-buffered saline (PBS) containing 0.02% sodium azide, pH 7.2, 0.5% bovine serum albumin (BSA), 2 mM EDTA, and Fc receptor blocking, rotated for 10 minutes, diluted in PBS (containing 2% BSA, 10% normal goat serum, 15 mM EDTA, 0.05% sodium azide), and dispensed into 96 well round bottom plates (1 $\times$ 10^5 cells/well). Sera are heat-inactivated (35 minutes at 56°C), diluted in PBS (containing 2% BSA, 10% normal goat serum, 15 mM EDTA, 0.05% sodium azide), and added to duplicate wells at 1:5 dilution. After shaking the plates (30 minutes at 300 rpm), cells are washed three times with PBS. Goat anti-human IgG (γ-heavy chain-specific, Alexafluor 647-conjugated) is added at 1:500 (diluted in PBS containing 2% BSA, 10% normal goat serum, 15 mM EDTA, 0.05% sodium azide). After shaking (30 minutes, 4°C), cells are washed three times with PBS and fixed in 4% paraformaldehyde (Electron Microscopy Sciences, Hatfield, PA), and analyzed by flow cytometry. Two populations are gated on the basis of GFP expression: positive (high AQP4 expression) and negative (low or no AQP4 expression). The median Alexafluor 647 fluorescence

intensity (MFI) for the GFP-positive population indicates relative abundance of human IgG potentially bound to AQP4 surface epitopes; MFI for the GFP-negative population indicates non-specifically-bound IgG. The IgG binding index is calculated as the ratio of average MFI for duplicate aliquots of each cell population, $\dfrac{\text{MFI}_{\text{GFP-positive}}}{\text{MFI}_{\text{GFP-negative}}}$.

Tissue-Based Assays

Patient serum and CSF and commercial monoclonal antibodies are tested on cryosections (4 μm) of adult mouse tissues: cerebellum, midbrain, cerebral cortex, hippocampus, kidney, and gut (**FIGURE 13–5**).[7] Sections are fixed using 4% paraformaldehyde for 1 minute, then permeabilized with 3-([3-cholamidopropyl] dimethylammonio)-1-propanesulfonate (CHAPS), 0.5%, in phosphate-buffered saline (PBS, for 1 minute), and then blocked for 1 hour with normal goat serum (10% in PBS). After PBS rinse, patient specimen is applied (serum is preabsorbed with bovine liver powder, 1:240 dilution, and CSF is nonabsorbed,

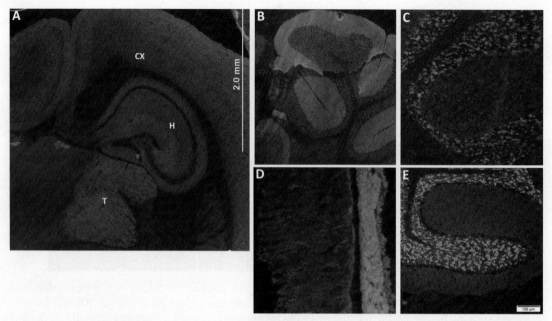

FIGURE 13–5 Indirect immunofluorescence assay, evaluating patient serum or CSF, utilizing a composite of mouse tissues (brain and gut shown here), as substrate for neural IgG-specific patterns of staining. Neural IgGs selectively stain brain tissue but spare non-neural tissues (e.g., gut, smooth muscle, and kidney). **(A)** GABA-B receptor-IgG stains the thalamus (T) more than the cortex (Cx) or hippocampus, and also stains the cerebellum **(B)**, with molecular layer (ML) staining being more intense than granular layer (GL). **(C)** In contrast to GAD65 antibody, stains the granular layer in a punctate synaptic fashion, more intensely than the molecular layer. **(D)** Smooth muscle antibody stains gastric smooth muscle but not brain (not shown). **(E)** In a patient with encephalopathy, DPPX-IgG has a unique pattern of staining of cerebellar cortex, with the granular layer being most intense.

Panels (a) and (b) reproduced from Jeffery, O. J., Lennon, V. A., Pittock, S. J., Gregory, J. K., Britton, J. W., & McKeon, A. (2013). GABAB receptor autoantibody frequency in service serologic evaluation. *Neurology*, 81(10), 882–887. doi:10.1212/WNL.0b013e3182a35271; Panels (c) and (d), Courtesy of Andrew McKeon MD; Panel (e) reproduced from Tobin, W. O., Lennon, V. A., Komorowski, L., Probst, C., Clardy, S. L., Aksamit, A. J., . . . McKeon, A. (2014). DPPX potassium channel antibody: frequency, clinical accompaniments, and outcomes in 20 patients. *Neurology*, 83(20), 1797–1803. doi:10.1212/WNL.0000000000000991.

1:2 dilution). After 40 minutes, and PBS wash, a human-specific secondary antibody conjugated with FITC is applied. Cover slips are mounted using antifade medium. Fluorescence images are captured using a microscope.

Immunoprecipitation Assay

AChR Ab testing for myasthenia gravis is often performed using immunoprecipitation assays. Immunoprecipitation assays employ synaptic membrane proteins solubilized from human limb muscle (Triton X-100) or human AChR-expressing cell lines, and are complexed with ^{125}I-α-bungarotoxin.[8] Goat antihuman IgG/IgM is used as a precipitant. Precipitates with gamma

emission higher than yielded by normal control sera are clarified by centrifugation and reassayed with ^{125}I-ligand with and without AChR. Values for ^{125}I-ligand precipitation (expressed as nmol/L) are subtracted from the mean value for AChR precipitation. Final results of 0.02 nmol/L or fewer at Mayo Clinic are considered negative.

ELISA

GAD65 (glutamic acid decarboxylase 65) antibody testing is often performed by ELISA for determining susceptibility to type 1 diabetes mellitus. For the purpose of this assay, GAD65 is expressed in yeast, purified and biotinylated. In this bridging ELISA format (Figure 13–2), advantage is taken of the bivalency of IgG binding to antigen on the solid phase (plate) and liquid phase (in solution).[9] To start, 25 µL of test sera is added to duplicate GAD65-coated wells (10 ng per well) and incubated with shaking (about 200 shakes per minute) for 1 hour at room temperature. The plate wells are then washed three times with wash buffer (150 mmol/L NaCl, 20 mmol/L Tris, 0.5 ml/L Tween 20, pH 8.0) and 100 µL (20 ng) of GAD65–biotin is added. After a further 1 h incubation with shaking, the plate wells are washed three times and incubated for 20 min with 100 µL of streptavidin peroxidase conjugate (Sigma-Aldrich, Poole, BH12 4QH, UK; 1 mg/L). A wash step is followed by adding tetramethylbenzidine (100 µL) and after 20 min, 0.5 mol/L H_2SO_4 (100 µL) to stop the color reaction, and measurement of absorbance is performed at 405 and 450 nm.

ANA Testing

ANA testing may also be performed using ELISA. Nuclear antigens from HEp-2 cells are adsorbed to the wells of a microtiter plate. In this indirect ELISA format, diluted sera, calibrator, or controls are added to the wells and incubated. After washing to remove unbound serum proteins, an enzyme-conjugated, antihuman-IgG antibody is added to detect IgG antibodies bound to the microtiter wells. After incubation and washing to remove unbound conjugate, substrate is added to the wells. After incubation, the enzyme-substrate reaction is stopped. The absorbance in each microtiter well is measured by an automated plate reader. The absorbances are proportional to the levels of antibodies to nuclear antigens present in the test sera, calibrator, or controls.

Cyclic Citrullinated Peptide (CCP) Antibody Testing

In this indirect ELISA format, a mixture of synthetic **citrullinated peptides** is adsorbed to the wells of a microtiter plate. Diluted sera, standards, or controls are added to the wells and incubated. After washing to remove unbound serum proteins, horseradish peroxidase-conjugated, monoclonal antihuman IgG antibody is added to detect IgG antibodies that have bound to the microtiter

wells. After incubation and washing to remove unbound conjugate, tetramethylbenzidine (TMB) substrate is added to the wells. After incubation, the enzyme-substrate reaction is stopped. The absorbance in each microtiter well is measured by use of an automated plate reader. The absorbances are proportional to the levels of CCP antibodies, and the concentrations of antibodies in the test sera and controls are determined by comparison to a multipoint standard curve.

Double-Stranded DNA (dsDNA) Antibody Testing

Microwells are precoated with calf thymus **double-stranded DNA (dsDNA)** antigen. The calibrators, controls, and diluted patient samples are added to the wells, and autoantibodies recognizing the dsDNA antigen bind during the first incubation. After washing the wells to remove all unbound proteins, purified peroxidase-labeled goat antihuman IgG conjugate is added. The conjugate binds to the captured human autoantibody, and the excess unbound conjugate is removed by an additional wash step. The bound conjugate is visualized with TMB substrate, which gives a blue reaction produce, the intensity of which is proportional to a concentration of autoantibody in the sample. Sulfuric acid is added to each well to stop the reaction. This produces a yellow endpoint color, which is read at 450 nm.

Confirmatory testing for borderline dsDNA by ELISA testing is performed by immunofluorescence assay (IFA).[10] Autoantibodies in a test sample directed against dsDNA bind to antigens in the substrate placed on the slide, which, in this case, is *Crithidia luciliae*. Classical dsDNA ELISA is accepted as the most sensitive but often less-specific method for SLE diagnostics. IFA using *Crithidia luciliae* has higher specificity. This test takes advantage of the tightly packed dsDNA and low protein levels within the kinetoplast of that anuclear organism. Sensitivities of the test for SLE range from 30 to 60%, with disease specificity of 95% or greater. Washing removes excess serum from the substrate. Fluorescein-conjugated (FITC) antiserum added to the substrate attaches to the bound autoantibody. After a second washing step to remove excess conjugate, the substrate is cover-slipped and viewed for fluorescent patterns with a fluorescent microscope. Observation of specific fluorescent patterns on the substrate indicates the presence of autoantibodies in the test sample.

Chemiluminescent Immunoassays

Autoimmune Thyroid Disease

Thyroglobulin is a large (600 kDa) glycoprotein to which the thyroid hormones thyroxine (T4) tri-iodothyroinine (T3) bind. Patient serum is added to a reaction vessel with paramagnetic particles coated with the thyroglobulin protein. The serum thyroglobulin antibody (TgAb) binds to the thyroglobulin. After incubation in a reaction vessel, materials bound to the solid phase are held in place by a magnetic field, while unbound materials are washed away. The thyroglobulin-alkaline phosphatase conjugate is added and binds to the TgAb. After the second incubation, materials bound to the solid phase are held in place by a magnetic field, while unbound materials are washed away. A chemiluminescent substrate is then added to the reaction vessel, and light generated by the reaction is measured with a luminometer. The light production is directly proportional to the concentration of thyroglobulin antibody in the sample.[11]

For **thyroid peroxidase (TPO)** antibody testing, patient serum is added to a reaction vessel with paramagnetic particles coated with TPO. TPO antibody binds to the thyroperoxidase. After incubation, materials bound to the solid phase are held in a magnetic field while unbound materials are washed away. Protein A-alkaline phosphatase conjugate is added and binds to the TPO antibody. After the second incubation, materials bound to the solid phase are held in a magnetic field while unbound materials are washed away. A chemiluminescent substrate is added to the vessel, and light generated by the-reaction is measured with a luminometer. The light production is directly proportional to the

concentration of TPO antibody in the sample. For TSHR stimulating or blocking antibodies, a competitive binding chemiluminescent assay can be undertaken. Patient specimen is treated with a reagent buffer consisting of a preformed complex of solubilized porcine TSH receptor and biotinylated anti-porcine TSH receptor mouse monoclonal antibody. TSHR antibody in patient serum is allowed to interact with the TSH receptor complex. After adding streptavidin-coated microparticles and a human thyroid-stimulating monoclonal autoantibody (M22) labeled with a ruthenium complex, bound TSHR Ab are detected by their ability to inhibit the binding of labeled M22. The entire complex becomes bound to the solid phase via interaction of biotin and streptavidin. This reaction mixture is aspirated into the measuring cell where the bound microparticles are captured onto the electrode surface and unbound substances are removed. Voltage is applied to the electrode, inducing a chemiluminescent emission, which is then measured against a calibration curve to determine the amount of thyrotropin receptor antibody in the patient specimen.[12]

To detect thyroid-stimulating antibodies, a cell-based bioassay may also be undertaken. Cyclic adenosine monophosphate (cAMP) production by thyroid-stimulating hormone (TSH)-responsive cells is measured upon exposure to patient serum and compared with that obtained in the same cells after exposure to normal control serum.[13] The assay employs Chinese hamster ovary cells permanently transfected with the human thyroid-stimulating hormone receptor (TSHR), and a luciferase expression construct under the control of a cAMP responsive promoter. Luciferase transcription in these cells is proportional to the concentration of intracellular cAMP. An aliquot of cells is incubated with each diluted patient serum. Cells are lysed at the end of incubation, luciferase substrate is added, and chemiluminescence is measured in a luminometer. The ratio of the light-units produced in the cell-lysate exposed to patient serum divided by a control cell-lysate light signal is the TSI index.

Multiplex Bead Assay: Connective Tissue Cascade

SS-A/Ro, SS-B/La, RNP, Sm, Scl 70, Jo 1, ribosome P, and centromere antibodies are measured by a commercial multiplex flow immunoassay system.[14] Recombinant or purified antigens are coupled covalently to polystyrene microspheres that are impregnated with fluorescent dyes to create unique fluorescent signatures, one microsphere type for each antigen. Diluted sera, calibrators, and controls are added to a mixture containing the antigen-coupled microspheres. Antibodies to each antigen bind to their homologous antigen-coupled microspheres (more than 10 can be measured at once). The microspheres are washed to remove extraneous serum proteins. Phycoerythrin-conjugated antihuman IgG antibody is then added to detect IgG antibodies bound to the microspheres. The microspheres are washed to remove unbound conjugate, and bound conjugate is detected by laser photometry. A primary laser determines the fluorescent signature of each microsphere, and a secondary laser reveals the level of phycoerythrin fluorescence associated with the microsphere surface. Results are calculated for each antigen-coated microsphere type by comparing the median fluorescence response to a series of multipoint calibration curves.

Microfluidics

A new technology with future potential for high throughput analysis is based on microfluidics and takes advantage of compact disks (CDs) in which the centrifugal force moves fluids through microstructures where sample and reagents are delivered to a mixing chamber on a nanoliter scale. More than 100 analyses can be carried out on one CD (analysis of antibodies against multiple proteins using a single CD or analysis for the same antibody in multiple patients).[15] Hydrophobic barriers separate different channels. Analyses are performed as a sandwich assay. The antigen is already captured to the column. The antibodies to be analyzed are applied onto the columns. Thereafter, fluorescently labeled secondary antibodies recognize the bound primary antibodies, and detection is carried out by laser-induced fluorescence.

Antibody Detection by Agglutination-PCR (ADAP)

ADAP combines methodologies from two distinct assay formats: the classic latex agglutination assay, where serum antibodies cluster antigen-latex particles into optically detectable complexes, and proximity ligation assays, in which protein–protein complexes are detected by PCR amplification.[16] The sample containing the target antibody analyte is incubated with a pair of antigen–DNA conjugates. Each conjugate bears an oligonucleotide sequence comprising either the 5' or 3' half of a full amplicon. Then antibodies within the sample agglutinate, the antigen–DNA conjugates and positions them for ligation upon the addition of a bridging oligonucleotide and DNA ligase. Finally, the newly generated amplicon is exponentially amplified with primers that bind their respective sites and are quantified by real-time qPCR. ADAP has been reported to produce comparable results for detection of thyroid disease and diabetes-pertinent antibodies.

Functional Assays

Measuring the ability of antibody to downregulate its target antigen, after cross-linking, from the surface of an expressing cell (modulation) has known clinical utility in myasthenia gravis ("high modulators" of AChRs frequently have thymoma) and in stiff-person syndrome (modulators of glycine receptor alpha 1 subunit are more likely to have a stiff-person diagnosis than those whose antibodies only bind to receptors).[8] Measurement of complement activation by antibody is informative for research but may have future clinical use.

GlyRα-IgG Modulating Assay

Twenty-four hours after transient transfection, patient or healthy control serum (heat inactivated [56°C] to deplete complement) is added to the

GlyRα1-transfected cells and is incubated for an additional 4 hours at 37°C. Slides are then washed twice at 4°C. Serum is diluted in 20% normal goat serum and added to the cells (on ice). After 30 minutes, cells are washed in cold PBS and goat anti-human IgG-FITC secondary antibody is added and incubated for 30 minutes. Cells are washed and fixed in 4% paraformaldehyde for 15 minutes. After further washing, cells are mounted and imaged. At 4°C, IgG in the serum of an affected patient binds to the surface of the live GlyRα1-transfected cells. After incubating for 4 hours at 37°C, IgG is no longer detected on the cell surface due to internalization (modulation) of the antigen by GlyRα-IgG.

CSF Testing

Further clues to an autoimmune or inflammatory etiology for a neurological disorder may be found on CSF evaluation. Elevated protein concentration (particularly if greater than 100 mg/dL), elevated numbers of white blood cells, abnormal numbers of CSF exclusive oligoclonal bands, and elevated IgG index and synthesis rate all support an autoimmune cause. These CSF findings are encountered in a variety of inflammatory CNS disorders also, including multiple sclerosis, and only rarely in pathologically proven neurodegenerative disorders (such as Alzheimer's disease) or infectious disorders (such as Creutzfeldt-Jakob disease). The **oligoclonal banding (OCB)** assay requires paired cerebrospinal fluid (CSF) and serum samples. Unconcentrated CSF and diluted serum are electrophoresed by isoelectric focusing. The separated IgG bands are visualized by an IgG immunoblot, separated electrophoretically, using isoelectric focusing. Oligoclonal bands that are present in the CSF (at least 4) and not in the serum are reported.[17] Kappa free light chain testing in CSF by nephelometry is a novel and promising method for CSF-specific Ig detection that does not require matched serum testing.[18]

Serum is the specimen type most commonly used to test for autoantibodies pertinent to autoimmune disease, although plasma can also be used. CSF is optimum for diagnosing certain autoimmune CNS disorders such as NMDA receptor encephalitis and autoimmune GFAP

astrocytopathy.[7] Antibody tests performed on serum alone might suffice for paraneoplastic antibody testing, although overall combined serum and CSF testing somewhat increase the diagnostic yield for classic paraneoplastic antibodies (such as collapsin response mediator protein-5 [CRMP-5] IgG). However, in the case of NMDA receptor antibodies, CSF is always more informative than serum. In contrast, VGKC complex antibodies are more readily detectable in serum than in CSF.

▶ Autoimmune Diseases and Pertinent Antibody Markers

Essentially, any organ in the body may be affected by autoimmune disease, although some are more commonly affected than others. Some diseases are generalized (non-organ-specific) while others are organ-specific. Common diseases and biomarkers are outlined in **TABLE 13–1**, with some examples of testing modalities in **TABLE 13–2**. Some classical examination findings are demonstrated in Figure 13–1.

Non-Organ-Specific Connective Tissue Diseases

Systemic Lupus Erythematosus (SLE)

Systemic lupus erythematosus (SLE, also known as lupus) is a systemic autoimmune disorder that can affect the skin, joints, lungs, kidneys, heart, hematologic system, and brain. A form limited to the skin is known as discoid lupus.[19] There are approximately 60 new cases of lupus per 1 million population per year. In the United States, the disease occurs more frequently among women and non-Caucasian racial groups, particularly adult black women, where the incidence is as high as 1 in 245. The course of the disease is variable, and most patients go through phases of remission and relapses (flares). Manifestations range from a short-lived illness with photosensitive rash and

TABLE 13–1 Common Systemic Autoimmune Diseases, Organs Affected, and Antibody Biomarkers

Disease	Organs Affected	Antibody Specificity
SLE	Nervous system, skin, kidney, joints, hematologic system	Nuclear antigens, DNA
Systemic sclerosis	Skin, upper gastrointestinal tract, lungs, kidneys, skeletal muscle, and pericardium	Centromeres, nucleoli, Scl-70, RNA polymerase III
Mixed connective tissue disease	Organs affected in SLE, systemic sclerosis, and dermatomyositis	Those relevant to SLE and also RNP antibody
Wegener's granulomatosis	Nervous system, respiratory tract, kidneys	cANCA, PR3
Microscopic polyangiitis, Churg Strauss syndrome	Respiratory tract (both), kidneys (microscopic polyangiitis)	pANCA, MPO
Rheumatoid arthritis	Joints (may have systemic complications also)	CCP
Sjogren syndrome	Eyes, mouth (may have systemic complications also)	SS-A (Ro), SS-B (La)
Graves' disease	Thyroid gland (excess hormone production)	Thyroid-stimulating hormone receptor
Hashimoto thyroiditis	Thyroid gland (diminished hormone production)	TPO, thyroglobulin
Type 1 diabetes	Endocrine pancreas	GAD65, IA2, insulin, ZnT8
Addison disease	Adrenal gland cortex	21-hydroxylase
Pernicious anemia	Gastric parietal cells	β subunit of H+/K+ ATPase, intrinsic factor
Immune thrombocytopenic purpura	Platelets	Platelet surface glycoproteins
Autoimmune hemolytic anemia	Red blood cells	Red blood cell antigens (temperature dependent [warm and cold agglutinins])
Antiphospholipid syndrome	Coagulation cascade	Phospholipids
Goodpasture's disease	Renal glomerular basement membrane	Alpha 3 chain of type IV collagen

(continues)

TABLE 13–1 Common Systemic Autoimmune Diseases, Organs Affected, and Antibody Biomarkers *(Continued)*

Disease	Organs Affected	Antibody Specificity
Autoimmune hepatobiliary diseases	Liver, biliary tract	Smooth muscle, nuclear antigens, mitochondria, liver/kidney microsomal antigens
Celiac disease	Intestinal villi	Transglutaminase 2, deamidated gliadin
Pemphigus	Epidermis	Desmogleins 1 and 3

Abbreviations: p/cANCA = perinuclear/cytoplasmic anticytoplasmic neutrophil antibody; CCP = citric citrullinated peptides; GAD65 = glutamic acid decarboxylase, 65 kilodalton isoform; IA2 = insulin antigen 2; MPO = myeloperoxidase; MuSK = muscle specific kinase; RNP = ribonucleoprotein; PR3 = proteinase 3; SS-A/SS-B = Sjogren syndrome antigen A or B; TPO = thyroid peroxidase.

TABLE 13–2 Examples of Common Autoimmune Diseases, Antigens and Testing Modalities Used for Diagnosis

Disease	Antigens	Cell-based IFA	Tissue-based IFA	ELISA	RIA	Western blot	Multiplex
Connective tissue	Nuclear, ds DNA, extractable nuclear antigens	+	−	+	−	+	+
RA	CCP	−	−	+	−	−	−
Thyroid	TPO, thyroglobulin	−	−	+	−	−	−
Myasthenia gravis	AChR MuSK	+	−	+	+	−	−
Paraneoplastic neurological disorders	Diverse	+	+	+	+	+	−
Celiac disease	Tg2 Deamidated gliadin	−	+	+	−	−	−
Diabetes	GAD65, IA2 insulin, ZnT8	−	−	+	+	−	−

Abbreviations: AChR = acetylcholine receptor; CCP = citric citrullinated peptides; ELISA = enzyme-linked immunosorbent assay; GAD65 = glutamic acid decarboxylase, 65 kilodalton isoform; IA2 = insulin antigen 2; IFA = (indirect) immunofluorescence assay; MuSK = muscle-specific kinase; RA = rheumatoid arthritis; RIA = radioimmunoprecipitation assay; TPO = thyroid peroxidase.

polyarthritis, to life-threatening illnesses affecting the kidney, brain, and cardiopulmonary system. Complement-mediated injury of the kidneys arises as a consequence of deposition of circulating immune complexes. Approximately 20% of patients with lupus develop antiphospholipid antibodies and are susceptible to venous thromboembolism and recurrent miscarriage. Biomarkers, including antinuclear antibody (ANA), Smith (Sm) antibody, and double-stranded DNA antibody are discussed further in the Testing Modalities section (D).

Scleroderma

Systemic sclerosis, otherwise known as **scleroderma**, is a rare connective tissue disorder (1:10,000 incidence) characterized by varying degrees of organ involvement, including fibrosis,

telangiectasias, and abnormalities of the digestive system.[20] The condition is classified using clinical and serological criteria into two major types: a diffuse, generalized, and more debilitating variant called systemic sclerosis or scleroderma; and a more localized variant characterized by CREST syndrome (Calcinosis, Raynaud's phenomenon, esophageal dysmotility, Syndactyly, and Telangiectasias). Diffuse systemic sclerosis is distinguished from CREST, mainly based on the extent of cutaneous fibrosis, which is more extensive in diffuse sclerosis. The organs most frequently affected by scleroderma are skin (**FIGURE 13–6C**), gastrointestinal tract, lungs, kidneys, skeletal muscle, and pericardium. Autoantibody profiles in systemic sclerosis assist in diagnosis, and the classification criteria include certain patterns of ANA binding to cell substrate (e.g., nucleolar). Specific autoantibodies include anticentromere (associated

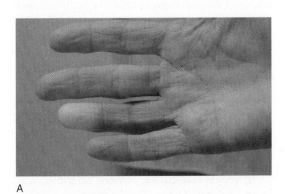

A

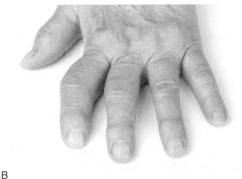

B

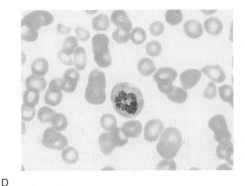

C   D

FIGURE 13–6 Examples of physical examination manifestations in autoimmune diseases. **(A)** Raynaud's phenomenon. **(B)** Hand deformities of rheumatoid arthritis. **(C)** Tight perioral skin in a patient with scleroderma. **(D)** Hypersegmented neutrophil and macrocytic red blood cells on blood film of a patient with pernicious anemia.

(a) © Barb Elkin/Shutterstock; (b) © Nataly Studio/Shutterstock; (c) © Karan Bunjean/Shutterstock; (d) © LindseyRN/Shutterstock.

with limited systemic sclerosis and pulmonary hypertension), anti-Scl-70 (associated with diffuse systemic sclerosis, lung fibrosis, and digital ulcers), and anti-RNA polymerase III (associated with diffuse systemic sclerosis, scleroderma renal crisis, and hand disability). The nucleolar pattern of ANAs is associated with progressive interstitial lung disease and pulmonary hypertension. A combination of one or more of indirect immunofluorescence, enzyme linked immunosorbent assay (ELISA), and multiplex bead immunoassays are commonly used diagnostic modalities. Some cases are ANA negative and generally have a distinct subtype and poor outcome. The main goal of treatment is to limit or prevent disease progression. This is most feasible when immunotherapy (usually mycophenolate mofetil or methotrexate) is initiated early in the disease course while internal organ fibrosis is minimal.

Mixed Connective-Tissue Disease

What **mixed connective-tissue disease (MCTD)** represents is controversial.[21] Some argue that MCTD is a distinct disease entity, while others contend that it represents an overlap syndrome, and others still feel that it is an early and nonspecific phase of an evolving, but more distinct disorder (such as SLE, systemic sclerosis, polymyositis, or dermatomyositis). In general, MCTD should be considered in a patient with antibody reactive, with the U1 small nuclear ribonucleoprotein particle (U1 snRNP) presenting with Raynaud's phenomenon (**FIGURE 13–6A**), diffuse hand fibrosis, and two or more of the following: arthritis, myositis, low white blood cell count, esophageal dysmotility, pleuritis, pericarditis, interstitial lung disease, or pulmonary hypertension. Population-based epidemiology data from Scandinavia have provided an estimate of MCTD prevalence (3.8 per 100,000) and incidence (2.1 per million per year). Genetic studies have demonstrated that MCTD is strongly HLA–linked. The HLA DRB1*04:01 and HLA-B*08 are risk factors for MCTD, while DRB1*04:04, DRB1*13:01, and DRB1*13:02 are protective. U1 snRNP antibodies were first described in sera from SLE patients, prior to MCTD being proposed as a separate entity. RNP antibodies bind three U1-specific proteins: A, C, and 70 kDa in the macromolecular U1 ribonucleoprotein complex. This complex also contains other connective-tissue, disease-relevant antigens such as the Sm antigen. Antibodies can be detected by ELISA or by a commercial multiplex flow immunoassay system.

Vasculitis

The vasculitides are a heterogeneous group of inflammatory disorders affecting blood vessels. In general, this diagnosis is made by pathological examination of biopsied tissue of an affected organ. Inflammation and necrosis of blood vessels (small, medium, or large sized) are observed histologically. The vasculitides have the potential to present with one or more of a wide variety of signs and symptoms and, if left untreated, can cause stroke, dementia, blindness, lung or gastrointestinal hemorrhage, destructive arthritis, skin ulceration, renal failure, or limb weakness (due to peripheral neuropathy), depending on the organs affected. There are three antineutrophil cytoplasmic antibody (ANCA)-associated vasculitides:[22] granulomatosis with polyangiitis (also known as Wegener's granulomatosis), microscopic polyangiitis, and eosinophilic granulomatosis with polyangiitis (also known as Churg-Strauss syndrome). All are necrotizing vasculitides, with few or no immune deposits, predominantly affecting small vessels (capillaries, venules, arterioles, and small arteries). These are relatively rare autoimmune diseases (46 to 184 per million of unknown cause). Perinuclear (pANCA) and cytoplasmic (cANCA) patterns of neutrophil staining by patient IgG on indirect immunofluorescence, and testing for their main specificities (myeloperoxidase [MPO] and proteinase 3 [PR3]) by ELISA, facilitate diagnosis when used in tandem with clinical features. Seropositivity may eliminate the need for tissue biopsy to make a diagnosis.

Wegener's granulomatosis is characterized by necrotizing granulomatous inflammation of small to medium vessels of the upper and lower respiratory tract, and often affects the kidneys (glomerulonephritis). Microscopic polyangiitis is characterized by nongranulomatous necrotizing vasculitis, with few or no immune deposits, predominantly affecting small vessels. Both renal and pulmonary involvement are common. Churg-Strauss syndrome is characterized by eosinophil-rich, necrotizing granulomatous inflammation of the respiratory tract and is associated with asthma and eosinophilia. Glomerulonephritis may also occur. The treatment for all of these disorders includes corticosteroids in conjunction with one or the other of cyclophosphamide or rituximab.

Organ-Specific Connective Tissue Diseases

Rheumatoid Arthritis

Rheumatoid arthritis (RA) is a systemic autoimmune disease characterized by inflammatory arthritis in all patients, and extra-articular manifestations in some.[23] There is a heritability risk of approximately 50%. RA has been associated with certain HLA-DRB1 alleles: HLA-DRB1*04, HLA-DRB1*01, and HLA-DRB1*10. Single nucleotide polymorphisms in non-HLA genes (PSORS1C1, PTPN2 and MIR 146A) have been associated with severe disease. Cigarette smoking is the strongest environmental risk factor associated with rheumatoid arthritis. Changes in the composition and function of intestinal microbiome have also been related to rheumatoid arthritis. In North America, 0.4 to 1% of the population is affected, and it is predominant in women (female:male ratio, 2.5:1). The prevalence of RA increases with age.

The most common clinical presentation of RA is polyarthritis of small joints of the hands (**FIGURE 13–6B**). Most commonly, joint involvement occurs insidiously over a period of months. Other commonly affected joints include wrists, elbows, shoulders, hips, knees, ankles, and metatarsophalangeal joints. Stiffness in the joints in the morning may last up to several hours, usually more than an hour. The patient may have a "trigger finger" due to flexor tenosynovitis. On examination, there may be swelling and tenderness of the affected joints (called synovitis), and there may be decreased range of motion. If untreated, later in the disease course, permanent joint deformities may develop.

Laboratory evaluation of patients with rheumatoid arthritis consists of obtaining rheumatoid factor (IgM antibody against the Fc portion of IgG). Approximately 45 to 75% of patients with RA test positive for rheumatoid factor. However, the presence of rheumatoid factor alone is not diagnostic of RA, and it is frequently detected in subjects without RA. It may be detected in connective-tissue disease, chronic infections, and healthy individuals, mostly in low titers.

Citrullinated protein (CCP) antibodies have the highest disease sensitivity and specificity. Citrulline is an amino acid generated by post-translational modification of arginyl residues by peptidyl arginine deaminases. CCP antibodies can be IgG, IgM, or IgA isotypes. The binding of antibodies leads to complement activation. The presence of antibodies in rheumatoid arthritis is associated with severe disease, joint damage, and an increase in mortality. Acute-phase reactants, erythrocyte sedimentation rate (ESR), and C-reactive protein (CRP) may be elevated in the active phase of arthritis. Plain film radiographs (X-rays), ultrasound, or MRIs of hands and feet can assist in detecting joint erosions. Disease-modifying, anti-rheumatic drugs (DMARDs) are initiated as soon as the diagnosis of rheumatoid arthritis is made. Traditional or conventional DMARDs include methotrexate, leflunonamide, sulfasalazine, and hydroxychloroquine. Biologic DMARDs include TNF (tumor necrosis factor) inhibitors (e.g., adalimumab, etanercept, and infliximab), and non-TNF inhibitors (e.g., tocilizumab [interleukin-6 inhibitor], abatacept (inhibits T-cell costimulation) and rituximab [anti-B cell]).

Sjogren Syndrome

Sjogren syndrome is a localized autoimmune disease causing dryness of the eyes (xerophthalmia), mouth (xerostomia), upper respiratory tract, and vagina and parotid enlargement (sicca symptoms).[24] Associated systemic features are known to arise in some patients. These include Raynaud's phenomenon, arthralgias, fatigue, and disorders of the liver, kidney, and lungs. Diagnostic antibodies include those reactive with extractable nuclear antigens, known as Sjogren syndrome (SS)-A (anti-Ro) and SS-B (anti-La). SS-A has highest sensitivity for Sjogren syndrome. These antibodies may be detected individually using an ELISA platform, or as part of a cascade of connective-tissue, disease-related antibodies, by latex bead-based multiplex technology, upon reflex from a positive ANA. However, 30% of patients with Sjogren syndrome can be SS-A and SS-B antibody negative. While other serological findings may be present in those individuals (e.g., polyclonal hypergammaglobulinemia, thyroid antibodies, and antinuclear antibody), none is specific for Sjogren syndrome. Additional diagnostic testing includes objective documentation of reduced tear production (Schirmer's test), saliva production, and radiological documentation of salivary gland dysfunction (such as salivary gland scintigraphy). The most specific test for Sjogren syndrome is demonstration of lymphocytic infiltration in a biopsy of a minor salivary gland. Treatments for dryness include artificial tears, eye lubricants, sugar-free gum, and vaginal lubricants. An oral medication, cevimeline, may also improve sicca symptoms. Systemic immunosuppressants may be required for severe, resistant anhidrosis and treatment of systemic symptoms.

Organ-Specific Endocrine Disorders

Hypophysitis

Autoimmune **hypophysitis**, or lymphocytic hypophysitis, is an inflammatory disorder affecting the anterior pituitary lobe, the posterior pituitary lobe, or both.[25] This is a rare disorder with incidence estimated at 1 in 9 million/year and female predominance (6:1). There is a strong association with pregnancy. Clinical findings vary according to the rapidity of progression of the disease process, which may be acute (over hours), subacute (over days to weeks), or chronic (over months to years). Acute manifestations (due to adrenocorticotropic hormone [ACTH] deficiency) are the same as adrenal insufficiency and hypothyroidism (due to TSH deficiency). Subacute manifestations typically occur during pregnancy or postpartum. In this scenario, signs and symptoms are those of a pituitary mass (headache and visual changes)

that resolve over time. Magnetic resonance imaging (MRI) of the pituitary gland typically demonstrates anterior pituitary swelling with evidence of inflammation. Hormonal changes occur but are less dramatic than in acute disease. The most widely used method to detect pituitary autoantibodies is indirect immunofluorescence utilizing cryosections of human or primate pituitary. This testing is limited by low clinical sensitivity (few affected patients are positive)[26] and low clinical specificity (many healthy subjects are positive also). Recent studies have reported IgG reactivities for pituitary cell types as having some specificity for autoimmune hypophysitis manifestations (e.g., antibody targeting ACTH-secreting cells being specific for patients with ACTH deficiency).

Autoimmune Thyroid Disease

Autoimmune thyroid diseases (Graves' disease causing hyperthyroidism and Hashimoto thyroiditis, causing hypothyroidism) are the most common autoimmune diseases in humans.[27] These disorders occur more commonly in patients with other established autoimmune diseases, and some patients without evidence of biochemical thyroid abnormalities are thyroid antibody positive (but presumably are at risk for those diseases). All forms of autoimmune thyrotoxicosis (Graves' disease, Hashimoto's thyroiditis, and neonatal thyrotoxicosis) are caused by the production of thyroid-stimulating hormone receptor (TSHR)-stimulating autoantibodies. Some patients with Graves' disease also have TSHR-blocking antibodies (see Section D for details on assay).

Graves' Disease

Common presenting symptoms include weight loss, weakness, dyspnea, palpitations, increased hunger and thirst, diarrhea, sweating, heat intolerance, tremor, irritability, and irregular menses. Thyroid metabolism is accelerated with faster plasma turnover, higher thyroid peroxidase (TPO) activity, excess thyroglobulin release, increased clearance of iodide from the plasma, and decreased retention of iodide in the thyroid, and usually increased gland volume.

Hashimoto's Thyroiditis. Hashimoto's thyroiditis may lead to overt hypothyroidism (causing one or more symptoms of fatigue, weight gain, cold sensitivity, attentional difficulties, dryness of skin, nails, and hair, constipation, muscle pain, and irregular menses). However, more patients have subclinical hypothyroidism with abnormal thyroid biochemical indices (increased TSH and normal thyroid hormone levels). More than 90% destruction of the thyroid gland usually occurs prior to onset of hypothyroidism. Although elevated thyroid antibody titers may provide an indication of the likelihood of overt hypothyroidism, no correlation of antibody titer and risk for hypothyroidism has been found to date. Thyroglobulin and TPO antibodies, detected by ELISA or chemiluminescent immunoassay, in addition to abnormal thyroid biochemistry, are diagnostic.

Hypoparathyroidism

Autoimmune hypoparathyroidism may occur as a stand-alone entity, or as one part of a multiorgan disorder known as autoimmune polyglandular syndrome.[28] The first direct evidence in support of an autoimmune basis for idiopathic hypoparathyroidism was provided in the 1960s when parathyroid antibodies were identified in patients with presumed autoimmune hypoparathyroidism by indirect immunofluorescence assay, using human parathyroid glands or parathyroid adenomas as substrate. In the 1990s, antibodies directed at the extracellular domain of the calcium-sensing receptor (CaSR) were found in patients with autoimmune hypoparathyroidism. CaSR antibodies have subsequently been found to either stimulate or inhibit the receptor, producing respectively, hypoparathyroidism or parathyroid hormone (PTH)–dependent hypercalcemia. Parathyroid hormone antibody detected by radio-binding assay is offered by some commercial laboratories.

Type 1 Diabetes Mellitus

Type 1 diabetes mellitus, also known as insulin-dependent diabetes, is an autoimmune disorder of deficient insulin production, caused by immune destruction of the β islet cells of the endocrine

pancreas.[29] Genetic susceptibility to type 1 diabetes has been linked to HLA-DR3, DR4, DQ2, and DQ8 antigens. HLA-DR2 may be protective against developing diabetes. Most patients develop this disorder in childhood or adolescence but it may occur at any age. Affected patients present with symptoms and signs of hyperglycemia (excessive thirst, increased urination, and weight loss). The diagnosis of any type of diabetes mellitus is achieved by detecting elevated fasting blood glucose ($\geq$126 mg/dL) or an elevated glycosylated hemoglobin (HbA1C, $\geq$ 6.5%), which is a measure of glycemia over a 3-month period. A diagnosis of autoimmune diabetes can be confirmed by detection of islet-cell antibodies, including glutamic acid decarboxylase, 65 kilodalton isoform (GAD65), insulin, IA-2, and zinc transporter 8, either by radioimmunoprecipitation assay (RIA) or ELISA. These autoantibodies also serve as biomarkers predicting future development of type 1 diabetes among certain high-risk groups, such as first-degree relatives of patients with diabetes and women with gestational diabetes. Seropositive diabetic patients are also predicted to require insulin earlier in the disease course than seronegative patients.

Addison Disease

Addison disease is an autoimmune-acquired form of primary adrenal insufficiency.[30] This is rare but potentially life-threatening. Bilateral adrenal cortex destruction leads to decreased production of adrenocortical hormones including cortisol and aldosterone. Although usually insidious in onset and progression, it can present acutely as adrenal crisis, usually in the context of intercurrent illness, such as infection. Addison disease can be an isolated finding or part of an autoimmune polyglandular endocrinopathy syndrome (type 1 and 2). Addison disease can occur at any age but most often presents during the second to third decade of life. The presentation is usually insidious in onset, and symptoms may be nonspecific. These include fatigue, weakness, weight loss, nausea, vomiting and abdominal pain, palpitations, and dizziness (due to low blood pressure). Hyperpigmentation of skin and mucous membranes can be seen later in the course of disease, resulting from elevated ACTH. The manifestations of addisonian crisis may include dehydration, refractory hypotension, and shock. Low-plasma sodium (hyponatremia) is the most common initial laboratory finding. Low-plasma potassium (hyperkalemia) may also develop. Hypoglycemia can occur because glucocorticoids are needed for gluconeogenesis. A cortisol level less than 18 μg/dL to 20 μg/dL is considered diagnostic. A high ACTH level is diagnostic of primary adrenal destruction. Adrenal antibodies (targeting 21-hydroxylase) serve as biomarkers of autoimmune destruction of the adrenal gland and are often detected by RIA assay utilizing I^{125} 21-hydroxylase as substrate. The first-line treatment is hydrocortisone (10 to 15 mg/m^2/day). Higher doses (so-called stress doses) of hydrocortisone are required in the setting of acute intercurrent illness to prevent an adrenal crisis. Mineralocorticoids should also be replaced in the form of fludrocortisone (0.05 to 0.2 mg/day).

Pernicious Anemia

Pernicious anemia is an autoimmune disease with hematologic (**FIGURE 13–6D**), gastric, and immunological abnormalities.[31] Diagnosis relies on histologically proven atrophic body gastritis, peripheral blood examination showing megaloblastic anemia with hypersegmented neutrophils, vitamin B$_{12}$ (cyanocobalamin) deficiency, and detection of intrinsic factor and gastric parietal cell (GPC) antibodies. The highest prevalence is encountered among Northern Europeans, and the prevalence increases with age, from 2.5 to 12%, as well as among those with other autoimmune diseases. HLA-DRB1*03 and DRB1*04 are known to be associated with other autoimmune disease as well as with pernicious anemia. Neurologic disorders occur as a result of vitamin B$_{12}$ deficiency. Disorders include encephalopathy, dementia, myelopathy, and peripheral neuropathy. The β subunit of the gastric enzyme H+/K+-ATPase is the target antigen. This proton pump is responsible for acid secretion in the stomach (from gastric parietal cells). It produces acid by secreting H+ ions in exchange with K+.

GPC antibodies are detected in 90% of affected patients. Intrinsic-factor antibodies are detected in 60% of affected patients. GPC antibodies are usually detected by indirect immunofluorescence performed on cryosectioned rodent stomach. Antibody positivity is characterized by a homogeneous and diffuse cytoplasmic staining of the GPCs. Several studies reported sensitivity and specificity of the ELISA method of 80 to 90%, with an excellent agreement with the immunofluorescence method. The analytical methods currently used to detect intrinsic-factor antibodies are immunoblotting, ELISA and chemiluminescent immunoassay. Highly purified H+/K+ATPase antigens from human or porcine stomach are used.

Hematologic Autoimmune Diseases
Immune Thrombocytopenia

Immune thrombocytopenia (ITP) is defined as a platelet count less than 100×10^9/L, caused by autoimmunity directed at platelets. ITP is an acquired form of thrombocytopenia, which can result in a variety of hemorrhagic states if platelets become very low ($< 50 \times 10^9$/L), or if the patient is taking antiplatelet therapy.[32] Most affected children have self-limited disease. In adults, ITP is usually a chronic disorder. The incidence of primary ITP in adults is 3.3/100,000 adults per year with a prevalence of 9.5 per 100,000 adults. Low platelets result from pathologic antiplatelet antibodies, T-cell–mediated destruction of platelets, and impaired synthesis of megakaryocytes. Most ITP occurs as a primary autoimmune hematologic disorder, although some patients can have ITP in the context of other autoimmune diseases (such as SLE and RA), or secondary to infections such as HIV. The majority of affected patients with ITP have IgG antibodies directed at platelet surface glycoproteins, GPIIb/IIIa and GP1b/IX/V. In addition, the presence of antiplatelet antibodies has been associated with increased risk of thrombosis. The diagnosis of ITP is generally made by obtaining a thorough history and examination from the patient, review of blood count, and peripheral smear. Antiplatelet antibody testing is not indicated for the diagnosis of ITP in most patients where other test results provide an unequivocal diagnosis. First-line therapy is corticosteroids (prednisone), although other immunosuppressants such as rituximab may also be used. Splenectomy is utilized in immunotherapy-refractory cases.

Autoimmune Hemolytic Anemia

Autoimmune hemolytic anemias are all characterized by shortened red blood cell (RBC) survival and the presence of autoantibodies reactive with autologous RBC antigens.[33] The latter is demonstrated by a positive direct antiglobulin (Coombs) test. These disorders are classified by the temperature at which autoantibodies bind optimally to RBCs. In warm antibody autoimmune hemolytic anemia, which constitutes 90% of adult cases, hemolysis is mediated by antibodies that bind to RBC antigens at body temperature (37°C). In cryopathic hemolytic syndromes, cold-reactive autoantibodies bind optimally to RBCs at lower temperatures. In children, cryoglobulins are generally of IgG isotype, while in adults, most are of the IgM isotype. Some patients have both warm and cold hemolysins. These diseases are further classified into primary and secondary causes. Secondary warm agglutinin disease may occur in the context of chronic lymphocytic leukemia, lymphomas, and autoimmune diseases, such as SLE. Secondary cold agglutinin disease is encountered in adolescents or young adults with *Mycoplasma pneumoniae* infections, infectious mononucleosis and sometimes in children with chickenpox. Certain drugs (usually second- or third-generation cephalosporin antibiotics) mediate secondary autoimmune hemolytic anemias, which are rare (incidence of about one per million). In contrast, warm antibody autoimmune hemolytic anemia has an incidence of 1 per 75,000 to 80,000 population, occurs in people of all ages, and accounts for about 80% of all autoimmune hemolytic anemia cases. Paroxysmal cold hemoglobinuria is most common in children, and accounts for about 2 to 5% of all cases of autoimmune hemolytic anemia.

The presenting symptoms of warm antibody autoimmune hemolytic anemia are commonly related to the anemia itself (weakness, fatigue, and pallor). Typically, onset of symptoms is insidious over months. Less often, a patient may notice sudden onset of symptoms of severe anemia and jaundice over a few days. Idiopathic (primary) chronic cold agglutinin disease (monoclonal IgM cold agglutinin-mediated) has its peak incidence after age 50 years. This disorder is considered a special form of monoclonal gammopathy, or low-grade lymphoproliferative malignancy. Most affected patients exhibit clonal B-lymphocyte proliferation and have chronic hemolytic anemia. Other patients have episodic, acute hemolysis with hemoglobinuria induced by chilling. In addition to symptoms of anemia, jaundice may be present. Livedo reticularis (a rash with a net-like appearance) are occasionally seen. Blue extremities (acrocyanosis) affecting the fingers, toes, nose, and ears, is caused by sludging of RBCs in the cutaneous microvasculature. Skin ulceration and necrosis are uncommon. Splenomegaly, a characteristic finding in lymphoproliferative diseases or infectious mononucleosis, may be observed.

On a blood film from a patient with hemolytic anemia, reticulocytosis (reflecting an increased production and egress of immature RBCs [reticulocytes] from the marrow), spherocytosis, RBC fragments, nucleated RBCs, and erythrophagocytosis by monocytes may be observed. Mild leukocytosis and neutrophilia are typical. RBC autoagglutination may be seen in the blood film, and in chilled anticoagulated blood from patients with cold-antibody autoimmune hemolytic anemia. Increased unconjugated plasma bilirubin and urinary urobilinogen are also characteristic.

Serum haptoglobin levels are low, and lactate dehydrogenase levels are increased.

The direct Coombs antibody test detects antibody, complement, or both on RBCs. A broad-spectrum antiglobulin reagent detects both immunoglobulin and complement components on patient RBCs. More specific reagents, which react selectively with IgG or with C3, are also utilized.

The autoantibodies in warm antibody autoimmune hemolytic anemia typically bind to all common types of human RBCs. Rather than being nonspecific, the autoantibodies from any given patient recognize one or more antigens common to almost all human RBCs. Cold agglutinins, reactive with precursors of ABH and Lewis blood group substances, cause RBC agglutination maximally at 0 to 5°C, which is reversible by warming. In paroxysmal cold hemoglobinuria, surviving RBCs are generally coated with complement. The direct antiglobulin reaction may be positive for complement during and briefly following an acute attack.

Antiphospholipid Syndrome

Antiphospholipid syndrome is characterized clinically by venous and arterial thromboses, miscarriage, and low platelets (thrombocytopenia).[34] The syndrome may be encountered in patients without or with other autoimmune diseases, primarily SLE. The syndrome is defined by the presence of at least one of these clinical disorders, and seropositivity for one or more of phospholipid antibodies (namely cardiolipin antibody, β2 glycoprotein-I antibody, and phosphatidylserine–prothrombin complex antibodies), or detection of lupus anticoagulant activity.

IgG and IgM phospholipid antibodies are readily detectable by ELISA. Detection of high titers of IgG antibodies, in particular, portends the highest risk for thrombosis. Lupus anticoagulant activity may be detected by measuring prolonged, activated partial thromboplastin time (APTT).

A more specific test for lupus anticoagulant activity is an in vitro, clot-based assay known as the Russell Viper Venom time, in which the common coagulation pathway is activated by a snake venom. In patients with antiphospholipid syndrome, the clotting time will be shortened. The advantage of this test over the APTT measurement is that other clotting disorders (hemophilia, antibodies to clotting factors VII and IX, or elevated factor VIII) will not produce a positive result. Prevalence of phospholipid antibodies in the general population ranges between 1 to 5%, although only a minority of these individuals develop antiphospholipid syndrome (prevalence, 40–50 cases per 100,000 persons). Although not necessary for a diagnosis of antiphospholipid syndrome, migraine, livedo reticularis (a rash with net-like appearance), and arthralgias are common clinical accompaniments. Immune suppression can prevent clinical manifestations from occurring in many cases. For patients who have already experienced a thrombotic event, lifelong treatment with an oral or subcutaneously administered anticoagulant is necessary.

Organ-Specific Renal Autoimmune Diseases

Goodpasture's disease, also known as anti-glomerular basement membrane (GBM) disease, is an autoimmune disease directed at the alpha 3 chain of type IV collagen, leading to glomerulonephritis and lung hemorrhage.[35] This can progress rapidly to organ failure and death if not recognized. There is some evidence of a genetic association with HLA-DR2. IgG antibody may be detected by Western blot and quantitated for disease surveillance by ELISA. In addition to serology, biopsied kidney tissue typically reveals widespread crescent formation in the glomeruli and linear IgG staining and C3 deposition along the GBM. Other forms of autoimmune nephritis are generally diagnosed by examination of biopsied kidney (direct immunofluorescence and immunohistochemistry) rather than by serology.

IgA nephropathy is the most common form of primary nephropathy worldwide. It is a chronic progressive disease characterized by IgA and C3 complement component in the mesangial area. Membranoproliferative glomerulonephritis (MGN) can be a manifestation of many different diseases, including systemic autoimmune diseases. Presenting disorders include proteinuria (nephrotic syndrome) and hematuria with proteinuria (nephritic syndrome). Low levels of complement components C1q, C3, and C4 and the presence of the C3 nephritic factor are supportive of the MGN diagnosis. Membranous nephropathy presents with severe proteinuria (nephrotic syndrome), and is characterized pathologically by deposition of immune complexes on the urinary side of the GBM.

Organ-Specific Gastrointestinal Disorders

Autoimmune Liver Diseases

Autoimmune liver diseases result from damage to hepatocytes or cholangiocytes, causing autoimmune hepatitis (AIH), primary biliary cirrhosis (PBC), and primary sclerosing cholangitis (PSC).[36] Some patients present without symptoms (increases in liver enzymes identified incidentally during routine physical examination). Other patients present with clinical evidence of liver disease, including fatigue, enlarged liver, abdominal fluid collection (ascites), hemorrhage (due to engorged esophageal veins, known as varices), and jaundice (yellowing of the skin due to hyperbilirubinemia).

Hypergammaglobulinemia is detected in affected patients. Autoantibody serology testing includes testing for smooth muscle antibodies (SMAs) and ANAs. Both SMAs and ANAs, along with other lab markers and biopsy evaluation, are included in the international diagnostic criteria for AIH. The SMAs (sensitivity and specificity both around 80%) associated with autoimmune hepatitis are generally specific for F-actin. In contrast, ANAs, although relatively sensitive for AIH, lack specificity, being associated with a variety of autoimmune diseases. Anti-mitochondrial antibodies (AMAs) are diagnostic markers for PBC. AMAs are found in >90% of patients with PBC, with a specificity of >95%. Anti-LKM-1 antibodies serve as a serologic marker for AIH type 2 and typically occur in the absence of SMA and antinuclear antibodies. These antibodies react with a short linear sequence of the recombinant antigen cytochrome monooxygenase CYP450 2D6. Exclusion of other causes of hepatitis and response to immunosuppressive treatment support the diagnosis of autoimmune hepatitis. The mainstay of autoimmune hepatitis treatment consists of corticosteroids (to induce remission) in combination with azathioprine (to maintain remission). Patients with AIH type 2 more often tend to be young, female, and have severe disease that responds well to immunosuppressive therapy.

Methodologies for detecting antibodies include indirect immunofluorescence of mouse stomach and kidney (for SMAs and AMAs) and HEp-2 cells (for ANAs). ELISA and multiplex platforms using HEp-2 (as substrate for ANAs) or M2 (as substrate for AMAs) are utilized in some laboratories. Although time consuming and lower throughput than ELISA or multiplex platforms, indirect immunofluorescence assay using rodent kidney, liver, and stomach tissue and HEp-2 cells as substrates, several antibodies characteristic for autoimmune hepatitis (ANAs, SMAs, liver-kidney microsomal antibody LKM) or for PBC (AMA), can be evaluated for simultaneously. Additional diagnostic information may be obtained by the fluorescent pattern of ANA on HEp-2 cells (e.g., multiple nuclear dots or nuclear rim) pointing to a variant syndrome of autoimmune hepatitis with features of PBC or PBC itself.

Celiac Disease

Celiac sprue (or celiac disease) is an autoimmune disease affecting the small bowel mucosa triggered by ingestion of gliadin protein of gluten in genetically susceptible individuals.[37] Gluten is enriched in wheat, rye, and barley, but not oats. The classical presentation is that of weight loss and fatty stools occurring because of malabsorption of fat from inflamed intestinal villi, which lose their typical finger-like architecture in the course of the disease. Other presentations include various malabsorption states such as anemia (from iron deficiency), rickets (from vitamin D deficiency), neurological disorders (from deficiency of one or more of vitamin B_{12}, folate, copper, and vitamin E) and skin disorders (due to zinc deficiency). In recent years, less overt gastrointestinal presentations have been encountered, particularly among affected adults, such as bloating, constipation, and weight gain. First-generation gliadin (wheat protein) antibody testing by ELISA had low specificity. Second-generation testing for endomysial antibody by tissue-based IFA had high specificity, but low sensitivity. Third-generation testing for tissue transglutaminase (Tg2) and deamidated gliadin antibodies, generally by ELISA, has >90% sensitivity and specificity for celiac disease. This is particularly true for the IgA isotype. IgG celiac antibody testing should be reserved for patients with IgA deficiency. The gold standard test remains duodenal biopsy to evaluate for inflammation and flattening of the small bowel villi. The treatment for celiac disease is a strict, lifelong, gluten-free diet. Evaluating patients self-treated with a gluten-free diet prior to diagnosis may be challenging; pertinent diagnostic antibodies may become undetectable and pathological changes in the small bowel mucosa may reverse. HLA-DQ2 and DQ8 testing is of value in those patients because it has a high negative predictive value. In a DQ2/DQ8-positive patient self-treated with a gluten-free diet, it may be necessary to have the patient undergo a gluten challenge followed by serological testing and small bowel biopsy.

Patients with celiac disease frequently have coexisting autoimmune disorders, including thyroid disease and type 1 diabetes. Occasionally, patients have accompanying autoimmune neurological disorders. Patients with cerebellar ataxia without celiac disease who are seropositive for first-generation gliadin antibodies, likely have a nonspecific serological finding only, rather than a gluten-initiated neurological disorder known as "gluten ataxia."

Inflammatory Bowel Disease

Inflammatory bowel disease (IBD) is a chronic intestinal inflammatory disorder of unknown etiology. The two major subtypes, Crohn's disease and ulcerative colitis, differ in their clinical courses, treatment responses, and prognoses.[26] The diagnosis of IBD is based on endoscopic, radiologic, and histopathologic criteria. At the time of writing, no single antibody marker could supplant invasive endoscopic and biopsy tests. In the future, antibody profiles may be helpful in one or more of diagnosis (particularly in early or undifferentiated IBD), predicting individuals at risk for developing one or other form of IBD, and determining subtypes of Crohn's disease. Potential markers of Crohn's disease include antibodies reactive with microbial targets such as glycans (mannan on the cell wall surface of baker's yeast [Saccharomyces cerevisiae], laminaribioside carbohydrate, chitobioside carbohydrate, and mannobioside carbohydrate), outer-membrane protein of E. coli, flagellin (a component of flagella on certain indigenous bacteria), and Pseudomonas fluorescens component I2. Each of these antibodies is detected in 50 to 70% of Crohn's disease cases and 10 to 20% of ulcerative colitis cases. In contrast, pANCA is detected in 60 to 70% of ulcerative colitis cases and 10% of Crohn's disease. In patients with indeterminate colitis, the combination of pANCA and S. cerevisiae antibody may be useful for predicting progression to either Crohn's disease or ulcerative colitis.

Autoimmune Cardiac Disorders

Antibodies reactive with monkey myocardium may be detected by indirect IFA in patients with autoimmunity targeting heart muscle (myocarditis), or after some other myocardial injury (e.g., within 2 to 3 weeks of a myocardial infarction). Neonates or fetuses of mothers seropositive for SS-A antibodies are at risk for various conduction defects, particularly complete heart block, with high mortality.[38] Potential antigenic targets in autoimmune cardiac channelopathies leading to dysrhythmias include sodium channel (e.g., $Na_v1.5$), potassium channels (e.g., Kv1.4), and calcium channels (L and T types). Patients with antibody targeting an accessory subunit of Kv4.2 channels, dipeptidyl-peptidase–like protein 6 (DPPX), have an autoimmune encephalomyelitis, but may also develop cardiac dysrhythmias.

Blistering Autoimmune Dermatoses
Pemphigus

Pemphigus is a group of rare autoimmune blistering diseases, characterized by the occurrence of autoantibodies against intraepidermal desmosomal structure proteins, such as desmoglein-1 and 3, causing loss of cell–cell adhesion between keratinocytes and intraepithelial blister formation called acantholysis.[39] Pemphigus is divided into three main types: pemphigus vulgaris, pemphigus foliaceus, and paraneoplastic pemphigus. These differ from one another in their clinical, histologic, and immunologic features and prognosis. In paraneoplastic pemphigus, autoantibodies can be directed against an antigen complex comprising the plakin family. Approximately 25% have a coexisting autoimmune disease affecting another organ. Paraneoplastic pemphigus is mostly associated with lymphoproliferative neoplasms, such as non-Hodgkin lymphoma, chronic lymphocytic leukemia, Castleman disease, and less commonly, thymoma and retroperitoneal sarcomas. Desmoglein 1 and 3 antibodies may be detected by ELISA.

Bullous Pemphigoid

pemphigoid is an autoimmune blistering disease targeting adhesion molecules, which are part of the hemidesmosomes at the dermal–epidermal junction. The immunohistologic hallmark is the formation of a subepidermal blister, and deposits of IgG and complement at the dermal–epidermal junction. Bullous pemphigoid is mediated by antibodies against structural components of the subepidermal basement membrane zone. These target a 230-kDa protein called BP antigen 1 (BPAG1) and a 180-kDa transmembrane protein known as BPAG2.

Organ-Specific Neurological Disorders

Autoimmune neurological disorders can occur on a basis that is either paraneoplastic (occurring alongside cancer), postinfectious, or idiopathic (of unknown cause).[40] Symptoms tend to be subacute in onset (over days to weeks), rather than hyperacute (over seconds to minutes), as in stroke, or insidious (over months to years), as in neurodegenerative disorders such as Parkinson's disease.

In broad terms, paraneoplastic neurological disorders arise as a peripheral immune response against one or more autoantigens in the nervous system that are also expressed in tumors. Tumor immune surveillance in affected patients usually results in neoplasia being confined to the primary organ and to regional lymph nodes. The neurological attack, in contrast, can be devastating, and can affect the central, peripheral, or autonomic nervous systems. Tumor-targeted immune responses are initiated by onconeural proteins expressed in the plasma membrane, nucleus, cytoplasm, or nucleolus of certain cancers. These

antigens are also expressed in neurons or glia and thus are coincidental targets (**TABLES 13–3** and **13–4**). Some antibodies (Table 13–3) have positive predictive values for very specific cancer types greater than 70%. Studies of autopsied tissues and experimental studies suggest that these types of paraneoplastic neurological disorders are caused by CD8+ cytotoxic T cells. The neurological deficits usually do not improve with treatment, although sometimes the clinical picture stabilizes postoncological therapy. Deaths from the complications of neurological disease (rather than from metastatic cancer) are common. Antibodies reactive with intracellular antigens are best detected by IFA using a composite of brain tissues (and non-CNS control tissues, such as kidney and gut) or Western blot.

The advent of "checkpoint" inhibitors, drugs that inhibit T-cell regulation via blockade of CTLA-4, PD-1, and PD-1 ligand, has been a breakthrough for the treatment of once rapidly fatal and incurable cancers such as metastatic melanomas and adenocarcinomas. Autoimmunity commonly develops in these patients (particularly thyroid disease). However, neurological autoimmunity is sometimes encountered in these patients also.

In contrast, antibodies directed at neural cell plasma membrane antigens (Table 13–4; e.g., NMDA receptors) are effectors through multiple mechanisms. Consistent with these antibodies being pathogenic, in vitro experiments and autopsy studies have demonstrated plasmablast, antibody, and complement deposition brain in perivascular and parenchymal distributions. These more-recently described antibodies have varying positive predictive values for cancer (e.g., <10% for glycine receptor antibody vs 50% or greater for antibodies targeting NMDA, AMPA, or $GABA_B$ receptors).

Examples of parainfectious autoimmunity include NMDA receptor encephalitis occurring 2 to 8 weeks post-HSV-1 encephalitis, and Guillain-Barre syndrome post campylobacter infection.

The response to one or more of steroids, intravenous immunoglobulin (IVIg) and plasma exchange is often excellent, with full neurological remission possible. These antibodies may be detected by one or more of tissue-based IFA

TABLE 13–3 Neuronal and Cytoplasmic Antibodies Commonly Encountered in Specimens

Antibody	Antigen	Oncological Association	Neurological Presentations
ANNA-1	ELAVL (Hu)	Small-cell carcinoma	Limbic encephalitis, brainstem encephalitis, sensory autonomic and other peripheral neuropathies
ANNA-2	NOVA 1, 2 (Ri)	Small-cell carcinoma, breast adenocarcinoma	Dementia, limbic encephalitis, brainstem encephalitis, myelopathy, opsoclonus-myoclonus syndrome, peripheral neuropathy
ANNA-3	Unknown	Aerodigestive carcinomas	Brainstem encephalitis, limbic encephalitis, myelopathy, peripheral neuropathy
AGNA	SOX-1	Small-cell carcinoma	Neuropathy, Lambert-Eaton syndrome, limbic encephalitis
Ma1, Ma2	PNMA1, PNMA2 (Ma1, Ma2)	Testicular (Ma2); breast, colon, testicular (Ma1)	Limbic encephalitis, hypothalamic disorder, brainstem encephalitis
NF-L	NF-L	Small-cell carcinoma, Merkel cell carcinoma Other neuroendocrine	Cerebellar ataxia, encephalopathy, myelopathy
PCA-1	CDR2	Mullerian/breast adenocarcinoma	Cerebellar ataxia, brainstem encephalitis, myelopathy, neuropathies
PCA-2	Unknown	Small-cell carcinoma	Limbic encephalitis, ataxia, brainstem encephalitis, Lambert-Eaton syndrome, peripheral and autonomic neuropathies
CRMP-5 IgG	CRMP-5	Small-cell carcinoma, thymoma	Cognitive disorders, depression, chorea, ataxia, myelopathy, radiculopathy, neuropathy, Lambert-Eaton syndrome
Amphiphysin IgG	Amphiphysin	Small-cell carcinoma, breast adenocarcinoma	Limbic encephalitis, aphasia, other subacute-onset dementias, stiff-person phenomenon, myelopathy, neuropathy
Recoverin antibody	Recoverin	Small cell carcinoma, neuroendocrine carcinomas	Retinopathy
GAD65 antibody*	GAD65	Thymoma; renal cell, breast or colon adenocarcinoma	Stiff-person syndrome, Stiff-person phenomena, ataxia, seizures, limbic encephalitis, brainstem encephalitis, ophthalmoplegia, parkinsonism, myelopathy
GFAP antibody	α/ε GFAP isoforms	Teratoma	Meningoencephalomyelitis

Findings among patients with neuronal, nuclear, or cytoplasmic antibodies and mostly classic paraneoplastic disorders.

TABLE 13–4 Plasma Membrane Antibodies Commonly Encountered in Autoimmune Disorders

Antibody	Antigen	Oncological Association	Neurological Presentation
VGKC-complex	LGI1, CASPR2	Small-cell lung carcinoma; thymoma; adenocarcinoma of breast, prostate	Limbic encephalitis, amnestic syndrome, executive dysfunction, personality change, disinhibition hypothalamic disorder, brainstem encephalitis, ataxia, extrapyramidal disorders, myoclonus, peripheral and autonomic neuropathy
NMDA receptor	GluN1	Ovarian teratoma	Anxiety, psychosis, seizures, amnestic syndrome, dyskinesia, hypoventilation, coma.
AMPA receptor	GluR1,2	Thymic tumors, lung carcinomas, breast carcinoma	Limbic encephalitis, nystagmus, seizures
GABA-B receptor	GABA-B receptor	Small-cell lung carcinoma, other neuroendocrine neoplasia	Limbic encephalitis, intractable seizures, orolingual dyskinesias
PCA-Tr	DNER	Hodgkin lymphoma	Cerebellar ataxia
*P/Q and N type calcium channel	P/Q and N-type calcium channels	Small-cell carcinoma, breast, or gynecological adenocarcinoma	Encephalopathies, Myelopathies, neuropathies, Lambert-Eaton syndrome
Muscle AChR	Muscle AChR	Thymoma, thymic carcinoma, lung carcinoma	Myasthenia gravis. Also sometimes observed in paraneoplastic CNS contexts.
Neuronal ganglionic AChR	Neuronal ganglionic AChR	Adenocarcinoma, thymoma, small-cell carcinoma	Dysautonomia, peripheral somatic neuropathies, encephalopathies.
NMO-IgG	Aquaporin-4	Some reports of thymoma and other solid tumors	Relapsing optic neuritis, transverse myelitis, encephalopathies
Glycine receptor	α1 subunit GlyR	Thymoma, lymphoma	Stiff-person syndrome and variants
Metabotropic glutamate receptor 1	mGluR1	Hodgkin lymphoma, prostate adenocarcinoma	Ataxia, dysgeusia, vertigo, cognitive symptoms, seizures
Metabotropic glutamate receptor 5 antibody	mGluR5	2 patients with Hodgkin lymphoma	Limbic encephalitis

Findings among patients with plasma membrane protein antibodies and autoimmune neurological disorders (Paraneoplastic or Idiopathic).

(or other immunohistochemical techniques) and cell-based assays (CBAs), where the cell-line is transfected to express the antigen of interest in its native conformational state on the cell surface. Testing for these kinds of antibodies using ELISA can result in nonspecific IgG binding to intracellular epitopes (false positives).

Neurological autoimmunity can occur at any level of the nervous system and may be multifocal. Disorders are discussed in craniocaudal anatomic order herein.

Optic Neuropathy

Subacute onset of painful vision loss is a typical presentation of **optic neuritis**. Many patients have a single episode of optic neuritis without sequelae or go on to develop other neurological manifestations of multiple sclerosis. Others with IgG antibody specific for aquaporin-4 or myelin oligodendrocyte glycoprotein (MOG) are at risk for recurrent autoimmune events affecting the optic nerve, spinal cord, and brain. Detection of one of these antibodies permits early intervention with immune-suppressing medication that can aid in relapse prevention. Because disease-pertinent IgGs are reactive with the extracellular domains of aquaporin-4 and MOG, optimum diagnostic specificity is achieved by using a live CBA format. Those cells, transfected with the molecule of interest (tagged with green fluorescent protein), express the antigen in its native conformational state, permitting detection of antibodies reactive with the extracellular domains only. The "read out" from IgG binding can be achieved by quantification of fluorescing cells with IgG bound by flow cytometry, or by observer-based indirect immunofluorescence.

A less-severe optic nerve disorder, known as optic papillitis, usually presents with painless blurring of vision, and a hazy-appearing optic disc on ophthalmologic examination. This phenomenon may be a clue to a more widespread autoimmune CNS disorder known as autoimmune glial fibrillary acidic protein (GFAP) astrocytopathy. Neurological problems may include meningitis, encephalitis, and myelitis. Symptoms tend to improve with corticosteroid treatment. This antibody can be identified by tissue-based indirect immunofluorescence assay and confirmed by GFAP-transfected, cell-based assay.

Uveitis

Uveitis is defined as inflammation of the vascular uveal tract of the eye, including the iris, ciliary body, and choroid. Adjacent structures including the retina, optic nerve, vitreous, and sclera may also be affected. There are no serological IgG antibody markers that assist in the diagnosis of uveitis, although there are some strong HLA associations. HLA-B27 is strongly associated with anterior uveitis occurring in the context of seronegative spondyloarthropathies (ankylosing spondylitis, psoriatic arthritis, Reiter syndrome). HLA-A29 is strongly associated with Birdshot chorioretinopathy. Uveitis may also occur as part of Vogt-Koyanagi-Harada disease, which is an exceedingly rare multiphasic, multisystem autoimmune inflammatory disorder with ocular, auditory, skin, and neurologic manifestations.

Retinopathy

Patients with autoimmune **retinopathy** present with gradual vision loss. In the early stages, patients complain of night-vision problems, narrow field of vision, and floaters. Patients may progress to complete vision loss. In some patients, the autoimmune response is triggered by an occult cancer, usually small cell carcinoma or melanoma. Recoverin antibody can be diagnostic of small cell carcinoma-related retinopathy. In patients with an inflammatory ophthalmitis (retinitis and inflammatory optic neuropathy), collapsin-response mediator protein 5 (CRMP-5) autoimmunity should be considered. Patients with CRMP-5 IgG detected should have radiological testing to search for small cell carcinoma and thymoma.

Hearing Loss

Acute sensorineural hearing loss (affecting the cochlea and VIIIth cranial nerve) without obvious external etiology is usually suspected to have an autoimmune cause and should prompt early treatment with corticosteroids. A triad of acute hearing loss, encephalopathy, and retinal vasculopathy is encountered in Susac syndrome. Although an autoimmune endothelial cell disorder has long been suspected in these patients, sensitive and specific antibody biomarkers are lacking.

Encephalopathy

Patients with autoimmune **encephalopathy** present with a rapid decline in mood, memory, and behavior, and also seizures. The classical clinical disorder encountered in an autoimmune context is limbic encephalitis, where there is inflammation of the limbic (mesial temporal regions) of the temporal lobes. Some patients have a more restricted presentation (seizures only, or rapidly progressive cognitive decline only). Either way, rapid identification of this diagnosis is paramount to ensure optimum response to immune therapies and early cancer nonneurological diagnosis, where applicable. Antibodies diagnostic of autoimmune encephalitis are numerous and are best tested for as part of a profile rather than on an individual basis. The latter practice may delay time to appropriate treatment or cancer diagnosis where the antibody has oncological significance. Evaluation of both serum and CSF for neural antibodies is required because the clinical sensitivity and specificity is optimum for different antibodies in different specimen types. For example, antibody targeting NMDA receptor is best tested for in CSF rather than in serum. In contrast, sensitivity for leucine-rich glioma inactivated 1 (Lgi1) antibody is most sensitively detected in serum, without loss of specificity. Responses to treatment vary and are best for Lgi encephalitis and NMDA receptor encephalitis, while responses to limbic encephalitis accompanying small cell carcinoma and ANNA-1 (anti-Hu) are usually limited.

Myelopathy

Autoimmune disorders of the spinal cord are characterized by weakness and numbness of the limbs, pain, and bowel and bladder dysfunction.

In some instances, the spinal cord can appear diffusely inflamed on MRI scan, and the spinal fluid (obtained by lumbar puncture) will have a markedly elevated white blood cell count. IgG antibodies tested for in the diagnostic laboratory are specific for aquaporin-4 and MOG. Patients with these antibodies detected are at risk for recurrence of autoimmune **myelopathy** (myelitis), optic neuritis, and sometimes encephalitis. The latter disorder is most common in children and is sometimes referred to as acute disseminated encephalomyelitis. Despite the severity of these disorders, they are treatable, making an early and accurate serological diagnosis important.

Myelopathy of a more insidious nature can occur in the context of a paraneoplastic neurological disorder. The pertinent antibodies are not myelopathy-specific, and overlap with those pertinent to encephalopathy. In fact, each antibody marker is cancer-specific, rather than neurological-phenotype specific. For example, patients with anti-Hu antibody (also known as anti-neuronal nuclear antibody type 1) detected can develop diverse neurological presentations (e.g., encephalopathy, myelopathy, or peripheral neuropathy, or sometimes a mixture of these), but the clinical syndrome is unified by the detection of small cell carcinoma (usually of lung) or another neuroendocrine tumor in all cases.

Stiff-person syndrome is an autoimmune disorder affecting inhibitory interneuronal pathways in the brainstem and spinal cord. GABA (synthesized by glutamic acid decarboxylase [GAD]) and glycine are neurochemicals critical for regulation of excitation. Autoimmunity targeting GABAergic and glycinergic inhibitory pathways have been described. Patients typically present with stiffness and spasms affecting the lower extremities and truncal regions. Neurological presentations may also be more limited (e.g., stiff-limb syndrome) or widespread (e.g., progressive encephalomyelitis with rigidity and myoclonus) than the classical stiff-person form. Among affected patients with glutamic acid decarboxylase (GAD65) antibody detected, coexisting autoimmune disease (most commonly thyroid disease or diabetes) is present in more than half. Stiff-person syndrome patients with glycine receptor antibody detected respond to immune therapies in 80% of cases (versus 40% for stiff-person syndrome generally).

Neuropathy

Peripheral **neuropathy** is one of the most common reasons for referral of a patient to a neurology clinic. Diagnosis is important as these disorders are generally treatable (unlike hereditary neuropathies or amyotrophic lateral sclerosis [ALS]). Symptoms are generally "stocking and glove" distribution sensory loss, pain, and distal limb weakness. Autoimmune neuropathies (unlike common diabetic and hereditary forms) tend to have subacute onset over weeks to months. There are several subtypes. Some are part of systemic disorders, which draw on knowledge from previous sections in this chapter. Vasculitic neuropathies usually lead to progressive weakness and sensory loss, due to nerve infarction. These may be diagnosed by biopsy of an affected nerve, or in the case of Wegener's granulomatosis, by serology for cANCA (PR3) antibody. Neuropathies may occur in the context of connective tissue diseases such as SLE and Sjogren syndrome, and can be one of the presenting disorders of a paraneoplastic syndrome. There are also inflammatory neuropathies without systemic or other neurological manifestations. These can be divided into demyelinating and axonal disorders, depending on whether the wiring (axon) or insulation (myelin) of the nerve is affected. Demyelinating neuropathies can be acute (known as acute inflammatory demyelinating polyneuropathy [AIDP] or Guillain-Barre syndrome) or chronic (known as chronic inflammatory demyelinating polyneuropathy [CIDP]). Weakness in AIDP can ascend quickly from distal to proximal, threatening upper extremity and respiratory function. Subtypes of these disorders are diagnosable by ELISA assay using ganglioside antigens as substrate. Gangliosides are glycosphingolipids found predominantly on cell surfaces of neurons. GQ1B antibody may assist in diagnosing the Miller-Fisher variant (cranial symptom predominant) of AIDP. Myelin associated glycoprotein (MAG) antibody may assist in diagnosing a distal-predominant form of CIDP. GM1 antibody is typically detected at high titers in patients with multifocal motor neuropathy with conduction block, which can mimic the universally fatal Lou Gehrig's disease (ALS). An axonal variant of these inflammatory neuropathies may be diagnosable by positivity for GM1 and Gd1a antibodies. Antibodies targeting paranode of Ranvier have recently been identified in some patients with CIDP, namely neurofascin (NF-155) antibody and contactin-1. NF-155 is detected in patients with a variant of CIDP that is accompanied by tremor, CNS demyelination, ataxia, and poor response to immunotherapy.

Autonomic Neuropathy

The autonomic nervous system regulates internal organ function (gut, bowel, bladder), heart rate, blood pressure, and sweating (thermoregulation). Autoimmune dysautonomia may be caused by antibody reactive with the alpha 3 subunit of the AChR, which is enriched in ganglia in the peripheral autonomic ganglia. These patients may remit with prolonged immune therapy. Other antibodies that may be detected in this context include ANNA-1.

Myasthenia Gravis

Myasthenia gravis is the prototypic autoimmune antibody-mediated neurological disorder. Affected patients present with fatigable weakness, meaning neuromuscular weakness that worsens with use and diurnally (symptoms worse later in the day). Any skeletal (striated) muscle can be affected, although common early presenting features include double vision, drooping eyelids (ptosis), and limb girdle weakness. A loss of cholinergic neuromuscular transmission occurs.

Ninety percent of cases can be attributed to antibody toward skeletal muscle acetylcholine receptor (AChR, α1 subunit expressing) in the postsynaptic muscle membrane. This autoimmune response may be triggered in the context of an anterior mediastinal neoplasm (thymoma, or thymic carcinoma). The risk for thymoma is highest among patients who produce antibodies with high capacity to produce downregulation (modulation) of the AChR from the surface of cells with muscle characteristics (such as the human rhabdomyosarcoma TE671 cell line), and with high titer antibodies reactive with skeletal muscle striational antigens. Striational antibodies can be detected using skeletal muscle as substrate in an ELISA format, or evaluating for subtypes of antibodies (against titin, ryanodine receptor, myosin, actin, and alpha actinin) using ELISA. Titin antibody may be predictive of thymoma.

Traditional AChR assays, still widely in use, take advantage of the ability of the snake venom neurotoxin, alpha bungarotoxin, to bind irreversibly to the α1 subunit of AChRs. AChR binding antibodies can be immunoprecipitated in a reaction tube containing solubilized human skeletal muscle whose AChR receptors are irreversibly bound to I-^{125} labelled alpha bungarotoxin. AChR modulation can be measured by incubating AChR expressing TE671 cells with patient serum and subsequently measuring bungarotoxin bound to remaining AChRs.

Approximately 4% of patients with myasthenia gravis have evidence of autoimmunity against muscle-specific kinase (MuSK), another protein in the postsynaptic membrane complex. Those patients with MuSK myasthenia often present with speech and swallowing difficulties.

Antibodies can be measured by RIA, ELISA or cell-based assays (Figure 13-2). Treatments can be directed at cholinesterase (increasing the amount of acetylcholine available to bind to AChRs) or the immune system. Common immunotherapies used include corticosteroids, plasma exchange, intravenous immunoglobulin, anti-CD20 monoclonal antibodies (e.g., rituximab), and purine analogues which interfere with DNA synthesis in lymphocytes (e.g., azathioprine).

Dermatomyositis

Dermatomyositis is an inflammatory disorder primarily affecting proximal limb muscles and skin. Patients present with weakness (difficulty standing up, climbing steps, or raising their arms above their heads). Patients with more severe disease may have difficulty lifting their heads off the bed because of neck flexor weakness, impaired swallowing due to pharyngeal muscle weakness, or shortness of breath due to diaphragmatic weakness. Dermatologic features include scaly erythematous lesions found on the extensor surfaces of the metacarpophalangeal, proximal interphalangeal, and distal interphalangeal joints known as Gottron papules. In addition, patients with dermatomyositis often experience a violaceous eruption on the upper eyelids, sometimes associated with periorbital edema, known as a heliotrope rash. Both of these skin features are pathognomonic for dermatomyositis. Mi-2 antibody is associated with severe skin manifestations.

Some patients have calcinosis, which is progressive deposition of calcium nodules in the subcutaneous tissues, which can erupt through skin and precipitate skin infection. Calcinosis is most common among those patients with nuclear matrix protein 2 (NXP2) autoantibody detected. Interstitial lung disease may also occur, particularly in those with antibodies reactive with Jo-1 or the melanoma differentiation-associated protein 5 (MDA5). Rarer complications include cardiomyopathy and arthritis. The diagnosis is based on clinical features and muscle tissue histology. The hallmark histologic feature of dermatomyositis is perifascicular atrophy, in which small atrophic fibers line the edges of fascicles that are otherwise composed of relatively normal-sized myofibers.

Necrotizing Myopathy

The hallmark of this disease is rapidly progressive limb weakness, leading to early disability, head, neck, and respiratory system, if untreated. Diagnosis may be supported by detection of signal recognition particle (SRP) antibody or HMG-CoA reductase antibody. Detection systems include Western blot and ELISA. SRP antibody has a distinct cytoplasmic antibody binding pattern by tissue IFA (including selective binding to cells in the proximal gastric mucosa). Sometimes HMG CoA reductase antibody latter is detected in patients who develop a rare autoimmune necrotizing myopathy in the context of HMG CoA reductase inhibitor (cholesterol-lowering "statin" therapy) exposure. Muscle biopsy reveals extensive necrosis, with macrophage infiltration, but little or no lymphocytic infiltration. Patients usually have responses to immune suppression, although the mortality of this disorder remains high.

Other Inflammatory Neurological Disorders Where Igg Measures (without Antigen Specificity) Are Biomarkers

Multiple Sclerosis

Although there is no antibody biomarker that unifies **multiple sclerosis (MS)** cases, and MS does not segregate with classical autoimmune diseases in terms of its occurrence in individuals and families, most would agree that MS is an immune-mediated disorder.[41] Data supporting this includes HLA genetic predisposition, a clear association with immunologically relevant risk factors (prior Epstein-Barr virus exposure and vitamin D deficiency), a relapsing and remitting inflammatory clinical and radiological course, inflammatory MRI head and spinal cord abnormalities, inflammatory spinal fluid findings, and remission maintenance by immunomodulating therapies.

Patients with relapsing-remitting multiple sclerosis may present with one or more of a diverse array of symptoms of central nervous system dysfunction in a subacute manner. Disease onset is usually in the second or third decade of life. Common manifestations include painful vision loss (optic neuritis), loss of balance, numbness, or weakness of the face or extremities. Symptoms tend to abate spontaneously, or after a course of corticosteroids, over weeks to months. Some patients develop a progressive course several decades after the onset of relapsing remitting disease (known as secondary progressive MS) or develop first manifestations insidiously in the 5th or 6th decade (primary progressive disease). Dissemination of disease in space (multifocal neurological and radiological manifestations) and time (multiple attacks) of symptoms are generally considered necessary for a diagnosis of MS. An MS-specific distribution of inflammatory-appearing lesions on MRI brain and especially MRI of the spinal cord are critical for making a diagnosis.

Exclusion of other diseases that may mimic MS is relevant on a case-by-case basis. For example, Lyme disease serology would be pertinent to evaluate in a patient who complained of tick bites before the onset of neurological symptoms. The detection of cerebrospinal fluid (CSF)-restricted immunoglobulin bands (known as oligoclonal bands) by electrophoresis is supportive of the diagnosis but may occur in other inflammatory CNS disorders. Other markers of inflammation may be detected in the CSF (elevations in protein, white blood cell count, IgG index, and IgG synthesis rate).

IgG4 and Related Autoimmune and Inflammatory Diseases

IgG4 is the least abundant Ig subclass (less than 5% of total IgG) in healthy subjects, and is unique in both structure and function. This molecule's production is controlled primarily by type 2 helper T (Th2) cells. IgG4 has been traditionally considered to play only a limited role in immune activation. It does not activate the classical complement pathway effectively, and because of its bispecificity (functionally monovalent), it is unable to cross-link antigens or form immune complexes. In certain autoimmune diseases, antigen-specific IgG4 molecules predominate. Examples of such diseases (and their biomarkers) include pemphigus vulgaris and pemphigus foliaceus (desmoglein IgG4), idiopathic membranous glomerulonephritis (podocyte M-type phospholipase A2 receptor IgG4), thrombotic thrombocytopenic purpura (ADAMTS13 IgG4), and a subset of myasthenia gravis (MuSK IgG4).

IgG4-Related Disease

Unrelated to these autoimmune diseases is a chronic infiltrative, inflammatory disorder, known as IgG4-related disease, which can affect one or more organs.[42] This is a rare disease affecting men more than women (3:1). Histopathological analysis of biopsy specimens is the cornerstone of diagnosis. Elevated IgG4 in tissue and serum are helpful in diagnosing IgG4-related disease. The key pathologic features include a dense lymphoplasmacytic infiltrate organized in a storiform (matted and irregularly whorled) pattern, obliterative phlebitis, and eosinophilic infiltrate. The inflammatory infiltrate is composed of an admixture of T and B lymphocytes. B cells are typically organized in germinal centers, while T cells are distributed diffusely throughout the lesion. All immunoglobulin subclasses may be represented within involved tissue, but IgG4 predominates. Tissues that may be affected include the meninges, lacrimal and salivary glands, thyroid gland, pancreas, long bones, and kidney. Pancreatic disease can mimic pancreatic cancer radiologically. Glucocorticoids are the mainstay of initial treatment. B lymphocyte depleting treatment with rituximab is also usually effective.

CASE STUDY

Case Reports

Case Report 1

A 41-year-old woman presented to her general practitioner (GP or family doctor) complaining of fatigue and numb feet. The patient had a history of patchy pigment loss from her skin (vitiligo) and Hashimoto thyroiditis. The latter had been diagnosed when the patient had presented to her doctor 5 years earlier with fatigue and menstrual irregularities. The GP had found elevated thyroid peroxidase (TPO) antibodies in her blood at that time, as well as elevated thyroid-stimulating hormone (TSH), and low free thyroxine plasma values. The patient also has a family history of autoimmune vitamin B_{12} deficiency (pernicious anemia) in her mother, and autoimmune thyroid disease in her mother and three sisters. She reported mixed Irish-Scandinavian ancestry. On this occasion, the GP rechecked her thyroid biochemistry and it was normal. Recognizing the strong personal and family history of autoimmunity, the GP subsequently evaluated for other autoimmune causes of fatigue. Pernicious anemia and Addison disease were excluded: vitamin B_{12} and methylmalonic acid levels were normal, and gastric parietal cell and intrinsic factor antibodies were negative. Early morning cortisol level was normal, and adrenal antibody (targeting 21-hydroxylase) was negative. Tissue transglutaminase IgA antibody was elevated, suggesting celiac disease. Upon further inquiry, the patient stated she had some mild to moderate loose stool and bloating for about 5 years, but this had not bothered her particularly, and so she had not reported this to a doctor. Iron, folate, vitamins D and E, and copper values were all low. A jejunal biopsy revealed flattening of the intestinal mucosa, with loss of normal villous architecture. The patient started a gluten-free diet and took daily oral supplements of the vitamins and minerals of which she was deficient. Within 12 weeks, her numbness had improved, and her fatigue had resolved.

Questions

1. What led the GP to think of autoimmune disease?
2. Is family history important or just coincidence in this patient?
3. Is doing all these complex tests for autoimmunity just an academic exercise?

Case Report 2

A 52-year-old man presented to a neurologist with insidious onset and slow progression of weakness in his lower extremities over 10 years. His father had difficulty walking, progressive from his 40s, although he

(continues)

CASE STUDY (Continued)

had not received a neurological diagnosis, and died from ischemic heart disease at age 60. The patient examination demonstrated spasticity and brisk reflexes in his lower extremities, consistent with spinal cord disease (myelopathy). Laboratory work demonstrated aquaporin-4 IgG by ELISA (20 IU/mL; normal, < 5 u/mL), potentially consistent with an autoimmune inflammatory disorder known as neuromyelitis optica. However, an MRI of the patient's spine demonstrated cord atrophy but no inflammatory changes. CSF demonstrated normal white cell count and protein. Because the clinical history was not suspicious for autoimmune myelitis, additional evaluations were undertaken. A serum protein electrophoresis demonstrated polyclonal hypergammaglobulinemia. Aquaporin-4 antibody testing by HEK293 live cell-based assay was negative.

Questions

1. Which antibody test result is to be believed?
2. Are some patients more prone to having false positive test results than others?
3. What is the likely diagnosis?

Case Report 3

A 59-year-old man presented for evaluation to a neurologist with gait problems. Examination revealed cerebellar ataxia. MRI head and spine imaging was normal. CSF revealed normal protein and cell count but elevated CSF-exclusive oligoclonal band numbers. The patient was diagnosed with multiple sclerosis (MS). Shortly afterward, the patient developed rapidly progressive memory decline. A repeat MRI of his head showed evidence of hippocampus inflammation bilaterally (limbic encephalitis). A paraneoplastic serum evaluation revealed ANNA-1 antibody (anti-Hu). Cancer imaging revealed a lung nodule, which revealed small cell carcinoma at biopsy. A paraneoplastic neurological disorder was the final diagnosis.

Questions

1. If the oligoclonal bands were positive in the CSF, surely this is MS?
2. What were the clues to a paraneoplastic disorder?
3. Should ANNA-1 be considered only when there is ataxia and limbic encephalitis?

▶ References

1. Theofilopoulos AN, Kono DH, Baccala R. The multiple pathways to autoimmunity. *Nat Immunol.* 2017;18(7): 716–724.

2. McKeon A, Tracy JA, Pittock SJ, et al. Purkinje cell cytoplasmic autoantibody type 1 accompaniments: the cerebellum and beyond. *Arch Neurol.* 2011;68(10):1282–1289.

3. Waters P, Woodhall M, O'Connor KC, et al. MOG cell-based assay detects non-MS patients with inflammatory neurologic disease. *Neurol Neuroimmunol Neuroinflamm.* 2015;2(3):e89.

4. Voigt J, Krause C, Rohwäder E, et al. Automated indirect immunofluorescence evaluation of antinuclear autoantibodies on HEp-2 cells. *Clin Dev Immunol.* 2012;2012:651058.

5. Honorat JA, Komorowski L, Josephs KA, et al. IgLON5 antibody: neurological accompaniments and outcomes in 20 patients. *Neurol Neuroimmunol Neuroinflamm.* 2017;4(5):e385.

6. Fryer JP, Lennon VA, Pittock SJ, et al. AQP4 autoantibody assay performance in clinical laboratory service. *Neurol Neuroimmunol Neuroinflamm.* 2014;1(1):e11.

7. Flanagan EP, Hinson SR, Lennon VA, et al. Glial fibrillary acidic protein immunoglobulin G as biomarker of autoimmune astrocytopathy: analysis of 102 patients. *Ann Neurol.* 2017;81(2):298–309.

8. Howard FM, Jr., Lennon VA, Finley J, et al. Clinical correlations of antibodies that bind, block, or modulate human acetylcholine receptors in myasthenia gravis. *Ann N Y Acad Sci.* 1987;505:526–538.

9. Amoroso M, Achenbach P, Powell M, et al. 3 Screen islet cell autoantibody ELISA: a sensitive and specific ELISA for the combined measurement of autoantibodies to GAD_{65}, to IA-2 and to ZnT8. *Clin Chim Acta.* 2016;462:60–64.

10. Gerlach S, Affeldt K, Pototzki L, et al. Automated evaluation of Crithidia luciliae based indirect immunofluorescence tests: a novel application of the EUROPattern-Suite Technology. *J Immunol Res.* 2015;2015:742402.

11. Thyroglobulin Antibody II Assay. In: Beckman Coulter I, Fullerton, CA ed 2011.

12. Roche Cobas Package Insert. In: Roche Diagnostics I, IN, ed.

13. Preissner CM, Wolhuter PJ, Sistrunk JW, et al. Comparison of thyrotropin-receptor antibodies measured by four commercially available methods with a bioassay that uses Fisher rat thyroid cells. *Clin Chem.* 2003;49(8):1402–1404.

14. Bardin N, Desplat-Jego S, Daniel L, et al. BioPlex 2200 multiplexed system: simultaneous detection of anti-dsDNA and anti-chromatin antibodies in patients with systemic lupus erythematosus. *Autoimmunity.* 2009;42(1):63–68.

15. Eriksson C, Agaton C, Kånge R, et al. Microfluidic analysis of antibody specificity in a compact disk format. *J Proteome Res.* 2006;5(7):1568–1574.

16. Tsai CT, Robinson PV, Spencer CA, et al. Ultrasensitive antibody detection by agglutination-PCR (ADAP). *ACS Cent Sci.* 2016;2(3):139–147.

17. Fortini AS, Sanders EL, Weinshenker BG, et al. Cerebrospinal fluid oligoclonal bands in the diagnosis of multiple sclerosis. Isoelectric focusing with IgG immunoblotting compared with high-resolution agarose gel electrophoresis and cerebrospinal fluid IgG index. *Am J Clin Pathol.* 2003;120(5):672–675.

18. Ladwig PM, Barnidge DR, Willrich MA. Quantification of the IgG2/4 kappa monoclonal therapeutic eculizumab from serum using isotype specific affinity purification and microflow LC-ESI-Q-TOF mass spectrometry. *J Am Soc Mass Spectrom.* 2017;28(5):811–817.

19. Doria A, Zen M, Canova M, et al. SLE diagnosis and treatment: when early is early. *Autoimmun Rev.* 2010;10(1):55–60.

20. Denton CP, Khanna D. Systemic sclerosis. *Lancet.* 2017;390(10103):1685–1699.

21. Gunnarsson R, Hetlevik SO, Lilleby V, et al. Mixed connective tissue disease. *Best Pract Res Clin Rheumatol.* 2016;30(1):95–111.

22. Yates M, Watts R. ANCA-associated vasculitis. *Clin Med (Lond).* 2017;17(1):60–64.

23. Atzeni F, Talotta R, Masala IF, et al. Biomarkers in rheumatoid arthritis. *Isr Med Assoc J.* 2017;19(8):512–516.

24. Mavragani CP, Moutsopoulos HM. Sjögren syndrome. *CMAJ.* 2014;186(15):E579–E586.

25. Falorni A, Minarelli V, Bartoloni E, et al. Diagnosis and classification of autoimmune hypophysitis. *Autoimmun Rev.* 2014;13(4-5):412–416.

26. Mitsuyama K, Niwa M, Takedatsu H, et al. Antibody markers in the diagnosis of inflammatory bowel disease. *World J Gastroenterol.* 2016;22(3):1304–1310.

27. Fröhlich E, Wahl R. Thyroid autoimmunity: role of anti-thyroid antibodies in thyroid and extra-thyroidal diseases. *Front Immunol.* 2017;8:521.

28. Brown EM. Anti-parathyroid and anti-calcium sensing receptor antibodies in autoimmune hypoparathyroidism. *Endocrinol Metab Clin North Am.* 2009;38(2):437–445.

29. Bingley PJ. Clinical applications of diabetes antibody testing. *J Clin Endocrinol Metab.* 2010;95(1):25–33.

30. Mitchell AL, Pearce SH. Autoimmune Addison disease: pathophysiology and genetic complexity. *Nat Rev Endocrinol.* 2012;8(5):306–316.

31. Bizzaro N, Antico A. Diagnosis and classification of pernicious anemia. *Autoimmun Rev.* 2014;13(4-5):565–568.

32. Lambert MP, Gernsheimer TB. Clinical updates in adult immune thrombocytopenia. *Blood.* 2017;129(21):2829–2835.

33. Packman CH. The clinical pictures of autoimmune hemolytic anemia. *Transfus Med Hemother.* 2015;42(5):317–324.

34. Cervera R. Antiphospholipid syndrome. *Thromb Res.* 2017;151(suppl 1):S43–S47.

35. Segelmark M, Hellmark T. Autoimmune kidney diseases. *Autoimmun Rev.* 2010;9(5):A366–A371.

36. Sebode M, Hartl J, Vergani D, Lohse AW, International Autoimmune Hepatitis Group (IAIHG). Autoimmune hepatitis: from current knowledge and clinical practice to future research agenda. *Liver Int.* 2018;38(1):15–22.

37. Snyder MR, Murray JA. Celiac disease: advances in diagnosis. *Expert Rev Clin Immunol.* 2016;12(4):449–463.

38. Brito-Zerón P, Izmirly PM, Ramos-Casals M, et al. Autoimmune congenital heart block: complex and unusual situations. *Lupus.* 2016;25(2):116–128.

39. Vassileva S, Drenovska K, Manuelyan K. Autoimmune blistering dermatoses as systemic diseases. *Clin Dermatol.* 2014;32(3):364–375.

40. McKeon A, Pittock SJ. Paraneoplastic encephalomyelopathies: pathology and mechanisms. *Acta Neuropathol.* 2011;122(4):381–400.

41. Lassmann H. Pathology and disease mechanisms in different stages of multiple sclerosis. *J Neurol Sci.* 2013;333(1-2):1–4.

42. Stone JH, Zen Y, Deshpande V. IgG4-related disease. *N Engl J Med.* 2012;366(6):539–551.

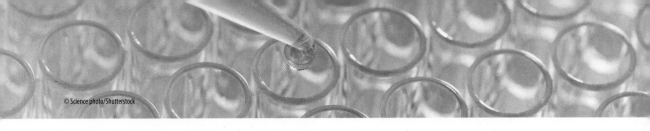

© Science photo/Shutterstock

CHAPTER 14

Tumor Immunology

Rosalie Sterner, MD, PhD

Aerobic
Anaerobic
Chimeric antigen receptor T cells
   (CAR-T cells)
Cytokine release syndrome (CRS)
Cytotoxic-T-lymphocyte-associated
   protein 4 (CTLA4)
Elimination
Enzyme-linked immunosorbent
   assay (ELISA)

Equilibrium phase
Escape phase
Etanercept
Flow cytometry
HCG (human chorionic
   gonadotropin)
Immunoediting
Immunohistochemistry (IHC)
Immunosurveillance
Metastases

Oxidative phosphorylation
Programmed death ligand 1 (PD-L1)
Programmed death protein 1 (PD-1)
Radioimmunoassay (RIA)
Tocilizumab
Tumor-associated antigens
Tumor markers
Tumor-specific antigens
Vaccines

LEARNING OBJECTIVES

Upon completion of this chapter, the reader should be able to:

1. Discuss the economic, morbidity and emotional impact of cancer.
2. Demonstrate awareness of the hallmarks of cancer.
3. Explain cancer's ability to evade immunosurveillance through immunoediting.
4. Order the three phases of immunoediting.
5. Compare and contrast tumor-specific and tumor-associated antigens.
6. Identify well-established tumor markers; correlate with disease presentation.
7. Review immunoassays utilized in cancer diagnosis.
8. Evaluate the use of immunotherapy in tumor treatment.
9. Describe advanced therapeutic approaches to cancer therapy including CAR-T and immune modulating antibody therapies.

▶ Introduction to Tumor Development and Immunology

According to the Centers for Disease Control and Prevention (CDC), cancer is the second leading cause of death in the United States.[1] It is highly likely that we or someone we know will be affected by cancer in our lifetimes. As a society, we have made a significant investment in trying to find better treatments for cancer. The National Cancer Institute's budget for 2019 is $5.74 billion.[2] Cancer takes a significant toll on us as a society in terms of morbidity, mortality, and financial cost. We have invested many resources into attempting to improve treatments and diagnostics, and to better understand the disease processes of cancer.

In this chapter, we will discuss the unique characteristics of cancer and the role of the immune system in cancer. We will describe the role of **immunosurveillance** and tumor-editing and the intricate interactions between cancer and the immune system. We will discuss tumor antigens and how they can potentially be used as targets in immunotherapy and used as tumor markers to potentially aid in clinical care ranging from diagnosis to management. We will explore different immunoassays that can potentially be used to measure these tumor markers in patients. Finally, we will discuss ways to engage the immune system to treat cancer.

Tumors and the Immune System

Classically, cancer cells are thought of as host cells that develop dysregulation in proliferation and homeostasis. There are six classical hallmarks of cancer,[3] self-sufficiency of growth, insensitivity to growth inhibitors, evasion of programmed cell death, limitless replication, sustained angiogenesis, and tissue metastasis (**TABLE 14–1**).

Normally, to move from a quiescent state to an active proliferative state, cells require mitogenic growth signals. Cancers often upregulate, or overexpress, the mitogen-activated protein kinase (MAPK), which can be triggered by common

TABLE 14–1 Classical Hallmarks of Cancer[3]

- Self-sufficiency in growth signals
- Insensitivity to growth-inhibitory (antigrowth) signals
- Evasion of programmed cell death (apoptosis)
- Limitless replicative potential
- Sustained Angiogenesis
- Tissue invasion and metastasis

Enabling Characteristics of Cancer[4]

- Genome instability and mutation
- Tumor-promoting inflammation

Emerging Hallmarks of Cancer[4]

- Reprogramming energy metabolism
- Evading immune destruction

mitogens, chemical substances that induce cell proliferation and growth. Many oncogenes mimic normal growth signals to allow cancer cells to develop self-sufficiency in growth signals. Cancer cells often acquire the ability to make growth factors to which they are able to directly respond.[3] For example, glioblastomas can produce platelet-derived growth factor (PDGF), and sarcomas can produce tumor growth factor α (TGFα).[3]

With normal cells in healthy tissues, quiescence and homeostasis are maintained by antiproliferative signals whereas cancer cells develop the ability to evade these antiproliferative signals, and develop insensitivity to growth-inhibitory (antigrowth) signals. In cervical cancer, for example, retinoblastoma protein (pRb) is sequestered by the viral oncoprotein E7 of human papillomavirus.[3] Disrupting the pRb pathway allows for the liberation of E2F transcription factors and makes the cells insensitive to antigrowth factors.[3]

Cancer cells not only often possess an enhanced ability to proliferate, but also are more resistant to programmed cell death, or apoptosis. For example, a chromosomal translocation in follicular lymphoma can result in upregulation of the bcl-2 oncogene, which is an anti-apoptotic protein.[3]

Evasion of programmed cell death (apoptosis) is yet another mechanism by which populations of malignant cells are able to expand.

However, growth signal autonomy, insensitivity to antigrowth signals, and resistance to apoptosis alone do not lead to large enough cell populations to produce large tumors. Normal cells possess an intrinsic programming that controls their multiplicity.[3] For cell populations to expand to large enough sizes to produce life-threatening tumors, this normal multiplicity control programming must be disrupted so that cells possess limitless replicative potential. One mechanism by which this occurs is via telomere maintenance, which is observed in nearly all cancers, and usually occurs via the upregulation of telomerase.[3]

Cells within tissues must lie within 100 μm of a capillary in order to receive sufficient nutrients and oxygen. Blood-vessel growth is very tightly regulated in normal tissues. Normal proliferating cells in tissue do not appear to possess the ability to intrinsically induce angiogenesis, blood vessel production.[3] Initially, aberrant proliferative cells lack the ability to produce blood vessels, which limits their proliferation. To grow in size, cancers must develop sustained angiogenesis.[3] In von Hippel Lindau (VHL) disease, patients can develop cancers such as kidney cancer among other disorders due to mutation of the VHL tumor suppressor gene, which can result in overexpression of vascular endothelial growth factor (VEGF).[3] VEGF is an angiogenesis-initiating signal.[3]

Most primary tumors produce pioneer cells that move out, invade adjacent tissues, and can travel to far off locations to produce their own colonies. These distant colonies are called **metastases**. Metastases are responsible for 90% of cancer deaths.[3] Tissue invasion and metastasis allow tumor cells to leave the primary tumor to find new spaces that are not so nutrient- and space-limited. These tumor cells will need to possess the other five hallmarks of cancer once they colonize a new location in order to successfully grow. In epithelial cancers, a common contributing mechanism to metastasis is loss of E-cadherin function. Normally, E-cadherin is expressed by epithelial cells and allows for cell-to-cell interaction that mediates transmission of antigrowth signals.

While cancer cells usually possess the six hallmarks described, the process by which they acquire them can vary markedly. In some instances, a certain mutation may only partially help to confer a single trait, whereas another single mutation may help confer several traits simultaneously.[3] However, it should be noted that these classical hallmarks of cancer are a reductionist view of cancer, focusing more on the genetically mutated cancer cells; but in reality, cancers are more complex, heterogeneous tissues where mutated cancers manipulate other normal cell types to help facilitate their growth and spread.

There are two "enabling characteristics" that are classically described in the context of cancer development[4]:

1. Genome instability and mutation
2. Tumor-promoting inflammation

There is variability in the mutations or alterations that impact genome maintenance and repair. However, there is ample destabilization of copy number and nucleotide sequence in human malignancies to implicate genome instability and mutation in cancer. These defects are advantageous to the defective cells and allow for tumor development, as they can accelerate the rate that premalignant cells develop the hallmarks of cancer.[4] Cancers often exhibit defects in DNA maintenance machinery, including DNA damage detection and repair activation, direct repair of damaged DNA, and inhibiting mutagenic agents before damage to DNA can occur.[4]

Inflammation is often evident at the earliest stages of cancer development. Immune cells, particularly of the innate immune system, can release mutagenic reactive oxygen species that can accelerate mutations.[4] Thus, tumor-promoting inflammation can help aid in the acquisition of the hallmarks of cancer. Interestingly, nearly every type of neoplastic lesion has been observed to contain immune cells.[4]

There are two further "emerging hallmarks" of cancer[4]:

1. Reprogramming energy metabolism
2. Evading immune destruction

Normally, healthy cells process glucose to pyruvate in glycolysis within the cytoplasm and then to carbon dioxide in the mitochondria in **aerobic** conditions (in the presence of oxygen) in a process called **oxidative phosphorylation**.[4] In **anaerobic** situations (the absence of oxygen), glycolysis is the main generator of energy, and processing with oxygen in the mitochondria does not occur. Reprogramming energy metabolism occurs in cancer cells. Even in the presence of oxygen, cancer cells rely heavily on glycolysis for metabolism. This is also referred to as the Warburg effect or aerobic glycolysis.[4] Interestingly, cancer cells have been noted to upregulate GLUT1 to increase glucose transport.[4] This increased uptake of glucose is exploited in positron emission tomography (PET) scans using a radiolabeled glucose analog to help find cancer.[4] Glycolytic fueling is associated with activated oncogenes including RAS and MYC and mutant tumor suppressors such as TP53.[4]

Normally, the immune system can eradicate incipient neoplasms before they become full-blown cancers.[4] The phenomenon is referred to as immunosurveillance and will be discussed in more detail below. Tumors manage to evade immune destruction by avoiding detection by the immune system, or by limiting immunologic killing, allowing them to survive and continue to grow. Interestingly, patients with more cytotoxic T lymphocytes and NK cells infiltrating colon or ovarian cancer tumors exhibit an improved prognosis compared with those that lack infiltrates.[4]

Immunosurveillance System for Tumor Recognition

Immunosurveillance is the mechanism by which the immune system, primarily lymphocytes, patrols for aberrant cells and eliminates them, preventing full-blown malignancy. Within the concept of immunosurveillance has evolved the advanced concept of **immunoediting** (FIGURE 14–1), which more broadly incorporates the protective properties of the immune system classically thought of in immunosurveillance, and the tumor-sculpting properties of the immune system in the development of cancer.[5] There are three phases in immunoediting[5,6]:

1. Elimination
2. Equilibrium
3. Escape

Elimination is the phase that encompasses the classical concept of immunosurveillance where the immune system detects and eliminates incipient neoplasm before the development of frank cancer.[5] In the elimination phase, abnormal cells are initially recognized by innate lymphocytes including NKT, NK, and γδ T Cells.[6] As more and more of these innate lymphocytes accumulate, they begin to produce IFN-γ (interferon gamma).[6] This causes the innate immune system to begin to produce several key chemokines, cellular products that induce cell motility and movement, including CXCL10 (IP10), CXCL9 (MIG), and CXCL11 (I-TAC).[6] These chemokines help to inhibit new blood vessel formation, and to attract immune cells including NK cells, dendritic cells, and macrophages.[6] The production of IFN-γ also helps to inhibit proliferation of the tumor. IFN-γ aids in the activation of NK cells and macrophages to kill tumor cells as they enter the tumor. The killing is mediated by these activated NK cells, and macrophages keep the growth of the tumor at bay until the adaptive immune system can respond. As tumor cells are killed via immunologic and nonimmunologic methods, dead cancer cell debris is taken up by dendritic cells, which then travel to the nearest draining lymph node where they can help cells from the adaptive immune system develop.[6] In the draining lymph node, tumor antigen-specific CD4+ and CD8+ T cells develop and then traffic to the tumor site via chemokine gradients.[6] These adaptive immune cells are able to recognize and help kill tumor cells that express the specific tumor antigen that they are able to recognize.

In immunosurveillance, the elimination phase of immunoediting, the immune system is able to destroy most neoplastic cells. In the **equilibrium phase**, the tumor is incompletely removed; however, the immune system has kept the tumor relatively controlled, producing a latency period.[5] Nonetheless, some neoplastic cells are able to survive

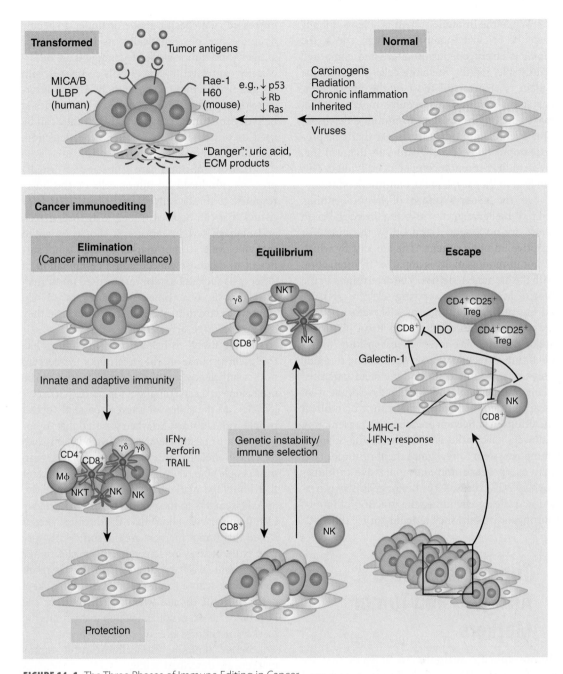

FIGURE 14–1 The Three Phases of Immune Editing in Cancer.

Reproduced from Dunn GP, Old LJ, Schreiber RD. The immunobiology of cancer immunosurveillance and immunoediting. *Immunity*. 2004;21(2):137–148.

the pressure of immunosurveillance and, eventually, clinically detectable disease becomes evident.[5] This equilibrium may be maintained chronically, or the selective pressure placed on the tumor cells by the immune system may result in sufficient "immunoediting" of the tumor so that some of these tumor cell variants can eventually evade the immune system and progress toward disease.[5]

While the immune system is able to initially keep the original tumor's growth in check, the tumor is heterogeneous in nature and composed of unstable, rapidly mutating cells. The immune system is able to kill most of the tumor cells, but some new variants acquire mutations that make them more resistant to immune defenses.[5] This eventually produces variants that can produce populations of malignant cells that can survive within an immunocompetent individual. This can lead to the escape phase of immunoediting.

In the **escape phase** of immunoediting, "edited" malignant cells surviving the equilibrium phase are no longer restrained by the innate or adaptive immune system.[5] The amount by which tumor immunogenicity is impacted by interaction with the immune system may be determined by the type of immune cells applying selective pressure during the equilibrium phase. Therefore, escape may vary mechanistically from tissue to tissue, and metastases may have the most striking immunoediting as they have been sculpted by immune pressure at the initial site and the metastatic site.[5] Many mechanisms aid in the development of escape. Tumor cells often gain direct or indirect mutations in antigen processing, and presentation pathways that make it difficult for the adaptive immune system to recognize them or tumor cells may overproduce immunosuppressive cytokines such as TGF-β or IL-10 or tumor cells may generate, activate, or encourage the function of immunosuppressive cells such as regulatory T cells.[5]

▶ Tumor-Associated Antigens and Tumor Markers

Tumor-specific antigens are antigens that are found only in malignant cells. **Tumor-associated antigens** are antigens found in malignant cells and in some normal tissue. Usually, cancer cells will express tumor-associated antigens to much higher levels than normal tissue, or the antigen is expressed only out of its normal context. For example, a particular antigen would normally be expressed in a specific tissue or under a specific circumstance physiologically. As tumor-specific antigens and tumor-associated antigens are differentially expressed in cancer cells compared with normal tissues, they can potentially be used as targets for immunotherapy to relatively specifically help destroy tumor cells. In addition, they can be used as tumor markers to aid in the detection, diagnosis, and management of cancer.[7]

Tumor markers are substances, usually proteins, produced by tumor cells or the host's response to tumor cells found in bodily fluids or tissues that can be used to help diagnose, detect, and manage certain cancers. It should be noted that an elevated tumor marker by itself is not sufficient to diagnose cancer, and a combination of other tests such as biopsy must be used to confirm the diagnosis.[7] Over time, tumor markers can help gauge response to treatment; after treatment, they can be used to test cancer recurrence.

While useful in helping to gauge things like treatment response or prognosis, tumor markers are not yet sufficiently sensitive or specific enough to be used alone as a screening tool for cancer.[7] Sensitivity refers to the ability of a test to correctly detect people with a disease. So when it is said that tumor markers are not sufficiently sensitive by themselves for cancer screening, this means tumor markers can miss people who really have the disease to an extent that limits the markers' usefulness by themselves. Specificity refers to the ability of a test to correctly identify people who don't have the disease. When it is said that tumor markers are not sufficiently specific by themselves for screening, this means tumor markers will give "false positives," or the test result comes back with a result that makes it look like a person has the disease when in reality he or she does not. This occurs often enough that it limits the markers' usefulness as a sole screening agent.

Some common, clinically relevant tumor markers are described below.

Carcinoembryonic Antigen (CEA)

Carcinoembryonic Antigen (CEA) is used as a prognostic indicator, to monitor response to therapy, and to detect recurrence in colon cancer.[8] This tumor marker lacks specificity. In addition to colon cancer, it can be elevated in smokers, cirrhosis, gastritis, inflammatory bowel disease, lung cancer, breast cancer, and other gastrointestinal cancers.[8] Thus, it is not used commonly in screening or diagnosis.

Alpha-1 Antitrypsin (α1-AT)

Alpha-1 antitrypsin (α1-AT) is a glycoprotein produced in numerous tissues including the liver, pancreas, gallbladder, lungs, and gastrointestinal tract.[9] It is nonspecific and is elevated in numerous cancers including but not limited to lung, thyroid, pancreatic, and other cancers.[9] Alpha-1 antitrypsin elevation is correlated with tumor stage and may also be able to serve as an indicator of treatment response.[9]

Prostate-Specific Antigen (PSA)

Prostate-specific antigen (PSA) is associated with prostate cancer. It can be used for prostate cancer screening in conjunction with a digital rectal exam.[8] Persistently elevated PSA levels with an otherwise negative workup can be used to diagnose occult malignancy.[8] PSA can be used as a prognostic indicator, can aid in the selection of imaging to determine staging, and can be used to determine recurrence. PSA can also be elevated in benign prostatic hyperplasia or prostatitis.[8]

Beta-2 Microglobulin

Beta-2-microglobulin (β2-microglobulin) is part of the major histocompatibility complex (MHC) I molecule. It serves as an important prognostic indicator in multiple myeloma with higher levels indicative of worse survival.[10] This is likely because higher levels correlate with higher tumor burden and renal failure.[10] In lymphoma, β2-microglobulin is associated with stage and tumor in chronic lymphocytic leukemia (CLL) with higher levels correlating with a worse prognosis.[10] Cytokines may regulate β2-microglobulin levels. Although the precise mechanisms for cytokine elevation are not known, vascular endothelium may release IL-6, which inhibits the death of CLL cells.[10] β2-microglobulin levels may also rise due to impaired kidney function. AIDS, hepatitis, and active tuberculosis can also raise β2-microglobulin levels.

hCG

A marker for testicular cancer is **hCG (human chorionic gonadotropin)**. It does not play a role in screening. It can aid in diagnosis by helping to distinguish seminomas from nonseminomatous germ cell tumors, with elevation in hCG more likely in nonseminomatous germ cell tumors.[8] It is also used as a prognostic indicator, aids in monitoring response to treatment, and helps detect recurrence of disease. Levels of hCG may also be elevated with marijuana use.

AFP

Another marker for testicular cancer and hepatocellular carcinoma (HCC) is AFP (α-fetoprotein). While AFP historically has been used in screening for HCC, it is no longer used in screening for HCC. It can aid in diagnosis of testicular cancer by helping to distinguish seminomas from nonseminomatous germ cell tumors, with elevation in AFP more likely in nonseminomatous germ cell tumors.[8] It is also used as a prognostic indicator, aids in monitoring response to treatment, and helps detect recurrence of disease of testicular cancer. AFP is not specific for testicular cancer, and may be elevated with hepatic steatosis or hepatic fibrosis.[8] HCC is primarily diagnosed with imaging, but elevated AFP in the presence of a mass is suggestive of HCC.[8] As a prognostic indicator, it can suggest portal vein thrombus, and can help detect the recurrence of disease in HCC. AFP is not specific for hepatic malignancy; as discussed above, AFP may be elevated in some testicular tumors as well as hepatic steatosis or hepatic fibrosis.[8] AFP may also be elevated with some ovarian tumors and in pregnancy.

CA 125

CA 125 is a marker for ovarian epithelial cancer. However, it serves no role as a screening test. In diagnosis, it can serve as an adjuvant to help distinguish whether an ovarian mass is benign or malignant. However, this is only effective in the case of epithelial ovarian cancers. CA 125 can aid in monitoring response to therapy and detecting recurrence of disease. CA 125 is not highly specific. It can also be elevated in lung cancer, breast cancer, pelvic inflammatory disease, endometriosis, and pregnancy.

CA 19-9

CA 19-9 is a marker associated with pancreatic cancer. CA 19-9 has neither a role in screening nor in diagnosis.[8] In the presence of a pancreatic mass, a CA 19-9 level above U/mL is highly indicative of malignancy.[8] Levels can help guide management of patients. CA 19-9 can serve as a prognostic indicator, aids in the assessment of resectability, helps assess response to treatment, and can be used to monitor for recurrence of disease.[8] CA 19-9 is not specific for pancreatic cancer. CA 19-9 levels may also be elevated in stomach cancer, lung cancer, colon cancer, breast cancer, pancreatitis, cirrhosis, and obstructive jaundice. CA 19-9 may result in false negatives for patients with the sialyl-negative phenotype, which is 5 to 10% of the population.

CA 15-3

CA 15-3 is a serum-based marker for breast cancer that detects the soluble moiety of the MUC1 protein. It can serve as a prognostic indicator where initial presentation with an elevated CA 15-3 level is associated with worse outcomes.[11] This is likely because CA 15-3 is a biomarker of micrometastases or occult metastases that cannot be detected radiographically.[11] CA 15-3 levels are not typically used to help determine prognosis in early breast cancer, however, due to its relatively low cost and ease, it may eventually be used preoperatively in combination with other prognostic factors to help optimize management. However, high levels of CA 15-3 at initial presentation should trigger investigation for metastases.

CA 27-29

CA 27-29 can be used to detect glycoprotein (MUC1) on the apical surface of epithelial cells. It is mainly associated with breast cancer. However,

it is also associated with colon cancer, gastric cancer, hepatic cancer, lung cancer, pancreatic cancer, ovarian cancer, and prostate cancer as well as benign conditions of the breast, liver, kidney, and ovarian cysts.[12] CA 27-29 is elevated in about one-third of patients with early-stage breast cancer and two-thirds of breast cancer patients with late-stage breast cancer.[12] Because of the poor predictive value in early breast cancer, CA 27-29 is not used for screening or diagnosing breast cancer but can aid in detecting preclinical metastases. CA 27-29 is often used in conjunction with CA 15-3.

▶ Immunoassays Used in Clinical Diagnosis of Circulating and Other Tumors

Tumor markers are often detected using immunoassays. Some common immunoassays include[13]:

1. Immunohistochemistry (IHC)
2. Enzyme-linked immunosorbent assay (ELISA)
3. Flow Cytometry
4. Radioimmunoassay (RIA)

A common thread of many immunoassays is that they utilize a monoclonal antibody to bind a tumor marker of interest. These antibodies are often either directly tagged with an identifiable marker, or the primary antibody is probed with a secondary antibody that is tagged with a marker.

Immunohistochemistry (IHC)

In **immunohistochemistry (IHC)**, these antibodies are often tagged with enzymes that can convert its substrate to a brightly colored marker. Sometimes the antibodies are fluorescently tagged. In IHC, the tissue (either solid tissue or cellular fluids such as blood) is collected. Tissue is often fixed to preserve it or frozen. Solid tissue is often paraffin embedded or frozen and sectioned to make slides. Smears can be produced from blood. The most widely clinically utilized technique is IHC.[13]

IHC can be used to categorize malignant solid tumors, leukemias, lymphomas, and to determine the origin of metastatic disease. It plays a critical role in helping to assess prognosis and markers of significance to therapeutic decisions. IHC can be performed on tumor tissue directly or, in some instances, from serum proteins in the blood.[14] IHC provides antibody-mediated specificity to help to identify cell types and tumor markers more specifically, compared with morphology alone conferred by regular histology.

Enzyme-Linked Immunosorbent Assay (ELISA)

In the **enzyme-linked immunosorbent assay (ELISA)**, the antibodies used to detect the molecule of interest are enzyme tagged. These enzymes can convert a substrate to produce a visible color change which can be quantified to determine concentrations. There are several different types of ELISA. One kind is described below. To detect an antigen of interest, the ELISA kit can have an antibody bound to the bottom of the plate that will detect the antigen of interest. The antigen of interest from the patient will stick to this bound antibody. A second antibody that is tagged with an enzyme is then added and binds the antigen. This forms an antibody "sandwich", with the antigen in the middle. Substrate can be added to detect the concentration of the antigen. ELISA is a good tool to identify serum proteins, such as tumor markers of interest. As a clinical example, ELISA is one method by which PSA can be measured. In the course of immunotherapy for cancer, techniques such as ELISA can aid in monitoring patient cytokine levels to help gauge response to treatment.

Flow Cytometry

In **flow cytometry**, the antibodies are fluorescently tagged. Flow cytometry requires cells to be in a suspension that can be run through the cytometer can then detect the presence of antibody bound cells. This makes analysis of hematological malignancies via flow cytometry a natural choice. In combination with morphological analysis, flow cytometry allows for fast and detailed assessment of antigen expression in hematological malignancies that can aid in making a diagnosis. Flow cytometry can be completed in a few hours, and in combination with morphologic analysis, can significantly narrow the diagnosis. Cytogenetic abnormalities in hematological malignancies are often associated with particular immunophenotypes, which can aid in selecting the most high-yield cytogenetic tests to perform.[15]

Radioimmunoassay (RIA)

In **radioimmunoassay (RIA)**, a known amount of radiolabeled antigen is mixed with antibody and produces a certain radioactive signal. This radiolabeled antigen/antibody mixture is then mixed with patient antigen. Radiolabeled antigen and unlabeled patient antigen will both compete for antibody binding. A second antibody is then used to bind to the primary antibody and precipitate the complex. The radioactive signal is then measured and can be used to calculate the concentration of antigen in the patient sample. This technique is most often applied to proteins found in the serum. As other nonradioactive technologies have developed, such as chemiluminescence as a substitute to radioisotopes, interest in classical RIA for tumor markers has become less popular, but historically, a few of the tumor markers queried by RIA include PSA, CA-125, and CA-15-3.[16]

▶ Tumor Immunotherapy

In order for the immune system to successfully combat a tumor, many steps must successfully occur (**FIGURE 14–2**). Initially, some tumor cells must die and release tumor antigens.[17] These tumor antigens then need to be taken up by dendritic cells in the right immune context to prevent peripheral tolerance. These dendritic cells present processed antigen to T cells to activate them. This must again occur in an immune context that favors effector T cells over regulatory T cells.[17] The T cells must traffic from the lymph node to the tumor site, infiltrate the tumor, recognize the cancer cells, and kill the tumor cells.[17]

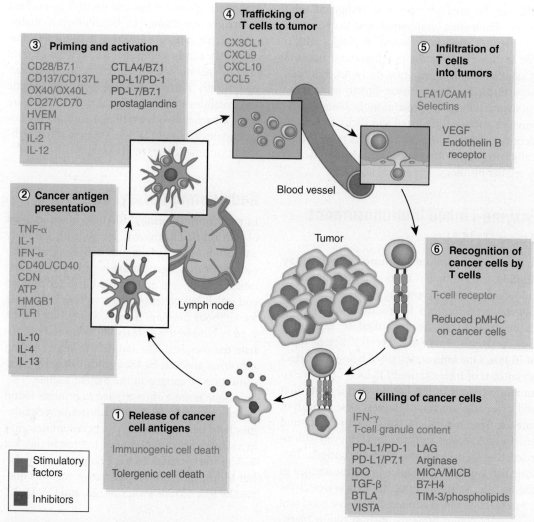

③ **Priming and activation**

CD28/B7.1	CTLA4/B7.1
CD137/CD137L	PD-L1/PD-1
OX40/OX40L	PD-L7/B7.1
CD27/CD70	prostaglandins
HVEM	
GITR	
IL-2	
IL-12	

④ **Trafficking of T cells to tumor**

CX3CL1
CXCL9
CXCL10
CCL5

⑤ **Infiltration of T cells into tumors**

LFA1/CAM1
Selectins

VEGF
Endothelin B receptor

② **Cancer antigen presentation**

TNF-α
IL-1
IFN-α
CD40L/CD40
CDN
ATP
HMGB1
TLR

IL-10
IL-4
IL-13

Blood vessel

Lymph node

Tumor

⑥ **Recognition of cancer cells by T cells**

T-cell receptor

Reduced pMHC on cancer cells

① **Release of cancer cell antigens**

Immunogenic cell death

Tolergenic cell death

⑦ **Killing of cancer cells**

IFN-γ
T-cell granule content

PD-L1/PD-1	LAG
PD-L1/P7.1	Arginase
IDO	MICA/MICB
TGF-β	B7-H4
BTLA	TIM-3/phospholipids
VISTA	

■ Stimulatory factors

■ Inhibitors

FIGURE 14-2 Stimulatory and inhibitory factors in cancer-immunity cycle.

Reproduced from Chen DS, Mellman I. Oncology meets immunology: the cancer-immunity cycle. *Immunity*. 2013;39(1):1–10.

Several obstacles block this process from occurring, however. Tumor antigen may not be effectively detected. Dendritic cells and T cells may treat antigens as self, encouraging tolerance and a regulatory T-cell response. Even if an appropriate response is initiated in the lymph node, the effector T cells may not traffic to the tumor appropriately, may be unable to infiltrate the tumor, or may be suppressed within the tumor microenvironment.

Thus immunotherapies focus on helping to overcome some of these obstacles to allow the host's immune system to help clear the tumor more effectively (**FIGURE 14-3**). Monoclonal antibodies that target the tumor, and bispecific antibodies that bind both the tumor and the T-cell have been developed and marketed for cancer immunotherapy.

Vaccines

Vaccines may be helpful in patients resistant to checkpoint blockade who lack T-cell infiltrates.[18] Cancer vaccines have been limited due to a lack

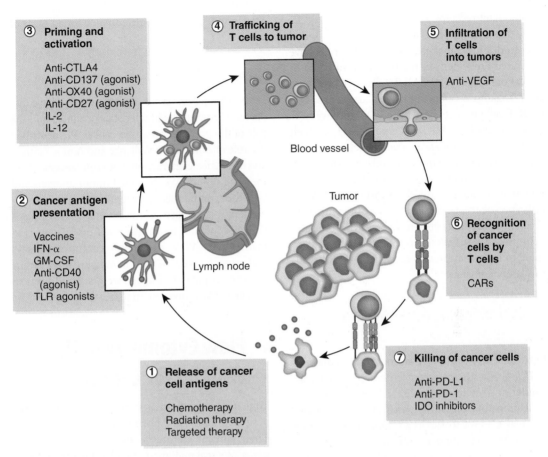

FIGURE 14–3 Therapies that interface with the cancer-immunity cycle.

Reproduced from Chen DS, Mellman I. Oncology meets immunology: the cancer-immunity cycle. *Immunity*. 2013;39(1):1–10.

of ability to potently stimulate T cells; remaining questions about optimization in which tumor antigens, delivery method, and adjuvants are best.[17] In addition, the immunosuppressive tumor microenvironment may inhibit antitumor responses.[17] Appropriate tumor antigens need to be identified and, even if identified, utilizing a single antigenic target (especially one that is not a main oncogenic driver) may be overcome by the cancer via antigenic drift.[17] However, developing multivalent vaccines is extremely difficult due to patient-to-patient variability, even intra-patient variability between tumor cells, and the difficulty in determining if predicted peptides will be generated and expressed by MHC.[17] Various, delivery methods have been attempted for vaccines, including

peptides in emulsified vehicles, direct dendritic cell targeting, adoptive transfer of antigen-loaded dendritic or tumor cells, recombinant viral vectors, and bacterial vectors.[17]

Chimeric Antigen Receptor T Cells

Chimeric antigen receptor T cells (CAR-T cells) are autologous patient T cells transduced with a chimeric antigen receptor that contains an antibody fragment which recognizes a surface marker found on a tumor. In the current clinical setting, this surface marker is usually CD19.[17] This antibody fragment is attached to T-cell signaling domains to make the chimeric antigen receptor. When the CAR-T cells are reinfused into the patient, this recombinant receptor allows them to more specifically target the antigen on the malignant cells and help to destroy the cancer cells. CAR-T cells have generated excitement in the treatment of hematological malignancy.[19,20] CAR-T cells have been successful against B-cell malignancies, and at least two CAR-T cell products have been FDA approved.[17,21] So far, successful CAR-T cell treatments have been limited to hematological malignancies as solid tumors have proved a more formidable challenge in part due to the tumor microenvironment.[17] There is potential for cancer to develop resistance to CAR-T cells specific to one antigen due to antigenic drift. Toxicities including cytokine release syndrome and neurotoxicity are serious side effects that must continue to be investigated to help bring CAR-T cells to a larger audience.[18,22,23]

Immunomodulating Antibody Therapies

Cytotoxic-T-lymphocyte-associated protein 4 (CTLA4) is a surface receptor on activated T cells similar in structure to CD28.[18] CD28 aids in T-cell activation by providing costimulatory signals, whereas CTLA4 works in an opposite fashion by raising the activation threshold for T-cell priming.[18] Ipilimumab is an anti-CTL4 antibody that inhibits the interaction of CTLA4, a negative regulator of T cells, with its ligands B7.1 and B7.2.[17] This aids in T-cell priming and activation, and allows for less selective T-cell expansion, affording the opportunity for more autoreactive T cells and, ideally, tumor-reactive T cells to expand. However, this can also result in toxicity to patients.

Programmed death protein 1 (PD-1), which is present on T-cells, binds with its ligand **programmed death ligand 1 (PD-L1)** on cancers, immune cells, or cells within the tumor microenvironment.[18] When binding with PD-L1 on an antigen-presenting cell, this can inhibit T-cell activation. When PD-L1 is bound on other cells, T-cell effector functions can be inhibited, T-cell migration can be blocked, T-cell proliferation can be reduced, and T-cell mediated killing can be impaired.[18] PD-L1 is expressed in 20 to 50% of cancers; thus anti-PD-1 and anti-PD-L1 antibodies help to block these T-cell inhibiting

effects and have shown efficacy in a broad array of cancers.[17]

Summary

In this chapter on tumor immunology, we have discussed the unique characteristics of cancer and the role of the immune system in cancer. We described the role of immunosurveillance and tumor-editing, and the intricate interactions between cancer and the immune system. We discussed tumor antigens and how they can be used as potential targets in immunotherapy and used as tumor markers to potentially aid in clinical care ranging from diagnosis to management. We explored different immunoassays that can potentially be used to measure these tumor markers in patients. Finally, we discussed ways to engage the immune system to treat cancer.

▶ Flow Cytometry in the Workup for Cancer

You are working in a clinical lab and receive peripheral blood and bone marrow from a patient. Their clinical picture is suspicious for an acute hematological malignancy, and initial morphological assessment of the samples you receive shows "blasts" consistent with an acute leukemia. Classically, morphological and cytochemical characteristics were utilized to diagnose hematological malignancy.[15] However, now immunophenotypic, cytogenic, and molecular assays are key tools in helping to refine the diagnosis.[15]

In combination with morphological analysis, flow cytometry allows for fast and detailed assessment of antigen expression in acute leukemia that can aid in making a diagnosis. Flow cytometry can be completed in a few hours, and in combination with morphologic analysis, can significantly narrow the diagnosis. Cytogenetic abnormalities in acute leukemias are often associated with particular immunophenotypes, which can aid in selecting the most high-yield cytogenetic tests to perform.[15] It is unrealistic to be able to test a comprehensive, undirected shotgun of the numerous genes that can contribute to hematological malignancies, especially in a timely manner. Thus, flow cytometry is critical in helping to narrow the list of likely genes involved based on immunophenotype. Certain antigens may also indicate prognosis or help direct therapy. The malignancy's immunophenotypic pattern can also aid in monitoring treatment response, minimal residual disease, and recurrence of disease.

To perform flow cytometry, fluid-based specimens work best, with peripheral blood and bone marrow being ideal candidates. Solid organ samples can also be analyzed with flow cytometry, but they must first be disaggregated and filtered, and the resulting samples may be more distorted than with cells from fluid.[15] In blood, for example, ammonium chloride is used to lyse red blood cells.[15] The remaining leukocytes are suspended in culture media and counted, so that when aliquoted

into tubes for staining, the number of cells is consistent.[15] The flow cytometer scans the samples, and histograms can then be analyzed. In the clinical labs, the data are often described by patterns of antigen expression in abnormal cell populations, in addition to an estimated percent of all cell types identified, including both normal and abnormal cells.[15] Initially, labs will typically "gate" on certain cell characteristics such as CD45 (leukocyte common antigen) and intrinsic light scatter properties to define populations that are further characterized by expression of particular antigens.

For this workup, you are typically provided a panel of markers detected by monoclonal antibodies to assess hematological malignancy, and a flow chart for acute leukemia diagnosis is also provided[15] (See **FIGURE 14–4**, **TABLE 14–2**, See also Chapter 8: Immunophenotyping).

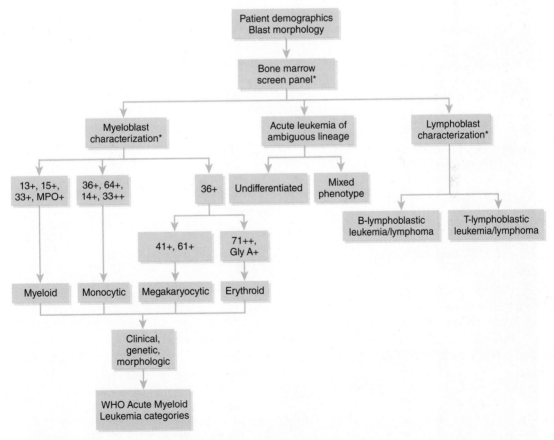

FIGURE 14–4 Flow Chart for Immunophenotyping Acute Leukemia.

Data from Peters JM, Ansari MQ. Multiparameter flow cytometry in the diagnosis and management of acute leukemia. *Arch Pathol Lab Med.* 2011;135(1):44–54.

TABLE 14–2 Subset of CD Markers Used in Immunophenotyping

Antigen	Myelo-blasts	Promy-elocytes	Matur-ing Grans	Mono-cytes	Eryth-roids	Mega-karyo-cytes	B Lym-phoid	T Lym-phoid	Comments
CD2	–	–	–	–	–	–	–	+	LFA-2; pan T-cell marker
CD3	–	–	–	–	–	–	–	+	OKT3; pan T-cell marker
CD4	–	–	–	–	–	–	–	Sub[b]	MHC-II associated; helper T cells
CD5	–	–	–	–	–	–	–	+	Leu-1; pan T-cell marker
CD7	–	–	–	–	–	–	–	+	Leu-9; pan T-cell marker
CD8	–	–	–	–	–	–	–	Sub	MHC-I associated; cytotoxic T cells
CD19	–	–	–	–	–	–	+	–	Leu-12; pan B-cell marker
CD20	–	–	–	–	–	–	+	–	L26; B-cell marker
CD22	–	–	–	–	–	–	+	–	BL-CAM; pan B-cell marker
CD79a[a]	–	–	–	–	–	–	+	–	MB-1; pan B-cell marker
CD13	+	+	+	+	–	–	–	–	Aminopeptidase N; pan myeloid marker
CD14	–	–	+	++	–	–	–	–	LPS receptor; bright on monocytes
CD15	–	+	+	–	–	–	–	–	LeuM1; maturing granulocytes
CD33	+	+	+	++	+	–	–	–	Sialic acid adhesion molecule; pan myeloid marker

Antigen	Comment								
CD36	GP IIIb/IV	–	–	+	+	+	–	–	–
CD117	c-kit; bright on mast cells	+	+	–	+	–	+	–	–
CD64	FC-γ receptor	–	–	+	+	–	–	–	–
MPO	Myeloperoxidase; definitive myeloid marker	Sub	+	+	–/+	–	Sub	–	–
CD71	Transferrin receptor; dim expression on activated cells	–	–	–	–	++	–	–	–
GlyA	CD235a; carries MN antigens on red cells	–	–	–	–	++	–	–	–
CD41	GP IIb; megakaryocytic	–	–	–	+	–	+	–	–
CD61	GP IIIa; megakaryocytic	–	–	+	+	–	+	Sub	–
CD10	CALLA, also expressed by hematogones	+	–	+	–	–	–	Sub	+
CD38	Broadly expressed	Var	Var	+	+	+	Var	Var	Var
CD45	Leukocyte common antigen	+	+	+	+	–	+	+	+
HLA–DR	Class II MHC component	+	–	+	+	–	+	+	–
CD34	Adhesion molecule; marker of immature cells	+	–	–	–	–	–	Sub	–
TdT	Nucleotide transferase; marker of immature cells	–	–	–	–	–	–	Sub	–

Abbreviations: CALLA, common acute lymphoblastic leukemia antigen; GlyA, glycophorin A; GP, glycoprotein; LPS, lipopolysaccharide; MHC, major histocompatibility complex; —, absence of expression on normal bone marrow populations; +, presence of expression on normal bone marrow populations; ++, bright expression.

Reprinted from Peters JM, Ansari MQ. Multiparameter flow cytometry in the diagnosis and management of acute leukemia. *Arch Pathol Lab Med.* 2011;135(1):44–54. Copyright 2011 College of American Pathologists.

The samples you receive and analyze show blasts that express B-cell lineage markers including CD19, CD22, and CD79a. CD10 is expressed brighter than in normal immature B-lymphocytes. PAX5 and TdT are also observed. In combination with morphology, these flow cytometry findings are consistent with acute lymphoblastic leukemia (ALL).[15] Your observations are reported and provided to the ordering physician who will use these data to make the patient's diagnosis.

CASE STUDY

The following case study is based on a real case report presented by Grupp et al.[22]

A 7-year-old female with relapsed and refractory pre-B cell ALL has relapsed multiple times and has exhausted traditional therapies. She had been treated with multiple chemotherapies including clofarabine, etoposide, and cyclophosphamide.

Having exhausted traditional therapies, she was enrolled in a trial. She received CAR-T cell therapy specific for CD19.

A few days after you treat her with CAR-T cells, she developed high fevers. She progressed to the point where she needed to be treated in the ICU, and required mechanical ventilation and blood-pressure support.

What was happening to the patient? How would you figure this out in the lab? In the lab, you have been using ELISA to follow cytokine levels. You note that there has been a dramatic increase in several cytokines in this patient including interleukin-6 (IL-6). You have also been tracking the number of CAR-T cells in the blood via flow cytometry and find that there has been a dramatic expansion of CAR-T cells. The patient has developed severe **cytokine release syndrome (CRS)**, which is a potentially life-threatening toxicity that can occur with CAR-T cell therapy due to an overly robust immune response. What can be done to help her?

To attempt to treat this severe toxicity, the physician gives her glucocorticoids, which can help decrease inflammation. However, this only briefly helps to control her fever and does not improve her hypotension.

As glucocorticoids do not appear to help much, the physician decides to get creative and to manipulate some of the dramatically elevated cytokines that you found, with medications already on the market for other purposes. She has tried treating her with **etanercept**, which is a TNF inhibitor classically used to treat autoimmune diseases like rheumatoid arthritis. Because you noted a particularly elevated IL-6 level, this helps the physician to decide to treat with **tocilizumab**, which is an IL-6 receptor-blocking antibody, classically used to treat rheumatoid arthritis.

Much to everyone's relief, the patient's fever reduces, and she is able to be weaned off of the ventilator and the blood pressure-stabilizing medication. As you continue to follow her progress by flow cytometry, you are even more pleased to see that these medications did not impair the ability of the CAR-T cells to proliferate, or to impair their efficacy in combating the cancer. The patient survived CRS, and her cancer is now in remission!

Critical Thinking Questions

1. What types of immunoassays would you use to monitor this patient's course: What types of tests could you use to monitor her for cytokine release syndrome? What types of tests would help you determine if the CAR-T cells are proliferating and persisting? How would you monitor the response of her cancer to treatment and check for disease recurrence?

2. Cytokine release syndrome is still a potentially dangerous toxicity associated with CAR-T cell therapy. Can you design a next-generation strategy to treat this toxicity: What other cytokine(s) would you potentially target? Would you target a specific cell type(s)? How would you do so, with antibodies… engineering an improved CAR-T cell…something else? Be creative. This is a real clinical problem. Your ideas could be highly useful!

3. While CAR-T cell therapy has shown to hold great promise for hematologic malignancies, results have not yet been as promising for solid tumors. Can you think of reasons why solid tumors have been more challenging in the context of CAR-T cell therapy?

▶ References

1. Soulet D, Rivest S. Bone-marrow-derived microglia: myth or reality? *Curr Opin Pharmacol.* 2008;8(4):508–518.

2. Chan WY, Kohsaka S, Rezaie P. The origin and cell lineage of microglia: new concepts. *Brain Res Rev.* 2007;53(2): 344–354.

3. Hanahan D, Weinberg RA. The hallmarks of cancer. *Cell.* 2000;100(1):57–70.

4. Hanahan D, Weinberg RA. Hallmarks of cancer: the next generation. *Cell.* 2011;144(5):646–674.

5. Dunn GP, Old LJ, Schreiber RD. The immunobiology of cancer immunosurveillance and immunoediting. *Immunity.* 2004;21(2):137–148.

6. Dunn GP, Bruce AT, Ikeda H, et al. Cancer immunoediting: from immunosurveillance to tumor escape. *Nat Immunol.* 2002;3(11):991–998.

7. Talbot K. Another gene for ALS: mutations in sporadic cases and the rare variant hypothesis. *Neurology.* 2009;73(15):1172–1173.

8. Reiter MJ, Costello JE, Schwope RB, et al. Review of commonly used serum tumor markers and their relevance for image interpretation. *J Comput Assist Tomogr.* 2015;39(6):825–834.

9. El-Akawi ZJ, Abu-Awad AM, Khouri NA. Alpha-1 antitrypsin blood levels as indicator for the efficacy of cancer treatment. *World J Oncol.* 2013;4(2):83–86.

10. Dasgupta AW, Amer. *Clinical Chemistry, Immunology and Laboratory Quality Control.* San Diego: Elsevier; 2014.

11. Duffy MW, Siun, McDermott, Enda, Crown, John. *Advances in Clinical Chemistry.* Vol 87. San Diego: Elsevier; 2015.

12. Perkins GL, Slater ED, Sanders GK, et al. Serum tumor markers. *Am Fam Physician.* 2003;68(6):1075–1082.

13. Sharma S. Tumor markers in clinical practice: general principles and guidelines. *Indian J Med Paediatr Oncol.* 2009;30(1):1–8.

14. Lindblom A, Liljegren A. Regular review: tumour markers in malignancies. *BMJ.* 2000;320(7232):424–427.

15. Peters JM, Ansari MQ. Multiparameter flow cytometry in the diagnosis and management of acute leukemia. *Arch Pathol Lab Med.* 2011;135(1):44–54.

16. Petitte B, Bialczak D, Fink L, Golightly D. Radioimmunoassay's Role in Patient Management. *Journal of Nuclear Medicine Technology.* 1991;19(3):155–159.

17. Chen DS, Mellman I. Oncology meets immunology: the cancer-immunity cycle. *Immunity.* 2013;39(1):1–10.

18. Palucka AK, Coussens LM. The basis of oncoimmunology. *Cell.* 2016;164(6):1233–1247.

19. Neelapu SS, Locke FL, Bartlett NL, et al. Axicabtagene ciloleucel CAR T-cell therapy in refractory large B-cell lymphoma. *N Engl J Med.* 2017;377(26):2531–2544.

20. Maude SL, Laetsch TW, Buechner J, et al. Tisagenlecleucel in children and young adults with B-cell lymphoblastic leukemia. *N Engl J Med.* 2018;378(5):439–448.

21. Schuster SJ, Svoboda J, Chong EA, et al. Chimeric antigen receptor T cells in refractory B-cell lymphomas. *N Engl J Med.* 2017;377(26):2545–2554.

22. Grupp SA, Kalos M, Barrett D, et al. Chimeric antigen receptor-modified T cells for acute lymphoid leukemia. *N Engl J Med.* 2013;368(16):1509–1518.

23. Porter DL, Levine BL, Kalos M, et al. Chimeric antigen receptor-modified T cells in chronic lymphoid leukemia. *N Engl J Med.* 2011;365(8):725–733.

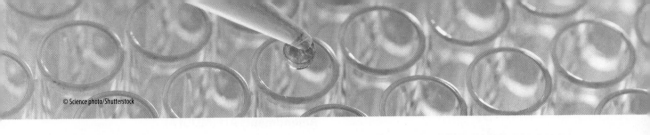

CHAPTER 15

Management, Regulation, and Clinical Translation in Immunodiagnostic Testing

Alexandra Greenberg-Worisek, PhD, MPH; **Shaheen Kurani**, ScM; and **Elitza S. Theel**, PhD

KEY TERMS

510(K)
Centers for Medicare and
    Medicaid Services (CMS)
Clinical laboratory improvement
    amendments (CLIA)
Code of federal regulations
Emergency use authorization
    (EUA)
Final rule

Food, drug, and cosmetic act (FD&C)
International organization for
    standardization (ISO)
In vitro diagnostics (IVDS)
Laboratory developed tests (LDTS)
Limited service laboratory
Medical device user fee
    amendments to the fda
    amendments act (MDUFA)

Medical device user fee and
    modernization act (MDUFMA)
Point-of-care tests (POCTS)
Premarket approval
Proficiency testing [PT]
Standard operating procedures
    (SOPS)

LEARNING OBJECTIVES

Upon completion of this chapter, the reader should be able to:

1. Review the history of regulation in clinical translation and immunodiagnostic testing.
2. Explain CLIA regulations in regard to laboratory standards for quality.
3. Identify sample tests that fit into the CLIA test complexity levels.
4. Identify the regulatory agencies in the United States for Point-of-Care Testing.
5. Describe the roles that point-of-care testing (PoCT) and lab developed Testing (LDT) have on the practice of medicine.

▸ History of Regulation of Serology and Immunodiagnostics in the United States

In the United States, **in vitro diagnostics (IVDs)** follow the same regulatory pathway as medical devices, rather than that of drugs and biologics. While the **Food, Drug, and Cosmetic Act (FD&C)** was ratified by Congress in 1938, devices were not regulated separately from other products until a recommendation was made from a special working group, the Study Group in Medical Devices, in 1970.[1] Dr. Theodore Cooper of the National Heart and Lung Institute led the group that issued a report which ultimately spurred the development and approval of the Medical Device Amendments of 1976.

The Medical Device Amendments set forth three regulatory classes for medical devices and were shortly followed by the implementation of new FDA processes for review of each device class. Briefly, each regulatory class is subject to different standards and controls. Class I devices generally pose the lowest risk to patients, and, therefore, undergo the lowest level of regulatory oversight. Class II devices are higher risk than Class I and require manufacturers to demonstrate device safety and effectiveness prior to market clearance. Class III devices pose the greatest risk to patients, as these are usually life-saving or life-sustaining, and undergo the most rigorous review. Depending on indication, IVDs, including immunologically- and serologically-based ones, may fall into any one of these categories. The FDA approval processes applicable to a particular IVD are dependent on the device classification (discussed in the next section, *Current Regulatory and Oversight Paradigms*).

In 2002, the FDA established "device user fees" through passage of the **Medical Device User Fee and Modernization Act (MDUFMA)**. This act required medical device companies to pay application submission and registration fees to the FDA as a means of providing funding for more staff to reduce turnaround time for product review. The user fees are reviewed and renewed every 5 years and are known as the **Medical Device User Fee Amendments to the FDA Amendments Act (MDUFA)**.

Parallel to the development of the FDA guidelines, the **Clinical Laboratory Improvement Amendments (CLIA)** were also created. These regulations apply specifically to clinical laboratories, including those conducting *in vitro* immunologic and serologic testing. The original iteration of CLIA, enacted in 1967 (Public Law 90-174), established the first paradigm for the licensing and monitoring of clinical laboratories.[2] Based on the specific tests performed within each laboratory, the license was granted at full, partial, or exempt monitoring levels; however, the emphasis was primarily on movement of samples between laboratories and states.

In light of myriad reports of inaccurate Pap smear tests, the Department of Health and Human Services' (DHHS) Office of the Assistant Secretary for Health for Planning and Evaluation (ASPE) undertook a study to determine the effectiveness of the initial CLIA regulations on clinical laboratories in the United States. In 1987, a report summarizing the findings from this study was submitted to ASPE, a version of which was subsequently published in the journal *Clinical Chemistry*.[3,4] This report made specific recommendations for revision of the original CLIA regulations from 1967. Four key recommendations were made: focus laboratory classification on function rather than geography; create a unified set of regulations applicable to all clinical laboratories; create an evaluation paradigm based on process as well as outcome; and focus on objective data in evaluation of laboratories.[4] These recommendations were evaluated and incorporated into what would become the Clinical Laboratory Improvement Amendments of 1988 (Public Law 100-578).[5] Since that time, implementation of CLIA has gone through several phases, all documented in the Federal Register as they were enacted; the most recent of which was the **Final Rule** submitted by the **Centers for Medicare and Medicaid Services (CMS)** (68 FR 3639), which included revisions to the **Code of Federal Regulations** (42 CFR 493).[6,7] These regulations continue to be in use today.

▶ Current Regulatory and Management Paradigms

Laboratory Oversight and Management

The primary objective of CLIA regulations is to create standards aimed at improving the quality of clinical laboratory testing provided to patients and ensuring the delivery of accurate test results. CLIA regulations are designed to oversee all clinical laboratories, including those that conduct testing on patient samples for any clinical purpose, including diagnosis, prevention, or guidance of treatment for any disease or condition.[8] As discussed briefly in the previous section, the requirements for CLIA '88 included a marked shift from categorization of laboratories based on geographic location and sample handling, to oversight based on complexity. It is important to note that CLIA sets the minimum standards for clinical laboratories and the tests they perform; laboratories should aim to go beyond those standards in their day-to-day operations. **TABLE 15–1** provides examples of immunological and serological tests in each level of complexity, per CLIA '88.[9]

Waived tests are exempt from almost all CLIA regulations, except for the rule regarding adherence to instrument and analyte manufacturers' instructions and maintenance.[10] Clinical laboratories performing any moderate or high complexity tests must meet the minimum standards for all CLIA regulations, including having quality control systems and processes in place. Additionally, they must participate in the "approved proficiency testing programs," which include objective external evaluations. These facilities must have on-site inspections at least every 2 years; such inspections may be conducted by one of several groups, including the Federal CLIA program or a CMS-approved organization (e.g., College of American Pathologists [CAP]).

In addition to classifying clinical laboratory tests by complexity, CLIA aims to ensure the quality of laboratory testing. This is accomplished through rules and regulations governing maintenance of laboratory manuals and **standard operating procedures (SOPs)**, operation of instruments, quality system essentials, and personnel training. Laboratories are required to keep current protocols and operating procedures in one collected volume or server, and ensure that these are updated and tracked appropriately using a document control system. Instruments used in clinical testing are required to be operated per manufacturer specifications, including regular maintenance, calibration, validation, and

TABLE 15–1 CLIA Test Complexity Levels and Examples of Serology and General Immunology Tests Reviewed and Classified by the FDA	
Test Complexity Level	**FDA-Reviewed Sample Tests**
Waived Tests (Class I)	▪ Influenza Type A and B (lateral flow immunoassay [LFA]) ▪ HIV-1 and HIV-2 in whole blood (LFA) ▪ Infectious mononucleosis (Epstein-Barr Virus [EBV], LFA)
Tests of Moderate Complexity (Class II)	▪ HSV Types 1 or 2 (enzyme immunoassay [EIA]) ▪ Hepatitis B surface antigen (EIA) ▪ *Toxoplasma gondii* IgM and IgG (EIA)
Tests of High Complexity (Class III)	▪ *Treponema pallidum* (syphilis) antibody assay ▪ Anti-mitochondrial antibody assay ▪ Anti-gliadin antibody assay

verification. Implementation and active utilization of a quality system for monitoring is also required; having the appropriate quality controls in place is critical for success. Finally, laboratories must train personnel according to established educational and training standards and ensure that personnel are retrained or have continuing education annually; this training must be clearly documented for each individual.

Responsibility for implementation of CLIA regulations falls primarily to CMS, including laboratories' testing samples from patients who are not enrolled in either Medicare or Medicaid programs.[10] The FDA and the Centers for Disease Control and Prevention (CDC) also share specific responsibilities for CLIA; collectively, these three agencies perform activities related to research, education, and regulation.[8] CMS is charged with collection of application and user fees, facility compliance inspections, issuing certification for laboratories, approval of accrediting organizations that perform compliance inspections, overseeing laboratory performance, and training programs (including **Proficiency Testing [PT]** programs), and updating and disseminating CLIA rules and regulations.[11] The FDA reviews and categorizes tests based on the level of complexity of the test and creates guidance for categorization of clinical laboratory tests; it is also responsible for reviewing Waiver by Application requests.[11] When applying to the FDA for any sort of **premarket approval** for tests, laboratories must concurrently apply for CLIA '88 categorization. One of the primary committees, the Clinical Laboratory Improvement Advisory Committee (CLIAC) is also housed within the CDC.[11]

CLIA oversight extends to the performance of clinical laboratories themselves. To become CLIA-certified, clinical laboratories must submit an application for certification. These applications include detailed information on the laboratory's testing practices (type of laboratory, tests performed, and specialty/subspecialty), operation (hours of operation, number of sites, laboratory ownership, affiliation of laboratory directors with other labs), and capacity (annual test volume). Certification applications also indicate the desired waiver status for each type of test as well as desired

accreditations and accrediting organizations for each test. Specific accreditations need to be in place for diagnostic immunology (e.g., syphilis serology) and general immunology. Furthermore, if a submitted test in another area (i.e., parasitology, virology) involves antibodies, it then falls under the purview of general and diagnostic immunology as well.[12]

Oversight of Laboratory Developed Tests

Laboratory developed tests (LDTs) are defined as IVD tests that are developed, manufactured, and used by a single clinical laboratory. As with other clinical IVDs, LDTs are classified as devices; however, regulation of these tests by either CMS's CLIA program or the FDA is dependent upon the scope of the use of the test.

While novel LDTs developed within a clinical laboratory with the intent of using the test only "in-house" do not necessarily require FDA clearance or approval, they are subject to CLIA regulations. CMS CLIA classifies all LDTs as "high complexity" tests, meaning that they are subject to the most rigorous of requirements.[13] Before the test can be used for clinical purposes, the individual laboratory must determine which performance characteristics need to be met for the test to be considered analytically validated. CMS' analytical validity review is context-dependent; that is, CMS views the test to be cleared or approved for use only within that one particular laboratory, under that laboratory's specific conditions (including staff, equipment, and patient populations). It is important to note, however, that CMS's review addresses analytical validity (e.g., How well does an LDT detect what it is supposed to detect?), not clinical validity (e.g., How accurate is the LDT for detection of the presence or absence of an indicated disease?).[14]

Additional voluntary standards have been put forth by several different accrediting organizations as well; these include those issued by The Joint Commission on Accreditation of Healthcare Organizations (JCAHO), The Commission on Office Laboratory Accreditation (COLA), and

CAP, among others.[15] JCAHO has the most comprehensive inspection checklist of these groups, as compared with COLA and CAP. All three have been granted "deemed" status by CMS, meaning that any clinical laboratory accredited by one of these organizations will hold both the accrediting organization's certificate as well as a CLIA Certificate of Accreditation. Therefore, accreditation by one of these organizations serves as an approved alternative to CLIA, as they go beyond the minimum standards established by CLIA.[15]

The FD&C Act requires that all IVDs, including LDTs, meet requirements for safety and effectiveness; however, the FDA generally exercises discretion with its oversight of LDTs and has not frequently enforced such regulations. In contrast to the CMS CLIA program's regulations, the FDA requirements address both issues of analytical and clinical validity, rather than analytical validity alone.

There are multiple international laboratory accreditation bodies and consumer protection agencies (**TABLE 15–2**). Many of these organizations use the standards for quality and safety set forth by the **International Organization for Standardization (ISO)** as the basis for their accreditation.[16] For medical laboratories, the focus is specifically on ISO 15189, which sets forth requirements for quality and competence within medical laboratories, including quality management systems, measurement management systems, auditing, and safety.[17]

Regulation and Management of Point-of-Care Testing

Point-of-care tests (PoCTs) are intended to be used at the patient's bedside, outside of the dedicated clinical laboratory space.[18] This is

---

TABLE 15–2 Examples of International Laboratory Accreditation Bodies and Consumer Protection Agencies

Country/Region	Laboratory Accreditation Bodies	Consumer Protection Agencies
United States	Clinical Laboratory Improvement Amendments (CLIA)/Centers for Medicare and Medicaid Services (CMS)	US Food and Drug Administration
European Union	European Co-operation for Accreditation (EA)	European Medicines Agency (EMEA)
United Kingdom	United Kingdom Accreditation Service (UKAS)	European Medicines Agency (EMEA)
Canada	Canadian Association for Laboratory Accreditation Inc. (CALA); Standards Council of Canada (SCC)	HealthCanada
Switzerland	Swiss Accreditation Service	Swissmedic
Australia	Australian Laboratory Accreditation Body (ALAB)	Therapeutic Goods Administration

particularly important in cases where rapid results are needed to make clinical decisions (i.e., under 15 minutes), although additional confirmatory testing may follow in the clinical laboratory at a later time. Examples of PoCTs include both "handheld" tests, such as those using immunostrip technologies; and larger "desktop" PoCTs, which include devices that measure specific chemical analytes.[18] Handheld and portable tests are also available for public health interventions in resource-limited settings where support or infrastructure for a full clinical laboratory does not exist.[19] Satellite laboratories (i.e., those that provide multiple services that may be delivered at point-of-care) must apply and be certified as "**limited service laboratories**."[20]

Much like tests performed within clinical laboratories, regulation and management of PoCTs fall under the purview of CMS and FDA. As with testing conducted within clinical laboratories, PoCTs have a variety of levels of complexity, from CLIA-waived to high complexity tests.[21] Regulation for PoCTs similarly emphasizes the training of the technologist or healthcare provider conducting the bedside testing, ensuring that the equipment and chemicals are used according to the manufacturers' protocols, and correctly maintaining the PoCT equipment.[22] Appropriate documentation of all machine validation and calibration must be completed in a consistent, controlled manner; additionally, all training of personnel must be documented and continuously updated as required for each PoCT offered through the program.

PoCT programs are required to meet the same standards as do clinical laboratories and must be accredited by COLA, CAP, or JCAHO, particularly if they are performing tests that are not eligible for a CLIA waiver.[9,23] PoCT programs that are considered extensions of a CLIA-certified laboratory (i.e., both are under the same CLIA number) must undergo facility and personnel inspection concurrently with the laboratory responsible for the program; if the program is independent of a permanent clinical lab, a separate CLIA inspection must be completed under a different CLIA number.[20]

Future Directions in Clinical Translation of Immunodiagnostic Tests

Extending Regulatory Oversight by the FDA

In light of reports regarding patient exposure to inappropriate or insufficient treatments as a result of unsupported LDT claims, the FDA announced in 2010 that it would undertake a thorough evaluation of whether it should continue with its policy of reinforcement discretion.[24,25] FDA oversight of all LDTs implies that individual laboratories developing their own tests would be required to demonstrate clinical validity of their testing system, similar to a manufacturer preparing for a premarket review.

Individual laboratories have resisted such oversight for multiple reasons.[26] First, many have argued that LDTs, such as the immunodiagnostic tests discussed in this textbook, fall under the purview of the "practice of medicine," and, therefore, should not require oversight by the FDA. Second, any device that undergoes the FDA review processes for premarket approval (including streamlined processes, such as the **510(k)**) incurs a great deal of cost, time, and administrative work. Many working in laboratory medicine argue that such processes would not only add additional burden to the process of developing LDTs, but would also lengthen the time to clinical translation of these tests, and would limit accessibility for patients as developers try to recoup cost via insurance payments.

On the other end of the spectrum sit manufacturers of IVDs, who are subject to FDA oversight and must meet safety, efficacy, and quality standards set forth by the agency.[26] Many manufacturers have supported the FDA's proposal of increasing oversight of LDTs, stating that IVDs are often held to higher standards for clinical validation than LDTs, including rigorous Good Manufacturing Practices (GMPs).[26] The stance of some companies is that streamlined processes through which many IVDs may go should not place too great of an expense or administrative burden upon individual laboratories.

The FDA hosted a public workshop in 2010 and reviewed hundreds of subsequent filed comments in an effort to better inform their published draft guidances for LDTs, released in 2014. In a similar fashion, a second public workshop was held in 2015 to review the draft guidances and to seek input from a broad array of experts and stakeholders. Additionally, FDA public health researchers worked to analyze events involving 20 LDTs, including immunodiagnostic tests, which met the minimum CLIA requirements but still resulted in harm to actual patients undergoing these tests.[27] Such harm included patients being told that they had a serious condition due to false-positive tests, resulting in unnecessary treatment and distress, as well as patients being informed that they did not have a serious life-threatening condition, which they did in fact have, resulting in failure to receive effective treatment for their condition.

After review of additional comments from the various workshops and systematic reports, the FDA published a discussion paper in 2017, with the hope of continuing the conversation surrounding LDT oversight beyond CLIA regulations.[28] While the FDA will continue its policy of enforcement discretion, which remains relatively vague, they have clearly identified the gaps in CLIA, which FDA's risk-based approach to oversight may help to fill.[27] This includes ensuring quality of the design and manufacture of devices and solvents, accurate labeling of laboratory tests and directions for use, removal of unsafe tests from the market, and the requirement for consent from patients participating in studies involving LDTs, among other needs and oversights.

Rapid Translation of LDTs and IVDs During Emergency Situations

Challenges that arise for developers and users of immunodiagnostic assays are epidemics of new or rare infectious diseases, such as Zika and Ebola viruses. As our world becomes increasingly connected, primarily through air travel, pandemics of infectious disease also become more frequent. In emergency situations such as recent outbreaks of the aforementioned diseases, it may be challenging to design, develop, and clinically validate such IVDs as would be done under non-emergency circumstances. Furthermore, many individual laboratories may not have the capacity or ability to develop these tests independently and may have to rely on tests that do not fall under the definition of LDTs.

In an effort to support rapid dissemination and implementation of needed immunodiagnostic and IVD tests during major public health events, the FDA has created special pathways for quick approval of IVDs and other therapeutics that fall under their jurisdiction. One key pathway is known as the **Emergency Use Authorization (EUA)**, which allows the FDA Commissioner to waive approval for medical products to be used in emergency situations to "diagnose, treat, or prevent serious or life-threatening diseases or conditions" when there are no approved products available for the outbreak at hand.[29] An EUA affords the opportunity for the newly developed tests or therapies to be used without the extensive testing and validation needed for a premarket approval during the time of a declared public health crisis; however, once the crisis ends or is declared complete, the product can no longer be used until it has been submitted through traditional FDA investigational and/or premarket approval pathways.

While EUAs may help to ease the regulatory burden associated with the clinical translation of a novel immunodiagnostic test during a public health emergency, further barriers to widespread clinical translation come in the form of administrative, political, and financial challenges. Many of these challenges may lie dormant until efforts for immunodiagnostic testing need to be scaled up to better serve populations affected by epidemics, when additional infrastructure, financial, and workforce needs make themselves known. This can be further complicated by the fact that barriers, such as cost and access, are country-dependent, and may be affected by international diplomatic efforts. There is, therefore, a need to determine a way to best equip laboratories to handle necessary scale-ups in testing internationally during emergency situations to better protect global public health.

CASE STUDY

Immunodiagnostics for Zika Virus

This case has been adapted from: Kurani S, Theel E, Greenberg-Worisek A. Diagnostic testing for Zika: a case study in rapid translation during a public health emergency. *Clin Trans Sci.* 2018;11(2):103–105.[30]

Situation and Background

The first reported cases of the mosquito-borne Zika virus (ZIKV) infection, which caught public attention, were diagnosed in Brazil in mid-2015, due in large part to the microcephaly phenotype exhibited by neonates infected with ZIKV through maternal-fetal transmission.[31] Although cases and smaller outbreaks had previously been reported in Africa, Asia, and Pacific Islands prior to 2014, due to the rapid spread and possible association with microcephaly, the World Health Organization (WHO) declared the ZIKV outbreak in Brazil and the Americas a Public Health Emergency of International Concern in 2016. The United States followed suit in 2016 as cases were being diagnosed stateside, specifically in Florida and later in Texas. The outbreak of ZIKV presented several problems, not only in the underlying biology but also in clinical care, diagnosis, management, and regulation.

Biological Challenges

ZIKV is a zoonotic disease initially detected in rhesus monkeys in Africa in the late 1940s and subsequently found to be transmitted to humans through the bite of infected *Aedes aegypti* or *Aedes albopictus* mosquitoes.[32] Two strains of ZIKV have been identified, referred to as the "African" and "Asian" lineages, based on their believed locations of origin.[32] It has been shown that the Asian strain, which results in a stronger infection, was predominantly responsible for the outbreak in 2015.[33]

Like other members of the *Flaviviridae* family (e.g., dengue virus [DENV], West Nile virus [WNV]), ZIKV is composed of a single-stranded RNA genome encapsulated within a protein-studded envelope.[34] Through these embedded proteins, ZIKV interacts with receptors on the surface of skin immune cells and neural progenitor cells to gain access and initiate infection.[31,34] Recent studies have suggested that some of these points of entry may be shared with DENV, which co-circulates with ZIKV in many of the same geographical regions.[34]

Clinical and Diagnostic Challenges

There are three primary challenges to clinical care of patients with ZIKV infections. First, the specific incubation period of the virus can vary significantly and is broadly estimated to be between 3 and 12 days.[35] Notably, the vast majority of infected individuals (~80%) remain entirely asymptomatic. Also, ZIKV can rapidly clear from the human body, often within 7 to 14 days of symptom onset.[34]

Second, ZIKV has multiple person-to-person routes of transmission, including sexual and materno-fetal. As with the majority of those infected, pregnant women may be asymptomatic; infection may, therefore, not be detected until a scheduled ultrasound or even birth, when the infant may exhibit the microcephaly phenotype and damage is irreparable.

A third complication is that the ideal window for detecting the virus is within the 7 to 14-day window.[33] Diagnostic testing methodologies developed for detection of ZIKV include reverse-transcription real-time polymerase chain reaction (RT-PCR) assays and IgM antibody capture enzyme-linked immunosorbent assays (MAC-ELISA). These methods have been used on urine, plasma, serum, and cerebrospinal fluid samples from patients.[32,36] Rapid development of clinical laboratory tests able to detect disease at or close to point-of-care has been particularly challenging. Part of the challenge has been due to the limited-in-duration, viremic period, and part has been due to the cross-reactivity of antibodies to ZIKV with antibodies to other closely related viruses such as DENV.

Management and Regulatory Challenges

One of the primary management problems that arose during the ZIKV outbreak was processing of the large volume of samples coming into the few labs, which had ZIKV testing capabilities; this resulted in a very slow turnaround time for confirmatory testing and a 3 to 4 week wait for patients to find out their results.[36] This delay was particularly concerning for pregnant women, especially those who lived in states that did not allow termination of pregnancy after 24 weeks of gestation. Timely development of the necessary IVDs was further compounded by limited initial funding for this work by the United States Congress.[37] Once greater levels of funding were secured, the CDC partnered with several national laboratories to expand their testing capacity during this time. Molecular and serologic testing were offered to patients through this laboratory network and through public health laboratories, which offered testing free of charge to the patient. Still, testing capacity and turnaround time remained slower than desired; reference laboratories charged for testing.

Once the United States government declared the ZIKV outbreak a public health emergency in 2016, the speed of translation of ZIKV diagnostic tests rapidly increased. This was due in part to the FDA's EUA process, which afforded companies developing diagnostic testing during such emergency the situations ability to commercialize their diagnostic assays with minimal FDA oversight, foregoing the traditional FDA review paradigms. This allowed for much-needed testing to be made available to the public in a matter of a few days to weeks, rather than months to years.[36] Diagnostic assays granted an EUA were considered cleared by the FDA until an end to the public health emergency was declared. At that point, diagnostic assays with EUA would be pulled from broad public use, reclassified as LDTs, and submitted through the FDA's 510(k) or Pre-Market Approval (PMA) processes for devices. Independent of the FDA's regulatory oversight during this time, the diagnostic tests utilized were required to meet the standards outlined by the Clinical Laboratory Improvement Amendments (CLIA).

Critical Thinking Questions for Discussion

1. What were the key infrastructure challenges in implementing and disseminating ZIKV diagnostic testing?
2. Imagine you had regulatory oversight during the time of the ZIKV outbreak (and an unlimited amount of funding). Would you have handled the management of this outbreak differently? How?
3. Given the long turnaround time for testing results, would you have prioritized certain patients? Would you consider doing so ethical? Why or why not?

▶ References

1. Gad SC. Regulatory aspects and strategy in medical device and biomaterials safety evaluation. In: Gad SC, ed. *Regulatory Toxicology, Second Edition*. Second ed. Boca Raton, FL, USA: CRC Press; 2001:85–102.
2. Chronology of CLIA Related Documents in the Federal Register & Code of Federal Regulations. 2017; https://wwwn.cdc.gov/CLIA/Regulatory/Chronology.aspx. Accessed 20 NOV, 2017.
3. Kenney ML. Quality assurance in changing times: proposals for reform and research in the clinical laboratory field. *Clin Chem*. 1987;33(pt 2):328–336.
4. Kenney ML, Greenberg DP. *Final report on assessment of clinical laboratory regulations*. Washington, DC: Office of the Assistant Secretary for Planning and Evaluation;1988.
5. Dingell RJD. Clinical Laboratory Improvement Amendments of 1988. In: Committee USHEaC, ed. *H.R. 5471* United States Library of Congress; 1988.
6. Medicare, Medicaid, and CLIA programs; laboratory requirements relating to quality systems and certain personnel qualifications. In: Centers for Medicare and Medicaid Services CfDCaP, and Department of Health and Human Services, ed. *68 FR 3639*. Washington, DC: United States Government Publishing Office; 2003.
7. Laboratory requirements. In: Centers for Medicare and Medicaid Services CfDCaP, and Department of Health and Human Services, ed. *42 CFR 493*. Washington, DC: United States Government Publishing Office; 2011.

8. Regulations for implementing the clinical laboratory improvement amendments of 1988: a summary In: Control CfD, ed. Atlanta, GA: MMWR; 1992:RR-2.

9. Tests granted waived status under CLIA. In: Centers for Medicare and Medicaid Services DoHaHS, ed. Washington, DC: Centers for Medicare and Medicaid Services; 2017.

10. CMS initiatives to improve quality of laboratory testing under the CLIA program. In: Centers for Medicare and Medicaid Services DoHaHS, ed. Washington, DC: Centers for Medicare and Medicaid Services; 2006.

11. Clinical laboratory improvement amendments (CLIA). 2017; https://www.fda.gov/MedicalDevices/DeviceRegulation andGuidance/IVDRegulatoryAssistance/ucm124105 .htm. Accessed November 20, 2017.

12. Director SaCG. Advance Copy—Revisions to State Operations Manual (SOM), Appendix C—Survey procedures and interpretive guidelines for laboratories and laboratory services (clinical laboratory improvement amendments (CLIA)). In: Centers for Medicare and Medicaid Services DoHaHS, ed. Baltimore, MD: Department of Health and Human Services; 2015.

13. LDT and CLIA FAQs. In: Centers for Medicare and Medicaid Services DoHaHS, ed. Baltimore, MD: Centers for Medicare and Medicaid Services; 2013.

14. How can consumers be sure a genetic test is valid and useful? *Genetics Home Reference* 2017; https://ghr.nlm .nih.gov/primer/testing/validtest. Accessed 20 NOV, 2017.

15. Immunology and Serology in Laboratory Medicine. In: Turgeon ML, ed: Elsevier Health Services; 2017: https://books.google.com/books?id=pEijDgAAQBAJ &pg=PA114&lpg=PA114&dq=serology+immunolo gy+clia&source=bl&ots=7jHYZ-yQjC&sig=Acgzvq _oTsbE5EngwohV09lJm9g&hl=en&sa=X&ved=0ahUKE wiExuvi4sPXAhXG6IMKHcCzDGQQ6AEIVTAI%20 -%20v=onepage&q=serology%20immunology% 20clia&f=false%20-%20v=snippet&q=serology%20 immunology%20clia&f=false#v=snippet&q=serology% 20immunology%20clia&f=false.

16. International Organization for Standardization. 2017; https://www.iso.org/home.html. Accessed 20 NOV, 2017.

17. ISO 15189:2012: Medical laboratories—requirements for quality and competence. 2014; https://www.iso.org /standard/56115.html. Accessed 20 NOV, 2017.

18. St John A, Price CP. Existing and emerging technologies for point-of-care testing. *Clin Biochem Rev.* 2014;35(3):155–167.

19. Drain PK, Hyle EP, Noubary F, et al. Diagnostic point-of-care tests in resource-limited settings. *Lancet Infect Dis.* 2014;14(3):239–249.

20. *CAP Accreditation Program: Point-of-Care Testing Checklist.* Northfield, IL: College of American Pathologists; 2011.

21. Clinical Laboratory Improvement Amendments (CLIA): Text Complexities. 2017; https://wwwn.cdc.gov/clia /resources/testcomplexities.aspx. Accessed 20 NOV, 2017.

22. Camacho-Ryan O, Bertholf RL. Monitoring point-of-care testing compliance. *Clinical Laboratory News* 2016; https:// www.aacc.org/publications/cln/articles/2016/february /monitoring-point-of-care-testing-compliance. Accessed November 20, 2017.

23. Carlson DA. Point of care testing: regulation and accreditation. *Clin Lab Sci.* 1996;9(5):298–302.

24. Laboratory developed tests. 2017; https://www.fda .gov/MedicalDevices/ProductsandMedicalProcedures /InVitroDiagnostics/LaboratoryDevelopedTests/default .htm Accessed 20 NOV, 2017.

25. The public health evidence for FDA oversight of laboratory developed tests: 20 case studies. 2015; https://www.fda .gov/medical-devices/vitro-diagnostics/laboratory -developed-tests. Accessed 20 NOV, 2017.

26. Gatter K. FDA Oversight of laboratory-developed Tests: where are we now? *Arch Pathol Lab Med.* 2017;141(6):746–748.

27. US Food and Drug Administration. The public health evidence for FDA oversight of laboratory developed tests: 20 case studies. November; 2015.

28. Discussion paper on laboratory developed tests (LDTs). Silver Spring, MD: United States Food and Drug Administration; 2017.

29. US Department of Health and Human Services, and Food and Drug Administration. Emergency use authorization of medical products and related authorities. *Guidance for industry and other stakeholders Google Scholar.* 2017.

30. Kurani S, Theel E, Greenberg-Worisek A. Diagnostic testing for Zika: observing rapid translation during a public health emergency. *Clin Transl Sci.* 2018;11(2):103–105.

31. Cugola FR, Fernandes IR, Russo FB, et al. The Brazilian Zika virus strain causes birth defects in experimental models. *Nature.* 2016;534(7606):267–271.

32. Theel ES, Hata DJ. Diagnostic testing for Zika virus: a postoutbreak update. *J Clin Microbiol.* 2018;56(4):e01972–01917.

33. Musso D, Gubler DJ. Zika virus. *Clin Microbiol Rev.* 2016;29(3):487–524.

34. Hamel R, Dejarnac O, Wichit S, et al. Biology of Zika virus infection in human skin cells. *J Virol.* 2015;89(17):8880–8896.

35. Krow-Lucal ER, Biggerstaff BJ, Staples JE. Estimated incubation period for Zika virus disease. 2017;23(5).

36. FDA. Emergency use authorizations. 2017; https://www .fda.gov/medicaldevices/safety/emergencysituations /ucm161496.htm#zika

37. Cohen J. U.S. officials welcome new Zika funding, but say delays hurt. 2016; http://www.sciencemag.org/news /2016/10/us-officials-welcome-new-zika-funding-say -delays-hurt

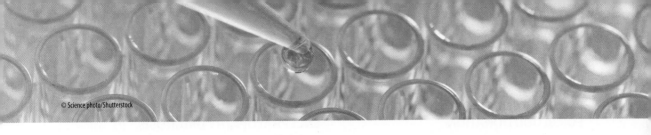

APPENDIX

Advanced Concepts

CONTENTS

The Properties of Other Chemical Diluents and Buffers Used in Serological Testing

Ian Clift, PhD MLS(ASCP)[CM]

All immunodiagnostic tests are performed in a background solution. In many cases, this solution is the patient's serum or other blood-based liquid. However, it is more often the case that these assays are performed in a physiologically similar solution, providing specific properties important for assay design or to enhance some part of the assay's mechanism. The most common physiologically similar solutions, recognizable if you have spent any time working in the laboratory, are described based on their properties within the laboratory's MSDS (Material Safety Data Sheet), described in Chapter 4: Safety and Standard Procedures. A few will be seen commonly throughout the laboratory field. Some of these common solutions are presented here.

▶ Saline Solutions

Water, along with electrochemical components, is the basis for all solutions used in serological and immunological studies. The so-called "normal saline," used in intravenous transfusions to make up for blood and hydration loss, is a simple combination of water and 0.9% sodium chloride, for example. It is also used to flush wounds and tissues. Saline solutions are also used for flushing, washing, diluting, and storing immunodiagnostic samples and reagents in the laboratory, with only subtle changes in the salt concentration.

The need for specimen storage or the maintenance of some specific physiological process in tissue or cells was the impetus for the development of more advanced saline solutions. Keeping cells in a physiologically similar state is the purpose of the commonly used anticoagulants as well. One of the first to develop a physiological saline solution was Ringer, whose Ringer's solution, which established the importance of sodium, potassium, calcium, chloride, and bicarbonate,[1] is still used today during dissections and tissue extractions on animals to keep the cellular components in useful working order, i.e., to reduce apoptosis and necrosis of cells. The saline buffering systems have since been improved in various ways. For instance, Krebs and Henseleit increased the concentration of bicarbonate, calcium, and potassium, and added phosphate and sulfate, which, in turn, created a solution that more closely resembled the physiological conditions found in human plasma.[1] Solutions such as this are often called **balanced salt solutions** and include commercially available products such as Earle's and Hank's balanced salt solutions, Eagle's minimum essential medium (MEM), Dulbecco's modified Eagle's medium (DMEM), as well as the Krebs-Henseleit buffer (KHB). They are commonly used today in medical and clinical research involving cell culture, in which case supplemental glucose is added as a fuel source for the cells.

Another use for saline solution is for the storage and washing of cells and analytes. One commonly used agent for this purpose is **phosphate buffered saline (PBS)**, which helps to maintain the pH of the assay components (**BOX AP-1**). PBS contains sodium chloride, sodium phosphate, and sometimes potassium phosphate. PBS is an isotonic solution (i.e., set to match the osmolality and ion concentration of the human body). PBS can be used for a variety of applications such as dilutions of specimens and rinsing of cells. It has also been used as a diluent in lyophilized (freeze-dried) reagents. The addition of EDTA to a PBS solution is useful for disengaging clumped cells. An alternative buffering solution called Tris buffered saline (TBS) is commonly used to create a slightly alkaline isotonic buffer. It is typically formed using 0.05 M Tris and 0.15 M sodium chloride and has a pH of 7.6, although there are several variants available and in common use. It is primarily used in immunoblotting and Western blotting during membrane washing and antibody dilution.

▶ Blocking Solutions

In many immunoassays, such as the popular ELISA assay, it is important to block unoccupied potential binding sites on solid-phase supports, such as plate wells. This nonspecific binding of protein will affect subsequent steps in the assay and may interfere with accuracy of results.[2] Blocking solutions should perform at least two roles increasing sensitivity of the assay and reducing background interference. While interference from endogenous antibodies is still sometimes unresolved, the use of blocking agents is recommended for reducing their effects.[3] Some of the most common blocking solutions include **bovine serum albumin (BSA)** and nonfat dry milk.

BSA is often used as a protein standard for many experiments, but it is more commonly used as a blocking agent. If antibodies are added directly to a sample, they are capable of binding to the antigen of interest (specific antigen) in addition to other proteins, nonspecifically, creating a high level of background staining. Blocking with BSA (typically 5%) prior to the addition of specific antisera will saturate these nonspecific binding sites thereby reducing background staining and increasing the visibility of the specific binding.

While BSA and nonfat dry milk are useful, some assays that require increased sensitivity may find interference from protein in the form of cross-reactivity and glycosylation. For example, nonfat dry milk is often added to a PBS, TBS, or TBS-T (TBS-Tween) solution as a cheap and widely available blocking method, but is not compatible with all antibodies. BSA is used for assays containing phospho-specific antibodies, as milk contains the protein casein, which is also a

---

BOX AP-1 Preparation of Stock **10×** Phosphate Buffered Saline (PBS)

Dissolve:

- 800 g NaCl
- 20 g KCL
- 144 g $Na_2HPO_4\ 2H_2O$
- 24 g KH_2PO_4
- In 8 L of distilled water

Using a stir bar on a magnetic mixer can ensure adequate mixing. Bring the solution volume up to 10 L with additional water. The pH of the stock solution will be approximately 6.8, but the diluted 1 × solution will be at 7.4. A pH meter should be used to measure pH directly. The pH can then be adjusted using hydrochloric acid or sodium hydroxide. To create **1×** PBS solution dilute 1:10.

phospho-protein and may lead to cross-reaction. In other cases, specific non-animal proteins are added to the blocking solution; however, these are less cost-effective and typically are tried as a later resort.[4] Blocking should be performed for between 1 and 1.5 hours at room temperature or overnight at 4 degrees C with rocking.

Other Reagents and Specific Additives

Cell culture media are commercially available for most immunodiagnostic tests that require a long-duration incubation involving living cells. They contain both a buffering system and numerous chemical additives that are useful for cellular survival including amino acids, sugar, and vitamins. One of the most commonly sold is the Roswell Park Memorial Institute (RPMI) medium. This formulation contains a large quantity of phosphate, and has been used traditionally for the growth of human lymphoid cells and also has found utility in examining the growth of human neoplasms and cancer cells. RPMI can be purchased commercially in a variety of formulations from a variety of vendors.

Many laboratories that conduct cell culture or long-term cellular studies will utilize **fetal calf serum (FCS)**, also known as fetal bovine serum. It is the most widely used serum supplement for *in vitro* cell culture. Similar to human sera, it is produced from clotted bovine blood and can maintain cells in culture where they can grow, divide, and flourish. One of the major components of this serum is BSA. It is also rich in growth factors, which are preserved by storage at frozen temperatures. Immunoassays, such as the indirect ELISPOT, requiring longer duration incubation phases, should be grown in a medium such as RPMI with a 10% FCS supplement.

Many other chemical agents are added to reagent and assay preparations for specific purposes. For example, **dimethylsulfoxide (DMSO)**, a widely available inexpensive liquid byproduct of the paper industry, is used as a vehicle for the delivery of drugs to cells, as a solvent, and in the fixation of cells. It is also used in many cryopreservation techniques in blood banking practice, including the preservation of platelets, other cells, and to prevent damage during hematopoietic stem cell cryopreservation.[5] **Sodium azide**, an inorganic molecule often found in commercial reagents such as antibodies, acts as a preservative and is useful for preventing the growth of organisms such as fungal and bacterial contaminants. Adding this reagent to a PBS solution will extend its shelf life considerably. However, caution should be used, as it is toxic to cells and is considered a biohazard.

Diagnostic Polyclonal and Monoclonal Antibody Development

Annika Lee, BS

Antibodies are immunoglobulin proteins that bind to a specific structural motif, or epitope, of another protein or molecule, an antigen. They coordinate the adaptive immune response, which is induced when the organism recognizes a substance as foreign or mounts an immune response that neutralizes and clears the foreign material. Immunoglobulins are able to bind specific protein structures because of their variable regions, which are rearranged in individual B-cell clones to produce different binding sites that can ultimately recognize and bind to almost any structure. Researchers can utilize this specific binding property to produce antibodies to their molecule of interest as a tool to localize, identify, or isolate the molecule studied. In a diagnostic setting, antibodies can be used to test serum or tissues for the presence of a pathological protein or toxin. Antibodies can be produced as either **polyclonal** or **monoclonal**.

▶ Polyclonal Antibodies

Polyclonal antibodies are specific to an antigen but are produced by multiple B-cell clones, leading to multiple antibodies that may target different epitopes on that same antigen. To produce polyclonal antibodies, we directly capitalize on the immune system's ability to recognize a foreign substance. To generate these antibodies, we immunize, through inoculation, an animal with the antigen of interest with the intent of raising an immune response against that antigen.[6] Any immune cell in this animal's body that can bind to this antigen will be activated to mount an immune response, leading eventually to B-cell conversion into plasma cells and serum antibody production against this antigen.[6] Because the body has an almost unlimited ability to recognize foreign proteins, multiple "recognitions" will most likely occur, and thus, a cocktail of antibodies will be secreted from every B-cell clone that recognizes an epitope. This serum provides the antibodies that will then be purified for use in research and/or diagnostic assay manufacturing.

Polyclonal Manufacturing

When inducing the immune response, it is important to ensure that antigen used to immunize the animal is pure; although purification is expensive and labor intensive, this will ensure the immune response provoked is against the desired antigen and not an impurity.[7] Reducing antigen and preparation toxicity (resulting from endotoxins, lipopolysaccharide, chemical residues, and/or high pH) ensures a robust immune response and lowers the risk to the animal host.[7] Often, following initial (or "prime") exposure to the antigen,

additional injections may be needed (a "boost" exposure) to sustain high levels of antibodies in the animal serum.[6]

Some substances, particularly small molecular-weight antigens, will not naturally produce a robust immune response, and so the antigen may need to be prepared with a substance that will ensure a robust immune response, an *adjuvant*, such as "Freund's adjuvant" or "keyhole limpet hemocyanin," to obtain antibody production. This biases the immune response against clearing the antigen.[7] Aseptic technique and preparing the antigen-adjuvant emulsion correctly protects animal health, allows a robust immune response, and prevents cross-contamination—ensuring response specificity.[7] One novel alternative to adjuvant is to "immunize" the animal with a gold-conjugated DNA molecule; this has proven successful in producing an immune response against classically nonimmunogenic membrane proteins.[8]

When choosing which animal to use for polyclonal antibody formation, there are multiple considerations. First, it is easier to induce an immune response in a species that is phylogenetically distant from the antigen (**BOX AP–2**).[7] It is best to use healthy, young animals, but because immune response will be unique to each animal, the lifespan of the animal or volume of collection must also be considered.[9] Ease of bleeding and antibody collection are other factors; rabbits, for instance, are larger, easier to bleed, and live longer

---

BOX AP–2 A Basic Method for Producing Polyclonal Antiserum in Sheep

1. Dissolve 150µg of antigen into 2mL of normal saline
2. Add 4mL of Freund's complete or incomplete adjuvant
3. Prepare a stable water in oil emulsion
4. Inject 2mL of emulsion into four subcutaneous sites per sheep
5. Bleed the animal 3 weeks later for testing.
6. Inject booster doses every 4 to 8 weeks until a satisfactory antiserum titer is achieved.

than mice or rats, but are still able to be kept in large numbers.[7] Chickens can be immunized to produce Igy, which will be concentrated in their eggs, providing an interesting alternative to collecting blood.[7] In any animal, the goal is to receive an immune response that gives a serum titer of antibody of 1:64,000.[7] This titer is determined by testing the serum against a control ELISA to check levels of antigen-antibody binding.

To use polyclonal antibody in the lab, blood is harvested from the animal and fractioned to isolate the portion containing the immunoglobulin proteins.[6] Because this fraction contains all of the immunglobulins produced by the animal, both specific to the antigen and not, purification is often needed—at maximum, it will contain only 10% antigen-specific antibodies.[10] The immunized serum is exposed to the desired antigen using an *in vitro* assay, which pulls out the desired antibody in order to determine the titer. When harvesting antibodies, 10% of circulating blood can be taken at any time, but because levels of antibodies will be very even within the same animal, often exsanguination is performed once the desired titer is achieved.[7,9]

A few problems with polyclonal antibodies include the variability of the product, in both production and final properties. The yield of antibodies is variable, in the same animal, as titer levels can vary with every bleed; and between animals, as the immune reaction strength is different among each animal. The death of one animal can impact antibody quality. This is specifically true in animals that are not immunologically identical (for example, larger model systems: rabbits, horses, sheep, goats), making it sometimes difficult to reproduce the antibody response to an antigen.[9,11] This variability is problematic if reproducibility is required between research findings, in diagnostics, or for use in clinical trials. Furthermore, no matter how specific to the antigen the antibodies produced are, they will never be as specific as a monoclonal antibody, which recognizes only one epitope.[6]

There are several reasons why polyclonal antibodies may still be preferable. First, they are quicker to develop, cheaper to produce, and will produce a more robust immune response when compared with monoclonal antibody production. Second, reactivity to multiple epitopes can be desired in research design. For instance, if the isotype of the antigen is not known, the cross-reactivity of a polyclonal antibody may help to ensure an antigen of interest is isolated in a new or different research application.[11] Binding to multiple epitopes allows enhanced detection or isolation in an ELISA or capture assay, which is useful if the concentration of the protein of interest is low.[6,11] Binding of antibodies to multiple epitopes on an antigen can confer specificity among samples with shared epitopes or amplify a weak signal.[11,12] Additionally, if using the polyclonal antibody for a therapy, it may allow greater efficacy by ensuring binding.[6] They have proven particularly useful as secondary antibodies, conjugated with a reporter molecule, where a highly specific epitope specificity is irrelevant.[12]

▸ Monoclonal Antibodies

Monoclonal antibodies, differing from polyclonal antibodies, are specific to a single epitope on a specific antigen. They are originally produced from one B-cell clone, which is isolated from an immunized animal and then transformed into a system that can support long-term production of that antibody. Historically, production of monoclonal antibodies was limited to culture of B cells, which could be maintained only for 10 to 14 days.[9] This was further complicated because most B cells tend to secrete IgM molecules, and the desired product is often IgG molecules.[7] Köhler and Milstein were the first to find a way to immortalize B-cell production by fusing a B-cell clone specific to one antigen, sheep red blood cells, with a myeloma line, a type of B-cell tumor, which is functionally immortal.[10,13] The new cell line is a fusion product, termed a *hybridoma*. This discovery earned them, along with Niels Jerne, the Nobel prize in physiology in 1984.[14]

Producing monoclonal antibodies traditionally involves inducing an immune response against the antigen of interest, purifying the B cells from the immune-responsive animal to fuse with an immortal cell line, selecting for successful fusion cells, confirming antibody production, and then upscaling production from those cell lines.[15] Initially, as in polyclonal antibody production, an animal is immunized with the antigen of interest to produce an immune response. The exact timeline is dependent on the antigen, but often the animal is immunized multiple times, with the final immunization being antigen only (i.e., no adjuvant), before the animal is killed to harvest the B cells from the spleen or other lymphoid tissue.[7] These B cells are then fused with a myeloma cell, typically from a BALB/c mouse, by culturing them together in polyethylene glycol, which causes the membranes to break. A BALB/c mouse is used because most myeloma cell lines are from BALB/c mice because injecting mineral oil into these mice induces myelomas.[7,9,10] Sendai virus or electric current is used to fuse the cells, creating a cell with double the nuclear material, which occasionally breaks down following fusion.[10,16] Because these are B-cell tumors, some will produce irrelevant antibodies, but specific clones can be selected.[9] Although other types of mice strains can be fused with a BALB/c myeloma, a completely BALB/c hybridoma, when injected back into the mouse will produce ascites (large amounts of fluid), which were traditionally used for upscaling antibody production.[10]

Fusion products are selected for, as they selectively grow in hypoxanthine-aminopterin-thymidine (HAT) medium; the fusion product contains an enzyme allowing them to process a toxin in this media, and each product is plated in its own separate culture well.[9,10] Following growth, cell culture supernatant is tested to see if it is producing the antibody specific to the antigen of interest, either by antibody capture, antigen capture, or functional screening.[9,10] Following hybridoma formation, it is possible to select for those secreting IgM or IgG isotypes by a magnetic cell sorting system, which can ensure isotype specificity as needed in the research setting.[17] The strain selected is then further cultured in wells to ensure enough cell product, and can be frozen for later use.[9] Successful hybridoma formation normally takes at least 2 months and may take up to a year.[10]

Monoclonal Manufacturing

To generate large amounts of monoclonal antibodies, hybridomas traditionally were injected into the abdominal cavities of mice, an optimal growth environment, to grow and secrete ascites into the abdominal cavity.[9] This fluid contains the desired antibodies, and after 1 to 2 weeks, would be collected.[7] Ascite production is the cheapest option for monoclonal antibody production.

A more expensive process is called "bulk tissue culture" hybridomas.[9] Bulk tissue has traditionally been limited by the ability to grow cells. However, optimizing media, bioreactive conditions, and cell lines can lead to 10g/L titers and 20 million cells/mL, meaning that it is feasible to scale production to commercial levels.[18]

Finally, for large scale production, "cloned antibody genes" are expressed "in high producing eukaryote systems such as plants or baculoviruses."[9] This animal-independent technique of antibody production utilizes recombinant technology to express the gene for an immunoglobin in a vector that then transcribes and translates the immunoglobulin product.[19] Again, antigen-specific cells are screened from an immunized animal by antigen binding, and the genetic material of these cells is processed to isolate the immunoglobin variable region.[20] Because variable regions include both a light and heavy chain, the expressed product is then screened to see which combination of light and heavy chains is antigen specific.[20] The genetic code can be amplified for the complete immunglobulin by reverse transcriptase PCR, to then directly clone it into vectors for mass production of immunoglobulin.[19] Following either method, the vector can then be cultivated to produce a large amount of antibodies. There is sometimes difficulty in producing functional mammalian or avian immunglobulin after producing them in a model organism, but this is being overcome as the understanding of this process is optimized.[20]

Monoclonal antibodies provide an immortal source of antibodies, which ultimately reduces the number of animals used in experiments if a constant source of antibodies is needed.[16] Their greatest benefit is this theoretically unlimited supply of a standardized product — the antibody produced has a known specificity and will be produced at a constant amount for as long as the culture is maintained, which provides a tool that can be consistently used in a reproducible manner.[9,11,12] The specificity of a single epitope outcompetes anything attainable by polyclonal antibody production, reducing "background noise and cross-reactivity."[12] If specifically detecting something with multiple epitopes, multiple monoclonal antibodies can be pooled to identify a product with all of the desired epitopes.[9] But, despite these improvements, development of a monoclonal antibody must still be well justified, as it is very expensive to produce, yield is still low compared with bleeding a large

animal, and development of a high-affinity monoclonal antibody can still be difficult. Furthermore, sometimes, the antibody produced is a low-affinity monoclonal antibody, which is cross reactive to many similar structural motifs in other proteins.[9]

One proposed way to harness increased specificity of antibodies without producing a monoclonal antibody is to purify polyclonal antibodies based on their epitope specificity.[21] To do so, the epitopes on the antigen are mapped, and a column with these epitopes at discrete levels on the column are synthesized.[21] As the serum passes through such a column, the specific epitopes elute out separately at different fractions, allowing better purification.[21]

Expanded Isolation Considerations for Blood Products

Ian Clift, PhD MLS(ASCP)[CM]

▶ Anticoagulants and Additives

Blood is subdivided into serum or plasma by the addition of anticoagulants. Multiple anticoagulants are commonly used in the clinical immunodiagnostic laboratory. Specifically, ethylenediaminetectraacetic acid (EDTA) and citrates (sodium and potassium) prevents coagulation by the chelation (binding) of calcium primarily used for testing hematological components such as hematocrits, hemoglobin, and cell differentiation. The patient's coagulation factors can then be tested later when calcium is restored to the blood product. Sodium fluoride is a weak anticoagulant used primarily for examining glucose specimens. Oxylates (ammonium and potassium) are still sometimes used when examining hematology specimens, but have been shown to interfere with some chemistry determinations and have, therefore, been replaced with EDTA in most cases. Finally, heparin (sodium, lithium, and ammonium) is considered

a very good anticoagulant because it is normally found in blood and only very little volume is needed. In most cases, these additives can be found in dry forms, commonly included in commercially manufactured vacuum tubes used for blood collection, and should be stored according to manufacturer recommendations. Color coding for vacuum tubes has been established, available through many Internet sources, and should be implemented and consulted when draws are conducted. In addition to additives, a nonadditive vacuum tube used predominantly in serology and blood banks allows for serum separation of clotted blood. Specifically, testing of the noncellular elements can be performed using red-topped and serum separator tubes. An examination of noncellular coagulation factors is usually tested from a light blue-topped tube containing sodium citrate or a lavender tube containing EDTA. Blood specimens collected for sterile culture are often collected in pale yellow tubes containing sodium polyanetholesulfonate (SPS), and blood bank personnel tend to use blood from bright yellow tubes containing acid citrate dextrose (ACD).

Whole Blood

The most commonly collected specimen is whole blood. Depending on the type of tube and anticoagulant additive, various testing from whole blood can be performed. When placed in a plain tube with no additives, blood will clot for serum extraction. Many manual serological tests still require the removal of serum from the blood clot; this is aided by centrifugation and tube systems for serum separation. In the former cases, a separate, clear plastic or glass tube is used to remove the serum fraction before testing. In the latter case, centrifugation forces the blood into a gel layer; after a short period (30 minutes), the gel rises and forms a hard barrier between the packed red cells and the serum. Many automated instruments can now remove serum from blood without the need for a specific separation step. With all blood and blood products, standard precautions should be observed. Whole blood does not last long in cold storage, as this leads to destruction/ rupturing of red cells; it should be separated into serum or plasma fractions for long-term frozen storage. Specialized collection and testing of various fractions of blood, including platelets, cryoprecipitate, and other donor units are commonly conducted in blood banking facilities but will not be discussed further here.

Serum and Plasma

While the primary use for serum is in serological testing, it can also be used in the chemistry lab for testing of electrolytes such as calcium, phosphorous, sodium, potassium, uric acid, cholesterol, and others. Serum or plasma should be separated from remaining blood cells using standard precautions including the use of protective gloves. During manual testing, tube stoppers must be removed carefully while covered with a protective gauze to prevent aerosols or splatter. Alternatively, a protective plastic shield can be used as a barrier. The serum or plasma can then be transferred to a glass or disposable plastic tube for further testing. After testing all remaining blood and body fluid,

products should be discarded in a biohazardous waste container.

The normal appearance of serum or plasma is a pale straw color. In blood bank practices, the plasma can be separated from the other components of blood through centrifugation or sedimentation. It is then frozen as fresh frozen plasma (FFP), or within 24 hours of phlebotomy in order to preserve coagulation factors, such as factor V and VIII, to be used in donations. The most common abnormal appearances of serum or plasma are caused by three conditions: hemolysis, jaundice, or lipemia.

A hemolyzed specimen appears with a redish hue caused by lysis of red cells and hemoglobin release. Hemolysis is often the result of improper preanalytical techniques, such as poor venipuncture (phlebotomy) in which trauma occurred to the blood vessel during the draw. However, other factors can lead to hemolysis as well, including freezing, prolonged exposure to heat, transfer of blood under excessive pressure, as well as adulterants such as alcohol. Hemolyzed blood is unsuitable for many chemistry tests due to the release of chemicals commonly confined to the cells, but can sometimes still be used for serology assays.

A brownish-yellow color to the serum or plasma is commonly caused by an increase in the bile pigments, specifically bilirubin. This can also be caused by the destruction of blood cells, at a time point prior to venipuncture, and could be a sign of liver damage or hepatitis; it may be accompanied by changes in skin tone, known as jaundice. Therefore, a brownish-yellow serum is called a jaundiced serum. A notation of the color of the serum should be written in any report, as this could be an indication of a medical issue needing attention.

Lipemia is caused by the buildup of excess lipids, or fats, in the serum or plasma. It is indicated by a milky, opaque appearance. While potentially indicative of a medical condition, lipemia does not interfere with many tests besides lipid panels such as triglycerides.

Serum and plasma should be separated only by trained individuals and safe practices, such as avoiding splashes and aerosols, and proper disposal of waste. Serum or plasma can be stored and frozen for preservation for extended periods of time but both are dependent on the type of assay to be performed, as long-term storage may lead to degradation or false elevation of some results.

▶ Erythrocytes

Erythrocyte, or red blood cell (RBC) markers are often the immunological target of blood bank serology testing. Blood collected for use in donor populations is regulated in the United States by the FDA, which mandates special containers such as sterile, pyrogen-free blood bags with specific lot number identification as well as a specific quantity of anticoagulant. For example, a 500mL blood bag contains 63mLs of anticoagulant. Along with acid citrate dextrose (ACD), used most often in tube draws and apheresis, citrate phosphate dextrose (CPD), citrate phosphate dextrose adenine (CPDA-1), and adenine-saline are all used as anticoagulants for whole blood to ensure longer shelf life; specifically 21, 35, and 42 days, respectively, when kept in a highly monitored refrigerated unit.

Erythrocytes can be separated from the whole blood through a differential centrifugation process that can also separate out platelets and plasma through variations in the centrifugation spin time and speed. In the blood bank, centrifugation can separate out the plasma and leave behind packed red cells. Other methods of separation can also be used, for example, to remove leukocytes, white blood cells, which can minimize the transmission of diseases such as cytomegalovirus (CMV), which reside in leukocytes. However, normal serological testing of erythrocyte antigens occurs within a typically anticoagulated whole blood unit. Erythrocytes are commonly screened for the common blood type antigens A, B, and H as part of pretransfusion testing. Typically, this can come from a venous blood draw in a heparin or EDTA tube, often drawn from the donor during the collection of the blood unit and from the patient during routine phlebotomy.

▶ Granulocytes/Leukocytes

Granulocytes and Leukocytes are collected, as part of a typical whole blood collection, but can be separated from the other components of blood via specialized separation techniques such as peripheral blood mononuclear cell (PBMC) isolation using Ficoll-Paque™ gradients,[22] through magnetic bead separation using specific antibodies, and via the lysis of erythrocytes, which are more susceptible to osmolysis. Reagents and solutions for white cell separation are commercially available. Using the Ficoll-Paque method, cells are centrifuged and white cells are present in a thin layer called the buffy coat, which can be extracted from the solution via careful pipetting (**FIGURE AP-1**). The Ficoll-Paque method of mononuclear cell isolation can be found in the Practical Applications section of this book.

Specific granulocyte populations can also be extracted from either a whole blood solution or an RBC lysed solution via fluorescence-activated cell sorting (FACS) using a flow cytometer and specifically associated surface antibody panels, such as CD11b+ Ly6G+ for neutrophils.

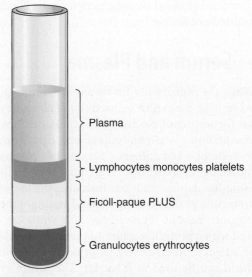

FIGURE AP-1 Separation of blood specimen via centrifugation using Ficoll-Paque.

Specimen Handling Outside the Laboratory

Annika Lee, BS

Patient samples are important tools in both diagnostic and research settings, but the validity of information gleaned from a sample ultimately depends on sample quality. If compromised, accuracy of results can suffer, which could inaccurately portray clinical outcomes in a research setting and lead to misdiagnosis and ineffective treatment planning in a clinical setting.[23] Quality control of patient samples initially begins with collection of that sample. Both patient and provider should pay careful attention to all stages of sample collection in which they are involved. This includes ordering the sample, preparing the patient for collection, collecting the sample from the patient, and processing, handling, labeling, storing, and transporting the sample to the proper laboratory setting for analysis.[24,25] Specimen collection is often performed by medical support staff, such as nurses, who are not trained in laboratory procedure and the rationale behind specific methodologies. As such, it is especially important to educate personnel and provide them with access to standardized reference material detailing the procedure associated with a specific sample.[26]

Sample collection begins with a lab requisition, or order. When a sample is ordered, the physician or nurse practitioner ordering should be specific about the testing needed. They should clearly identify which patient the sample was ordered from, who is ordering the sample, when the sample should be collected, which tests should then be taken from the sample, the location on the patient where the sample should be taken, and what symptoms have led them to order the sample and testing.[27] This level of communication helps to avoid confusion among personnel who order the sample and those who perform sample collection; helps to determine proper sample handling according to standardized reference materials; and will eventually allow the laboratory to process the sample correctly.

Next, properly preparing the patient for sample collection reduces redundant repeat sampling. This is the step where the patient is most directly involved in sample quality—providers should clearly inform patients of any preparation needed for the sample taken, most commonly fasting or provocation, and confirm that the patient understands those instructions.[27] For instance, when taking "serum, plasma, or whole blood," especially when testing for "lipids, triglycerides, and lipoproteins," the patient should often perform an overnight fast to avoid lipemia or contamination of fat droplets.[24,28] For a glucose challenge, the patient will need to be "provoked," or ingest a high concentration of glucose prior to sample taking.[24] The patient is responsible for adhering to those requirements once they are given, and, immediately prior to sample collection, the provider should confirm with the patient that preparations were followed. Providers should also note other physiological states that could impact sample quality, such as adequate water intake and normal emotional or physical stress, which can impact biological profiles, to determine if the sample will be compromised.[23] Finally, the timing of collections is important—there are normal fluctuations of certain biomarkers, such as serum ion, with circadian rhythm, and often, the first of the morning samples give a most accurate picture of a patient's basal state.[23] Taking compromised samples can be an invasive waste of resources, and mistakes in collection cannot often be "fixed;" instead, they will simply require retesting following the appropriate procedure.[25]

Now that the patient is prepared, collecting the specimen should begin with confirming the patient's identity. This can be accomplished by confirming the patient's name and birth date against the order form verbally, from patient or guardian, or via valid ID if the patient is compromised.[28,29] Following this, the provider should clearly arrange the supplies for specimen taking, and place the patient physically to ease sample taking and reduce cross contamination e.g., placing an arm correctly with a closed fist for venipuncture, or lying back to expose the genital region for a microbial culture.[29] The provider preparing to take the sample should wash his or her hands and correctly don the proper personal protection; this prevents cross-contamination of the sample and protects both patient and sample taker from communicable diseases.[25,29] The site of sample collection should be prepped as needed by the provider—for instance, the collection site may be sterilized.[29] In general, the tools for collection of samples should be either sterile, single-use, or sterilized before and after every use, to protect the patient and prevent sample contamination.

Collection methodology is specific to each sample, and adhering to this methodology increases sample quality. For blood samples, the method of collection needs to consider hemolysis, lipemia, inadequate draw/"quantity not sufficient," clotting, and order of draw.[27] Hemolysis, or breaking red blood cells, compromises sample quality, and can be avoided by appropriate needle selection, gentle technique in blood drawing, making sure that the alcohol used to sterilize the sight has dried, and being gentle with sample treatment following collection.[23] Many blood samples have additives that require immediate sample processing—the provider must invert a tube an appropriate amount to create a correct ratio of additives to sample, and prevent micro-clotting in samples with an anticoagulant, although not so forcefully as to destroy the integrity of the sample.[23,27] Because the tubes are pretreated with additives, a sample draw order is important to reduce cross contamination. This order is well delineated in most lab manuals and specified by the color-coded caps used in that specific facility.[29,30] It is good practice for the provider to confirm this methodology and check that the material used is correct at each use, confirming the correct color tube as well as checking the label to ensure the tube, contains the correct additives needed for the specific sample drawn.[27] The correct volume of blood drawn is important in blood draws, both because the ratio of additive to sample is pre-set and because requested volumes are needed for a certain number of assays—often, two performances, either singly or in duplicate, are required to ensure validity of results.[23,24] Minimum volumes account for instrument dead volume, and so a lesser volume may mean an insufficient sample quality.[24] Finally, using unexpired tubes is important, as is storing tubes at a proper temperature.[23,29]

In a microbiology setting, preferences for certain specimen collection methodologies should be noted, such as sample taking versus swabbing. For wounds, tissue aspirates are preferred, as swab volume is small and swab design increases the chance of microbial cross-contamination.[25] Again, the provider should clarify the specific methodology for each specimen collected before taking the sample to avoid repeat sampling.[23] In the case of a urine culture, how or whether a patient should cleanse him- or herself before collecting the stream should be noted.[27] Because microbiology culture technique is a bit harder to ensure quality, the physician should identify which specific screening he or she is interested in and the rationale behind it, and then contact the lab to confirm the way they prefer the sample to be collected to ensure quality of culture.[27] For certain samples, such as cerebral spinal fluid (CSF), there is an increased need to label the sample as it is taken; the order of the draw determines which panels can be run on the sample. The first fluid collected is used for chemistry and serology, the second for microbiology, the third for cell counts, and the fourth for anything extra.[27] CSF is considered irreplaceable as a high risk sample procedure and requires rapid transport to the lab to prevent sample deterioration.[27]

Following sample collection, provider handling of the specimen is very important. The sample should be legibly labeled on the container itself (labeling on the lid or transport container could separate the sample from its label).[27,29] Proper labeling could include indelible ink and a label material that can withstand storage conditions such as freezing.[31] For sample identification, the provider should include at least two patient identifiers, one biographic, such as patient name, and one numeric, such as a medical record number, test order number, or date of birth.[26,29] It is good practice to also label the sample with the name of the provider who collected the sample, the age of the patient from which the sample is taken, the reason for collection, and the site of collection.[24,28] This can prevent misinterpretation between what was collected and what is being tested in the lab, ensures the sample is compared with the correct age-sensitive reference values, and provides a contact if any clarification is needed.[24,25,28] Labeling ensures proper diagnosis, sample processing in a detached facility, and decreases the creation of an unknown biohazard.

Finally, the proper container must be selected for transit, especially when the lab is not in the same facility as the site of collection.[32] When packaging, the sample should be in a container that will not cause it to break in transit and potentially expose the transporter to hazardous bodily fluid.[24] This includes initially closing the caps securely, and for increased precaution, capping containers with Parafilm after sealing or using vials with internal O-rings in addition to external seals.[25,31] Whether the container for collection needs to be sterile depends on the sample taken; in most cases, except stool, sterility is important.[25] Finally, for transport, samples must be placed in a labeled, plastic leakproof biohazard bag, and with something to contain potential spilled material. Request forms should be stored separately from the sample itself; this prevents it from becoming contaminated biohazardous material.[26,28,30,32] Sharps or needles should not be transported with specimens, but should be disposed of in proper containers.[24,28]

When providers and patients note the importance of following the standard methodology for sample collection, doing so provides a laboratory with a high-quality sample to analyze. This protects the information that results from this analysis, as well as keeping the patient and staff safe in a setting with potentially hazardous biomaterial.

Determining Cost Structure for Manual and Automated Systems

Ian Clift, PhD MLS(ASCP)[CM]

Multiple factors must be considered when determining the cost per unit test run in a diagnostic operation. The conversion from manual testing to automated testing requires a cost calculation to be performed for determining a break-even and cost-benefit analysis. Included in this estimation are the start-up expenses, the labor costs, and the resources (reagents and supplies) required to perform an individual test. Globally, these factors define the cost for a billable procedure, i.e., the cost billed to a payer. All nonbillable costs in the laboratory must be allocated to the cost of a billable procedure to ensure that total operational expenses are covered. The costs associated with manual and automated tests are different, and estimates should form the basis for any long-term assay design change in the laboratory. In general, these factors must be calculated for financial purposes and are performed in association with the financial affairs office (or similar entity) within the institution. Depending on the purpose of the data, multiple models can be utilized to assess the value of a laboratory assay. For example, cost-effectiveness analysis and cost-utility analysis are used to determine whether a health intervention provides a value; they are used by insurance and government agencies to determine reimbursement rates of laboratory tests.[33] These complex analyses require multiple forms of data, but require at their root the estimated direct costs of a performed test. More commonly employed within an institution, activity-based management, which focuses on the consumption of resources through activity, provides the basis for Activity-Based Costing (ABC), which lumps revenues under the category of Products and Services and costs under Resources. Under this structure, both costs and revenues, i.e., Resources, and Produces and Services, are the

TABLE AP–1 Categories of Laboratory Assay Expenses		
Category	**Definition**	**Examples**
Direct Costs	Attributable to an individual test	Reagents
Indirect Costs	Not Attributable to an individual test	Utilities, regulatory fees, management fees
Fixed Costs	Constant costs, not dependent on test volume	Maintenance contracts, regulatory fees
Variable Costs	Dependent on test volume	Reagents
Semi-Fixed Costs	Step-like variation in cost	Labor costs, multi-use equipment, and supplies

result of Activity, such as a test order from a provider leading to associated technologist time.

Test charges do not equate to test revenue directly; instead, one must first subtract expenses to perform the test (test costs) from income earned from performing the test. While income, profit, and revenue are all determined primarily outside of the laboratory unit, the estimation of test expenses is best performed within it, by knowledgeable members of the laboratory team. The following section describes some of the standard assessments used for determining the cost structure (expenses) (**TABLE AP–1**) for a generic diagnostic test when transitioning from manual to automated analysis. Furthermore, costs, primarily labor costs, are described in terms of activity utilizing ABC Analysis.

▶ Start-Up and Indirect Expenses

Large-instrument acquisition typically requires a capital equipment purchase, which comes with its own set of requirements regarding cost. The overall cost of capital equipment is determined through a depreciation schedule, typically a straight-line depreciation in most hospital and laboratory operations. This means the instrument is said to lose the same amount of value over a

finite time period in which the cost of the instrument is accounted for by the finance department. These equipment costs should be part of any assessment of compared costs for manual and automated methods. It is determined by accounting for the cost of the instrument and dividing it first by the expected years of service on the depreciation schedule, and then by the estimated number of assays run on the instrument during the year. This provides an instrument-related cost per test performed that can then be factored into the total cost per test. Alternatively, if the equipment is leased or rented, these costs should be associated similarly with the cost per test.

Additional equipment costs should be part of any assessment of compared costs for manual and automated methods as well. For example, is there a maintenance plan for the instrument? If so, how much does it cost per year? If not, how much should be allocated to instrument maintenance year to year to keep it in working order? Additionally, what costs are associated with validation of the new assay? With Activity Based Costing, these equipment costs are allocated and divided by the number of assays performed as of overhead equipment costs.

Start-up costs, such as comparison analysis, validation studies, and development of new standard operating procedures, may or may not be included in an ABC, break-even, or cost-benefit analysis. For most FDA-approved assays,

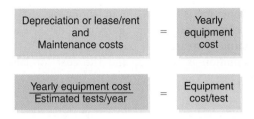

FIGURE AP-2 Association of equipment cost into test cost.

rigorous testing for clinical use has already been performed; however, verification of claimed assay performance characteristics are still necessary as well as a comparison of all clinically reportable aspects of the assay.

The cost of instrumentation and equipment is reduced per test as the test volume increases.

▶ Labor Costs

The major advantage expected from the conversion from manual to automated analysis is found in the labor saving per unit test performed. In general, automated assays require less hands-on time and therefore can provide economic savings related to the amount of time laboratorians are required to focus on an individual assay. The labor involved in running a manual test is distinct to the test performed, method employed, and standard operating procedure in place at the individual institution. Labor costs are calculated through estimates of the number of tests performed by a single technologist in a given work day divided by the number of tests, or through an estimate of the actual time to perform all steps in a single assay. This technologist time is converted to a cost-per-minute based on the technologist's average rate of pay, as measured by their total compensation package, not just their take-home pay. Simultaneous testing via manual methods should be considered when making a cost estimate for labor. In one study of cost for performing ABO/Rh blood typing, this labor cost was nearly halved when estimated, based on running 12 tests simultaneously versus one test at a time.[34] Some tests do not require a significant additional amount of time per test up to a certain volume of tests performed

simultaneously, depending on the number of tests that can be performed together. However, a step-wise doubling of labor costs occurs over this amount of tests.

Other factors that may be reduced in automated analysis include maintenance and calibration times, which are often onboard the analyzer and require less hands-on time. These additional costs are sometimes called nonvalue added steps as they do not directly lead to a patient result.

Depending on the test performed, labor costs tend to increase in a step-wise fashion.

▶ Additional Resource Costs

The cost of materials, including reagents, diluents, and consumables, is typically higher for automated analysis due to the use of proprietary (or rare) materials and must also be calculated into a total cost estimate. Calculating reagent costs is typically performed using a simple line-by-line approach in which the reagent cost per volume is divided by the volume used per assay. Similarly, the cost of running calibrators and controls is based on the unit cost to run the calibrator divided by the average number of tests that use that control in a specified time period. Technologist time to perform these calibrations and controls may or may not be included in the analysis, or may simply be estimated as negligible when the cost is amortized by the number of tests performed, sometimes in the thousands or tens of thousands depending on the test.

The cost of a test is converted into a revenue rate using the surcharge/cost plus method, in which the actual cost is multiplied by a factor of 1.5 to determine the price expected from the payer. These prices are often not set by the laboratory organization but by external third-party price fixing, such as the price reimbursed for specific text codes through Medicare and Medicaid in the United States and through agreements with insurance companies. Standardized reimbursement rates may influence the revenue from a given test and be important in the determination of break-even and cost-comparison analysis.

Ultimately, however, the determination as to whether to initiate a conversion from manual to automated methods is based on two important factors: the cost of equipment and the cost of labor. Traditionally, the tradeoff for automation is a reduction in labor costs with an increase in instrument/equipment costs. As test volume increases, the cost per assay for instrumentation is reduced, and the cost for labor increases.

B- and T-Cell Deficiencies

Brittney Dinkel, PhD

The adaptive immune response is critical for protection against pathogens. B-cell and T-cell defects cause a weak immune response leading to chronic bacterial and viral infections. While the lack of B cells and T cells leads to immunodeficiencies and increased infections, improper development or uncontrolled B-cell and T-cell responses can result in autoimmune disorders where the B cells and T cells are attacking the host's tissues.

▶ B-Cell Deficiencies

B-cell immunodeficiencies can be caused by mutations in the BCR signaling pathway, or mutations that inhibit receptor rearrangement, class-switching, or affinity maturation.[35] X-linked agammaglobulinemia (XLA) is a primary immunodeficiency that is caused by a mutation on the X chromosome that causes a defect in Burton's Tyrosine Kinase (BTK). BTK is a B-cell signaling molecule that is required for signaling from the pre-BCR for B-cell development. Symptoms of XLA typically do not begin to appear until about 6 months of age due to the maternal IgG transferred through the placenta. As the maternal IgG is cleared from the infant, the infant will have recurrent, severe, bacterial infections, especially in the upper respiratory tract. Typical diagnostic tests for XLA include nephelometry to determine antibody levels, and flow cytometry to determine the number of B cells present. Genetic testing can also confirm the diagnosis.

Hyper IgM syndrome occurs when B cells are unable to class switch due to mutations in the class switch machinery or due to their inability to receive T-cell help.[36] Patients with hyper IgM syndrome have normal or even high levels of IgM but lack IgG, IgA, or IgE antibodies. This means that they have only low-affinity antibodies and are more susceptible to extracellular pathogens. Hyper IgM is most often caused by a mutation in CD40 ligand, thereby preventing T cells from providing the necessary signals to the B-cell to induce class switching. Their B cells are also unable to form germinal centers in order to undergo affinity maturation. Hyper IgM syndrome is often diagnosed by testing antibody concentration for the various isotypes. If the patient is lacking IgG, IgA, and IgE antibodies, flow cytometry can be performed on the T cells to measure CD40L levels on the T cells. Genetic testing is also used to confirm the diagnosis.

▶ T-Cell Deficiencies

T-cell immunodeficiencies are characterized by a lack of T cells or the inability of T cells to carry out effector functions. One well characterized T-cell deficiency is Wiskott-Aldrich syndrome.[37,38] Wiskott-Aldrich syndrome is caused by a mutation in the WAS protein (WASP). WASP is activated downstream of TCR signaling and is required for cytoskeletal rearrangements. WASP also has the role of a transcription factor and regulates T-cell differentiation. Symptoms of the Wiskott-Aldrich system include increased bleeding due to impaired development of platelets; recurrent bacterial, viral, and fungal infections; and eczema of the skin. Although Wiskott-Aldrich syndrome is classified as an immunodeficiency, it also has symptoms associated with autoimmune diseases resulting in the T-cell mediated destruction of red blood cells or other organs. Patients are also more susceptible to developing cancer. Wiskott-Aldrich is often suspected when a young boy has unusual bleeding or bruising and platelet anomalies along with immune defects resulting in recurrent infections at about 2 years of age. A diagnosis of Wiskott-Aldrich relies heavily on genetic testing and quantitative PCR to determine WASP expression levels.

▶ B- and T-Cell Deficiencies

Severe combined immunodeficiencies (SCID) are characterized by a dramatic decrease of both B and T cells. One of the most common causes of SCID is X-linked SCID, resulting in a mutation in the IL-2R subunit common γ (IL2Rγ).[39] IL-2 common gamma chain is required for expression of the cytokine receptors for IL-2, IL-4, IL-7, IL-19, IL-15, and IL-21. Development of B cells, T cells, and NK cells require signaling through the cytokine receptors. Patients with SCID are extremely susceptible to bacterial, viral, and fungal infections. Infants suspected of having SCID are diagnosed if they have low counts of B cells, T cells, and NK cells, as well as altered antibody concentration in serum. The patient will also lack pathogen-specific antibodies after having recurrent infections. Genetic testing and flow cytometry can be used to determine the specific cause of SCID.

▶ Autoimmune Diseases

Autoimmune diseases are caused by an inborne or acquired failure to cull self-reactive lymphocytes. Systemic lupus erythematosus is a chronic inflammatory disease where the immune system targets the patient's own tissues as though they are a foreign pathogen.[38,40] Lupus may attack various tissues including the skin, kidneys, brain, heart, lungs, and blood. Depending on which tissues are targeted, the symptoms can vary. Symptoms may include a butterfly-shaped rash on the face, fatigue, joint pain, chest pain and shortness of breath, dry eyes, or headaches. Diagnostic tests include whole blood cell counts, kidney and liver tests, urinalysis to look for increased protein levels, and an antinuclear antibody (ANA) test. ANA tests look for the presence of antibodies that react to various components of the cell nucleus. ANA testing is the strongest indication of lupus.

Another example of an autoimmune disease is type I diabetes.[41] Type I diabetes occurs when the cytotoxic T cells attack the β-cells of the pancreas that produce insulin, or autoantibodies are produced that result in the damage of the pancreas. Type I diabetes results in the inability to break down sugar into energy. Symptoms include increased thirst and urination, extreme hunger, blurred vision, and weight loss. Diagnosis of Type I diabetes includes the routine tests to diagnose diabetes: glycated hemoglobin (A1C) test, random blood sugar test, and fasting blood sugar test. To distinguish a diabetes diagnosis between type I and type II, a blood test for autoantibodies that are commonly associated with type I diabetes is performed.

▶ Cancers

Immune cells have the ability to rapidly proliferate in response to pathogen stimulation. However, if there is a mutation that allows for the rapid proliferation of B cells or T cells without antigen stimulation, cancer can develop. One common malignancy of B cells is multiple myeloma.[38,42] Multiple myeloma is the uncontrolled growth of a single clone of a plasma cell. The cancer cells produce high levels of their monoclonal abnormal antibody, called M proteins, and take over the bone marrow to prevent the production of healthy blood cells. Symptoms of multiple myeloma include bone pain due to the tumor growth and frequent infections due to the lack of pathogen-specific antibodies. Diagnostic tests include blood and urine tests to look for M proteins, and examination of the bone marrow. The doctor will remove a small sample of the bone marrow (a bone biopsy) which will be used for immunohistochemistry staining and fluorescence in situ hybridization (FISH) to determine chromosome abnormalities.

The adaptive immune system is a complex system that requires careful balance. A defect in

B or T cells can lead to an immunodeficiency, resulting in recurrent infections. A break in tolerance can also result in B and T cells recognizing self-antigen as pathogens, causing tissue damage. Many more dysfunctions of the adaptive immune system occur that were not covered here.

Clinical Utility of Characterizing Stem-Cell Markers

Ian Clift, PhD MLS(ASCP)[CM]

Stem cells can be found in most tissues and fluids of the human body; however, they are present more numerously during development. In adulthood, they are predominately isolated to select locations, such as the bone marrow, under normal physiological conditions. Beyond some well-established implications for stem cells in therapy, their localization and presence in clinical specimens has begun to be crucially scrutinized in diagnosis of disease and management of therapies within many advanced practice spaces. A stem cell is differentiated from mature cells functionally via its potential to become a variety of cell types through the process of maturation; it is capable of both self-renewal and differentiation. However, many markers of stem cell populations can be detected on the surface of cells through common immunodiagnostic approaches such as flow cytometry (**FIGURE AP-3**). Most well studied in the immune system, both stem cells and progenitor cells are often closely associated with many human diseases, most notably human cancers. Importantly, the reemergence of stem-cell markers on the surface of cells often occurs in cancer. Furthermore, populations of stem cells have been used in the development of novel therapies for treating a multitude of diseases, including lymphomas and leukemia.

All stem cells are not the same, and the classifications of stem cells can be segregated rudimentarily into three populations of interest for the diagnostician; specifically, we will look at markers of embryonic, adult, and cancer stem cells.

▶ Embryonic Stem Cells

Embryonic stem cells (ESCs) are defined as cells that derive from the inner cell mass of the early-stage embryo. Although ESCs have been used in therapeutic applications, controversy exists over the usage of these cells due to their source of origin. Early work with embryonic stem cells, however, led to the characterization of numerous surface and other markers that differentiate them from other non–self-renewing cell populations.

Of note, three Stage Specific Embryonic Antigens (SSEAs) recognizing carbohydrate epitopes involved in controlling cell surface interactions during development were found on ESCs, and subsequently found on the surface of cancer stem cells, such as teratocarcinoma and some adult tissue cells.[43] SSEA-1, for example, is also known as Lewis x and CD15. In addition, a multitude of CD markers has been associated with both human and mouse ESCs including CD9, CD24, and CD133.[43] Some of these CD markers are also found on mature cells and tumor stem cells as well.

FIGURE AP-3 Phenotypic marker locations.
Reproduced from Zhao W, Ji X, Zhang F, Li L, Ma L. Embryonic stem cell markers. *Molecules.* 2012;17(6):6196–6236.

TABLE AP–2 Stem Cell Surface Markers	
Some Common Stem Cell Markers	
Marker	**Importance**
CD9 (MRP1, TM4SF, DRAP-27, p24)	Embryonic stem cells
SSEA-1 (CD15/Lewis x), SSEA-3, SSEA-4	Human germ line, embryonic stem cell
CD29 (β1 integrin)	Stem cells, muscle cells
CD31 (PECAM-1)	Bone marrow-derived stem cells
CD34	Hematopoietic stem cells, bone marrow cells
CD59 (Protectin, MAC-inhibitory protein)	Epithelial cells, epithelial cancer stem cells, other stem cells
CD117 (c-KIT, SCFR)	Blood progenitor cells and stem cells
CD133	Hematopoietic and other stem cells
CD324 (E-Cadherin)	Embryonic stem cells, carcinoma stem cells
Nestin	Neural stem cells
STRO-1	Mesenchymal and stromal stem cells

▶ Adult Stem Cells

Adult stem cells, also known as somatic stem cells, are found in isolated organ-specific locations throughout the body. Their CD marker profile is similar to those found in ESCs. They are responsible for producing new organ-specific cells when cells of this organ or tissue are damaged or die. They are also regarded favorably for potential therapeutic uses as the ethical concerns regarding the use of embryonic stem cells are removed. One of the earliest uses of adult stem cells was in the process of stem cell transplantation that occurred by replacing the bone marrow of a diseased individual with healthy cells from a donor.[44] Two commonly isolated stem cells are hematopoietic stem cells, those that are responsible for all of the cells of a hematological fate including RBCs, WBCs, and platelets, as well as mesenchymal stem cells (MSCs). Both of them can be derived from the bone marrow; however, MSCs are also commonly extracted from adipose (fat) tissue. MSCs have been shown in culture and in vivo to differentiate into bone, cartilage, fat, and brain tissues.[45] Although MSCs have been found to be important for recovery from tissue and cellular damage, they have also been implicated in the progression toward diseases such as cancer. Traditionally, mesenchymal stem cells lose the ability to migrate and proliferate as they acquire a more epithelial cell structure. However, epithelial to mesenchymal transition (EMT) is a critical process in development during the process of tissue and organ formation.[46,47]

▸ Cancer Stem Cells

Cancer stem cells, which are thought to give rise to many hematological cancers, have been observed for more than 20 years when researchers induced acute myeloid leukemia in mice after transplanting cells exhibiting the CD34+CD38+ phenotype.[46] Aging may play a key role in the development of adult cancers and myeloproliferative disease through the differentiation of stem-cell populations as a result of an increase in cell death caused by tissue damage, reactive oxygen species, and inflammation.[48] As cells age and die, cellular homeostasis is shifted toward proliferative pathways, pushing previously quiescent stem-cell populations toward maturation; errors to this maturation process are thought to be a contributing factor in the formation of cancer. Supporting this argument, cancers are often seen during times of extreme cellular proliferation, including infancy, and as individuals age. The transition from mature back to immature cells is often characterized by a shift from an epithelial profile to a mesenchymal profile, which is accompanied by the re-emergence of stem-like traits that allow for rapid proliferation, invasion, and migration; the hallmarks of a cancerous cell. Indeed, several studies have indicated that the process of EMT is correlated with highly aggressive breast cancer variants.[46]

▸ From Diagnostics to Therapy

Recent advances in our understanding of stem cells have led to their increased utility in medical interventions. In order to achieve sufficient numbers of cells for clinical and commercial goals, increasingly systematic approaches to stem-cell culturing and bioprocessing have occurred.[44] The early success of bone marrow stem-cell transplant has spurred research into growth and development of stem cells in culture.

In one procedure, stem cells were harvested from the iliac crests during reconstructive surgery, grown in culture, and first characterized by their adherence to a plastic microwell dish.[45] Cells were then stained with fluorescent markers for CD14, CD45, CD54, and CD90 and visualized using confocal microscopy. These cells were then induced to differentiate in culture to a variety of cell types including osteocytes (bone cells), adipocytes (fat cells), and Schwann cells typically found in the neural crest.[45] Surface and internal markers of these fats were also used to track the success of their growth and development. Basic research has shown that stem cells, once implanted, can lead to in vivo development of new bone and skin tissue among others that have an effect on growth acceleration.[49] A series of clinical trials using mesenchymal stem cells was started in the early 2000s and focused on diseases of the bones, such as arthritis, fractures, and osteoarthritis; diseases of the nervous system, such as autism, Parkinson's, multiple sclerosis, and spinal cord injury, and heart disease.[49] As these therapeutic approaches continue to reach the clinical space, cellular tracking and monitoring will be an emerging laboratory role. A major part of this tracking will be the examination of changes in cellular numbers based on their immunophenotypic profiles.

Immune Organ Dysfunction

Barsha Dash, BS

This section is focused on immune organ dysfunction, i.e., aberrant or loss of function of primary and secondary immune organs that can compromise immunity in humans, and methods to diagnose these disorders and approved treatments.

▶ Thymic Disorders

As you may recall, the thymus is the primary organ of T-cell development and is composed of an epithelial framework that directs the development and selection of T cells. T cells are indispensable for adaptive immune responses, which include direct killing of infected cells, potentiation of B-cell mediated, humoral immunity by helper T cells. Partial or total loss of thymus function can alter or inhibit T-cell development, resulting T-cell-dependent immunodeficiency. DiGeorge syndrome is a congenital disorder of thymic aplasia or failure leading to total or partial loss of T-cell development and hence, recurrent infections in patients are common.[50] Patients with DiGeorge syndrome harbor a deletion on the long arm of chromosome 22 (22q11.2). This deletion prevents the formation of embryonic pharyngeal structures such as pharyngeal pouches, resulting in thymic and thyroid aplasia or deficiency along with other developmental defects such as congenital

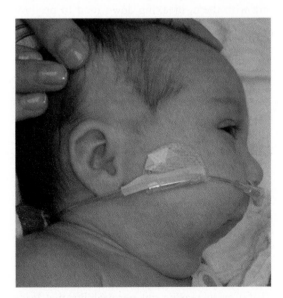

FIGURE AP–4 Child with DiGeorge syndrome. In addition to craniofacial defects, such as hypertelorism and microstomia, thought to arise as a result of defects in neural crest development, these individuals have partial or complete absence of the thymus as well, leading to significant immunological impairment.

Reproduced from Thomas W Sadler, Langman's Medical Embryology, 12e, LWW Wolters Kluwer.

heart defects, learning difficulties, and altered facial features, which are used to detect DiGeorge syndrome (**FIGURE AP–4**). Chromosomal deletion is detected using FISH, and T-cell numbers can be gauged using flow cytometry. Nude severe combined immunodeficiency (Nude SCID) is a very rare congenital genetic defect that prevents the development of thymic epithelial cells as a result of a mutation in the winged-helix-nude (WHN) gene.[51] This gene is expressed in thymic epithelial cells but not cells of hematopoietic lineage in the thymus. WHN-deficient thymic epithelial cells do not support T-cell development and are associated with recurrent infections. Mutations in genes can be determined by sequencing techniques and RT-PCR.

Thymic dysfunction can lead to tolerance breakdown as a result of aberrant T-cell activation. APECED (autoimmune polyendocrinopathy-candidiasis-ectodermal dystrophy) is a rare systemic autoimmune disease and is caused by AIRE mutations.[52,53] AIRE is critical for the expression of tissue-restricted antigens by mTECs. Loss of AIRE function prevents mTECs from expressing tissue-restricted antigens, causing defects in negative selection. This, is turn, allows autoreactive T cells to escape the thymus, resulting in multiorgan autoimmunity, as well as increased occurrence of: opportunistic candida infection as a result of increased damage to mucosal surfaces, and production of antibodies that neutralize Th17-dependent cytokines; diabetes due to pancreas beta cell damage; vitiligo due to melanocyte damage; as well as endocrine gland damage causing numerous problems such as hypothyroidism. Thus, appropriate thymic function is fundamental to creating a repertoire of T cells that can recognize a broad array of antigens without causing harm to itself.

It is important to note that the thymus is acutely sensitive to stress, which may result in thymic atrophy. Physiological stressors such as autoimmunity alter thymic function leading to alterations in T-cell development. Thus, optimal functioning of the thymus is also secondary to overall immune system homeostasis.[54,55] Thymic involution has been observed as a result of autoimmune diseases such as Myasthenia Gravis, Graves' disease, and Systemic Sclerosis. Myasthenia Gravis is also associated with thymic carcinomas originating from epithelial cells that make up the thymus.

Immune Disorders Arising in Bone Marrow

Bone marrow is the primary site of hematopoiesis in young and adult humans. Normal hematopoiesis gives rise to myeloid and lymphoid cells. Aplastic anemia is a bone marrow failure disorder, specifically, hematopoietic failure in humans.[56] Although now treatable with bone marrow transplantation and immune suppressants, aplastic anemia caused fatality only a few decades ago. It is thought to be an outcome of environmental triggers and genetic predisposition. An inflammatory trigger causes aberrant T-cell activation (Th1 cells), resulting in immune-mediated destruction of hematopoietic stem cells (HSCs) and hindering hematopoiesis. The exact reasons for aberrant T-cell activation is not known. However, aplastic anemia patients have an overrepresentation of HLA-DR2 molecules and other polymorphisms in genes associated with exuberant immune activation. Reduction in hematopoietic stem cells can be detected using flow cytometry examination of cell composition and numbers of bone marrow aspirates, or by a bone marrow biopsy.

Aberration in hematopoiesis may also arise because of oncogenic events. An example of this is chronic myeloid leukemia (CML). CML occurs due to a reciprocal translocation event between chromosome 9 and 22 in an HSC. The altered chromosome, 22 is called the Philadelphia chromosome and confers survival and proliferative advantage to the HSC by encoding a fusion tyrosine kinase called BCL-ABL. The malignant HSC gives rise to granulocyte myeloid progenitors, which acquire the capacity of self-renewal, thus resulting in abnormal expansion of the myeloid progenitor compartment. In addition, these progenitors do not reach terminal differentiation, thus immature granulocytes take over bone marrow space. Tyrosine kinase inhibitors have been used to treat the disease in many patients; additionally, bone marrow transplantation has been used. Together, these examples illustrate the importance of stringent regulation of hematopoiesis for sustenance of bone marrow environment and immune system.

Mucosa-Associated Immune Pathology

The mucosal surface is constantly exposed to food antigens and microbes and is a critical area of constant surveillance by the immune system. Homeostasis of the mucosal surfaces is dependent on tolerance of the immune system of food and commensal bacteria (microbiota). Commensal bacteria and their host organism share a symbiotic relationship. There are a number of benefits of harboring commensal bacteria: preventing colonization by pathogenic bacteria by competing with them, breaking down food to produce metabolites for the host, as well as the maturation of the immune system by various kinds of cross-talk. Much of this cross-talk is carried out by epithelial cells of the mucosa, such as intestinal epithelial cells and bacteria. Although typically these epithelial cells are not considered immune cells, they express many pattern recognition receptors that allow them to communicate with the microbiota. These cells play the role of segregating commensals from the host by secreting mucus and other protective molecules such as defensins. Epithelial barrier integrity is dependent on tight junction interactions between adjacent cells. Disruption of these interactions as a result of defects in proteins that mediate tight junction formation can result in dysbiosis of the gut. Dissolution of these interactions results in inflammatory bowel disease (IBD) by increasing gut permeability that leads to increased translocation of bacteria. Recent studies indicate that gut homeostasis is critical for preventing other diseases such as arthritis and multiple sclerosis. Irritable bowel disease (IBD) is detected by colonoscopy, and magnetic resonance imaging (MRI).

Red Cell Diseases Contraindicated for Blood Donation

Ian Clift, PhD MLS(ASCP)^{CM}

In addition to an appropriate type and screen crossmatch, certain donor populations are contraindicated for acceptance within most blood donor systems. Specifically, two questions on the AABB and FDA approved Donor History Questionnaire (DHQ) ask the potential donor if he or she has been diagnosed with any type of cancer, including leukemias, and if he or she has a bleeding disorder or blood disease.[57] Those donors who self-report most cancers, including leukemias and lymphomas, are indefinitely deterred from donating blood, as are patients who report a blood disease such as hemophilia, sickle cell anemia, thalassemia, and polycythemia. In addition, the physical examination of the potential donor includes both a blood pressure and hemoglobin test in order to flag donors who did not report or were not aware of a preexisting exclusionary condition. For example, a patient with a hemoglobin level below 12.5 g/dL will be deferred from donation, as it may be an indicator of anemia or other hemoglobinopathy such as thalassemia. The most common cause of temporary deferral is low hemoglobin (46%) with a major subset of these as a result of anemia (18%).[25] Nonetheless, undiagnosed individuals may still enter the donor pool. Below are some of the most common hematological conditions that have an impact on blood donation and transfusion.

Hemoglobinopathies and Thalassemia

Hemoglobinopathies are genetic or acquired abnormalities in the production of hemoglobin. Thalassemia, considered the most common inherited disease in the world, and found often in populations of middle-eastern origin, includes two varieties based on production imbalance in hemoglobin A1 globin chains. Specifically, α-thalassemia is caused by a mutation in one of the four genes that end codes the two α-globin chains of hemoglobin A1 and β-thalassemia is caused by a mutation in one of the two genes encoding the two β-globin chain. Primary laboratory indicators of thalassemia include hematological analysis of red cell indices and morphology, which can be followed by genetic testing for differential diagnosis.[26] Thalassemias are of importance to the blood bank practice, not only because of their roles in donor deferral, but also because treatment for thalassemia is often performed through therapeutic blood donation, sometimes as often as twice per month in these patients.

Polycythemia Vera

Polycythemia vera (PV) is a disease that mediates erythrocyte destruction (erythrocytosis), primarily in older male patients. These patients are often characterized by increased red blood cell production and coagulopathy. However, the patients may be asymptomatic. Although not considered a cancer, it can progress to myelodysplasic syndrome and acute leukemia in up to 5% of cases. Diagnosis of a PV is made through a combination of clinical and laboratory findings.[27]. Laboratory indicators include an increased hematocrit, increased neutrophil populations, and thrombocytosis. It may also progress toward other hematological malignancies. Blood safety is a major rationale for the deferral of donors with known PV, based on its association with malignancies and RBC functional disorders.

Autoimmune Hemolytic Anemia

RBC destruction can occur as a result of IgG and IgM responses to antigens on the surface of erythrocytes in a cluster of diseases called autoimmune hemolytic anemia (AIHA). The interaction between Ig Fc or complement can lead to the removal of erythrocytes from the circulation through macrophage phagocytosis within the spleen. The most common AIHA is caused by warm-reactive autoantibodies, which occur at physiological temperatures (37°C). While warm-reactive autoantibodies can be detected in the immunohematology laboratory through DAT testing, donor populations are often excluded from donation due to the presence of low hemoglobin and hematocrit values.

▶ Pernicious Anemia

Another anemia with potential immune detection is pernicious anemia, a megaloblastic anemia caused by a patient's inability to secrete intrinsic factor (IF) that results in a vitamin B12 deficiency. Specific assays detect antibodies toward IF. The presence of these antibodies, and antibodies against parietal cells of the gastrointestinal track, have been suggestive that pernicious anemia is an autoimmune disorder.

An Approach to Autoimmune Encephalopathy Diagnosis, Including Neural Antibody Testing Algorithms

Andrew McKeon, MD, D (ABMLI)

▶ Neural-Specific Autoantibody Profiles

Detection of certain neural autoantibodies in serum or CSF is consistent with a diagnosis of an autoimmune encephalopathy and helps direct a search for cancer.[41] Screening tests for these autoantibodies include immunofluorescence (tissue-based or cell-based) and immunoprecipitation assays. In some instances, reflex testing may be indicated to confirm antigen-specificity (by Western blot) or to quantitate an endpoint value or titer. The testing algorithms for the three disease states are similar. Some autoantibodies are more readily detected in serum (e.g., Lgi1-IgG) and others in CSF (e.g., NMDA receptor antibody); thus, the diagnostic yield is maximized by testing both serum and CSF, simultaneously or sequentially.

Seropositivity for non-neural antibodies warrants detailed investigation for an autoimmune pathogenesis for encephalopathy, dementia, or epilepsy. Informative non-neural autoantibody specificities may be organ-specific (such as thyroid autoantibodies) or nonorgan specific (such as antinuclear, anti-smooth muscle, or antimitochondrial antibodies). These markers per se lack specificity for neurological autoimmunity. The detection in CSF of elevated protein, white cell count, CSF-exclusive oligoclonal bands, IgG index, or IgG synthesis rate also support an autoimmune etiology. However, these parameters lack specificity for an autoimmune cause and may be detected in other inflammatory CNS disorders for which there are no specific biomarkers, e.g., multiple sclerosis, sarcoidosis.

▶ Oncological Significance

Algorithmic testing for autoantibody profiles is a more sensitive diagnostic strategy than nominal physician-selected, single antibody testing. For example, seropositivity for amphiphysin-IgG predicts either small-cell carcinoma or breast adenocarcinoma, but the presence or absence of coexisting antibodies narrows that differential diagnosis. Among 63 Mayo Clinic patients with amphiphysin antibody and a known history of cancer, 33 had small-cell lung carcinoma. Of those 33 patients, 27 had one or more coexisting neural-specific autoantibodies, which also predicted small-cell carcinoma. In contrast, no coexisting autoantibody was detected among 30 amphiphysin-IgG-positive patients in whom breast adenocarcinoma or other cancer type was found.

The frequency of cancer detection in seropositive patients varies from 20% for VGKC-complex IgG, to 80% for ANNA-1 (pulmonary or extra-pulmonary small–cell carcinoma in almost all cases). Suspicion of a paraneoplastic cause may be raised by risk factors obtained from the clinical history. This suspicion may be honed to a search for a specific cancer based on the profile of autoantibodies detected. A thorough physical examination and computerized tomography (CT) of chest, abdomen, and pelvis are commonly undertaken as primary screening tests. Other tests may be required depending age, sex, and other risk factors. Pelvic ultrasound (including transvaginal imaging) or MRI and gynecological examination are required to evaluate for ovarian carcinoma or teratoma. Mammography and breast examination are required to evaluate for breast carcinomas. Testicular ultrasound, prostate-specific antigen (PSA) testing and prostate examination by digital rectal examination are required to evaluate for testicular and prostate carcinomas, respectively. When neuroblastoma is suspected, and CT body imaging is negative, a radiolabeled MIBG (metaiodobenzylguanidine) body scan should be considered. Endoscopic examination of the upper and lower gastrointestinal tracts and bronchial tree should also be considered where appropriate. Positron emission tomography coregistered with CT (PET CT) imaging increases the diagnostic yield for cancer by 20% for patients in whom standard evaluations have not revealed cancer.[42]

▶ Implications for Treatment

The profile of antibodies detected may guide immunotherapy, and may also be informative for neurological prognosis. Studies suggest that autoimmune neurological disorders for which the antigens of marker IgGs are intracellular, such as Hu, rarely improve with antibody-depleting therapies. On the other hand, IgGs targeting neural cell surface receptors (such as the NMDA receptor IgG) do have a pathogenic role in effecting autoimmune CNS disorders, which may remit after antibody-depleting immunotherapy. Serial trials of corticosteroids, intravenous immune globulin, and plasma exchange are considered first-line treatments to establish immunotherapy responsiveness. Some patients, such as those with autoimmune NMDA receptor encephalitis, may require many months of treatment. Early use of immunosuppressants such as rituximab or cyclophosphamide may be required to maximize recovery.

▶ References

1. Tas AC. The use of physiological solutions or media in calcium phosphate synthesis and processing. *Acta Biomater.* 2014;10(5):1771–1792.

2. *Thermo Scientific Pierce Assay Development Technical Handbook.* United States. 2011.

3. Schiettecatte J, Anckaert E, Smitz J. Interferences in Immunoassays. In: Chiu NHL, ed. *Advances in Immunoassay Technology*: InTech; 2012.

4. Bass JJ, Wilkinson DJ, Rankin D, et al. An overview of technical considerations for Western blotting applications to physiological research. *Scand J Med Sci Sports.* 2017;27(1):4–25.

5. Santos NC, Figueira-Coelho J, Martins-Silva J, et al. Multidisciplinary utilization of dimethyl sulfoxide: pharmacological, cellular, and molecular aspects. *Biochem Pharmacol.* 2003;65(7):1035–1041.

6. Chan WY, Kohsaka S, Rezaie P. The origin and cell lineage of microglia: new concepts. *Brain Res Rev.* 2007;53(2):344–354.

7. Leenaars M, Hendriksen CF. Critical steps in the production of polyclonal and monoclonal antibodies: evaluation and recommendations. *ILAR J.* 2005;46(3): 269–279.

8. Hansen DT, Robida MD, Craciunescu FM, et al. Polyclonal antibody production for membrane proteins via genetic immunization. *Sci Rep.* 2016;6(21925).

9. Campbell AM. *Monoclonal Antibody and Immunosensor Technology: The production and application of rodent and human monoclonal antibodies.* Amsterdam: Elsevier; 1991.

10. Greenfield EA. Generating Monoclonal Antibodies. *Antibodies: A Laboratory Manual, Second Edition.* Second ed. Cold Spring Harbor: Cold Spring Harbor Laboratory Press; 2014:201–221.

11. Alphabetical Index: monoclonal & polyclonal antibodies. 2017;http://www.sigmaaldrich.com/life-science/cell-biology /antibodies/antibody-products.html?TablePage=14574648.

12. Sephton CF, Good SK, Atkin S, et al. TDP-43 is a developmentally regulated protein essential for early embryonic development. *J Biol Chem.* 2009;285(9): 6826–6834.

13. Köhler G, Milstein C. Continuous cultures of fused cells secreting antibody of predefined specificity. *Nature.* 1975;256(5517):495–497.

14. The Nobel Prize in Physiology or Medicine 1984. 2014; https://www.nobelprize.org/prizes/medicine/1984 /summary/.

15. R Edwards SB, I Howes. Principles of Immunodiangostics tests and their development: with specific use of radioisotopes as tracers. In: Edwards R, ed. *Immunodiagnostics: A Practical Approach*: Oxford University Press; 1999.

16. Methods of Producing Monoclonal Antibodies. In: Committee NRCU, ed. Washington DC: National Acadamies Press; 1999.

17. Apiratmateekul N, Phunpae P, Kasinrerk W. A modified hybridoma technique for production of monoclonal antibodies having desired isotypes. *Cytotechnology.* 2009;60(1–3):53.

18. Li F, Vijayasankaran N, Shen AY, et al. Cell culture processes for monoclonal antibody production. *MAbs.* 2010;2(5):466–479.

19. Kurosawa Yoshioka MN, Isobe M. Target-selective homologous recombination cloning for high-throughput generation of monoclonal antibodies from single plasma cells. *BMC Biotechnol.* 2011(11):39–47.

20. Kivi G, Teesalu K, Parik J, et al. HybriFree: a robust and rapid method for the development of monoclonal antibodies from different host species. *BMC Biotechnol.* 2016;16(2).

21. Hjelm B, Forsström B, Igel U, et al. Generation of monospecific antibodies based on affinity capture of polyclonal antibodies. *Protein Sci.* 2011; 20(11): 1824–1835.

22. Ficoll-Paque PLUS: Instructions 71-7167-00 AG. *Cell Preparation.* www.gelifesciences.com/cellprep: GE healthcare Bio-Sceince AB; 2007:16.

23. Sample handling guide. 2013. http://www.lencolab.com /doctors/sample_handling_guide.html. Accessed June 10, 2017.

24. General guidelines. 2017. http://www.questdiagnostics .com/home/physicians/testing-services/specialists /hospitals-lab-staff/specimen-handling/general.html. Accessed June 10, 2017.

25. Nucifora K. The importance of proper specimen collection and handling. 2015; https://www.labtestingmatters.org/the -importance-of-proper-specimen-collection-and -handling/. Accessed June 12, 2017.

26. Laboratories MM. Specimen Collection and Preparation Guide. In: Clinic M, ed. Rochester. 2016.

27. Specimen Labeling, Storage & Handling Guidelines. 2017; https://www.cdc.gov/urdo/downloads/specstoragehandling .pdf.

28. Austria G. Specimin Collection & Handling Manual, Laboratory. In: Health P, ed. 8 ed. 2014.

29. Geisinger. Blood Specimen Collection and Processing. 2016; https://www.geisingermedicallabs.com/catalog/blood _specimens.shtml. Accessed Jun 10, 2017.

30. Laboratories A. General Specimen Handling. ACL Laboratories 2017.

31. Centers for Disease Control and Prevention (CDC.) Specimen Labeling, Storage, & Handling. Georgia: CDC.

32. Clatworthy AL. Neural-immune interactions—an evolutionary perspective. *Neuroimmunomodulation.* 1998; 5(3–4):136–142.

33. Fang C, Otero HJ, Greenberg D, et al. Cost-utility analyses of diagnostic laboratory tests: a systematic review. *Value Health.* 2011;14(8):1010–1018.

34. Shin KH, Kim HH, Chang CL, et al. Economic and workflow analysis of a blood bank automated system. *Ann Lab Med.* 2013;33(4):268–273.

35. Smith CI, Islam KB, Vorechovský I, et al. X-linked agammaglobulinemia and other immunoglobulin deficiencies. *Immunol Rev.* 1994;138:159–183.

36. Qamar N, Fuleihan RL. The hyper IgM syndromes. *Clin Rev Allergy Immunol.* 2014;46(2):120–130.

37. Cotta-de-Almeida V, Dupré L, Guipouy D, et al. Signal integration during T lymphocyte activation and function: lessons from the Wiskott-Aldrich syndrome. *Frontiers Immunol.* 2015;6:47.

38. Geier CB, Piller A, Linder A, et al. Leaky RAG deficiency in adult patients with impaired antibody production against bacterial polysaccharide antigens. *PLoS One.* 2015;10(7):e0133220.

39. Allenspach E, Rawlings DJ, Scharenberg AM. X-Linked Severe Combined Immunodeficiency. In: Pagon RA, Adam MP, Ardinger HH, et al., eds. *GeneReviews(R).* Seattle (WA)1993.

40. Nicolaou O, Kousios A, Hadjisavvas A, et al. Biomarkers of systemic lupus erythematosus identified using mass

spectrometry-based proteomics: a systematic review. *J Cell Mol Med.* 2017;21(5):993–1012.

41. Gomez-Tourino I, Arif S, Eichmann M, et al. T cells in type 1 diabetes: instructors, regulators and effectors: a comprehensive review. *J Autoimmun.* 2016;66:7–16.

42. Touzeau C, Moreau P, Dumontet C. Monoclonal antibody therapy in multiple myeloma. *Leukemia.* 2017;31(5): 1039–1047.

43. Zhao W, Ji X, Zhang F, et al. Embryonic stem cell markers. *Molecules.* 2012;17(6):6196–6236.

44. Placzek MR, Chung IM, Macedo HM, et al. Stem cell bioprocessing: fundamentals and principles. *J R Soc Interface.* 2009;6(32):209–232.

45. Brohlin M, Mahay D, Novikov LN, et al. Characterisation of human mesenchymal stem cells following differentiation into Schwann cell-like cells. *Neurosci Res.* 2009;64(1): 41–49.

46. Chiotaki R, Polioudaki H, Theodoropoulos PA. Cancer stem cells in solid and liquid tissues of breast cancer patients: characterization and therapeutic perspectives. *Curr Cancer Drug Targets.* 2015;15(3):256–269.

47. Kerosuo L, Bronner-Fraser M. What is bad in cancer is good in the embryo: importance of EMT in neural crest development. *Seminars Cell Dev Biol.* 2012;23(3):320–332.

48. Vas V, Wandhoff C, Dörr K, et al. Contribution of an aged microenvironment to aging-associated myeloproliferative disease. *PLoS One.* 2012;7(2):e31523.

49. Nery AA, Nascimento IC, Glaser T, et al. Human mesenchymal stem cells: from immunophenotyping by flow cytometry to clinical applications. *Cytometry A.* 2013;83(1):48–61.

50. Davies EG. Immunodeficiency in Digeorge syndrome and options for treating cases with complete athymia. *Front Immunol.* 2013;4:322.

51. Markert ML, Marques JG, Neven B, et al. First use of thymus transplantation therapy for FOXN1 deficiency (nude/ SCID): a report of 2 cases. *Blood.* 2011;117(2):688–696.

52. Pitkänen J, Peterson P. Autoimmune regulator: from loss of function to autoimmunity. *Genes Immun.* 2003;4(1):12–21.

53. Bansal K, Yoshida H, Benoist C, et al. The transcriptional regulator Aire binds to and activates super-enhancers. *Nat Immunol.* 2017;18(3):263–273.

54. Dooley J, Liston A. Molecular control over thymic involution: from cytokines and microRNA to aging and adipose tissue. *Eur J Immunol.* 2012;42(5):1073–1079.

55. Lio CWJ, Hsieh CS. A two-step process for thymic regulatory T-cell development. *Immunity.* 2008;28(1): 100–111.

56. Young NS, Calado RT, Scheinberg P. Current concepts in the pathophysiology and treatment of aplastic anemia. *Blood.* 2006;108(8):2509–2519.

57. Blood Donor History Questionnaires. 2018; http://www.aabb.org/tm/questionnaires/Pages/dhqaabb.aspx. Accessed September 28, 2018.

Glossary

12/23 Rule A V(J)D recombination rule in which genes with a 12 nucleotide spacer can be combined only with genes that have a 23 nucleotide spacer.

510(k) A type of Food and Drug Administration premarket submission that demonstrates that a new device is at least as safe and effective as a predicate (existing approved) device on the market.

A

Acoustic dispensing Also known as acoustic droplet ejection; a technique used in the engineering of noncontact liquid dispensers. Uses a pulse of ultrasound to move low volumes without physical contact.

Acquired immunodeficiency syndrome (AIDS) Caused by the HIV-1 or HIV-2 virus; is characterized by the inactivation or destruction of T-lymphocytes of the CD4 subset leading to increased susceptibility to infection and disease.

Activation-Induced Cytidine Deaminase (AID) Enzyme that converts cytidine (C) residues in DNA into Uridine (U) in single-stranded DNA.

Acute An early infection/disease period wherein a higher than normal or initial increase in antibody production is observed. Early phase of antibody detection.

Acute hemolytic transfusion reaction (AHTR) a type of HTR associated with rapid hemolysis within 24 hours of transfusion.

Addison disease An autoimmune acquired form of primary adrenal insufficiency.

Adenovirus A common group of double stranded DNA viruses that infect the eyes, lungs, intestine and nervous system. A causative agent for the cold. Used in viral immune therapies due to board infectivity.

Adjuvant A substance that enhances the immune response to an antigen.

Adsorption The process of adhesion of molecules to a surface for the separation of products.

Aerobic Involving or requiring oxygen.

Aerosolization Spreading through the air.

Affinity A bond at a single binding site, or a single antigen with a single Fab region of an antibody.

Affinity maturation A process by which activated B cells produce antibodies of increased affinity to an antigen through TfH cell stimulation.

Agglutination The formation of large complexes from the association of particulate antigens, i.e., attached to particles or cells, with specific antibodies.

Agglutination inhibition A competitive assay in which patient antigens and particulate kit antigens compete for antibody. The lack of agglutination is seen as positive for antigenic presence in the patient.

Agglutinogen A substance that produces an agglutinin; antibody that agglutinates cells, acting as an antigen.

Aliquots The portions of a larger sample or stock reagent used for separate storage or individual analysis.

Alternative pathway Antibody-independent activation of the complement system.

Amoebiasis Also known as amoebic dysentery; infection with amoebas from the Entamoeba group.

Amorph A gene that does not produce a detectable antigen, such as the O blood group.

Anaerobic Not involving or requiring oxygen.

Analyte A general term for any substance being measured or identified.

Anamnestic response Also an immune response; a defensive reaction in the body after recognition of foreign substances in which antibodies against antigens are formed.

ANAs Anti-nuclear antibodies; are tested in patient serum or CFS as a nonspecific indicator of autoimmune diseases and used in the diagnosis of systemic lupus erythematosus.

Antibodies Also known as soluble immunoglobins (Igs); they are specific glycoproteins produced in response to antigenic stimulus. They have a range of specificities determined through V(J)D rearrangement and are found in serum, plasma, and other body fluids.

Antibody-antigen complex A fixed amount of antibody combined with antigen in a structured array.

Antibody titer Also referred to as titer; it is the lowest concentration of an antibody that can elicit a detectable reaction during an immunoassay. Reported as the inverse of the dilution factor, i.e., a titer of 8 is reported for a 1:8 dilution.

Antiglobulin An antibody directed against gamma globulin (Ig), used to bind human Ig in immunoassays. See Direct and Indirect antiglobulin tests.

Antiphospholipid syndrome A syndrome defined by the presence of at least one of these clinical disorders, and seropositivity for one or more of phospholipid antibodies (namely cardiolipin antibody, β2 glycoprotein-I antibody, and phosphatidylserine–prothrombin complex antibodies), or detection of lupus anticoagulant activity.

Antiserum Serum containing antibodies against specific antigens.

Antithrombin (AT) is a glycoprotein in the coagulation pathway that inactivates a number of enzymes including thrombin.

Apurinic/apyrimidinic endonuclease (APE1) An enzyme involved in DNA base excision repair activated during class switching.

Arbovirus A generalized name for any viruses that are passed or transmitted by arthropods; most commonly the tick, the culex, and the aedes mosquito; members include the flaviviridae, togaviridae, bunyaviridae, and reoviridae families.

Arthroconidia A type of fungal spore produced by hyphae segmentation.

Autoimmune regulator (AIRE) A transcription factor that is expressed in the thymus, which drives transcription of tissue-specific genes so that more diversity of self-antigen is present in the thymus for negative selection of T cells.

Avidity The overall strength of binding between an antibody and antigen.

Axonemes Microtubule cytoskeleton at the core of cilium or flagellum.

B

Bacillus anthracis The etiologic agent of anthrax.

Balanced salt solutions Saline buffering systems for long-term storage of cellular components.

Basophils Granulocytes involved in decreasing clotting through heparin and in the allergic immune response.

B-cell Lymphoid cell containing the BCR and responsible for antibody production, produced in the bone marrow.

BCR The defining receptor of the B-cell, which is structurally identical to the antibody from the same B-cell; ostensibly a membrane-bound antibody.

Biohazardous Pertaining to biohazards; any biological substance that may pose a risk to the health of a living organism.

Biosensor An analytical tool for the detection of biological substances through a physicochemical detector. Includes three parts: analyte recognition signal, signal transducer, and readout device.

Blastoconidia A unit of asexual reproduction in budding yeast and other fungi; seen physically via microscopy.

Blastomycosis Infection caused by the soil fungus Blastomyces.

Bombay Phenotype A phenotype in individuals with normal A and B genes but no A and B antigen expression resulting from a missing H antigen. They may have anti-H in their serum.

Bovine serum albumin Used as a protein standard for many experiments, but it is more commonly used as a blocking agent.

Bullous pemphigoid An autoimmune blistering disease targeting adhesion molecules that are part of the hemidesmosomes at the dermal–epidermal junction.

Burkitts Lymphoma A form of non-Hodgkin's lymphoma, which starts in the B-cell leading to impaired immunity.

C

Calcium release-activated channels (CRAC) Specialized calcium channels in the cell membrane that replenish calcium in the cell.

Calibrators A device or series of substances used to adjust the accuracy of an assay or instrument.

California Encephalitis Group Viral group including pathogenic members such as La Cross Virus. Transmitted by mosquito.

Candidiasis A fungal infection due to the yeast candida.

CD3 Cluster of differentiation 3; a portion of the TCR and the defining immune marker for all T lymphocytes.

CD4 Cluster of differentiation 4; the defining immune marker of T helper cells; also called CD4 T cells.

CD8 Cluster of differentiation 8, the defining immune marker of cytotoxic T cells; also called CD8 T cells.

CD markers Cluster of differentiation (or cluster designation) markers are any of several hundred cellular antigens used for immunophenotyping.

Celiac sprue Also known as celiac disease; an autoimmune disease affecting the small bowel mucosa triggered by ingestion of gliadin protein of gluten in genetically susceptible individuals.

Centers for Medicare and Medicaid Services (CMS) Part of the United States Department of Health and Human Services that is responsible for management of several federal healthcare-related programs, including Medicare and Medicaid.

Centroblasts An enlarged B-cell proliferating in a germinal center.

Centrocytes A nondividing centroblast that functions to test the affinity of BCRs.

Chemiluminescence The emission of light from chemical reaction that does not produce significant heat.

Chemokines Subset of cytokines, both soluble and insoluble, that provide molecular cues for cellular migration.

Chikungunya virus A disease causing virus spread by mosquitoes. Commonly causes fever and joint pain.

Chimeric antigen receptor T cells (CAR-T cells) Autologous patient T cells transduced with a chimeric antigen receptor that contains an antibody fragment that recognizes a surface marker found on a tumor. In the current clinical setting, this surface marker is usually CD19.

Chromotrope An acid dye.

Cilia Plural for cilium; short hairline vibrating appendages found on many cell types including bacteria and protozoa, which provide motility.

Citrullinated peptides A peptide modification that commonly forms autoantibodies seen in rheumatoid arthritis.

Classical pathway Complement activation through an antibody-dependent trigger.

Class switching A process occurring in mature B cells in which the immunoglobin isotype is changed to best respond to the infection or pathogen.

Class switch recombination (CSR) See Class switching.

Clinical Laboratory Improvement Amendments (CLIA) Federal regulations that apply specifically to the management and oversight of quality and safety of clinical laboratories in the United States.

Clonal expansion An adaptive immune system process in which a small number of precursor lymphocytes differentiate into specific effector and memory phenotypes.

Clot A mass of coagulated blood.

Cluster of Differentiation (CD) Also known as cluster of designation or classification determinant; is a process for defining immune cells in immunophenotyping through the use of cell surface marker profiles.

CNS Central Nervous System.

Coagglutination The specific name of a series of reverse passive agglutination tests in which bacteria, most commonly *Staphylococcus aureus*, are used as the inert particle.

Coccidian coccidia-like. Single-celled intracellular parasites.

Coccidioidomycosis Infection caused by inhaling spores of Coccidiodes immitis or posadasii.

Code of Federal Regulations A master document containing all of the permanent rules and regulations issued by the government of the United States of America; it includes all rules and regulations published in the Federal Register by departments and agencies within the government.

Colonize In microbiology, the establishment of a microorganism in a specific location, followed by its growth and proliferation.

Common lymphoid progenitors Immature cells of the lymphocyte lineage leading to B and T lymphocytes.

Competitive Assay Also known as hemophilic; a binding assay based on competition between labeled and unlabeled tracers for a limited number of antibody binding sites.

Complement-dependent microcytoxicity (CDC) Also complement-dependent cytotoxicity assay and lymphocyte cytotoxicity test; an assay performed for serological typing of HLA as well as for antibody screening and characterization prior to transplant.

Complement fixation The process of binding serum complement to an antibody-antigen complex. A complement fixation test is an immunoassay in which complement is added to detect the presence of a specific antibody or antigen based on whether cell lysis occurs; lysis occurs in the absence of the specific analyte examined.

Confocal microscopy A microscopic imaging technique for increasing optical resolution via a spatial pinhole to block out-of-focus light; forms include confocal laser scanning and confocal scanning microscopy.

Conidia A fungal spore formed at the end of hyphae for asexual reproduction.

Conidiophores A hypha containing a conidium; asexual fungal body.

Conjugated A chemical linking of two molecules; e.g., antibodies are conjugated to tracer molecules for use in the assay design.

Constant region Portion of the immunoglobulin heavy and light chain that determines the immunoglobin class. It is connected to two variable regions.

Continuing education Learning activities designed to keep healthcare professionals up-to-date on advances and specialization areas after formal education has ended.

Convalescent Later or postinfection period wherein an increased level of antigen-specific antibody can be found in a host. Later-phase antibody detection.

Coronaviruses A common virus type that infects the nose, sinuses, and throat.

Cryptococcosis An infection of the pulmonary system caused by inhalation of Cryptococcus neoformans or gattii.

Cyst A typically noncancerous growth filled with liquid that may contain pathogens.

Cytokine release syndrome (CRS) A potentially life threatening toxicity caused by massive cytokine release that can occur with CAR-T cell therapy due to an overly robust immune response.

Cytokines Soluble messengers that bind receptors on cell surface and initiate gene expression changes.

Cytomegalovirus (CMV) Member of the herpes virus family that causes mononucleosis-like syndromes and must be differentiated serologically from Epstein Barr.

Cytotoxic-T-lymphocyte-associated protein 4 (CTLA4) A surface receptor on activated T cells similar in structure to CD28 that adds in T-cell activation.

Cytotoxic T cells CD8+ cells; also known as killer T cells; involved in the destruction of infected and cancerous cells.

D

D-dimer A fibrin degradation product consisting of two fibrin proteins and used as a clinical indicator of fibrinolysis.

Delayed hemolytic transfusion reaction (DHTR) A type of HTR associated with hemolysis seen days to months after transfusion.

Dendritic cells (DCs) Antigen presenting cells (APCs) that act at the interface of innate and adaptive immune responses.

Dengue virus A single-positive RNA virus in the Flaviviridae family that is the causative agent for Denque Fever.

Diluent The major component of a solution. In physiological assays, this may often be a saline solution in which a solute is dissolved for dilution studies or in reagent prep.

Dimethyl sulfoxide (DMSO) A widely available, inexpensive liquid byproduct of the paper industry; is used as a vehicle for the delivery of drugs to cells, as a solvent, and in the fixation of cells.

Direct agglutination The use of serum antibodies to detect specific cells through their agglutination. One variant is hem-agglutination.

Direct agglutination assay An assay in which a cell (bacterial or mammalian) is the agglutinin in a response.

Direct antiglobulin test (assay) (DAT) Also direct Coombs test; used in blood bank serology to indicate if a red blood cell has been coated in vivo with antibody or complement; the addition of anti-human globulin and visual indication of agglutination is considered positive. It maintains limited utility clinically in cases of autoimmune hemolytic anemia.

Direct fluorescent antibody technique (DFA) A fluorescently conjugated antibody binds directly to the antigen of interest in a specimen for detection.

Direct transmission Also contact transmission; a pathogen spread directly through physical interaction with an infected host.

Double-stranded DNA (dsDNA) Is a common target of ANAs found in autoimmune disease.

Double diffusion Also known as Ouchterlony; a precipitation method in which both antigen and antibodies are placed in separate wells within a soft agar or agarose. Used for identification and quantification of antigens or antibodies.

Double negative (DN) cells Immature T cells that lack both CD4 and CD8 expression.

Double positive (DP) cells Immature T cells that still contain both CD4 and CD8 expression.

Dysjunctor cells A fungal cell structure that undergoes lysis to release conidium.

E

Eastern Equine Encephalitis A viral mediated brain infection spread via mosquitoes infected with Eastern Equine Encephalitis Virus (EEEV).

EDTA Acronym for ethylenediaminetetraacetic acid, a common anticoagulant to prevent the coagulation of blood via calcium chelation.

Electrophoresis Separation of molecules such as proteins, in an electrical field based on differences in charge and size.

Elimination phase The phase of immunoediting that encompasses the classical concept of immunosurveillance where the immune system detects and eliminates incipient neoplasm before the development of frank cancer.

Emergency Use Authorization (EUA) A tool/process through which the FDA Commissioner may allow unapproved medical products to be used publicly during an emergency related to the diagnosis, treatment, or prevention of serious or life-threatening conditions.

Encephalopathy A general term for brain disease, injury, malfunction, and damage.

Endemic A disease or infection type found regularly in an area or group.

Enterovirus A genus of RNA viruses with 71 distinguished serotypes that are named for their transmission through the intestine. Includes the polio virus and Coxsackie viruses.

Enzyme-linked immunosorbent assays (ELISA) Commonly considered a backbone method for diagnostic testing in infectious disease; the sample is exposed to the antibody-enzyme complex, allowing Ab-Ag specific binding to occur, bound molecules are immobilized, and unbound antibody and sample are washed; levels of the patient antigen are quantified by enzymatic activity through reactions with a colored substrate.

Enzyme A substance that acts as a catalyst for a biochemical reaction.

Enzyme immunoassay (EIA) Analogous to the RIA but instead using an enzyme-linked reagent where measurement is determined by examining the turnover of substrate into product.

Enzyme Multiplied Immunoassay Technique (EMIT) Also known as EMIA, is a variation on the EIA; in this assay, an excess of antibody is added and followed by an antigen-enzyme complex in which the unbound complex acts on the colored substrate.

Epitope In immunology, the portion of an antigen with which an immune response is directed. Generally, the specific binding domain involved in a coupling/interaction. Modifications to the domain can increase or decrease affinity.

Epstein Barr Virus (EBV) Member of the herpes virus family that causes classical infectious mononucleosis, and is thought to be involved in malignancies such as Burkitts Lymphoma.

Equilibrium constant $K = K1/K2 = [AgAb]/[Ab][Ag]$; where bracketed quantities represent the concentration of complex (AgAb), antibody (Ab), and antigen (Ag). The constant K is a measure of goodness of fit and depends on the avidity and total strength of molecular interactions between the antibody and antigen. High affinity and high avidity both push toward an increase in complex or the rate of K1.

Equilibrium phase The phase of immunoediting in which the tumor is incompletely removed; however, the immune system has kept the tumor relatively controlled, producing a latency period.

Equimolar Containing the same number of moles of products in a solution, i.e., antibodies to antigen.

ERK Extracellular signal-regulated Kinase; part of the MEK/ERK pathway of intracellular signaling leading to gene transcriptional changes after TCR stimulation. Often used as an indication of TCR activation in cellular assays.

Erythrocyte Another name for red blood cells (RBCs); normally a biconcave disc without a nucleus, they transport hemoglobin throughout the body and get their color from the iron within.

Escape phase The phase of immunoediting in which "edited" malignant cells surviving the equilibrium phase are no longer restrained by the innate or adaptive immune system.

Etanercept A TNF inhibitor classically used to treat autoimmune diseases like rheumatoid arthritis.

Ethymic progenitors (ETP) The first defined stage of T-cell lineage specification from the common lymphoid progenitor (CLP) stage.

Eukaryotic An organism/cell that has an enclosed nucleus and cytoplasmic organelles.

Event In flow cytometry, this is one recorded measurement reading, typically from a single cell and fluorescence sensor.

Excyst To emerge from a cyst.

F

Fab A fragment of an immunoglobulin molecule cleaved by the enzyme papain. Includes one light chain and half of a heavy chain bound by a disulfide bond. Two Fab fragments are obtained from each immunoglobulin during papain cleavage. Includes the antigenic binding domain.

Factor XIII Also known as fibrin stabilizing factor, it is an enzyme that crosslinks with fibrin during coagulation.

Fc A fragment of an immunoglobulin molecule cleaved by the enzyme papain. Includes two halves of a heavy chain bound by a disulfide bond. The fragment of an immunoglobulin that binds to the Fc receptors.

Febrile nonhemolytic transfusion reaction (FNHTR) A transfusion reaction associated with fever but not hemolysis.

Fetal calf serum Also known as fetal bovine serum; the most widely used serum supplement for in vitro cell culture.

Fibrinogen Also known as Factor I, one of the most clinically important coagulations factors, it produces fibrin through the enzyme thrombin.

Final Rule Detailed rules and regulations in final draft form, published by various agencies and departments of the government of the United States of America; usually published or announced within the Federal Register.

Flagella Whip-like appendages on a cell or microorganism providing motion.

Flagellates A microorganism that has flagella.

Flaviviruses Viruses of the Flaviviridae family. RNA viruses found in arthropods that can infect humans.

Flocculation Formation of fluffy masses of precipitate that occur within a narrow range of antigen concentration.

Flow cell A chamber through which cells/particles pass in single file for sample acquisition via laser-stimulated light emission.

Flow cytometry A technology used to analyze surface and subsurface components of cell populations in a specimen through fluorescence antibody detection recorded as events in computerized plots. Important in the immunophenotyping of cells for changes in population density as well as antigenic expression levels.

Fluorescein A commonly used fluorochrome used in microscopy and flow cytometry; it absorbs light at 494 nm and emits light at 512 nm.

Fluorescein isothiocyanate (FITC) A derivative of fluorescein functionalized with an isothiocyanate reactive group; the most widely used fluorochrome tracer.

Fluorescence immunoassays (FIA) Also known as fluoroimmunoassays; this assay is analogous to the RIA but uses a fluorophore label.

Fluorescence polarization immunoassays (FPIA) A fluorescent homogenous assay that does not require the separation of the free and complexed tracers.

Fluorescence Stimulated emission of light radiation as a result of incident light radiation.

Fluorochomes Also fluorophores; a fluorescent chemical, which, when stimulated by light of a specific wavelength spectrum, can re-emit light at a different wavelength.

Follicular T cells (Tfh) Specialized CD4+ T cells that stimulate better antibody production through their interaction with B cells.

Fomites Materials likely to carry infections such as clothing, utensils, and other objects.

Food, Drug, and Cosmetic Act (FD&C) Laws passed in 1938 by the government of the United States of America that charge the FDA with oversight of safety of food, drugs, and cosmetics.

Food and Drug Administration (FDA) The federal agency within the government of the United States of America responsible for oversight of safety of food, drugs, and cosmetics.

G

GAD65 Glutamic Acid Decarboxylase 65; is a biomarker of autoimmune central nervous system (CNS) disorders and other autoimmune disorders.

Germinal center Location within secondary lymphoid tissues, such as lymph nodes, where B cells differentiate, proliferate, and undergo antibody rearrangement.

Giardiasis Infection with *Giardia duodenalis.*

Goodpasture's disease Also known as anti-glomerular basement membrane (GBM) disease; an autoimmune disease directed at the alpha 3 chain of type IV collagen, leading to glomerulonephritis and lung hemorrhage.

Graft-versus host disease (GVHD) A transplant disorder in which the grafted tissue attacks the host tissue resulting from grafted immune cells; particularly common in stem cell and bone marrow transplants.

Granulocyte Leukocytes with secretory granules in the cytoplasm, including basophils, neutrophils, and eosinophils. Related to and/or derived from myelocytes.

Granulomatous A disease indication characterized by the formation of a granuloma; a cluster of immune cells, predominantly macrophages; caused by bacterial and fungal species.

Guillain-Barre A rare disorder (or syndrome) in which the immune system attacks the nervous system; leading to tingling, weakness, and eventual paralysis.

H

Hapten A small molecule that can act as an immunogen when coupled with a larger carrier molecule.

hCG Human chorionic gonadotropin; a hormone produced during pregnancy but also upregulated in some cancers.

Helminth eggs Eggs of the parasite worm known as helminths.

Hemagglutination The specific agglutination of red cells from specific antibody binding to antigens on their cell surface.

Hematopoietic stem cells (HSCs) Stem cells that give rise to all other blood cells in a process called hematopoiesis. Source of all erythrocytes, myelocytes, and lymphocytes.

Hemolysin A substance found in the blood that destroys red blood cells.

Hemolysis The lysis of red blood cells.

Hemolytic disease of the fetus and newborn (HDFN) A disease caused by maternal IgG antibodies crossing the placenta and attacking fetal RBCs.

Hemolytic transfusion reactions (HTR) A transfusion reaction leading to blood cell destruction caused by patient antibody to donor RBCs.

Hepatitis viruses Including viruses named hepatitis A, B, C, D, and E, they are named for causing diseases of the liver but have little else in common. The serologic approach, rather than direct detection, remains the approach of choice.

Herpes Simplex Virus (HSV) Including HSV type 1 (HSV-1) and HSV type 2 (HSV-2); causes blistering infections with HSV-1 more common in oral infections (cold sores, fever blisters) and HSV-2 more common in genital infections.

Heterogeneous Assays Assay requiring separation steps; typically requiring a solid-phase support to distinguish between bound and free fractions.

High complexity Tests that are most difficult to perform or are most subject to error and require quality control, quality assurance, proficiency testing and stricter personnel requirements. Require a CLIA certificate of compliance. The Joint Commission and CLIA indicated that high complexity testing be

performed by individuals with documented sufficient training to perform the tests; typically, a bachelors degree in a biological science including a medical laboratory science program.

Histology The study of microscopic structures in biological tissues.

Histoplasmosis One of the most common systemic fungi infections seen in the Midwest and South United States, including around the Mississippi River, the Ohio River valley, and the Appalachian Mountains. Caused by *Histoplasma capsulatum*.

Homogeneous Assays Assay requiring no separation; depends on a change in signal between bound and free fractions for detection.

Human embryonic kidney cells (HEK-293) A cell line derived from human embryonic kidney grown in culture and one of the most common used in cell biological testing.

Human epithelial type 2 cell (HEp-2) A cell line commonly used in the detection of ANAs from patient serum or CFS.

Human Immunodeficiency Virus (HIV) Including HIV-1 and HIV-2; retroviruses that lead to AIDS in undiagnosed and untreated patients. Targets CD4 T cells selectively, inactivates and destroys them.

Human leukocyte antigens (HLA) Antigen presenting MHCs of human origin. Compatibility indicators for transplant recipients.

Human T-cell lymphotropic viruses (HTLV) Retroviruses are the cause of ATLL, TSP/HAM, HAU including HTLV-1 and HTLV-2. Similar to HIV viruses but found most prominently in Southeast Asia.

Hybridization The process of combining different organisms to create a hybrid. Used as a technique for cellular studies; may occur naturally, creating resistant organisms.

Hyphae Branching filaments that make up the growing parts of a fungus.

Hypophysitis A rare condition of acute or chronic inflammation, including the autoimmune-mediated lymphocytic hypophysitis.

I

IκB An inhibitor, or one of a group of inhibitors, of the NF-κB signal transduction cascade.

Immune complexes A combination of antigen, antibody, and complement found in the blood and lymph and taken up by B cells.

Immune organs Also known as lymphoid organs; consist of both the primary and secondary lymphoid tissues.

Immune thrombocytopenia (ITP) A platelet count less than 100×10^9/L, caused by autoimmunity directed at platelets.

Immunocompromised A host with a reduced ability to fight infections.

Immunodeficient A host that lacks the ability to fight infections.

Immunodiffusion A method of detecting/measuring antibodies and antigens via precipitation after diffusion in a gel.

Immunodominant sugar Referring to a glycoprotein or glycolipid sugar that provides antigen specificity.

Immunoediting An interaction between immunosurveillance and tumor response. Made up of three phases: elimination, equilibrium, and escape.

Immunoelectrophoresis (IEP) A two-step process in which proteins are first separated by electrophoresis and then allowed to diffuse through an adjacent gel, producing precipitin arcs.

Immunofixation electrophoresis (IFE) A semiquantitative method of gel precipitation to identify abnormal bands seen in serum or other body fluid in which electrophoresed proteins are coupled to antibodies added directly to the gel in search of monoclonal antibodies.

Immunofluorescence (IF) A laboratory method in which specific antibodies are conjugated chemically to fluorescent dyes for use in fluorescence immunoassays and other antigen-binding assays.

Immunogenicity The ability of a particular antigen or other substance to initiate an immune response.

Immunoglobulins (Ig) Any of a class of proteins utilized by the immune system for antigen detection. Found in serum and other body fluids as well as associated with immune cells; e.g., BCR, IgG, IgM, IgE, IgD, and IgA. Both soluble and membrane-bound Igs are also known as antibodies.

Immunohistochemistry (IHC) Common form of immunostaining of tissues. Used to identify antigenic targets in a tissue section.

Immunophenotyping The process of specifying immune cell lineage and sublineages on the basis of cellular markers.

Immunoreagents A generalized term describing all reagents that are used in an immunoassay.

Immunosurveillance The process in which cells of the immune system look for and detect foreign particles.

Indirect agglutination assay Also passive agglutination assay, latex fixation assay; a type of agglutination assay in which the agglutination is an indicator of antibody binding to some antigen found in the specimen and bound to reagent detection particle.

Indirect antiglobulin test (IAT) Also indirect Coombs test; more common of the two antiglobulin tests performed in blood bank serology, it is used in prenatal testing of pregnant women and prior to blood transfusion for the detection of antibodies against foreign blood cells in the serum. Patient serum is incubated with foreign red cells and then has anti-human globulin added before inspection for agglutination.

Indirect fluorescent antibody technique (IFA) A secondary fluorescently conjugated antibody binds to a primary antibody bound to the antigen of interest in the specimen for detection.

Indirect transmission The spread of pathogen without direct contact with an infected host. Examples include: aerosol and interaction with fomites.

Inflammatory bowel disease (IBD) A chronic intestinal inflammatory disorder of unknown etiology.

Influenza virus Including type A and type B influenza virus, is the causative agent of the flu.

International Organization for Standardization (ISO) An international body responsible for setting standards for industrial and commercial standards.

In Vitro Diagnostics (IVDs) Laboratory tests conducted *ex vivo* that are able to detect disease or infection. Some IVDs are available for either laboratory or home use.

ITAMs (immuno-receptor tyrosine-based activation motifs); A conserved region of adaptor proteins on the cytoplasmic face of the cell membrane critical for intracellular signaling; most notably part of the TCR complex.

K

Kinases An enzyme that catalyzes the transfer of phosphates to other molecules from ATP, producing ADP and phosphorylating the molecule.

L

Laboratory Developed Tests (LDTs) IVDs that are developed, manufactured, and used by a single clinical laboratory.

Larvae Plural of larva. An immature form of an insect including various parasites.

Lateral flow immunoassay A paper-based device used in the detection of a target analyte visualized through a color change on the paper. A common design for point-of-care immunoassays.

LAT Linker for activation of T cells; A membrane protein associated with many signaling molecules involved in T-cell activation.

Law of mass action A mathematical law that describes the equilibrium relationship between soluble reactants and insoluble products that has been applied to antibody-antigen interactions.

LCK Lymphocyte-specific protein tyrosine kinase; a 56 kDA protein tyrosine kinase that specifically phosphorylates tyrosine residues in lymphocytes during intracellular signaling.

Lectin pathway Complement activation via mannan-binding lectin (MBL)

Leukocyte Another name for white blood cell (WBC); a number of pathogens and infection-activated, motile cells involved in the immune response; found throughout the body but circulating extensively in the peripheral blood.

Limited Service Laboratories Clinical laboratories that conduct a limited number of tests, primarily CLIA-waived tests. These may be an extension of a larger clinical laboratory or health system or may be stand-alone laboratories.

Linked recognition A process by which B cells are activated by helper T cells that respond to the same antigen.

Liquid-phase In contrast to solid phase, does not require a structure for separation steps and instead uses a secondary soluble reagent for byproduct removal and analyte determinations, i.e., a secondary antibody.

Lyme disease An infection caused by *Borrelia burgdorferi*; a spirochete, carried by the deer tick causing flu-like symptoms and joint pain. Characterized by a distinctive bull's eye pattern rash.

Lymphocyte A cluster of related small leukocytes (white blood cells) with a round nucleus that is responsible for most adaptive immune responses; includes both T and B lymphocytes.

Lymphoid Related to the tissues and cell lineages involved in T and B lymphocyte development.

Lymphoid tissue inducer cells (LTi) Cells involved with the formation of lymph nodes during development in the presence of appropriate molecular signals.

Lysis The degradation or destruction of a cell through cell membrane rupture.

Lysosome A cellular compartment that houses enzymes used to degrade or digest substances.

M

Macrophages An antigen-presenting cell that phagocytizes bacteria and others for removal from the host.

Major histocompatibility complex MHC; a fundamental structure used for the presentation of antigens in mammalian cells; analogous to HLA complex in humans.

Mast cells A resident connective tissue cell containing granules involved in the immune response.

Material Safety Data Sheet (MSDS) Also known as a safety data sheet (SDS), is a document that lists information relating to occupational safety and health; guidelines are regulated by OSHA in the United States.

Measles Formerly known as rubeola; a highly contagious virus that causes fever, cough, conjunctivitis, an oral rash of bluish-white lesions of the buccal mucosa (Koplik spots), and a maculopapular rash on the skin lasting 6 or more days.

Medical Device User Fee Amendments to the FDA Amendments Act (MDUFA) The portion of the MDUFMA referring to collection of user fees associated with submission and registration of products and companies; reviewed and renewed every 5 years.

Medical Device User Fee and Modernization Act (MDUFMA) Passed I 2002, the MDUFMA enables the FDA to provide better and more efficient review services for devices submitted for evaluation to make regulatory changes to improve the safety and efficacy of devices available to United States citizens and to charge user fees upon submission of a product to support these services.

Merozoites A stage of intracellular parasitic infection in which the parasites rupture cell walls to infect other cells. Seen in *Plasmodium* species.

Metastases The distant spread of a malignancy (cancer).

Method validation Also known as assay validation; a process implemented during the adoption of a new method, assay, or test to confirm suitability for its intended use. Typically requires extensive comparison testing with pre-existing methodologies and statistical analysis of the sensitivity and specificity of a method.

Microbiome The entire community of microorganisms in an environment; including a body location.

Microbiota See microbiome; microorganisms found at a particular site.

Microfluidics Using a network of channels to manipulate the flow of liquids at the microliter-to-picoliter range.

Microsporidia A fungal group of spore-forming single-celled parasites.

Middleware Computer software that interfaces with and provides a function to other software applications and instruments.

Mixed connective tissue disease (MCTD) A term used to indicate any number of arthritic disorders including SLE and scleroderma resulting from autoimmunity.

Mode of transmission Also method of transmission; the various ways by which a pathogen moves from a reservoir to a host.

Moderate complexity More complex than waived tests; much of the testing performed in clinical laboratories falls into this category, subject to biannual proficiency testing. Requires a CLIA certificate of compliance. The Joint Commission and CLIA indicated that moderate complexity testing be performed by individuals with sufficient training documented to perform the tests; commonly, graduation from a medical laboratory science program.

MOG Myelin oligodendrocyte glycoprotein; a glycoprotein important in the myelination of nerves that is commonly detected nonspecifically in patients with diverse CNS diseases.

Monoclonal antibodies Antibodies that are specific to a single epitope on a specific antigen. The product of hybridomas, a fusion of a single B-cell clone and a myeloma.

Monocytes The largest peripheral blood leukocyte involved in bacterial defense.

mRNA Messenger RNA; conveys genetic information from DNA to the ribosome for protein productions.

Multiple sclerosis (MS) An immune-associated disorder sometimes referred to as autoimmune; although no antibody marker has yet been found, it is a demyelinating disease that affects nerve transmission from the brain and affects the brain, spinal cord, and peripheral nerves.

Myasthenia gravis The prototypic autoimmune antibody-mediated neurological disorder attributed to antibody toward skeletal muscle acetylcholine receptor (AChR, α1 subunit expressing) in the postsynaptic muscle membrane in 90% of cases.

Mycobacterium tuberculosis The infectious bacteria responsible for the lung disease tuberculosis.

Mycotic Infected by fungus.

Myelocyte An immature granulocyte found in the bone marrow and sometimes released into the peripheral circulation during disease. In hematopoiesis, myelocytes derive from a common myeloid precursor and can develop into all granulocyte types.

Myeloid Any tissues and systems related to the bone marrow and spinal cord. Erythrocytes, platelets, and granulocytes derive from a common myeloid progenitor.

Myelopathy Any compression injury to the spinal cord.

N

Nephelometry An immunological technique used to determine the levels of blood plasma/serum proteins. A measure of the angled light transmitted due to the scattering of particles suspended in a solution.

Neuromyelitis optica (NMO) A rare inflammatory disease that mimics MS; the ratio of affected women to men is 9:1 and is caused by an autoantibody toward the AQP4 receptor on astrocytes.

Neuropathy Also known as peripheral neuropathy; refers to a condition that affects the activity of peripheral nerves.

Neutrophils A polymorphonuclear leukocyte containing granules involved with pathogen killing through phagocytosis.

Non-contact dispensing Also known as jetting; a form of liquid dispensing used in automated clinical instruments that reduces the risk of specimen cross-contamination via various pressures, pulses, and other methods.

Noncompetitive Assay Also known as heterophilic; including traditional sandwich assays in which an unknown antigen binds to a reagent antibody or vice versa.

Normal flora Also known as normal microbiota; microorganisms normally found in a body location not causing illness or disease.

Noroviruses A contagious virus that causes diarrhea and vomiting. Common cause of stomach flu in population-confined areas such as cruise ships.

O

Oligoclonal banding Bands of immunoglobulin seen in CSF or serum and are indicative of various neurological diseases such as MS, and are indicative of inflammation of the CNS.

Oocysts A cyst containing a zygote of a protozoan parasite.

Opportunistic An infection that occurs in an immunocompromised or vulnerable host.

Optic neuritis Inflammation that damages the optic nerve, a bundle of nerve fibers that transmits visual information from the eye to the brain.

Oxidative phosphorylation The cellular process in which ATP is formed resulting from a transfer of electrons involving oxygen.

P

Pathogens Microorganisms or virus that causes illness or disease.

Pattern recognition receptors (PRR) Cell surface receptors that detect a limited and conserved set of molecular patterns present on microbes and usually absent on mammalian cells.

Pemphigus A group of rare autoimmune blistering diseases.

Peripheral blood The fluid of the venous and arterial vasculature with which most serological and immunological studies are performed.

Pernicious anemia An autoimmune disease with hematologic, gastric, and immunological abnormalities.

Personal Protective Equipment (PPE) Items used by laboratory personnel to protect against infectious agents; e.g., gloves, lab coat, safety glasses, and ventilation devices.

Petechiae Tiny, circular, unraised, discolored patches on the skin that appear in clusters and result from various causes including arboviral infection.

Phagocytes Any of several cell types; typically leukocytes, that are capable of engulfing and absorbing bacteria and other cells or particles, e.g., macrophage.

Phagolysosome A cellular compartment that results from the fusion of the phagosome and lysosome in which a microorganism or foreign particle is degraded.

Phagosome A cellular compartment that houses engulfed microorganisms or foreign particles.

Phosphatases Specifically, a protein phosphatase; an enzyme that removes a phosphate group from a protein.

Phosphate buffered saline A solution used to maintain the pH of the assay components.

Photomultiplier tubes (PMTs) Transducers that convert the photon energy from fluorescent markers into an electronic signal that is then recorded in association with a single cell as part of a data packet.

Phylogenetic The evolutionary relationship between organisms.

PKCθ Protein Kinase C θ, is one of the calcium-independent serine/threonine kinases in the PKC subfamily that is restricted to cell types, such as T cells, and involved in the NF-κB signal cascade and formation of the immunological synapse.

Plasma The liquid fraction of anticoagulated whole blood used in a variety of clinical and biological assays; a source of proteins, antibodies, and antigens.

Plasma cells A mature B-cell that produces and releases into circulation a single type of antibody; upregulated during a repeat infection with a pathogen.

Plasmablasts Short-lived B-cell type that migrates to infection sites and releases antibody.

Plasmin An enzyme involved in the destruction of the fibrin clot.

PLCγ Phospholipase C gamma (γ) is one of a class of membrane-associated enzymes that cleave phospholipids as part of a signal transduction cascade.

Point-of-care tests (PoCTs) IVD tests usually used at the patient's bedside or in the clinical office, outside of dedicated laboratory space.

Polyclonal antibodies Antibodies specific to an antigen, but produced by multiple B-cell clones, leading to multiple antibodies that may target different epitopes on that same antigen.

Postzone The lack of a visible reaction resulting from an excess of antigen. May lead to a false negative in an assay.

Pre-Market Approval (PMA) The process by which the FDA reviews Class III (high-risk) medical devices for safety and efficacy prior to approving the device to market.

Precipitation A visible insoluble product formed from the interaction of a soluble antigen and a soluble antibody.

Precipitation curve A graph of the precipitate formed during the titration of an antibody to a given antigen.

Primary lymphoid tissues The bone marrow and thymus; locations of lymphocyte development and maturation.

Proficiency testing The testing of unknown specimens provided by outside agencies to monitor laboratory quality; required for all CLIA-compliant clinical moderate and high complexity testing in the United States.

Proficiency Testing (PT) The process by which a CMS-approved program sends unknown samples to a laboratory for testing and requires the clinical laboratory to submit their sample results to the program for review. This allows the PT program to score each laboratory according to CLIA criteria.

Proglottids A segment of a tapeworm that can sexually reproduce.

Programmed death ligand 1 (PD-L1) The ligand for PD-1, a protein used in normal cells to reduce the incidence of autoimmunity by downregulating the immune response and stimulating self-tolerance; upregulated on cancers to avoid immune destruction.

Programmed death protein 1 (PD-1) Also CD279; a protein on the surface of cells that regulates the immune system's response by downregulating activity.

Protein C Also known as autoprothrombin IIA and Factor XIV, it plays a role in regulation of anticoagulation pathways.

Protein S Or S protein, a plasma glycoprotein which binds which aids in the complement cascade and counteracts coagulation.

Prozone The lack of a visible reaction resulting from an excess of antibody. May lead to a false negative in an assay.

Pseudohyphae Similar to hyphae but fragile and lacking connections between cells; fungi.

Pyriform Pear shaped.

Q

qRT-PCR Quantitative reverse transcription polymerase chain reaction; a variant of PCR, a technique that first reverse transcribes RNA to DNA from a specimen and then amplifies the DNA to give a quantification of the initial levels of RNA based on the number of cycles needed to reach detection compared with a control.

Quality assurance The overall process of assessing quality patient results, which involves continuous monitoring of all pre- to postanalytical variables in a clinical laboratory for quality.

Quality Controls Materials or processes used for continuous monitoring of laboratory test reliability.

Quality indicators The measurements used by a laboratory to ensure compliance with quality.

R

Radial immunodiffusion (RID) Also called the Mancini method and single radial immunodiffusion. A precipitation technique in which antibody is distributed within a gel and antigen is added to a well to determine the concentration of antigen based on a measurement of the zone of equivalence.

Radioallergosorbent test (RAST) A variant of the RIA, performed by binding the antigen of interest, i.e., an allergen or parasite, to gel filtration media, such as Sepharose or other solid-phase support.

Radioimmunoassay (RIA) One of the earliest labeled immunoassay designs; a sensitive competitive immunoassay that employs readiolabeled antigens that compete with sample antigens.

RAG genes Recombination Activating Gene (RAG-1 and RAG-2); genes coding for enzymes that play a significant role in the development of the T- and B-cell receptor rearrangement, including antibodies.

Recombination signal sequences (RSSs) Noncoding DNA sequences recognized by the RAG1/RAG2 enzyme complex during recombination of immature T and B cells.

Refractile Ability of granules to scatter light.

Reservoir A source location of a pathogen.

Resident colonizers Microorganisms colonized in an ideal or normal body location.

Respiratory Syncytial Virus (RSV) Virus that infects the lungs predominant in young children. May lead to coughing, wheezing, and be implicated in asthma.

Retinopathy A complication caused by the damaging of blood vessels in the eyes; increased in diabetics.

Retroviruses An RNA virus that inserts a DNA copy of their genome into a host cell to replicate; includes HIV.

Rheumatoid arthritis A systemic autoimmune disease characterized by inflammatory arthritis in all patients, and extra-articular manifestations in some.

Rhinoviruses The most common infectious agent in humans and the primary cause of the common cold. Member of the Picornaviridae family.

Rocket immunoelectrophoresis The most common variant of immunoelectrophoresis used in the clinical laboratory; a one-dimensional assay for the quantification of serum proteins.

Rotavirus A contagious virus of the stomach and intestines that leads to watery diarrhea, vomiting, fever, and abdominal pain; predominately affecting infants and toddlers.

Rubella The agent of "German measles" or "three-day measles." The virus is transmitted from person to person through aerosols and is highly infectious.

Rubeola See Measles.

S

Sandwich assay Generally, an immunoassay based on the ability of antibody to bind with more than one antigen.

Saprobe An organism that lives off dead or decaying material.

Scleroderma Also known as systematic sclerosis; a chronic disease of the connective tissue resulting from autoimmunity.

Secondary lymphoid organs The lymph nodes, spleen, and other immune cell accumulation areas involved in immune responses. Sites of antigen presentation cellular activation, proliferation, and differentiation.

Secondary lymphoid tissues Including the lymph nodes and spleen, they help maintain mature lymphocytes until an infection initiates their migration.

Septation The formation of a septum; dividing wall, in fungi.

Septum A dividing wall seen in fungus with microscopy.

Serial dilution A stepwise dilution of a substance to create a logarithmic reduction of solute in diluent during each step.

Serology The study of serum and products of the serum, predominantly antibodies and antigens.

Serotypes Closely related microorganisms distinguished by sets of antigens.

Serum An amber colored fluid containing proteins, including antibodies and antigens, which results from the separation of clotted blood.

Sharps Devices and objects that can puncture or lacerate the skin; safely disposed of in puncture-resistant sharps containers.

Sheath fluid A concentrated fluid that creates a laminar flow that pushes cells into a single file for entry into the flow cell of a flow cytometer.

Single diffusion One method of immunodiffusion, used to detect antigens or antibodies in soft agar or agarose, in which diffusion is measured in one dimension only; also called the Oudin procedure after its originator.

Sjogren syndrome A localized autoimmune disease causing dryness of the eyes (xerophthalmia), mouth (xerostomia), upper respiratory tract, and vagina and parotid enlargement (sicca symptoms)

SLP76 SH2 domain containing leukocyte protein of 76 kDa; an adaptor protein that binds to many enzymatic proteins involved in T-cell activation.

Sodium azide An inorganic molecule often found in commercial reagents such as antibodies, acts as a preservative and is useful for preventing the growth of organisms such as fungal and bacterial contaminants.

Solid-phase A platform for an immunoassay; association of an immunoreagent to a structure such as a tube, well, or slide, for the purpose of analyzing unknown products.

Solid-phase support A structure such as a tube, well, or slide used in the design and conduct of an assay.

Solute The minor component of a solution. In clinical assays, it is typically the component of interest and is dissolved in a diluent.

Sporozoites Spore-like stage of a parasitic organism such as malaria.

Standard Operating Procedures (SOPs) Detailed, step-by-step instructions written to help employees and technicians conduct complex tasks and protocols in a repeatable and reliable fashion and to assist in compliance monitoring.

Standard operating procedures (SOP) A procedure or process that has been approved for systematic use and must be followed exactly to ensure safety, quality, and reliability of a laboratory test or operation within an institution.

Switch regions (S regions) Two regions enzymatically cleaved during class switching to form staggered double-strained DNA breaks, which lead to sequence excision and repair.

Syphilis A common sexually transmitted disease caused by the spirochete *Treponema pallidum*. Once a major health threat, it is now treated with penicillin successfully.

Systemic lupus erythematous (SLE) A systemic autoimmune disorder that can affect the skin, joints, lungs, kidneys, heart, hematologic system, and brain.

T

T-cell Lymphoid cells containing the TCR, which matures in the thymus; involved in the immune response.

TCR The defining receptor on the T-cell, which can detect antigen if presented in association with the MHC.

Teleomorph A sexual reproduction stage of fungi also called a fruiting body. Contrast to anamorph; asexual reproductive stage.

Terminal pathway Also referred to as the membrane attack pathway, begins with the cleavage of the molecular C5 on the surface of the target cell and is common to all pathways of complement activation.

Th1 One of two main classes of helper T cells; involved in responses to intracellular parasites, viruses, and bacteria.

Th2 One of two main classes of helper T cells, involved in responses to extracellular parasites, and helminth infections.

Th17 A recently discovered helper T-cell lineage involved in the induction of tissue inflammation and tissue destruction as seen in immune-mediated inflammatory disease.

T helper cells (T$_H$) CD4+ cells, which help the immune response by stimulating other cells through cytokine release.

Thrombin An enzyme that produces fibrin from fibrinogen during coagulation of blood.

Thrush A mouth infection caused by Candida.

Thyroid disease Autoimmune thyroid diseases such as Graves' Disease and Hashimoto thyroiditis are the most common autoimmune diseases in humans caused by the production of thyroid-stimulating hormone receptor (TSHR)-stimulating autoantibodies.

Thyroid peroxidase (TPO) Higher levels of this enzyme are seen in autoimmune thyroid diseases such as Graves' disease.

Tocilizumab An IL-6 receptor-blocking antibody used to treat rheumatoid arthritis.

Toll-like receptors (TLRs) A class of single, membrane-spanning proteins that play an important role in innate immunity.

Toxoplasmosis A disease caused by *Toxoplasma gondii*, a common parasite found in undercooked meat and in cat feces.

Transducers A device that converts variations in signal, such as light, into an electrical signal.

Transfusion-associated circulatory overload (TACO) A common transfusion reaction resulting from excess blood volume causing overload indicated by edema, rapid increase in blood pressure, cough, and tightness of the chest.

Transfusion-related acute lung injury (TRALI) A rare syndrome characterized by sudden respiratory distress following transfusion in which lung injury occurs.

Transient colonizers Microorganisms in a nonideal or temporary body location.

Tregs Regulatory T cells; maintain homeostasis by suppressing the immune response.

Trophozoites A stage of growth for sporozoan parasites in which nutrients are being aquired from the host.

Tumor-associated antigens Antigens found in malignant cells and in some normal tissue typically at much higher levels than normal tissue.

Tumor-specific antigens Antigens that are found only in malignant cells.

Tumor markers Substances, usually proteins, produced by tumor cells or the host's response to tumor cells found in bodily fluids or tissues that can be used to help diagnose, detect, and manage certain cancers.

Turbidimetry The measure of the reduction of direct transmitted light due to scattering of particles suspended in a solution. When compared with a control solution and standard curve, can be used to determine the concentration of an analyte.

Type 1 diabetes mellitus Also known as insulin-dependent diabetes; is an autoimmune disorder of deficient insulin production, caused by immune destruction of the β islet cells of the endocrine pancreas.

U

Unicellular A single-celled organism.

Uracil DNA glycosylase (UNG) An enzyme that removes uracil from DNA and initiates base-excision repair.

Uveitis Inflammation of the vascular uveal tract of the eye, including the iris, ciliary body, and choroid.

V

V(D)J recombination A mechanism of genetic recombination that occurs exclusively in developing lymphocytes leading to the antigenic specificity of antibodies and receptors produced by these cells.

Vaccines A manufactured preparation to stimulate an immune response and protect against pathogens by using a weakened, altered, or dead version of the disease-causing agent.

Variable region Amino terminal portion of the immunoglobulin molecules that determines antigenic specificity. Two are associated with a single constant region.

Varicella Zoster Virus (VZV) Also known as varicella or herpes zoster; member of the herpes virus family that causes childhood chickenpox and adult-onset shingles.

Vulvovaginitis Infection of the vagina and vulva.

W

Waived Referring to Waived Testing. The least regulated, and least complex, set of laboratory assays designated by the Clinical Laboratory Improvement Act of 1988.

Western blotting A technique for protein identification widely used in immunogenetics and other cell and serum studies that requires a prior protein electrophoresis for separation followed by a blotting to nitrocellulose paper and addition of labeled antibodies toward suspected sample antigens.

Western equine encephalitis virus (WEEV) A virus passed to humans and horses through mosquitoes, similar to EEEV, it leads to brain infections.

West Nile Virus An arborovirus in the Flaviviridae family that is the leading cause of mosquito-borne disease.

Z

ZAP70 Zeta-chain–associated protein kinase 70; a kinase associated with the TCR and involved in its intracellular signaling.

Zika virus Causative agent of the rapidly emerging zika fever; a member of the flaviviridae family and serologically identified via IgG and IgM antibody presentation in patients.

Zone of equivalence Also known as equivalence zone; a location in which antibody and antigen are at the same concentration.

Index